Stedman's

DERMATOLOGY & IMMUNOLOGY

WORDS

INCLUDES

RHEUMATOLOGY, ALLERGY, & TRANSPLANTATION

SECOND EDITION

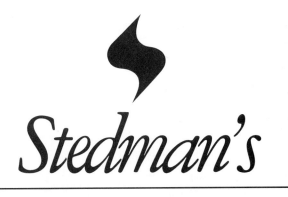

Stedman's

DERMATOLOGY & IMMUNOLOGY WORDS

INCLUDES RHEUMATOLOGY, ALLERGY, & TRANSPLANTATION

SECOND EDITION

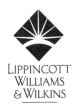

LIPPINCOTT
WILLIAMS
& WILKINS

Publisher: Rhonda M. Kumm
Senior Manager: Julie K. Stegman
Associate Managing Editor: Trista A. DiPaula
Associate Managing Editor: William A. Howard
Art Director: Jennifer Clements
Production Coordinator: Kevin Iarossi
Typesetter: Peirce Graphic Services, Inc.
Printer & Binder: Malloy Litho, Inc.

Printed in the United States of America

Second Edition, 2002

Library of Congress Cataloging-in-Publication Data

Stedman's dermatology & immunology words.—2nd ed.
    p. cm.
  ISBN 0-7817-3059-7 (alk. paper)
    1. Dermatology—Terminology. 2. Immunology—Terminology. 3. Allergy—
Terminology. 4. Rheumatology—Terminology. 5. Communicable diseases—
Terminology. I. Title: Stedman's dermatology and immunology words. II. Title:
Dermatology & immunology words.

RL41 .S74 2001
616.5′001′4—dc21
                                                              2001050427
                                                                    01
                                              1 2 3 4 5 6 7 8 9 10

Contents

Acknowledgments

An important part of our editorial process is the involvement of medical transcriptionists—as advisors, reviewers, and editors.

We extend special thanks to Sandy Kovacs, CMT, and Patricia White, CMT, for editing the manuscript, helping to resolve many difficult content questions, and contributing material for the appendix sections. We also extend special thanks to Helen Littrell, CMT, for performing the final prepublication review.

We are also grateful to our MT Editorial Advisory Board members, including Marty Cantu, CMT; Patricia Gibson; Renee Hentz, RRA; Robin Koza; and Peg Nelson, CMT. These medical transcriptionists and medical language specialists served as important editors and advisors.

Other important contributors include Darcy Johnson, who focused on the appendix sections; Susan Bartolucci, CMT; Rose M. Berry; Donna C. Brosmer, CMT; Sherry Crawford, CMT; Janice Deal, RN, BSN; Shemah Fletcher; Susan Forste, CMT; Vicki Hawhee; Heather Little, CMT; Kathryn C. Mason, CMT; Pamela Maykulsky; Miriam Miller, CMT; Judy Moody; Wendy Ryan, RHIT; Cheri Sawyer, CMT; Suzanne Taubert, CMT; Dora Vasquez; Jenifer Walker, MA; Judi Walls, CMT; Linda Warren; and Annette Weiland, CMT.

Barb Ferretti played an integral role in the process by reviewing the content files for format, updating the database, and providing a final quality check.

As with all our *Stedman's* word references, this resource incorporates the suggestions and expertise of our many contacts in the medical transcriptionist community. Thanks to all of our advisory board participants, reviewers, and editors; AAMT meeting attendees; and others who have written us with requests and comments—keep talking, and we'll keep listening.

Editor's Preface

Responding to needs of medical transcriptionists. . .what a novel idea! With this updated version of *Stedman's Dermatology & Immunology Words,* Lippincott Williams & Wilkins has once again listened to our suggestions and risen to the occasion.

In today's rapidly changing world of patient information documentation, a knowledgeable medical transcriptionist is an extremely valuable asset to any healthcare organization that maintains records. This book responds to the needs of transcriptionists by covering terms from new and evolving areas in dermatology and immunology, including allergy and rheumatology, as well as organ transplantation. Additionally, it includes useful appendix sections, such as illustrations, sample reports, and lists of common terms by procedure. I recommend that you become familiar with this book's appendices, so that you know exactly how much and what kind of information is available to you. Knowing where to look is half the battle in the quest for finding the "right word."

My sincere thanks goes to Patty White, CMT, for being the second editor. We have worked on a few books together, and we make a good team. I can always count on her to catch what I miss. I also had the pleasure of meeting Patty at the AAMT meeting in Arlington, Virginia this year. Technology is our greatest asset, but nothing can replace personal contact to make a job come together.

The editorial staff is also a valuable group of people who help put this book together. Thanks to Will Howard for his role as associate managing editor and for coordinating the timeline and logistics. It is an honor to be part of a team of intelligent and hardworking individuals.

This book is designed to help you find your unfamiliar word. I always smile when I find my word, and hopefully this book will make you smile too.

Sandy Kovacs, CMT

Publisher's Preface

Stedman's Dermatology & Immunology Words, Second Edition, offers an authoritative assurance of quality and exactness to the wordsmiths of the healthcare professions—medical transcriptionists, medical editors and copyeditors, health information management personnel, court reporters, and the many other users and producers of medical documentation.

We received many requests for updates to *Stedman's Dermatology & Immunology Words.* As the requests continued to accumulate, we realized that medical language professionals needed a current, comprehensive reference for these specialties.

In *Stedman's Dermatology & Immunology Words, Second Edition,* users will find thousands of terms related to dermatology, immunology, rheumatology, allergy, and transplantation. Included are terms for problems like acne, contact dermatitis, alopecia, eczematous dermatoses, autoimmune diseases, allergies, allergic asthma, and rheumatologic disorders. Transplantation terms, including words for tissue engineering, HLA typing, and antirejection drug therapies, have also been added. Included in this edition are terms for diagnostic and therapeutic procedures, new techniques, and lab tests, as well as equipment names and abbreviations with their expansions. The appendix sections provide anatomical illustrations with useful captions and labels; normal lab values; sample reports; common terms by procedure; and drugs listed by indication. For quick reference, we have also included lists of common allergens and transplant organizations.

This compilation of more than 75,000 entries, fully cross-indexed for quick access, was built from a base vocabulary of approximately 45,000 medical words, phrases, abbreviations, and acronyms. The extensive A-Z list was developed from the database of *Stedman's Medical Dictionary, 27th Edition,* and supplemented by terminology found in current medical literature (please see list of References on page xvi).

We at Lippincott Williams & Wilkins strive to provide you with the most up-to-date and accurate word references available. Your use of this word book will prompt new editions, which we will publish as often as updates and revisions justify. We welcome your suggestions for improvements, changes, corrections, and additions—whatever will make this *Stedman's* product more useful to you. Please complete the postpaid card at the back of this book, and send your recommendations care of "Stedman's" at Lippincott Williams & Wilkins.

Explanatory Notes

Medical transcription is an art as well as a science. Both approaches are needed to correctly interpret the dictation of a physician, whose language is a product of education, training, and experience. This variety in medical language means that there are several acceptable ways to express certain terms, including jargon. *Stedman's Dermatology & Immunology Words, Second Edition,* provides variant spellings and phrasings for many terms. These elements, in addition to complete cross-indexing, make *Stedman's Dermatology & Immunology Words, Second Edition,* a valuable resource for determining the validity of terms as they are encountered.

Alphabetical Organization
Alphabetization of main entries is letter by letter as spelled, ignoring punctuation, spaces, prefixed numbers, or other special characters. For example:

aminosidine sulfate
21-aminosteroid
aminotransferase

All Greek characters are spelled out except when used in an abbreviation. For example:

alpha
> a. adrenergic stimulation
> a. fetoprotein
> a. hemolysin
> a. thalassemia

In subentry alphabetization, the abbreviated singular form or the spelled-out plural form of the noun main entry word is ignored.

Format and Style
All main entries are in **boldface** to expedite locating a sought-after term, to enhance distinction between main entries and subentries, and to relieve the textual density of the pages.

Irregular plurals and variant spellings are shown on the same line as the singular or preferred form of the word. For example:

dermatitis, pl. dermatitides

curette, curet

Hyphenation

As a rule of style, multiple eponyms (e.g., Chauffard-Still syndrome) are hyphenated. Also, hyphens have been added between a manufacturer and one or more eponyms (e.g., Vital-Metzenbaum dissecting scissors). Please note that in many cases, hyphenation is a question of style, not of accuracy, and thus is a matter of choice.

Possessives

Possessive forms have been dropped in this reference for the sake of consistency and conformance with the guidelines of the American Association for Medical Transcription (AAMT) and other groups. Please note, however, that in many cases, retaining the possessive, like hyphenating, is a question of style, not of accuracy, and thus is a matter of choice. To form the possessive of a word, simply add the apostrophe or apostrophe "s" to the end of the word.

Cross-indexing

The word list is in an index-like main entry-subentry format that contains two combined alphabetical listings:

(1) A *noun* main entry-subentry organization, which is typical of the A-Z section of medical dictionaries like *Stedman's*:

dermatosis
    acantholytic d.
    acquired d.
    ashy d.
    industrial d.

nail
    brittle n.
    convex n.
    parrot-beak n.
    reedy n.

(2) An *adjective* main entry-subentry organization, which lists words and phrases as you hear them. The main entries are the adjectives or modifiers in a multiword term. The subentries are the nouns around which the terms are constructed and to which the adjectives or modifiers pertain:

congenital
    c. ectodermal defects
    c. dysphagocytosis
    c. hypomelanotic macule
    c. syphilis

nevus
    n. comedonicus
    n. fibrosus
    n. flammeus
    n. pigmentosus

This format provides the user with more than one way to locate and identify a multiword term. For example:

dissemination
    skin d.

skin
    s. dissemination

disease
    Quincke d.
    Raynaud d.

Quincke
    Q. disease
    Q. edema

It also allows the user to see together all terms that contain a particular descriptor, as well as all types, kinds, or variations of a noun entity. For example:

laser
    alexandrite l.
    argon l.
    l. Doppler velocimetry
    l. plume
    ruby l.

membrane
    basal cell m.
    Bruch m.
    m. ruffling
    synovial m.
    tympanic m.

Wherever possible, abbreviations are separately defined and cross-referenced. For example:

FUO
    fever of unknown origin

fever
    f. of unknown origin (FUO)

origin
    fever of unknown o. (FUO)

References

In addition to the manufacturers' literature we gather at various medical meetings, scientific reports from hospitals, and the lists created by our MT Editorial Advisory Board members from their daily transcription work, we used the following sources for new terms in *Stedman's Dermatology & Immunology Words, Second Edition:*

Books

Arndt KA. Manual of Dermatologic Therapeutics, 5th Edition. Philadelphia: Lippincott Williams & Wilkins, 1995.

Austen KF, Frank MM, Atkinson JP, Cantor HI. Samter's Immunologic Diseases. Philadelphia: Lippincott Williams & Wilkins, 2001.

Bowden RA, Ljungman P, Paya C, eds. Transplant Infections. Philadelphia: Lippincott-Raven, 1998.

Cush JJ, Kavanaugh AF. Rheumatology: Diagnosis and Therapeutics. Baltimore: Lippincott Williams & Wilkins, 1999.

Drake E. Sloane's Medical Word Book, 4th Edition. Philadelphia: Saunders, 2002.

Emery RW, Miller LW, eds. Handbook of Cardiac Transplantation. Philadelphia: Hanley & Belfus, Inc., 1996.

Hall JC. Sauer's Manual of Skin Diseases, 8th Edition. Philadelphia: Lippincott Williams & Wilkins, 2000.

Koopman WJ. Arthritis and Allied Conditions: A Textbook of Rheumatology, 14th Edition. Philadelphia: Lippincott Williams & Wilkins, 2000.

Lahita RG, ed. Textbook of the Autoimmune Diseases. Philadelphia: Lippincott Williams & Wilkins, 2000.

Lance LL. Quick Look Drug Book 2001. Baltimore: Lippincott Williams & Wilkins, 2001.

Maddrey WC, Schiff ER, Sorrell MF, eds. Transplantation of the Liver, 3rd Edition. Philadelphia: Lippincott Williams & Wilkins, 2001.

Odom RB, James WD, Berger TG. Andrews' Diseases of the Skin: Clinical Dermatology, 9th Edition. Philadelphia: Saunders, 2000.

Patterson R, ed. Allergic Diseases: Diagnosis and Management, 5th Edition. Philadelphia: Lippincott-Raven, 1997.

Ratz JL, ed. Textbook of Dermatologic Surgery. Philadelphia: Lippincott Williams & Wilkins, 1997.

Rietschel RL, Fowler JF, eds. Fisher's Contact Dermatitis, 5th Edition. Philadelphia: Lippincott Williams & Wilkins, 2001.

Sheehan C. Clinical Immunology: Principles and Laboratory Diagnosis, 2nd Edition. Philadelphia: Lippincott-Raven, 1997.

Stedman's Medical Dictionary, 27th Edition. Baltimore: Lippincott Williams & Wilkins, 2000.

Vera Pyle's Current Medical Terminology, 8th Edition. Modesto, CA: Health Professions Institute, 2000.

CD

UpToDate Clinical Reference Library on CD, Version 8:3. Wellesley, MA: UpToDate, 2000.

Journals

The American Journal of Dermatopathology. Baltimore: Lippincott Williams & Wilkins, 1999–2000.

Archives of Dermatology. Chicago: American Medical Association, 1999–2000.

Arthritis & Rheumatism. New York: John Wiley & Sons, 1999–2000.

Current Opinions in Organ Transplantation. Philadelphia: Lippincott Williams & Wilkins, 1999–2000.

Immunology Today. London: Elsevier Science, 2000.

JCR: Journal of Clinical Rheumatology. Baltimore: Lippincott Williams & Wilkins, 2000–2001.

Journal of Allergy and Clinical Immunology. St. Louis, MO: Mosby, 1999–2000.

The Latest Word. Philadelphia: Saunders, 1999–2000.

Transplantation. Baltimore: Lippincott Williams & Wilkins, 1999–2000.

Websites

http://centerwatch.com/patient

http://edcenter.med.cornell.edu/CUMC_PathNotes/Dermpath/Dermpath_02.html

http://www.arthritis.org/answers/drugguide/default.asp

http://www.fda.gov/cder/rdmt/internetflap.htm

http://www.hpisum.com

http://www.medicaledu.comp/absorptv.htm

http://www.mtdesk.com

http://www.mtmonthly.com

http://www.niaid.nih.gov/publications/transplant/glossary.htm

http://www.organdonor.gov

http://www.virtualdrugstore.com

A

   Aristocort A
   A and D Ointment
   hepatitis A (HA)
   A 2M

A5

   Peroxin A5, A10

A-200

   A. Pyrinate
   A. Shampoo

Å

  angstrom
   Å unit

a

   a collarette of epidermis
   a disintegrin and matrilysin
    (ADAM)

5a8

   monoclonal antibody to CD4, 5a8

A1 test

AA

  arachidonic acid
   AA, AL amyloidosis

AAD

  acroangiodermatitis
  American Academy of Dermatology

AADI

  anterior atlantodental interval

AAE

  acquired angioedema

AAI

  American Association of Immunologists

A-alpha nerve fiber

AAP

  American Academy of Pediatrics

Aarskog-Scott syndrome

Aastrom Replicell System

AAV

  adeno-associated virus
  ANCA-associated vasculitis

AAVT

  acral arteriovenous tumor

Ab

  antibody

abacavir

abalone

Abbott HIVAG-1 monoclonal antigen

ABC

  avidin-biotin-horseradish peroxidase
   complex
   ABC method

ABCD

   ABCD rule of dermatoscopy
   ABCD sign

ABE

  acute bacterial endocarditis

Abelcet

Abelson murine leukemia virus

Abernethy sarcoma

aberrant glycosaminoglycan metabolism

ABG

  arterial blood gas

ABH

  angina bullosa haemorrhagica

abigne

AbioCor implantable replacement heart

abiotrophy

abirritant

ablastin

ablation

ablative

abnormal

   a. DNA repair
   a. loricrin crosslinking

abnormality

   biochemical a.
   calcinosis cutis, osteoma cutis,
    poikiloderma, and skeletal a.'s
    (COPS)
   dental a.
   a.'s of genitalia, retardation of
    growth, and deafness
   immunochemical a.
   microvascular a.
   nail fold capillaroscopy a.
   nail fold capillary loop a.
   oral cavity a.
   pigmentary a.
   skeletal a.

abnutzung pigment

ABO

   ABO antigen
   ABO incompatibility
   ABO mismatch

ABO-incompatible kidney transplantation

abortive

   a. neurofibromatosis
   a. transduction

abortus

   Bacillus a.

ABP

  ambulatory blood pressure

ABPA

  allergic bronchopulmonary aspergillosis
   ABPA panel

abradant

abrade

abraded wound

abrasion
> brush burn a.
> mechanical a.
> pleural a.

abrasive

Abrikosov tumor

abscess
> brain a.
> Brodie a.
> cheesy a.
> cold a.
> conglobate a.
> crypt a.
> cutaneous a.
> Dubois a.
> eosinophilic a.
> filarial a.
> follicular a.
> gas a.
> intraepidermal a.
> metastatic tuberculous a.
> mixed aerobic/anaerobic a.
> Munro a.
> mycobacterial a.
> Paget a.
> parafrenal a.
> Pautrier a.
> phlegmonous a.
> pneumococcic a.
> protozoal a.
> pulp a.
> pulpal a.
> pyemic a.
> pyogenic a.
> recurrent cutaneous a.
> spirillar a.
> staphylococcal a.
> stellate a.
> sterile a.
> strumous a.
> subepidermal a.
> subungual a.
> sudoriferous a.
> sudoriparous a.
> tuberculous a.
> verminous a.

abscessus
> *Mycobacterium a.*

absent
> a. dermal component
> a. reaction
> a. tonsil

Absidia

absolute
> a. blood eosinophil count (AEC)
> oak moss a.

absorbable mesh

absorbent
> a. gelling material (AGM)
> a. ointment

Absorbine
> A. Antifungal Foot powder
> A. Jock Itch
> A. Jr. Antifungal

absorptiometry
> dual-beam photon a.
> dual-energy x-ray a. (DEXA, DXA)
> photon a.

absorption
> cutaneous a.
> external a.
> fluorescent treponemal antibody a. (FTA-ABS)
> nonspecific a.
> parenteral a.
> percutaneous a.

abtropfung

ABX-CBL monoclonal antibody

ABX-IL8

ACA
> acrodermatitis chronica atrophicans
> anticardiolipin antibody
> anticentromere antibody
>> ACA antibody

acacia
> a. tree
> a. tree pollen

ACAD
> allograft coronary artery disease

ACADERM patch test

ACAID
> anterior chamber-associated immune deviation

acanthamebiasis

Acanthamoeba
> *A. astronyxis*
> *A. castellani*
> *A. culbertsoni*
> *A. glebae*
> *A. hatchetti*
> *A. palestinensis*
> *A. polyphaga*
> *A. rhysodes*

Acanthaster
> *A. planci*

Acanthocheilonema
> *A. viteae*
> *A. viteae* excretory-secretory antigen

acanthocyte

acanthoid

acantholysis
> suprabasilar a.

acantholytic
> a. dermatosis

a. dyskeratoma
a. dyskeratosis
a. squamous cell carcinoma
acanthoma, pl. **acanthomata, acanthomas**
a. adenoides cysticum
basosquamous-cell a.
clear cell a.
Degos a.
epidermolytic a.
a. fissuratum
a. inguinale
intraepidermal a.
pale cell a.
pilar sheath a.
a. tropicum
a. verrucosa seborrheica
acanthorrhexis
acanthosis
a. nigricans (AN)
a. palmaris
a. papulosa nigra
a. seborrheica
acanthotic epidermal proliferation
acarian
acariasis
demodectic a.
psoroptic a.
sarcoptic a.
acaricide
acarid
acaridiasis
Acarina
acarine
a. dermatosis
acarinosis
A-Caro-25
acarodermatitis
a. urticarioides
acaroid
acaroides
acarophobia
acarotoxic
Acarus
A. *balatus*
A. *folliculorum*
A. *siro*
acatalasemia
acatalasia
accelerated
a. graft atherosclerosis (AGAS)
a. phase (AP)

a. reaction
a. rejection
Accelerator cannula
Ac'cents permanent lash liner
Accents system
accentuation
acrosyringeal a.
follicular a.
perifollicular a.
accessory
a. auricle
a. molecule
a. muscle
a. tragus
accident
serum a.
accidental host
acclimatization
Accolate
accommodation
accordion hand
Accuderm punch
Accuhair needle
AccuProbe system
Accu-set System
AccuSite injectable gel
Accutane
AccuTrax Peak Flow Meter
Accuzyme
A. enzymatic debrider
A. enzymatic debriding agent
ACD
allergic contact dermatitis
ACE
Aerosol Cloud enhancer
angiotensin-converting enzyme
Ace bandage
Acedapsone
Acel-Imune
acellular
a. pannus tissue
a. pertussis vaccine combined with
diphtheria and tetanus toxoid
(DTaP)
Acephen
acephylline
aceracear
acervuline
Aceta
acetabular dysplasia
acetabuli
protrusio a.

NOTES

3

acetabulum
acetamidine
acetaminophen
>chlorpheniramine,
>>phenylpropanolamine, and a.
>a., chlorpheniramine, and
>>pseudoephedrine
>a. and diphenhydramine
>a. and isometheptene mucate
>a. and phenyltoloxamine
>phenyltoloxamine,
>>phenylpropanolamine, and a.

acetanilide
acetarsol
acetarsone
Acetasol HC Otic
acetate
>aluminum a.
>betamethasone a. (BA)
>cortisone a.
>Cortone A.
>cyproterone a.
>dexamethasone a.
>Florinef A.
>fludrocortisone a.
>hydrocortisone a.
>Hydrocortone a.
>mafenide a.
>m-cresyl a.
>megestrol a.
>methylprednisolone a. (MPA)
>octreotide a.
>paramethasone a.
>pirbuterol a.
>sermorelin a.

acetazolamide
acetic
>a. acid
>a. acid, propanediol diacetate, and
>>hydrocortisone

acetin
acetone-insoluble antigen
acetonide
>fluocinolone a.
>triamcinolone a. (TAA)

Acetoxyl
acetylation
>a. of cellular protein
>a. of serum protein

acetylcholine
>a. depletion
>a. receptor antibody (AChRAb)

acetylcholinesterase deficiency
acetylcysteine
acetyl ethyl tetramethyl tetralin (AETT)

acetylhydrolase
>platelet-activating factor a. (PAF-
>>AH)

acetylsalicylic acid (ASA)
acetyltransferase
>chloramphenicol a. (CAT)

Achard-Thiers syndrome
Achenbach syndrome
Aches-N-Pain
Achilles
>A. bursitis
>A. tendon

achlorhydria
Acholeplasma laidlawii
achondrogenesis type II
Achorion schoenleinii
AChRAb
>acetylcholine receptor antibody

achromasia
achromatosis
achromia
>consecutive a.
>a. parasitica
>a. unguium

achromians
>incontinentia pigmenti a.

Achromobacter
>*A. xylosoxidans*

achromoderma
achromotrichia
Achromycin
>A. Ophthalmic
>A. Topical
>A. V
>A. V Oral

acid
>acetic a.
>acetylsalicylic a. (ASA)
>adenylic a.
>a. agglutination
>all-*trans*-retinoic a.
>alpha-hydroxy a. (AHA)
>aluminum acetate and acetic a.
>amino a.
>aminobenzoic a.
>amino levulinic a. (ALA)
>5-aminolevulinic a.
>aminosalicylic a.
>amoxicillin and clavulanic a.
>a. anhydride
>arabic a.
>arachidonic a. (AA)
>arylalcoanoic a.
>azelaic a.
>battery a.
>benzoic acid and salicylic a.
>bichloracetic a.
>boric a.

branched chain deoxyribonucleic a. (bDNA)
cantharic a.
chemiluminescent in situ hybridization for detection of cytomegalovirus deoxyribonucleic a.
chenodeoxycholic a.
cholic a.
13-*cis*-retinoic a.
citric a.
clavulanic a.
coal tar and salicylic a.
complementary deoxyribonucleic a. (cDNA)
cytidine monophospho-*N*-acetyl neuraminic a. (CMP-NANA)
delta-aminolevulinic a.
deoxyribonucleic a. (DNA)
dichloroacetic a.
a. dye
eicosapentaenoic a.
enteric-coated acetylsalicylic a. (ECASA)
essential fatty a. (EFA)
ethylenediaminetetraacetic a. (EDTA)
exogenous polyunsaturated fatty a.'s
fibric a.
flufenamic a.
folic a.
folinic a.
a. fuchsin
fusidic a.
gamma-aminobutyric a. (GABA)
gamma-linolenic a.
glucuronic a.
glycolic a.
glycyl-transfer ribonucleic a.
gold 4-amino-2-mercaptobenzoic a.
guanylic a.
holmium ethylenediamine tetramethylene phosphonic a.
homogentisic a. (HGA)
hyaluronic a.
hydrochloric a.
hydroperoxyeicosatetraenoic a.
hydroquinone USP and glycolic a.
hydroxyeicosatetraenoic a. (HETE)
5-hydroxyindoleacetic a.
iduronic a.
infectious nucleic a.

inosinic a.
kojic a.
lactic a.
L-ascorbic a.
linoleic a.
lipoteichoic a. (LTA)
malic a.
a. maltase
A. Mantle
A. Mantle Creme
mefenamic a.
monochloroacetic a.
N-acetylneuraminic a.
nalidixic a.
octulosonic a.
oleic a.
omega-3, -6 fatty a.
paraaminobenzoic a. (PABA)
paraaminosalicylic a.
phytanic a.
plicatic a.
podophyllin and salicylic a.
pseudomonic a.
pyruvic a.
retinoic a.
ribonucleic a. (RNA)
salicylic a. (SA)
salicylic acid-lactic a. (SAL)
salicylic acid and lactic a.
a. Schiff stain
serum uric a.
a. skin
sodium citrate and citric a.
stearic a.
sulfuric a.
sulfur and salicylic a.
tartaric a.
Tc-dimercaptosuccinic a. (DMSA)
tenoxicam a.
tiaprofenic a.
ticarcillin and clavulanic a.
tranexamic a.
transfer ribonucleic a. (tRNA)
trichloroacetic a. (TCA)
undecylenic a.
uric a.
Acidaminococcus fermentans
acidase
  antideoxyribonucleic a.
acid-fast bacillus (AFB)
acidic fibroblast growth factor (a-FGF)

NOTES

acidification
 endosomal a.
acidophilus
 Lactobacillus a.
 a. milk
acidosis
 lactic a.
 metabolic a.
 respiratory a.
acid-Schiff test
acid-secreting gastric parietal cell
aciduria
 orotic a.
acinar cell
Acinetobacter
 A. anitratus
 A. calcoaceticus
 A. calcoaceticus-baumannii complex
 A. lwoffi
Acintomadura
ACIP
 Advisory Committee on Immunization
 Practice
ACIS
 Automated Cellular Imaging System
 ACIS immunohistochemical stain
acitretin
aCL
 anticardiolipin
 aCL antibody
ACLAb
 anticardiolipin antibody
ACLE
 acute cutaneous lupus erythematosus
Aclovate
 A. topical
acmes
 stadium a.
acne
 A. Aid cleansing bar
 a. albida
 apocrine a.
 a. arthritis
 a. artificialis
 a. atrophica
 a. bacillus
 bromide a.
 a. cachecticorum
 a. cheloidalis
 chlorine a.
 a. ciliaris
 ClearLight treatment for a.
 colloid a.
 comedo a.
 common a.
 a. conglobata
 conglobate a.
 corynebacterium a.

 a. cosmetica
 cystic a.
 a. cystica
 a. decalvans
 a. detergicans
 a. disseminata
 a. dorsalis
 epidemic a.
 a. erythematosa
 a. estivalis
 excoriated a.
 a. excoriée des jeunes filles
 a. frontalis
 a. fulminans
 a. generalis
 halogen a.
 a. hypertrophica
 a. indurata
 infantile a.
 a. inversa
 iodide a.
 keloid a.
 a. keloid
 a. keloidalis (AK)
 a. keloidalis nuchae
 a. keratosa
 lupoid a.
 Mallorca miliary actinic a.
 a. mechanica
 mechanical a.
 a. medicamentosa
 menstrual a.
 a. mentagra
 miliary a.
 Mudd a.
 a. necrotica
 a. necrotica miliaris
 a. necroticans et exulcerans
  serpiginosa nasi
 neonatal a.
 a. neonatorum
 nodulocystic a.
 occupational a.
 oil a.
 papular a.
 a. papulosa
 petroleum a.
 picker's a.
 pomade a.
 premenstrual a.
 propionibacterium a.
 a. punctata
 pustular a.
 a. pustulosa
 pyogenic sterile arthritis, pyoderma
  gangrenosum and a. (PAPA)
 a. rosacea
 a. scrofulosorum

a. seborrheica
a. simplex
steroid a.
summer a.
a. surgery
a. syphilitica
systemic a.
tar a.
a. tarsi
a. telangiectodes
a. tetrad
trade a.
tropical a.
a. tropicalis
a. urticata
a. varioliformis
a. venenata
a. vulgaris
acné chéloïdique
acneform, acneiform
a. dermatitis
a. eruption
a. lesion
a. syphilid
acneforme, acneiforme
erythema a.
acnegen
acnegenic
acneic
acneiform (*var. of* acneform)
acneiforma
ulerythema a.
acneiforme (*var. of* acneforme)
acne-pustulosis-hyperostosis-osteitis
acnes
Bacillus a.
Corynebacterium a.
Propionibacterium a.
acne-seborrhea complex
Acnex
acnitis
Acnomel
A. Acne Mask
A. BP 5
A. cream
acomia
Acorn classification
acoustic
a. reflex threshold
a. rhinometry (AR)
ACPA
anticytoplasmic antibody

acquired
a. agammaglobulinemia
a. angioedema (AAE)
a. biotin deficiency
a. C1 inhibitor deficiency
a. cornification disorder
a. dermatosis
a. digital fibrokeratoma
a. dyskeratotic leukoplakia
a. generalized lipodystrophy
a. hemolytic anemia
a. hemolytic icterus
a. hemophilia
a. hyperostosis syndrome (AHYS)
a. hypertrichosis lanuginosa
a. hypogammaglobulinemia
a. ichthyosis
a. immune deficiency syndrome (AIDS)
a. immunity
a. immunodeficiency
a. immunodeficiency syndrome (AIDS)
a. immunodeficiency syndrome-related complex (ARC)
a. immunodeficiency syndrome-related virus (ARV)
a. intrathymic tolerance
a. leukoderma
a. leukopathia
a. melanocytic nevus
a. partial face-sparing lipodystrophy
a. pellicle
a. progressive lymphangioma (APL)
a. sensitivity
a. trichoepithelioma
a. tufted angioma (ATA)
a. vascular disorder
acquisita
alopecia a.
epidermolysis bullosa a. (EBA)
acquisitum
ACR
American College of Rheumatology
ACR criteria
Acradinium-ester-labeled nucleic acid probe
acral
a. arteriolar ectasia
a. arteriovenous tumor (AAVT)
a. erythema
a. fibrokeratoma

NOTES

acral *(continued)*
 a. lentiginous melanoma (ALM)
 a. persistent papular mucinosis
 a. vitiligo
Acremonium
acrex
acridine
acriflavine
acrisorcin
acritochromacy
acrivastine and pseudoephedrine
acroangiodermatitis (AAD)
acroasphyxia
acrocephalosyndactyly
acrochordon
acrochordonectomy
 Strother a.
acrocyanosis
 orthostatic a.
 remitting necrotizing a.
acrodermatitis
 a. chronica
 a. chronica atrophicans (ACA)
 a. continua
 a. continua of Hallopeau
 a. enteropathica
 Hallopeau a.
 a. hiemalis
 papular a.
 a. papulosa infantum
 a. perstans
 pustular a.
 a. pustulosa
 a. vesiculosa tropica
acrodermatosis
acrodynia
acrodynic erythema
acrofacial vitiligo
acrogeria
acrohyperhidrosis
acrokeratoelastoidosis
acrokeratosis
 a. neoplastica
 paraneoplastic a.
 a. paraneoplastica
 a. verruciformis
 a. verruciformis of Hopf
acrokeratotic poikiloderma
acrolein
acrolein-induced cystitis
acroleukopathy
acromegalic
 a. arthropathy
acromegaly
acromelalgia
acromelanosis progressiva
acromicria

acromioclavicular
 a. articulation
 a. degeneration
 a. joint
acromiodeltoideus
acroosteolysis
acropachy
 thyroid a.
acropachyderma
acroparesthesia
 Nothnagel-type a.
 Schultze a.
 Schultze-type a.
acroparesthesias
acropigmentatio
 a. reticularis
 a. reticular of Kitamura
acropigmentation
 a. of Dohi
 Kitamura reticulate a.
acropurpura
acropustulosis
 a. of infancy
 infantile a.
acroscleroderma
acrosclerosis
acrospiroma
 eccrine a.
 giant eccrine a.
 malignant clear cell a.
acrosyringeal accentuation
acrosyringium
acroterica
 morphea a.
acroteric morphea
Acrotheca aquaspera
acrotrophodynia
AcryDerm
 A. border island dressing
 A. hydrogel sheet
 A. Strands
 A. Strands filler
acrylate
acrylic acid allergy
acrylonitrile
Acsorex
act
 Coinage A.
 throwing a.
 Toxic Substance Control A.
Actagen
 A. Syrup
 A. Tablet
actamar
actarit
ACTH
 adrenocorticotropic hormone
 ACTH therapy

Acthar
ActHIB vaccine
Acticel wound dressing
Acticin Cream
Acticoat
    A. burn dressing
Acticort Topical
Actiderm
actidione
Actifed
    A. Allergy Tablet
    A. 12 Hour
Actimmune
actin
    filamentous a.
    A. FSL
    A. monomer
actin-binding protein
Actinex
    A. topical
actinic
    a. burn
    a. cheilitis
    a. dermatitis
    a. elastosis
    a. granuloma
    a. keratosis
    a. light
    a. porokeratosis
    a. prurigo
    a. purpura
    a. reticuloid
    a. reticuloid syndrome
actinica
    cheilitis a.
    dermatitis a.
actinicity
actinicus
    lichen planus a.
actinism
actinobacillosis
Actinobacillus
    A. actinomycetemcomitans
    A. equuli
    A. hominis
    A. lignieresii
    A. suis
    A. ureae
actinodermatitis
actinodermatosis
actinoides
    Thysanosoma a.

actinolyte
Actinomadura
    A. madurae
    A. pelletieri
actinometer
actinometry
actinomycelial
Actinomyces
    A. bovis
    A. hominis
    A. israelii
    A. naeslundii
actinomycetemcomitans
    Actinobacillus a.
actinomycetoma
actinomycin
actinomycoma
actinomycosis
    cervical a.
    cervicofacial a.
actinomycotic
    a. mycetoma
actinomycotin
actinoneuritis
actinophage
actinophytosis
actinoquinol sodium
actinotherapeutics
actinotherapy
    foil bath pulsed ultraviolet a.
    ultraviolet a.
action
    mechanism of a.
Actiprofen
activated
    a. charcoal
    a. macrophage
    a. partial thromboplastin time (APTT)
    a. vitamin K-dependent factor
activation
    complement a.
    lymphocyte a.
    natural killer cell a.
    NK cell a.
activation-induced cell death (AICD)
activator
    plasminogen a.
    polyclonal a.
    a. protein 1 (AP1)
active
    a. anaphylaxis

NOTES

active *(continued)*
    a. carrier
    A. Dry Lotion
    a. immunity
    a. immunization
    a. joint
    Labello A.
    a. nevus
    a. pinocytosis
    a. prophylaxis
    a. range of motion
    a. sensitization
    a. serum
    a. specific immunotherapy (ASI)
    a. transport
activin
activity
    adenosine triphosphatase a.
    amidolytic a.
    ATPase a.
    complement a.
    hyaluronidase a.
    IL-2 receptor-b and cytotoxic a.
    immunophilin isomerase a.
    increased sympathoadrenal a.
    kallikrein a.
    lymphocyte chemoattractant a.
    patient global assessment of
      disease a.
    physician global assessment of
      disease a.
    recombinational a.
    rheumatoid factor-like a. (RFLA)
    vitiligo disease a. (VIDA)
actomyosin
Actos
Actron
acuity
    LogMAR visual a.
Acular Ophthalmic
acuminata
    verruca a.
acuminate
    a. papular syphilid
    a. wart
acuminatum, pl. **acuminata**
    condyloma a. (CA)
    papilloma a.
    verruca acuminata
acuminatus
    lichen ruber a.
acupuncture needle dermatitis
Acuson 128XT ultrasound
Acusyst-Xcell
    A.-X. monoclonal antibody
    A.-X. monoclonal antibody
      culturing system

acuta
    parapsoriasis lichenoides et
      varioliformis a.
    pityriasis lichenoides et
      varioliformis a. (PLEVA)
    pustulosis vacciniformis a.
    urticaria a.
acute
    a. allergic urticaria
    a. anaphylactic reaction
    a. anterior poliomyelitis
    a. asthma attack
    a. atrophic oral candidiasis
    a. atrophic paralysis
    a. bacterial endocarditis (ABE)
    a. bronchopulmonary aspergillosis
      panel
    a. bulbar poliomyelitis
    a. cellular xenograft rejection
    a. contagious conjunctivitis
    a. crescentic glomerulonephritis
    a. cutaneous leishmaniasis
    a. cutaneous lupus erythematosus
      (ACLE)
    a. decubitus ulcer
    a. disseminated encephalitis (ADE)
    a. disseminated encephalomyelitis
      (ADEM)
    a. disseminated histiocytosis
    a. disseminated myositis
    a. epidemic conjunctivitis
    a. epidemic leukoencephalitis
    a. epiglottitis
    a. febrile neutrophilic dermatosis
    a. flaccid paralysis (AFP)
    a. follicular conjunctivitis
    a. generalized exanthematous
      pustulosis (AGEP)
    a. hemorrhagic edema (AHE)
    a. hemorrhagic glomerulonephritis
    a. herpes zoster
    a. herpetic gingivostomatitis
    a. humoral rejection (AHR)
    a. hypersensitivity pneumonitis
    a. idiopathic polyneuritis
    a. idiopathic thrombocytopenic
      purpura
    a. infectious disease
    a. infectious nonbacterial
      gastroenteritis
    a. inflammation (AI)
    a. intermittent porphyria (AIP)
    a. interstitial nephritis
    a. intravascular hemolysis
    a. laryngotracheobronchitis
    a. lupus pneumonitis
    a. lymphoblastic leukemia (ALL)
    a. lymphocytic leukemia (ALL)

a. meningococcemia
a. myelogenous leukemia (AML)
a. myeloid leukemia (AML)
a. necrotizing encephalitis
a. necrotizing ulcerative gingivitis (ANUG)
a. otitis media (AOM)
a. paranasal sinusitis
a. paronychia
a. peritonitis
a. phase protein
a. phase reactant (APR)
a. phase reaction
a. physiology and chronic health evaluation (APACHE)
a. poststreptococcal glomerulonephritis (APSGN)
a. primary hemorrhagic meningoencephalitis
a. pulmonary reaction
a. radiation pneumonitis
a. radiodermatitis
a. respiratory failure (ARF)
a. retinal necrosis (ARN)
a. retroviral syndrome
a. rheumatic arthritis
a. rheumatic fever (ARF)
a. rheumatoid arthritis
a. rhinitis
a. scalp cellulitis
a. seroconversion syndrome
a. transfusion reaction
a. tubular necrosis
a. vascular purpura
a. vascular xenograft rejection (AVXR)
acutum
  ulcus vulvae a.
acutus
  pemphigus a.
acyclovir
acyl chain
AD
  atopic dermatitis
ADA
  adenosine deaminase
  ADA deficiency
Adagen
ADAM
  a disintegrin and matrilysin
Adamantiades-Behçet syndrome
adamantinoma

Adams-Oliver syndrome
adapalene
  a. cream
  a. gel
Adapin
adaptor
  bi-luer lock a.
  ENTsol a.
ADASI
  Atopic Dermatitis Area and Severity Index
ADCC
  antibody-dependent cell-mediated cytotoxicity
  antibody-dependent cellular cytotoxicity
addicted scrotum syndrome
Addison
  A. disease
  A. keloid
  A. morphea
  A. pigmentation
Addison-Gull disease
addisonian
  a. dermal pigmentation
  a. melanosis
addisonism
addition-deletion mutation
additive
  a. arthritis
  food a.
  impermeant solution a.
  substrate solution a.
addressin
addressing ligand
adductor digiti quinti
ADE
  acute disseminated encephalitis
adefovir
ADEM
  acute disseminated encephalomyelitis
Aden
  A. fever
  A. ulcer
adenine
  a. arabinoside
adenitis
  Bartholin a.
  syphilitic inguinal a.
  vestibular a.
adeno-associated virus (AAV)
adenocarcinoma
  colonic a.

NOTES

11

adenocarcinoma (*continued*)
eccrine a.
Lucké a.
sebaceous a.
adenoepithelioma
adenoid
a. cystic carcinoma
adenoidal facies
adenoidal-pharyngeal-conjunctival (A-P-C)
a.-p.-c. virus
adenoidectomy
adeno-like
gallus a.-l. (GAL)
adenolipoma
adenolipomatosis
adenoma
aggressive digital papillary a. (ADPA)
apocrine a.
papillary eccrine a.
sebaceous a.
a. sebaceum
adenomatoid
adenomatosis oris
adenopathy
hilar a.
adenosatellite virus
adenosine
a. deaminase (ADA)
a. deaminase deficiency
a. diphosphate (ADP)
a. monophosphate (AMP)
a. triphosphatase (ATPase)
a. triphosphatase activity
a. triphosphate (ATP)
adenosylcobalamin
adenoviral
a. gene transfection
Adenoviridae
adenovirus (AdV)
canine a. 1
a. fiber knob
gutless a.
immunogenetic wild-type a.
adenovirus-mediated gene transfer
adenovirus-reactive T cell
adenylate cyclase toxin
adenylic acid
adenylosuccinic acid synthetase
ADEPT
antibody-directed enzyme prodrug therapy
adequate
a. hydration
a. urine output
adermal

adermia
a. congenita
adermic
adermogenesis
Ad fiber-knob
ADG
adjustable-length gauge needle
ADG needle
adherence
a. assay
immune a.
adhesin-receptor interaction
adhesins
adhesion
a. aid
cell-cell a.
corneocyte a.
homophilic cell-cell a.
integrin-mediated a.
keratinocytic a.
a. molecule
a. molecule cascade
a. phenomenon
a. protein
a. test
adhesional and glide friction
adhesive
Biobrane a.
a. capsulitis
Indermil tissue a.
Indermil topical a.
Scanpor acrylate a.
a. serositis
adiaphoresis
adiaphoretic
adiaspiromycosis
Adie tonic pupil
adipofibroma
adipogenic
adipogenous
adipometer
adiponecrosis subcutanea neonatorum
adiposa
blepharoptosis a.
seborrhea a.
adiposalgia
adipose infiltration
adiposis dolorosa
adipositis
adiposity
painful a.
adiposum
sclerema a.
adjustable-length
a.-l. gauge
a.-l. gauge needle (ADG, ADG needle)

adjuvant
    Freund complete a.
    Freund incomplete a. (FIA)
    immunologic a.
    a. vaccine
ADL 2-1294
Adlone Injection
administration
    Food and Drug A. (FDA)
adnata
    alopecia a.
adnexal
    a. carcinoma
    a. tumor
adnexum, pl. adnexa
    ocular adnexa
adolescent eczema
adoptive
    a. immunity
    a. immunotherapy
ADP
    adenosine diphosphate
ADPA
    aggressive digital papillary adenoma
ADR
    adverse drug-induced reaction
adrenal
    a. cortex disorder
    hypothalamo-pituitary a. (HPA)
    a. insufficiency
Adrenalin
    A. Chloride
adrenergic
    a. drug
    a. urticaria
adrenocortical
    a. failure
    a. insufficiency
adrenocorticosteroid
    a. therapy
adrenocorticotropic
    a. hormone (ACTH)
    a. hormone therapy
adrenoleukodystrophy
Adriamycin
Adrucil injection
ADS
    antibody-deficient syndrome
ADSI
    Atopic Dermatitis Severity Index

Adson
    A. test
    A. toothed forceps
adsorbed
    tetanus toxoid, a.
adsorbent
Adsorbotear Ophthalmic solution
adsorption
    immune a.
adsorptive voltametry
adult
    a. bullous dermatosis
    a. eczema
    latent autoimmune diabetes of a.'s (LADA)
    a. respiratory distress syndrome (ARDS)
    a. T-cell leukemia (ATL)
    a. T-cell leukemia/lymphoma (ATLL)
    a. T-cell lymphoma
    a. T-cell lymphoma-leukemia
    a. tuberculosis
adult/adolescent spectrum of HIV disease (ASD)
adulterated rapeseed oil-associated toxic oil syndrome
adult-onset systemic Still disease
adultorum
    scleredema a.
    a. scleroderma
adult-type rheumatoid arthritis
AdV
    adenovirus
Advair
advanced
    A. Formula Oxy Sensitive Gel
    a. glycation end-product (AGE)
advancement flap
adventitia
adventitial dermis
adventitious cyst
adverse
    a. drug-induced reaction (ADR)
    a. drug reaction
Advil
    Children's A.
    A. Cold & Sinus Caplets
Advisory Committee on Immunization Practice (ACIP)
AEA
    allergic extrinsic alveolitis

NOTES

AEC
> absolute blood eosinophil count
> ankyloblepharon, ectodermal defect, and
>   cleft lip and/or palate
> AEC syndrome

AECA
> antiendothelial cell antibody
> antiendothelial cell autoantibody

AECP
> antiepiligrin cicatricial pemphigoid

Aedes albopictus

aegleria invadens

Aeroaid

aeroallergen
> mold a.

Aerobacter

aerobe
> obligate a.

aerobic

AeroBid-M Oral Aerosol Inhaler

AeroBid Oral Aerosol Inhaler

aerobiology

Aerochamber nebulizer

aerodigestive

AeroEclipse Aerosol Delivery Device

aerofaciens
> *Eubacterium a.*

aerogen

aerogenes
> *Pasteurella a.*

aerogenesis

aerogenic tuberculosis

aeroirritant

Aerolate
> A. III
> A. Jr
> A. SR

aerometric study

Aeromonas
> A. caviae
> A. hydrophila
> A. septicemia
> A. shigelloides
> A. sobria
> A. veronii

aerophil

aerophilic

aeroplankton

Aeroseb-Dex

Aeroseb-HC Topical

aerosol
> Brethaire Inhalation A.
> A. Cloud enhancer (ACE)
> DEY albuterol inhalation a.
> Duo-Medihaler A.
> Fluro-Ethyl A.
> ipratropium bromide a.
> monodisperse a.

> Nasalide Nasal A.
> a. sensitization (AS)
> a. spray
> Tilade Inhalation A.
> Virazole A.

aerosolization

aerosolized pollutant exposure

AeroSonic personal ultrasonic nebulizer

AeroTech II nebulizer

AeroZoin

Aertemia Salinas sequence

aeruginosa
> *Pseudomonas a.*

aestival (*var. of* estival)

aestivale (*var. of* estivale)

aestivalis (*var. of* estivalis)

AETT
> acetyl ethyl tetramethyl tetralin

AEU
> allercoat enzyme allergosorbent unit

AF
> Diprolene AF

AF-1, -2 antigen

AFB
> acid-fast bacillus

AFC
> allergic fungal sinusitis
> antibody-forming cell

afferent
> a. arterioles
> a. nerve fiber

affinity
> a. antibody
> functional a.
> intrinsic a.
> a. labeling
> a. maturation

affinity-purified antiidiopeptide antibody

a-FGF
> acidic fibroblast growth factor

afibrinogenemia

A-Fil

AFIP
> Armed Forces Institutes of Pathology

Afipia felis

Aflexa

AFO
> ankle-foot orthosis

AFP
> acute flaccid paralysis

Africa
> Out of A.

African
> A. Burkitt lymphoma
> A. cutaneous Kaposi sarcoma
> A. endemic relapsing fever
> A. Gold
> A. hemorrhagic fever

A. histoplasmosis
A. honeybee
A. horse sickness
A. horse sickness virus
A. lymphadenopathic Kaposi sarcoma
A. meningitis
A. swine fever
A. swine fever virus (ASFV)
A. tick typhus
A. tick virus
A. trypanosomiasis
Africanized honeybee sting
African-variety Kaposi sarcoma
Afrin
A. Children's Nose drops
A. Nasal Solution
A. Tablet
Afrinol
AFS
aldehyde-fuchsin stain
Aftate
after
before and a. (B&A)
aftosa
AFX
atypical fibroxanthoma
afzelii
Borrelia a.
Ag
antigen
AGA
androgenetic alopecia
agalactiae
Streptococcus a.
*a*Gal epitope
agammaglobulinemia
acquired a.
Bruton a.
secondary a.
Swiss type a.
transient a.
X-linked a.
agar
BCYE a.
buffered charcoal yeast extract a.
corn meal a.
a. diffusion assay
a. gel diffusion
Kirby-Bauer a.
Löwenstein-Jensen a.

Mueller-Hinton a.
Sabouraud a.
agarose gel
AGAS
accelerated graft atherosclerosis
AGE
advanced glycation end-product
Agency
Regional Organ Procurement A. (ROPA)
Agenerase
agenesia
agenesis
pilorum a.
pulmonary a.
agent
Accuzyme enzymatic debriding a.
alkylating a.
alpha-adrenergic blocking a.
antifibrinolytic a.
antifoaming a.
antihypertensive a.
antihyperuricemic a.
antimalarial a.
antipruritic a.
antirheumatic a.
Bittner a.
chelating a.
chemical a.
chemotherapy a.
chimpanzee coryza a. (CCA)
cholinergic a.
coloring a.
comedolytic a.
cooling a.
cytoprotective a.
cytotoxic a.
delta a.
denaturing a.
dispersing a.
Eaton a.
emulsifying a.
entire body imaging a.
epsilon-aminocaproic a.
F a.
fertility a.
foamy a.
gastroprotective a.
hemostatic a.
immunosuppressive a.
keratolytic a.
lactic dehydrogenase a.

NOTES

15

agent *(continued)*
LDH a.
LeukoScan diagnostic a.
macrolide antimicrobial a.
MS-1, -2 a.
noncorticosteroid antiinflammatory a.
Norwalk a.
Norwalk-like a.
Panafil enzymatic debriding a.
Panafil-White enzymatic
debriding a.
prophylaxis a.
psychotropic a.
Reovirus-like a.
Santyl enzymatic debriding a.
sclerosing a.
skin exposure reduction paste
against chemical warfare a.'s
(SERPACWA)
topical hemostatic a.
transforming a.
virus-inactivating a.
Wor Ditchling a.
AGEP
acute generalized exanthematous
pustulosis
age pigment
age-related osteoporosis
agglutinate
agglutinating antibody
agglutination
acid a.
bacteriogenic a.
cold a.
cross a.
false a.
group a.
immune a.
indirect a.
latex particle a.
mixed a.
nonimmune a.
passive a.
reversed passive latex a.
spontaneous a.
agglutinative
agglutinin
blood group a.
chief a.
cold a.
cross-reacting a.
febrile a.
flagellar a.
group a.
H a.
immune a.
incomplete a.
major a.

minor a.
O a.
partial a.
plant a.
saline a.
serum a.
somatic a.
warm a.
Yersinia pseudotuberculosis a.
agglutinogen
blood group a.
T a.
agglutinogenic
agglutinophilic
agglutinoscope
agglutogen
agglutogenic
aggrecanase-induced aggrecan neoepitope
aggrecan CS/KS
aggregate
a. anaphylaxis
IgG-RF complement a.
immunoglobulin G rheumatoid
factor complement a.
link-protein-stabilized a.
snowball a.
snowbank a.
aggregated human IgG
aggregation
familial a.
aggregometry
aggressin
aggressive
a. cell cluster
a. digital papillary adenoma
(ADPA)
a. hepatitis
a. infantile fibromatosis
aging
photo a.
premature a.
AgiSite alginate wound cover
AGM
absorbent gelling material
agminata
agminated follicle
agminate folliculitis
agnails
agnogenic myeloid metaplasia (AMM)
agonist
alpha-adrenergic a.
beta-adrenergic a.
bronchoactive a.
histamine H_1 a.
agranulocytosis
feline a.
agrarius
Apodemus a.

agretope
agria
>protoporphyria prurigo a.
>prurigo a.

agrius
>lichen a.

Agrobacterium
>*A. radiobacter*
>*A. tumefaciens*

AH50 assay
AHA
>alpha-hydroxy acid

AHE
>acute hemorrhagic edema

AHG-CDC
>antiglobulin-enhanced complement-
>dependent cytotoxicity

AHGXM
>antihuman globulin crossmatch

AHR
>acute humoral rejection
>airway hyperresponsiveness

A-hydroCort
AHYS
>acquired hyperostosis syndrome

AI
>acute inflammation
>allergy and immunology
>>apo AI
>>>apolipoprotein AI
>>>apolipoprotein AI (apo AI)

AI-502
AIA
>antigen-induced arthritis
>aspirin-intolerant asthma

AIC
>aminoimidazole carboxamide

AICAR
>aminoimidazole carboxamide ribotide

AICA-riboside
>aminoimidazole carboxamide-riboside

AICD
>activation-induced cell death

aid
>adhesion a.
>Compoz Nighttime Sleep A.
>Congest A.
>Sleep A.
>Travel A.

AIDS
>acquired immune deficiency syndrome
>acquired immunodeficiency syndrome

>transfusion-associated AIDS (TA-
>AIDS)
>AIDS vaccine

AIDS-related
>A.-r. complex (ARC)
>A.-r. virus (ARV)

AIF-1
>anemia-inducing factor-1

AIH
>autoimmune hepatitis

AIHA
>autoimmune hemolytic anemia

AIL
>angioimmunoblastic lymphadenopathy

AILD
>angioimmunoblastic lymphadenopathy
>with dysproteinemia

Ailos nebulizer
AIMS
>arthritis impact measurement scale

ainhum
ainhumoides
>sclerodactylia annularis a.

AIP
>acute intermittent porphyria

air
>a. bronchogram
>a. cleaner
>a. coil
>a. conditioning
>high-efficiency particulate a.
>(HEPA)
>liquid a.
>a. pollution
>a. pollution control
>a. spora
>a. trapping

airborne
>a. contact dermatitis
>a. spore
>a. transmission

Airet
air-fluidized bed
airspace
>a. consolidation
>peripheral a.
>a. process

Airstrip composite dressing
AirWatch Asthma monitor
airway
>a. bacterial colonization
>a.'s disease

NOTES

airway *(continued)*
a. eosinophilia
a. hyperresponsiveness (AHR)
a. pressure release ventilation (APRV)
a. reactivity
a. resistance
a. responsiveness
a. smooth muscle (ASM)
AITP
autoimmune thrombocytopenia
Ajellomyces
A. dermatitidis
AK
acne keloidalis
Akabane virus
akamushi
a. disease
Leptotrombidium a.
Trombicula a.
akari
Rickettsia a.
AK-Chlor Ophthalmic
AK-Cide Ophthalmic
AKD
atypical Kawasaki disease
AK-Dex Ophthalmic
AK-Dilate Ophthalmic solution
akeratosis
AK-Homatropine Ophthalmic
AK-Mycin
AK-Nefrin Ophthalmic solution
Akne-Mycin topical
AK-Neo-Dex Ophthalmic
AK-Poly-Bac Ophthalmic
AK-Pred Ophthalmic
Akrinol Cream
AkroTech mattress
AK-Spore
A.-S. H.C. Ophthalmic Ointment
A.-S. H.C. Ophthalmic suspension
A.-S. H.C. Otic
AK-Sulf Ophthalmic
AK-Tate
AKTob Ophthalmic
AK-Tracin Ophthalmic
AK-Trol Ophthalmic
AKU
alkaptonuria
Akwa Tears solution
AL
AL protein
ALA
amino levulinic acid
antilymphocyte antibody
ALA dehydratase deficiency porphyria

gamma-ALA dehydratase deficiency porphyria
AlaBLOT kit
Ala-Cort Topical
Aladdin infant flow system
alae nasi
Alagille syndrome
Alamast
alanine aminotransferase
alanyl-transfer ribonucleic acid synthetase
alanyl-tRNA synthetase
Ala-Quin topical
alar ligament
Ala-Scalp Topical
AlaSTAT
A. allergy immunoassay system
A. assay
A. latex allergy test
alastrim
alastrimic
Alatest Latex-specific IgE allergen test kit
AlaTOP inhalant allergy screen
alba, pl. **albae**
lepra a.
linea a.
miliaria a.
morphea a.
phlegmasia a.
pityriasis a.
stria a.
albedo unguium
albendazole sulfoxide
Albenza
albicans, pl. **albicantes**
Candida a.
linea a.
Monilia a.
stria a.
albida
acne a.
albidum
atrophoderma a.
albimanus
Anopheles a.
albinism
Amish a.
autosomal dominant oculocutaneous a.
autosomal recessive ocular a. (AROA)
brown oculocutaneous a.
circumscribed a.
complete imperfect a.
complete perfect a.
cutaneous a.
Forsius-Eriksson-type ocular a.

a. I, II
localized a.
minimal-pigment oculocutaneous a.
Nettleship-Falls ocular a.
Nettleship-Falls-type ocular a.
ocular a. (OA)
oculocutaneous a. (OCA)
partial a.
piebald a.
red a.
rufous oculocutaneous a.
temperature-sensitive
  oculocutaneous a.
type I, IA, IB, II
  oculocutaneous a.
type I, II ocular a.
type I-MP, I-TS oculocutaneous a.
tyrosinase-negative
  oculocutaneous a.
tyrosinase-positive oculocutaneous a.
tyrosinase-related oculocutaneous a.
X-linked ocular a. (XOAN)
yellow mutant a.
yellow oculocutaneous a.
albinismus
  a. circumscriptus
  a. conscriptus
  a. universalis
albino
albinoidism
albinotic
alboatrum
  Verticillium a.
Albolene
albopictus
  Aedes a.
Albright
  A. dimpling sign
  A. disease
  A. hereditary osteodystrophy
  A. sign
  A. syndrome
albumin
  amoxicilloyl-human serum a. (AX-HSA)
  ampicillin-human serum a. (AMP-HSA)
  Bence Jones a.
  low plasma a.
  penicillin-penicilloyl human
    serum a. (PPO-HSA)
  Q a.

albumin-autoagglutinating factor
albus
  lichen a.
  Staphylococcus a.
albuterol sulfate syrup
Alcaligenes
  A. denitrificans
  A. faecalis
  A. odorans
  A. piechaudii
  A. xylosoxidans
Alcian blue stain
alclometasone
  a. dipropionate
alcohol
  benzyl a.
  cinnamic a.
  ethyl a.
  isopropyl a.
  a. pledget
  wool wax a.
alcoholic white shake lotion
alcohol-related liver disease (ALD)
Alcyonidrium
ALD
  alcohol-related liver disease
Aldara cream
aldehyde
  cinnamic a.
aldehyde-fuchsin stain (AFS)
alder
  red a.
  a. tree
  a. tree pollen
aldesleukin
Aldrich syndrome
alendronate sodium
Aleppo boil
aleukemic leukemia
Aleutian
  A. mink disease
  A. mink disease virus
Aleve
alexandrite laser
alexin unit
Alexion anticomplement C5a
ALEXlazr laser
Alezzandrini syndrome
alfa
  epoetin a. (EPO)
alfa-2a
  interferon a.

NOTES

alfa-2b
> interferon a.

alfalfa
> a. grass
> a. weed pollen

alfa-n3
> interferon a.-n.

Alferon N

ALG
> antilymphocyte globulin

AlgiDerm
> A. alginate dressing
> A. alginate wound cover
> A. wound dressing

algid stage

alginate
> a. dressing
> a. wound cover

AlgiSite
> A. alginate dressing
> A. wound dressing

Algisorb wound dressing

alglucerase

algodystrophy

algofunctional Lequesne index

algorithm
> Dermatologic Diagnostic A.
> diagnostic a.
> Needleman-Wunsch a.
> problem-oriented a.
> Relpal a.

Algosteril
> A. alginate dressing
> A. alginate wound cover

ALHE
> angiolymphoid hyperplasia with eosinophilia

Alibert
> A. disease
> A. keloid
> A. mentagra

Alibert-Bazin syndrome

Alibour solution

Alimentum formula

aliphatic
> a. hydrocarbon
> a. residue

aliquant

aliquot

alitretinoin

alizarin red S stain

Alkaban-AQ

alkaline phosphatase and pyrophosphate

alkalinization

alkalinizer
> urinary a.

alkali patch test

alkaloid
> *Vinca* a.

alkanolamineborate

alkaptonuria (AKU)

Alka-Seltzer Plus Cold Liqui-Gels Capsule

alkyarylsulfonate

alkyl
> a. aryl ether
> a. phenoxyl polyethoxy ethanol

alkylamine

alkylating
> a. agent
> a. therapy

ALL
> acute lymphoblastic leukemia
> acute lymphocytic leukemia

Alldress composite dressing

alleaceae

Allegra

Allegra-D

allele
> blank a.
> DR1 a.
> DR3 a.
> DR5 a.
> HLA a.
> a. HLA DQw7
> a. HLA-DR4
> a. HLA-DR7
> HLA-DRB1 a.
> a. HLA DRw53
> human leukocyte antigen a.
> a. human leukocyte antigen DQw7
> a. human leukocyte antigen DRw53
> null a.
> permissive MHC a.
> promotor a.

allelic
> a. exclusion
> a. polymorphism

Aller-Aide

AllerCare allergy control product

Aller-Chlor Oral

allercoat enzyme allergosorbent unit (AEU)

Allercon Tablet

Allerderm Protective Glove System

Allerdryl

Allerest
> A. 12 Hour Nasal Solution
> A. Maximum Strength

Allerfrin
> A. Syrup
> A. Tablet

Allergan Ear drops

allergen
> a. contact

environmental a.
epidermal a.
a. exposure
flux a.
inhalant a.
a. inhalation challenge test
Lolium perenne a.
Lol p a. (I-III)
occupational a.
recombinant a.
a. specific nasal challenge
20-allergen Hermal screening series
allergenic
    a. epitope
    a. extract
allergen-induced
    a.-i. asthma
    a.-i. mediator release
allergic
    a. angiitis
    a. angioedema
    a. apostematous cheilitis
    a. asthma
    a. bronchopulmonary aspergillosis
    (ABPA)
    a. conjunctivitis
    a. contact dermatitis (ACD)
    a. contact stomatitis
    a. coryza
    a. crease
    a. diathesis
    a. eczema
    a. eczematous contact-type
    dermatitis
    a. encephalomyelitis
    a. eosinophilic gastroenteritis
    a. eosinophilic gastroenterocolitis
    a. extract
    a. extrinsic alveolitis (AEA)
    a. facies
    a. fungal sinusitis (AFC)
    a. gold dermatitis
    a. granulomatosis
    a. granulomatous arteritis
    a. importance
    a. inflammation
    a. manifestation
    a. nonthrombocytopenic purpura
    a. orchitis
    a. phlyctenulosis
    a. reaction
    a. rhinitis

a. rhinobronchitis
a. rhinoconjunctivitis
a. salute
a. sensitivity
a. shiner
a. urticaria
a. vasculitis
allergin
allergist
allergization
allergize
allergized
allergoid
allergologic
allergologist
allergology
allergosis
Allergy
    A. Elixir
    A. Relief
allergy
    acrylic acid a.
    atopic a.
    bacterial a.
    Benylin for A.'s
    car a.
    cerebral a.
    cold a.
    contact a.
    cow's milk a. (CMA)
    delayed a.
    drug a.
    durable-press a.
    food a.
    gelatin a.
    hereditary a.
    IgE-mediated food a.
    immediate a.
    immunoglobulin E-mediated food a.
    a. and immunology (AI)
    insulin a.
    intrinsic a.
    Japanese sargassum a.
    latent a.
    latex a.
    nasal a.
    natural rubber latex a.
    nickel a.
    ocular a.
    physical a.
    polyvalent a.
    propylene glycol a.

NOTES

allergy *(continued)*
    Rowe elimination diet for food a.'s
    seasonal a.
    spina bifida-associated latex a.
    spontaneous a.
    a. tablet
    a. unit (AU)
    universal a.
    a. vaccine
AllerMax Oral
Allernix
Allerphed Syrup
Allerprick needle
AllerSpray
Allescheria boydii
Allevyn
    A. adhesive foam dressing
    A. cavity foam dressing
    A. island foam dressing
    A. synthetic dressing
    A. tracheostomy foam dressing
all-fours maneuver
alligator skin
Allis forceps
alloantibody
alloantigen
alloantigenicity
alloantigen-independent risk factor
alloatherogenesis
allochromasia
Allochrysine
AlloDerm
    Cymetra micronized A.
    A. processed tissue graft
    A. universal dermal tissue graft
Allodermanyssus sanguineus
allogenic, allogeneic
    a. antigen
    a. bone marrow cell infusion
    a. bone marrow transplantation
    a. dendritic cell
    a. effect
    a. effect factor
    a. graft
    a. hematopoietic stem cell transplantation (allo-HSCT)
    a. inhibition
    a. transplant
allograft
    cardiac a.
    a. coronary artery disease (ACAD)
    double renal a.
    heart a.
    a. irradiation
    kidney a.
    liver a.
    lung a.
    neonatal skin a.
    a. pathology
    a. rejection
allographic stem cell transplant (mini-allo)
allogroup
allo-HSCT
    allogenic hematopoietic stem cell transplantation
alloimmunization
AlloMune
allopeptide
    donor a.
allophenic
alloplast
Alloprin
allopurinol
alloreactive cell
alloreactivity
allosensitization
allotope
allotoxin
allotransplantation
    cardiac a.
    liver a.
allotrichia circumscripta
allotype
    Am a.
    Gm a.
    InV a.
    Km a.
    latent a.
    nominal a.
    simple a.
    a. suppression
allotypic
    a. determinant
    a. marker
Allovectin-7 DNA/lipid complex
Allpyral
allscale
all-*trans*-retinoic acid
allylamine
allyl isothiocyanate
ALM
    acral lentiginous melanoma
Almeida disease
almond
Alnus glutinosa
Alocort
aloe
    Cortaid with A.
    Dermtex HC with A.
    Fruit of the Earth Moisturizing A.
    A. Vesta antifungal ointment
aloetic
Alomide Ophthalmic

alone

    pancreas transplant a. (PTA)

alopecia

    a. acquisita

    a. adnata

    a., nail dystrophy, ophthalmic complication, thyroid dysfunction, hypohidrosis, ephelides and enteropathy, and respiratory tract infection (ANOTHER)

    androgenetic a. (AGA)

    a. androgenetica

    androgenic a.

    a. capitis totalis

    Celsus a.

    central centrifugal scarring a. (CCSA)

    cicatricial a.

    a. cicatrisata

    cicatrizing a.

    a. circumscripta

    congenital sutural a.

    congenital triangular a.

    a. disseminata

    drug a.

    drug-induced a.

    favic a.

    favid a.

    female pattern a.

    follicular a.

    a. follicularis

    frontal fibrosing a. (FFA)

    a. furfuracea

    a. generalisata

    a. hereditaria

    hot comb a.

    Jonston a.

    a. leprotica

    a. liminaris

    a. liminaris frontalis

    lipedematous a.

    lupus a.

    male pattern a.

    marginal a.

    a. marginalis

    a. marginata

    mechanical a.

    a. medicamentosa

    moth-eaten a.

    a. mucinosa

    a. neoplastica

    a. neurotica

    noncicatrizing a.

    nonscarring a.

    a. orbicularis

    patterned a.

    physiologic a.

    pityriasic a.

    a. pityrodes

    postmenopausal frontal fibrosing a.

    postoperative pressure a.

    postpartum a.

    a. prematura

    premature a.

    a. presenilis

    pressure a.

    pseudopelade-type a.

    roentgen a.

    scarring vertex a.

    a. seborrheica

    senile a.

    a. senilis

    a. symptomatica

    syphilitic a.

    a. syphilitica

    tick bite a.

    toxic a.

    a. toxica

    traction a.

    traumatic a.

    a. traumatica

    a. triangularis

    a. triangularis congenitalis

    a. universal areata

    a. universalis

    x-ray a.

alopecic

Aloprim Injection

ALP

    antileukoproteinase

alpha

    a. adrenergic stimulation

    a. cell

    a. chain

    a. chain disease

    a. fetoprotein

    a. Gal antibody

    a. hemolysin

    interferon a. (IFN-alpha)

    A. Keri lotion

    a. lactalbumin

    a. nerve fiber

    a.-nonrapid eye movement (alpha-NREM)

NOTES

alpha *(continued)*
    PGF_2 a.
    A. 1 pump
    5 a. reductase
    a. thalassemia
    tumor necrosis factor a.
    a. wave intrusion
$alpha_1$
    a. antitrypsin deficiency panniculitis
    a. proteinase deficiency
alpha-2 globulin
alpha-adrenergic
    a.-a. agonist
    a.-a. blocking agent
alpha-amino-p-toluene sulfonamide
alpha2-antiplasmin
alpha-antitrypsin
    serum a.-a.
$alpha_1$-antitrypsin ($alpha_1$-AT)
    a.$_1$-a. deficiency
$alpha_1$-AT
    $alpha_1$-antitrypsin
alpha, delta sleep anomaly
alpha-difluoromethylornithine
alpha-enolase
alpha-glutathione S-transferase assay
alpha-heavy-chain disease
alpha-helix
alpha-hydroxy acid (AHA)
alpha-interferon 3
Alpha-Keri
    A.-K. oil
    A.-K. soap
alpha-lactalbumin
alpha-latrotoxin
alpha-melanocyte-stimulating hormone (alpha-MSH)
alpha-methyldopa
alpha-MSH
    alpha-melanocyte-stimulating hormone
$alpha_2$-neuraminoglycoprotein
alpha-nonrapid eye movement sleep
alpha-NREM
    alpha-nonrapid eye movement
    alpha-NREM sleep
5-alpha-R
    5-alpha-reductase
5-alpha-reductase (5-alpha-R)
    5-a.-r. type 1, 2
5-alpha reductase inhibitor
alpha-1-thymosin
Alphatrex Topical
$alpha_1$-trypsin inhibitor
Alphavirus
alphoides
    lepra a.
alphos
    lepra a.

alprazolam
ALPS
    autoimmune lymphoproliferative syndrome
Alrex
AL-Rr Oral
ALS
    amyotrophic lateral sclerosis
    antilymphocyte serum
Alström syndrome
Alteon
alteration
    ecologic a.
    glucocorticoid-mediated stress-induced immune a.
    metabolic a.
    red cell membrane a.
Alternaria
    A. alternanta fungus
    A. alternata
    A. mold
    A. tenuis
alternariosis
alternata
    Alternaria a.
alternate-day therapy
alternative
    a. pathway of complement cascade
    a. polyadenylylation
Al-Test
Alti-Flunisoline
Altinac
aluminum
    a. acetate
    a. acetate and acetic acid
    a. chloride
    a. chloride hexahydrate
    a. chloride solution
    a. chlorohydrate
    a. density step scale
    a. Finn chamber
    a. lactate
    a. oxide
    a. salt
alum-precipitated
    a.-p. antigen
    a.-p. preparation
    a.-p. pyridine-extracted pollen extract
Alupent
alvei
    Bacillus a.
    Hafnia a.
alveolar
    a. capillary
    a. fluid clearance
    a. infiltration by histiocyte
    a. macrophage

A

a. ventilation
a. ventilation per minute
alveolar-arterial oxygen gradient
alveolar-septal amyloidosis
alveoli (*pl. of* alveolus)
alveolitis
allergic extrinsic a. (AEA)
cryptogenic fibrosing a. (CFA)
diffuse fibrosing a.
extrinsic allergic a.
fibrosing a.
occupational allergic a.
alveolointerstitial
alveolus, pl. **alveoli**
ventilated a.
ALW
arch-loop-whorl system
ALX1-11
alymphoplasia
Nezelof type of thymic a.
thymic a.
Am
A. allotype
A. antigen
AMAD
Assessment Measure for Atopic
Dermatitis
amalgam
dental a.
a. tattoo
amantadine
a. hydrochloride
Amapari virus
amaranth
green a.
Amaranthaceae
amaranth-chenopod
amastigotes
amatol
amber
Baltic a.
Ambi
A. 10
A. Skin Tone
AmBisome
Amblyomma
A. americanum
A. cajennense
A. hebraeum
amboceptor
a. unit
Amboyna button

ambrette
musk a.
Ambrosia
A. artemisiifolia
A. psilostachya
A. trifida
ambulans
ulcus a.
ambulant erysipelas
Ambulator shoe
ambulatory blood pressure (ABP)
ambustiforme
ulcus a.
ambustion
ambustionis
dermatitis a.
amcinonide
Amcort Injection
amdinocillin
Ameba histolytica
amebiasis cutis
amebic
a. granuloma
a. ulcer
amebicide
ameboma
Amechol
amegakaryocytic thrombocytopenia (AT)
amelanosis
amelanotic
a. melanoma
a. nevus
amelioration
leukapheresis-induced a.
ameloblastoma
melanotic a.
peripheral a.
pigmented a.
America
Dystrophic Epidermolysis Bullosa
Research Association of A.
(DEBRA)
Infectious Disease Society of A.
(IDSA)
Americaine
American
A. Academy of Dermatology
(AAD)
A. Academy of Pediatrics (AAP)
A. Association of Immunologists
(AAI)

NOTES

25

American *(continued)*
    A. Association of Textile Chemicals & Colorists
    A. cockroach
    A. College of Rheumatology (ACR)
    A. elm
    A. elm tree
    A. leishmaniasis
    A. Rheumatism Association (ARA)
    A. Rheumatism Association index
    A. Society of Transplant Surgeons (ASTS)
    A. trypanosomiasis
    A. Type Culture Collection (ATCC)
americana
    leishmaniasis a.
americanum
    Amblyomma a.
americanus
    Necator a.
Amerigel
    A. topical ointment
    A. topical ointment hydrogel dressing
amerospore
Amersol
Amesec
A-methaPred Injection
Amevive
amiantacea
    pityriasis a.
    tinea a.
amiantaceous crust
Amico
    A. extractor
    A. nail nipper
amicrobic
amide compound
amidolytic activity
amidophosphoribosyltransferase
amifloxacin
amikacin sulfate
Amikin injection
amine
    biogenic a.
    a. precursor uptake and decarboxylation (APUD)
amino
    a. acid
    a. acid metabolism
    a. ethyl ethanolamine
    a. levulinic acid (ALA)
aminoacetonitrile
aminoacyl-tRNA synthetase

aminobenzoate
    a. ester
    ethyl a.
para-**aminobenzoate (PAB)**
aminobenzoic acid
aminoglutethimide
aminoglycoside
aminoimidazole
    a. carboxamide (AIC)
    a. carboxamide-riboside (AICA-riboside)
    a. carboxamide ribotide (AICAR)
5-aminolevulinic acid
Amino-Opti-E Oral
aminopenicillin
aminophylline, amobarbital, and ephedrine
aminopterin syndrome
Aminoquinoline
aminosalicylate sodium
aminosalicylic acid
aminosidine sulfate
aminosteroid
21-aminosteroid
aminotransferase
    alanine a.
amiodarone pigmentation
amiprilose HCl
Amish albinism
Ami-Tex LA
Amitril
amitriptyline hydrochloride
AML
    acute myelogenous leukemia
    acute myeloid leukemia
AMM
    agnogenic myeloid metaplasia
ammonia
    a. dermatitis
    a. rash
ammoniated mercury
ammonium
    a. lactate
    quaternary a.
amnioma
A-mode ultrasound
amorolfine
amorphous
    a. parenchymal opacification
    a. substance
AMO Vitrax
amoxicillin/clavulanate (AMX/CL)
    a. suspension
amoxicillin and clavulanic acid
amoxicilloyl-human serum albumin (AX-HSA)
Amoxil

AMP
adenosine monophosphate
Amp
Jaa A.
amphimicrobe
amphiphysin
amphiregulin (AR)
Amphocil
amphophilous
Amphotec
amphotericin
a. B
a. B cholesteryl sulfate complex
a. B colloidal dispersion
a. B lipid complex
a. B lipid complex injection
a. B liposomal formulation
amphotropic virus
AMP-HSA
ampicillin-human serum albumin
ampicillin
a. and probenecid
a. and sulbactam
ampicillin-human serum albumin (AMP-HSA)
Ampicin
A. Sodium
Ampilean
amplicon
deoxyribonucleic acid a.
DNA a.
Amplicor viral load test
amplification
a. assay
chirp-pulse a.
HBV bDNA signal a.
hepatitis B virus branched chain deoxyribonucleic acid signal a.
human immunodeficiency virus DNA a.
nucleic acid sequence based a. (NASBA)
Amplified Mycobacterium Tuberculosis Direct Test
amplifier host
Ampliwax PCR Gem
amprenavir
amprolium hydrochloride
amputating ulcer
amputation neuroma
amstelodamensis
typhus degenerativus a.

amstelodami
Aspergillus a.
Amvisc
A. plus
AMX/CL
amoxicillin/clavulanate
AMX/CL suspension
Amycolatopsis orientalis
amyctic
amylin
IAPP a.
amyloid
a. A protein
articular a.
cutaneous a.
a. degeneration
a. disease
a. fibril
a. fibril protein
a. P component
primary a.
a. Q
secondary a.
a. structure
a. syndrome
systemic a.
a. tumor
amyloidosis
AA, AL a.
alveolar-septal a.
bullous a.
cerebral a.
a. cutis
cystatin C a.
dialysis-related a.
endocrine a.
familial a.
fibrogen-associated a.
focal a.
gelsolin a.
hemodialysis-associated a.
hereditary cardiopathic a.
heredofamilial a.
immune-derived a.
immunocyte-derived a.
lichen a.
lichenoid a.
localized cutaneous a.
lysozyme-associated a.
macular a.
mediastinal a.
neuropathic a.

NOTES

amyloidosis *(continued)*
    nodular pulmonary a.
    nonneuropathic systemic a.
    oculoleptomeningeal a.
    parenchymal a.
    pleural a.
    polyneuropathic a.
    primary cutaneous a.
    primary localized a.
    primary systemic a.
    pseudotumoral mediastinal a.
    pulmonary a.
    secondary systemic a.
    secondary tumor-associated
      cutaneous a.
    systemic visceral a.
    tracheobronchial a.
    transthyretin a.
amyloidotic nephropathy
amyopathic
    a. dermatomyositis
amyotrophic
    a. lateral sclerosis (ALS)
    a. syphilitic myelitis
AN
    acanthosis nigricans
ANA
    antinuclear antibody
    speckled-pattern ANA
anabolic steroid
anabrosis
anabrotic
Anacardium
    A. melanorrhoea
    A. occidentale
Anacin
anaemicus *(var. of* anemicus*)*
anaerobe
    facultative a.
anaerobic
    a. bacterial arthritis
    a. *Bifidobacterium*
    a. cellulitis
Anaerobiospirillum
anaerobius
    Peptostreptococcus a.
anaesthetica
    lepra a.
Anaflex 750
Anafranil
anagen
    a. effluvium
    a. growth phase
anagrelide
Ana-Guard
Anahelp
AnaKinra
Ana-Kit

anal fissure
anallergic
analog, analogue
    purine a.
    semisynthetic a.
analogous
Analpram
analysis, pl. **analyses**
    antigenic a.
    bioelectrical impedance a. (BIA)
    displacement a.
    dual-fluorescence a.
    gait a.
    genome-side linkage a.
    genomic a.
    Griess a.
    immunofluorescence a.
    latent class a.
    limiting dilution a. (LDA)
    Northern blot a.
    post hoc a.
    power spectral a.
    quantitative immunoglobulin a.
    saturation a.
    spectral a.
    ultrastructural a.
    univariate regression a.
    a. of variance (ANOVA)
    a. of variance test
analyte
analyzer
    Electra 1000C coagulation a.
    Gemini automated centrifugal a.
    Malvern a.
    MiniOX 1A oxygen a.
    Opti 1 portable pH/blood gas a.
    SPART a.
Anamine Syrup
anamnesis
anamnestic
    a. reaction
    a. response
ananaphylaxis
ANAP
    anionic neutrophil-activating peptide
anaphylactic
    a. antibody
    a. crisis
    a. desensitization
    a. hypersensitivity reaction
    a. intoxication
    a. shock
    a. state
    a. syndrome
anaphylactica
    enteritis a.
anaphylactogen
anaphylactogenesis

anaphylactogenic
anaphylactoid
    a. crisis
    a. phenomenon
    a. purpura
    a. reaction
    a. shock
anaphylatoxin
    C3 a. (C3a)
    a. inactivator
    a. peptide
anaphylaxis
    active a.
    aggregate a.
    antiserum a.
    bird nest a.
    chronic a.
    complement-mediated a.
    controlled a.
    drug a.
    eosinophil chemotactic factor of a.
      (ECF-A)
    exercise-induced a. (EIA)
    fire ant a.
    food-associated exercise-induced a.
    generalized a.
    heterocytotropic a.
    homocytotropic a.
    Hymenoptera venom a.
    immediate active cutaneous a.
      (IACH)
    inflammatory factor of a. (IF-A)
    inverse a.
    local a.
    passive cutaneous a. (PCA)
    penicillin-induced a.
    pharmacologic mediators of a.
    reversed passive a.
    slow-reacting factor of a. (SRF-A)
    slow-reacting substance of a. (SRS-
      A)
    systemic a.
    undifferentiated somatoform IA a.
anaphylaxis-angioedema-frequent
    idiopathic a.-a.-f. (IA-A-F)
anaphylaxis-angioedema-infrequent
    idiopathic a.-a.-i. (IA-A-I)
anaphylaxis-generalized-frequent
    idiopathic a.-g.-f. (IA-G-F)
anaphylaxis-generalized-infrequent
    idiopathic a.-g.-i. (IA-G-I)

anaphylaxis-questionable
    idiopathic a.-q. (IA-Q)
anaphylaxis-variant
    idiopathic a.-v. (IA-V)
anaphylotoxin
anaplasia
Anaplex Liquid
Anaprox
Ana-Sal HIV test
anatomic
    a. tubercle
    a. wart
anatomical
    a. tubercle
    a. wart
anatoxic
anatoxin
anatripsis
anatriptic
Anatuss
Anavar
ANCA
    antineutrophil cytoplasmic antibody
    antineutrophilic cytoplasmic antibody
ANCA-associated vasculitis (AAV)
ANCA-positive vasculitis (APV)
Ancef
anchor
    glycophosphatidylinositol a.
Ancobon
Ancotil
Ancylostoma
    A. braziliense
    A. caninum
    A. duodenale
ancylostoma dermatitis
ancylostomiasis
    cutaneous a.
    a. cutis
Anderson-Fabry disease
andersoni
    Dermacentor a.
Anderson sampler
Andes virus
Andrews disease
androgen
androgen-dependent syndrome
androgenetica
    alopecia a.
androgenetic alopecia (AGA)
androgenic alopecia

NOTES

androstane
androstanediol
androstanedione
androstene
androstenedione
androsterone
anemia
>acquired hemolytic a.
>aregenerative a.
>autoimmune hemolytic a. (AIHA)
>Blackfan-Diamond a.
>chronic hemolytic a.
>congenital a.
>Cooley a.
>dermatopathic a.
>drug-related immunohemolytic a.
>equine infectious a.
>Fanconi a.
>fish tapeworm a.
>hapten mechanism of hemolytic a.
>hypochromic normocytic a.
>iron deficiency a.
>Leishman a.
>megaloblastic a.
>microangiopathic hemolytic a.
>neonatal a.
>a. neonatorum
>pernicious a.
>severe aplastic a. (SAA)
>sickle cell a.

anemia-inducing factor-1 (AIF-1)
anemic halo
anemicus, anaemicus
>nevus a.

anemone
>sea a.

anemophilous
anergic
>a. leishmaniasis
>a. T cell

AnergiX.RA
anergy
>cutaneous a.
>native a.
>natural a.
>negative a.
>nonspecific a.
>a. panel
>peripheral a.
>positive a.
>specific a.
>in vitro a.

Anestacon
anesthesia
>Madajet XL local a.

anesthetic
>eutectic mixture of local a.'s
>(EMLA)

>intradermal a.
>a. leprosy
>preoperative a.
>topical a.

anetoderma
>a. of Jadassohn
>Jadassohn a.
>Jadassohn-Pellizzari a.
>a. of prematurity
>Schweninger-Buzzi a.
>a. of Schweninger-Buzzi
>a. scleroatrophy

aneuploidy
>deoxyribonucleic acid a.
>DNA a.

aneurin hydrochloride
ANF
>antinuclear factor

ANGEL
>angiolipoma, posttraumatic neuroma,
>glomus tumor, eccrine spiradenoma,
>and leiomyoma cutis
>ANGEL tumor

angel
>a. kisses lesion

Angelman syndrome
angel-wing deformity
angiectodes
>nevus a.

angiitis
>allergic a.
>choroidal a.
>Churg-Strauss a.
>granulomatous a.
>hypersensitivity a.
>leukocytoclastic a.
>a. livedo reticularis
>necrotizing a.
>nonnecrotizing a.
>systemic hypersensitivity a.

angina
>Bretonneau a.
>a. bullosa haemorrhagica (ABH)
>herpetic a.
>Ludwig a.
>Vincent a.

anginose scarlatina
angioblastic lymphadenopathy
angiocentric lymphoma
Angiocol
angiodermatitis
>disseminated pruriginous a.

angiodestructive lymphoma
angioedema
>acquired a. (AAE)
>allergic a.
>episodic a.
>hereditary vibratory a.

a. profile
vibratory a.
angioedema-induced urticaria
angioedema-urticaria-eosinophilia
syndrome
angioendothelioma
endovascular papillary a.
angioendotheliomatosis
malignant a.
neoplastic a.
a. proliferans
proliferating systematized a.
reactive cutaneous a. (RCA)
systemic proliferating a.
angiofibroma contagiosum tropicum
angiogenesis
a. factor
a. inhibitor
angiogranuloma
angiography
angiohistiocytoma
multinucleate cell a.
angioid streak
angioimmunoblastic
a. lymphadenopathy (AIL)
a. lymphadenopathy with
dysproteinemia (AILD)
angioinvasive lesion
angiokeratoma
circumscriptum a.
a. corporis diffusum
a. corporis diffusum universale
Fabry a.
a. of Fordyce
Fordyce a.
localized a.
Mibelli a.
a. of Mibelli
solitary a.
verrucous a.
angiokeratosis, pl. **angiokeratoses**
angioleiomyoma
angiolipoma, posttraumatic neuroma,
glomus tumor, eccrine spiradenoma,
and leiomyoma cutis (ANGEL)
angiolupoid
angiolymphatic invasion
angiolymphoid
a. hyperplasia
a. hyperplasia with eosinophilia
(ALHE)

angioma
acquired tufted a. (ATA)
capillary a.
a. cavernosum
cavernous a.
cherry a.
hereditary hemorrhagic a.
infectious a.
keratotic a.
plane a.
plexiform a.
senile a.
serpiginosum a.
a. serpiginosum
a. simplex
spider a.
stellate a.
strawberry a.
sudoriparous a.
superficial a.
tuberous a.
tufted a.
angiomatodes
nevus a.
angiomatoid Spitz nevus
angiomatosis
bacillary a.
cutaneomeningospinal a.
meningooculofacial a.
Sturge-Weber encephalotrigeminal a.
universal a.
angiomatous nevus
angiomyoneuroma
angioneuromyoma
angioneurotic
a. dermatosis
a. edema
angioneurotica
purpura a.
angioproliferative lesion
angiosarcoma (AS)
angiosperm
Angiostrongylus costaricensis
angiotensin-converting enzyme (ACE)
angle
center-edge a.
Lovibond a.
angry
a. back phenomenon
a. back reaction
a. back syndrome

NOTES

Angström
Å. unit (Å unit)
angstrom (Å)
Angström unit (Å unit)
angular
a. cheilitis
a. conjunctivitis
a. stomatitis
anhidrosis
thermal a.
thermogenic a.
anhidrotic ectodermal dysplasia
anhydride
acid a.
phthalic a.
terpine a.
trimellitic a.
anhydrous
a. facial foundation
a. lanolin
a. theophylline
ani
pruritus a.
anicteric virus hepatitis
anidrosis
anidrotic
animal
control a.
conventional a.
a. dander
a. dander sensitivity
a. hair
Houssay a.
normal a.
a. scabies
sentinel a.
a. toxin
a. virus
anion
superoxide a.
anionic
a. detergent
a. neutrophil-activating peptide (ANAP)
anisa
Legionella a.
anisakiasis
gastrointestinal a. (GIA)
Anisakis
A. simplex
anitratus
Acinetobacter a.
Anitschkow myocyte
ANKENT
ankylosis and ankylosing enthesopathy

ankle
annular atrophic connective tissue panniculitis of the a.
retinacula of a.
ankle-foot orthosis (AFO)
ankyloblepharon, ectodermal defect, and cleft lip and/or palate (AEC)
ankylosing
a. enthesopathy
a. hyperostosis
a. spondylitis (AS)
ankylosis
a. and ankylosing enthesopathy (ANKENT)
bony a.
a. nonunions
anlage
Ann Arbor staging
annexin V
annual bluegrass
annular
a. atrophic connective tissue panniculitis of the ankle
a. distribution of lesion
a. elastolytic giant cell granuloma
a. erythema
a. erythematous plaque
a. lichen planus
a. lipoatrophy
a. syphilid
annulare
erythema a.
generalized granuloma a.
granuloma a. (GA)
localized granuloma a.
perforating granuloma a.
subcutaneous granuloma a.
annularis
leukotrichia a.
lichen planus a.
lipoatrophia a.
livedo a.
psoriasis a.
annularity
annulata
psoriasis a.
thrix a.
annulatus, pl. annulati
pilus a.
pseudopilus a.
annulus
a. fibrosus
a. migrans
ano
fistula in a.
anogenital
a. disorder
a. epidermal cyst

a. pilar cyst
a. sebaceous cyst
a. vestibular cyst
a. vestibular papilla

anomaly
alpha, delta sleep a.
DiGeorge a.
Jordan a.
morning glory a.
nevoid a.
reticulate pigmented a.
Rieger a.
sleep a.

anonychia
Anopheles
A. *albimanus*
A. *freeborni*
A. *funestus*
A. *gambiae*

anorexia
anorexigenic
ANOTHER
alopecia, nail dystrophy, ophthalmic complication, thyroid dysfunction, hypohidrosis, ephelides and enteropathy, and respiratory tract infection
ANOTHER syndrome

ANOVA
analysis of variance
ANOVA test

anoxia
focal a.

Ansaid Oral
anserina
cutis a.

anserine bursitis
Answer
Herbal A.

ant
a. bite
black a.
fire a.
red imported fire a.
a. sting

Antabuse
antagonism
bacterial a.

antagonist
calmodulin a.
insulin a.
leukotriene a.

nonselective adenosine receptor a.
recombinant human interleukin-1 receptor a.

antalgic gait
antazoline phosphate
Antazone
antecubital fossa
antemortem
antenna, pl. **antennae**
Antense antitension device
anterior
a. atlantodental interval (AADI)
a. chamber-associated immune deviation (ACAID)
a. spinal artery syndrome
a. synechia formation
a. uveitis

anteriores
limbi palpebrales a.

anteversion
femoral a.

anthelix
elastotic nodules of a.

anthelminthic
anthelmintic
anthelotic
anthema
anthesis
Anthopsis deltoidea
anthracic
anthracis
Bacillus a.

anthracoid
anthraconecrosis
Anthra-Derm
Anthraforte
anthralin
anthramucin
anthranilate
Anthranol
anthrarobin
Anthrascalp
anthrax
cutaneous a.
a. toxin

anthropi
Ochrobacterium a.

anthroponosis
anthroponotic cutaneous leishmaniasis
anthropophaga
Cordylobia a.

anti-70K antibody

NOTES

anti-A antibody
Anti-Acne
    A.-A. Control Formula
    A.-A. Formula for Men
    A.-A. Spot Treatment
antiadhesin antibody
antiagglutinin
antialexin
antiallergic
anti-alpha-fodrin antibody
antianaphylaxis
antiandrogen
antianthrax serum
antiantibody
antiantitoxin
antiapoptotic
    a. effect
    a. molecule
antiarachnolysin
antiautolysin
anti-B4 blocked ricin
anti-B7-1 monoclonal antibody
antibacterial therapy
anti-B antibody
antibasement
    a. membrane antibody
    a. membrane antibody-induced
      glomerulonephritis
    a. membrane nephritis
    a. membrane zone autoantibody
antibiogram
antibiont
antibiosis
AntibiOtic
    A. Otic
antibiotic
    a. enterocolitis
    fluoroquinolone a.
    a. protein
    a. sensitivity
    a. sensitivity test
antibiotic-associated colitis
antibiotic-resistant
anti-BMZ autoantibody
antibody (Ab)
    ABX-CBL monoclonal a.
    ACA a.
    acetylcholine receptor a. (AChRAb)
    aCL a.
    Acusyst-Xcell monoclonal a.
    affinity a.
    affinity-purified antiidiopeptide a.
    agglutinating a.
    alpha Gal a.
    anaphylactic a.
    anti-A a.
    antiadhesin a.
    anti-alpha-fodrin a.

anti-B a.
antibasement membrane a.
anti-B7-1 monoclonal a.
antibody excess a.
anticardiolipin a. (ACA, ACLAb)
anti-CD3 a.
anti-CD4 a.
anti-CD18 humanized a.
anti-CD54 a.
anticentromere a. (ACA)
antichemokine a.
antichromatin a.
anti-CMV a.
anticolon a.
anticyclic citrullinated peptide a.
anticytoplasmic a. (ACPA)
anti-D anti-Rh a.
anti-DNA a.
anti-DNA-topoisomerase I a.
anti-dsDNA a.
anti-EA a.
anti-EBV a.
antiendomysial a.
antiendothelial cell a. (AECA)
anti-Epstein-Barr virus a.
anti-Fas a.
antifibrin a.
antifilaggrin a.
anti-GAD a.
antigliadin a.
anti-HA a.
anti-HAV a.
anti-HB$_c$ a.
anti-HB$_e$ a.
anti-HB$_s$ a.
antihistone a.
antihistone-(H2A-
  H2B)/deoxyribonucleic acid
  complex a.
anti-HLA class I a.
antiidiotype a.
anti-IgA a. (IgE class)
anti-IgE humanized monoclonal a.
anti-Jo-1 a.
anti-Jp-1 a.
anti-70K a.
antikeratin a.
anti-Ku a.
anti-La a.
antilactoferrin a.
anti-La/SSB a.
antilymphocyte a. (ALA)
antimelanocyte a.
anti-Mi-2 nuclear a.
antimitochondrial a.
anti-MPO a.
    antimyeloperoxidase antibody

antimyeloperoxidase a. (anti-MPO antibody)
antimyosin a.
antineuronal a.
antineutrophil cytoplasmic a. (ANCA)
antineutrophilic cytoplasmic a. (ANCA)
antinuclear a. (ANA)
antinuclear matrix a.
antinucleosomal a.
anti-P a.
antiparvovirus 19 a.
antipeptide a.
antiphospholipid a. (APA, APLA)
anti-PM-Scl a.
antipneumococcal a.
anti-Ri a.
antiribonucleoprotein a.
antiribosomal a.
antiribosomal-P a.
antiribosome a. *anti-Ro a.*
anti-RNA pol I a.
anti-RNP a.
anti-Ro a.
anti-Ro/SSA a.
antirubella a.
anti-S a.
anti-Scl-70 a.
antiscleroderma-70 a. (anti-Scl-70)
antisignal recognition particle a.
anti-Sjögren syndrome A, B a.
anti-Sm a.
anti-Smith a.
antismooth muscle a.
antisperm a.
anti-SRP a.
anti-SS-A a.
anti-SS-B a.
antisynthetase a.
anti-Th a.
antithymocyte a.
antithyroid microsomal a.
antitopoisomerase I a.
anti-tTG a.
antityrosinase a.
anti-U1, -U3 RNP a.
anti-VEGF a.
anti-Yo a.
auto-antiidiotypic a.
autologous a.
avidity a.
basement membrane zone a.
Bexxar radiolabeled monoclonal a.
bispecific a.

bivalent a.
blocking a.
a. blocking assay
blood group a.
BMZ a.
BR96-doxorubicin monoclonal a.
2C3 anti-VEGF a.
CC49 monoclonal a.
CD1a a.
CD5 a.
CD5+ a.
CD10 a.
CD11a a.
CD11b a.
CD11c a.
CD14 a.
CD15 a.
CD18 a.
CD19 a.
CD20 a.
CD21 a.
CD22 a.
CD24 a.
CD28 a.
CD29 a.
CD38 a.
CD43 a.
CD44 a.
CD49a a.
CD49b a.
CD49c a.
CD49e a.
CD49f a.
CD54 a.
CD106 a.
CD3 monoclonal a.
CD4 monoclonal a.
CD8 monoclonal a.
CD16 monoclonal a.
CD25 monoclonal a.
CD56 monoclonal a.
CD69 monoclonal a.
CD71 monoclonal a.
cell-bound a.
CF a.
C100-3 hepatitis C virus a.
chimeric a.
chromatin a.
cold a.
cold-reactive a.
combining-site a.
a. combining site
complement-fixing a.
complete a.

NOTES

antibody *(continued)*

cross-reacting a.
cryptosporidiosis a.
cytophilic a.
cytoplasmic antineutrophil cytoplasmic a. (C-ANCA, c-ANCA)
CytoTAb polyclonal a.
cytotropic a.
dacliximab monoclonal a.
a. deficiency
a. deficiency disease
Diffistat-G polyclonal a.
direct fluorescent a. (DFA)
Donath-Landsteiner a.
a. dysfunction
E5 monoclonal a.
7E3 monoclonal antiplatelet a.
enhancing a.
Epstein-Barr virus-induced early a.
Escherichia coli polysaccharide a.
a. excess
fluorescent antimembrane a. (FAMA)
Forssman a.
Gal a.
group A carbohydrate a.
Ha-1A monoclonal a.
hemagglutinating a.
a. to hepatitis B core antigen (HB$_c$Ab, HBcAb)
a. to hepatitis B e antigen (HB$_e$Ab, HBeAb)
a. to hepatitis B surface antigen (HB$_s$Ab, HBsAb)
heteroclitic a.
heterocytotropic a.
heterogenetic a.
heterophil a., heterophile a.
histone a.
histone-DNA a.
HIV neutralizing a.
homocytotropic a.
human anti-CMV a.
human anticytomegalovirus a.
human leukocyte a. (HLA)
humoral a.
hybrid a.
hybridoma a.
I-B1 radiolabeled a.
idiotype a.
IgA a.
IgA antiendomysial a.
IgA antigliadin a.
IgE a.
IgG a.
IgM anticardiolipin a.
immobilizing a.

ImmuRAIT-LL2 monoclonal a.
incomplete a.
indirect fluorescent a.
infliximab monoclonal a.
inhibiting a.
inhibition fluorescent a.
islet cell a. (ICA)
isophil a.
Jo-1 a.
LDP-02 humanized monoclonal a.
LeuTech radiolabeled a.
lupus anticoagulant a. (LAC)
LymphoCide a.
lymphocyte function-associated a.-1 (LFA-1)
lymphocyte function-associated a.-2 (LFA-2)
lymphocyte function-associated a.-3 (LFA-3)
lymphocytotoxic a.
MAb-170 monoclonal a.
MabThera monoclonal a.
Mi-2 a.
monoclonal a. (MAB, MoAb)
monoclonal antiendothelial cell a. (mAECA)
myositis-specific a.
native type anti-DNA a.
natural a.
neutralizing murine monoclonal antitumor necrosis factor a.
nonprecipitable a.
nonprecipitating a.
nonprecipitation a.
normal a.
nucleosome a.
OKT3 a.
Oncolym radiolabeled monoclonal a.
opsonizing a.
ornithine-ketoacid transaminase 3 a.
Orthoclone OKT3 anti-CD3 monoclonal a.
Orthomune monoclonal a.
Ovarex MAb monoclonal a.
palivizumab a.
panel-reactive a. (PRA)
panreactive monoclonal a.
percent reactive antibody/panel reactive a. (PRA)
perinuclear antineutrophil cytoplasmic a. (P-ANCA)
P-K a.
PM 81 monoclonal a.
polyclonal a.
polynucleotide a.
Prausnitz-Kustner a.
precipitating a.

preexisting a.
preformed a.
prophylactic a.
ProstaScint monoclonal a.
r24 a.
rabbit antithymocyte globulin
   polyclonal a.
RATG polyclonal a.
reaginic a.
ReoPro monoclonal a.
Rituxan monoclonal a.
Scl-70 a.
serum antiglomerular-basement-
   membrane a.
single-stranded anti-DNA a.
SJ441 a.
skin-sensitizing a.
speckled-pattern antinuclear a.
Thomsen a.
thyroid-blocking a. (TBAB)
thyroid-stimulating a. (TSAb)
thyroid-stimulating hormone-
   displacing a.
thyroid-stimulating hormone
   receptor a.
thyroperoxidase a.
TI-23 cytomegalovirus
   monoclonal a.
treponema-immobilizing a.
treponemal a.
TSH-displacing a.
TSH receptor a. (TRAb)
type I, IIb antineuronal a.
univalent a.
U1 RNP a.
Vi a.
vitiligo a.
warm-reactive a.
Wassermann a.
WinRho SD a.
xenoreactive natural a. (XNA)
XMMEN-OE5 monoclonal a.
Y12 monoclonal a.
antibody-deficient syndrome (ADS)
antibody-dependent
   a.-d. cell-mediated cytotoxicity
      (ADCC)
   a.-d. cellular cytotoxicity (ADCC)
**antibody-directed enzyme prodrug
   therapy (ADEPT)**
antibody-forming cell (AFC)

antibody-phage display
antibotulinus serum
antibromic
anti-C3 assay
anticalpastatin autoantibody
anticardiolipin (aCL)
   a. antibody (ACA, ACLAb)
   a. antibody syndrome
   a. autoantibody
anti-CD3
   a.-CD3 antibody
   SMART a.-CD3
anti-CD18 humanized antibody
anti-CD4 antibody
anti-CD54 antibody
**anti-CD11a humanized monoclonal
   antibody for psoriasis**
anticentromere antibody (ACA)
anti-Centruroides antivenin
antichemokine antibody
anticholera serum
anticholinergic drug
antichromatin antibody
alpha$_1$-antichymotrypsin
anti-CMV
   anticytomegalovirus
      anti-CMV antibody
anticoagulant
   circulating a.
   lupus a. (LA)
anticolon antibody
anticomplement
anticomplementary
   a. factor
   a. serum
anticontagious
anticonvulsant
   hydantoin a.
anticrotalus serum
anticyclic citrullinated peptide antibody
anticytokine
anticytomegalovirus (anti-CMV)
anticytoplasmic antibody (ACPA)
anticytotoxin
anti-D
   a.-D. anti-Rh antibody
   a.-D. enzyme-linked immunosorbent
      assay
   a.-D. immunoglobulin
Anti-Dandruff
   Neutrogena Healthy Scalp A.-D.

NOTES

Anti-Dandruff *(continued)*
    Satinique A.-D.
    A.-D. Shampoo
antideoxyribonuclease B (anti-DNase B)
antideoxyribonucleic acidase
antidepressant
    heterocyclic a.
    tricyclic a.
antidimer DNA
anti-DNA antibody
anti-DNase B
    antideoxyribonuclease B
anti-DNA-topoisomerase I antibody
Antidote
    H-F A.
antidouble-stranded DNA
anti-dsDNA antibody
anti-EA antibody
anti-EBV
    anti-Epstein-Barr virus
    anti-EBV antibody
anti-EGF receptor antibody for cancer
antielastase
antiendomysial antibody
antiendothelial
    a. cell antibody (AECA)
    a. cell autoantibody (AECA)
antiendotoxin
    XXMEN-OE5 a.
antienzyme
antiepidermal growth factor receptor
  antibody for cancer
antiepiligrin cicatricial pemphigoid
  (AECP)
antiepithelial serum
anti-Epstein-Barr
    a.-E.-B. virus (anti-EBV)
    a.-E.-B.-virus antibody
antiestrogenic
anti-Fas antibody
antifibrin antibody
antifibrinolytic agent
antifilaggrin antibody
antifoaming agent
antifungal
    Absorbine Jr. A.
    Breezee Mist A.
    EcoNail a.
    a. therapy
anti-GAD antibody
antigen (Ag)
    Abbott HIVAG-1 monoclonal a.
    ABO a.
    Acanthocheilonema viteae excretory-
      secretory a.
    acetone-insoluble a.
    AF-1, -2 a.
    allogenic a.

    alum-precipitated a.
    Am a.
    antibody to hepatitis B core a.
      (HB_cAb, HBcAb)
    antibody to hepatitis B e a.
      (HB_eAb, HBeAb)
    antibody to hepatitis B surface a.
      (HB_sAb, HBsAb)
    antigen excess a.
    Au a.
    Aus a.
    Australia a.
    autologous a.
    bacterial a.
    Be^a a.
    Becker a.
    Bi a.
    Bile a.
    bivalent a.
    blank a.
    blood group a.
    bullous pemphigoid a. (BPA)
    cancer-testis a.
    capsular a.
    carcinoembryonic a. (CEA)
    C carbohydrate a.
    CDE a.
    centromere a.
    Chido-Rodgers a.
    chlordiazepoxide a.
    cholesterinized a.
    Chr^a a.
    cicatricial pemphigoid a.
    class I, II, III a.
    cold-induced skin a.
    commercial a.
    common acute lymphocytic
      leukemia a. (CALLA)
    complete a.
    conjugated a.
    cutaneous lymphocyte a. (CLA)
    D a.
    delta a.
    Dharmendra a.
    Di a.
    differentiation a.
    Dsg3 a.
    Duffy a.
    ENA a.
    endogenous a.
    epidermolysis bullosa acquisita a.
    Epstein-Barr nuclear a. (EBNA)
    a. excess
    exogenous a.
    extractable nuclear a. (ENA)
    Fas a.
    Fer a.
    flagellar a.

food a.
Forssman a.
Frei a.
Fy a.
G a.
Ge a.
glycophorin a.
Gm a.
Good a.
Gr a.
group a.'s
H a.
H-2 a.
He a.
heart a.
hepatitis A a. (HAA)
hepatitis-associated a. (HAA)
hepatitis B core a. (HB$_c$Ag, HBcAg)
hepatitis B e a.
hepatitis B surface a. (HB$_s$Ag, HBsAg)
heterogenetic a.
heterogenic enterobacterial a.
heterophil a.
heterophile a.
hexon a.
high molecular weight-melanoma-associated a. (HMW-MAA)
histocompatibility a.
HLA a.
Ho a.
homologous a.
Hu a.
human leukemia-associated a.
human leukocyte a. (HLA)
human lymphocyte a. (HLA)
human thymus lymphocyte a.
I a.
Ia a.
idiotypic a.
incomplete a.
a. interferon
InV group a.
isophile a.
Jk a.
Jobbins a.
Js a.
K a.
KF-1 a.
KI a.

killer inhibitor receptors-human leukocyte a. (KIR-HLA)
Km a.
Kveim a.
Kveim-Stilzbach a.
La a.
Lan a.
LDA-1 a.
Le a.
leukocyte common a.
Levay a.
LH 7:2 a.
Lu a.
luminal a.
Ly a.
Lyb a.
lymphocyte function-associated a. (LFA)
lymphogranuloma venereum a.
Lyt a.
M a.
M$_1$ a.
Mas a.
melanoma-specific a.
microchimeric a.
Mitsuda a.
mixed vespid a.
MNSs a.
Mu a.
multivalent a.
mumps skin test a.
noninherited maternal a. (NIMA)
nonspecific cross-reacting a. (NCA)
O a.
oncofetal a.
organ-specific a.
Ot a.
OVA a.
ovalbumin a.
OX-K proteus a.
Oz a.
P a.
p24 a.
pancreatic oncofetal a. (POA)
partial a.
P blood group a.
penton a.
peptide a.
PM-Scl a.
pollen a.
polymerized a.
polymyositis-scleroderma a.

NOTES

39

antigen *(continued)*
polysaccharide a.
pp65(UL83) a.
private a.
proliferating cell nuclear a.
(PCNA)
proliferation-associated a.
protein a.
public a.
QA a.
R a.
red cell a.
Rh a.
Rhus toxicodendron a.
Rhus venenata a.
ribonucleoprotein a.
ribonucleoprotein a.
RNP a.
Ro a.
S a.
sensitized a.
shock a.
sialoglycoprotein a.
skin-specific histocompatibility a.
Sm a.
Smith a.
soluble liver a. (SLA)
somatic a.
species-specific a.
specific a.
Stobo a.
streptococcal M a.
Streptococcus M a.
Su a.
surface a.
Sw^a a.
Swann a.
synthetic a.
T a.
Tac a.
T-dependent a.
theta a.
thymus-independent a.
tissue-specific a.
Tj a.
Tr^a a.
transplantation a.
tumor a.
tumor-associated a.
tumor-associated transplantation a.
(TATA)
tumor-specific transplantation a.
(TSTA)
a. unit
V a.
Vel a.
Ven a.

very late activation a. (VLA-1
antigen)
vespid a.
Vi a.
viral capsid a.
VLA-1 a.
very late activation antigen
Vw a.
Webb a.
Wr^a a.
Wright a. (Wr^a)
Xg a.
Yersinia a.
YKL-40 a.
Yt^a a.
antigen-1
leukocyte factor a. (LFA-1)
lymphocyte function a. (LFA-1)
lymphocyte function-associated a.
(LFA-1)
antigen-3
lymphocyte function-associated a.
(LFA-3)
antigen-4
cytotoxic T lymphocyte a. (CTLA-
4)
very late a. (VLA-4)
antigen-antibody
complement-activating a.-a.
a.-a. complex
a.-a. reaction
antigen-binding
a.-b. diversity
single-chain a.-b. (SCA)
a.-b. site
antigen-combining site
antigenemia
cytomegalovirus a.
a. test
antigenemically cross-reacting food
antigenic
a. analysis
a. antibody lattice formation
a. binding receptor
a. competition
a. complex
a. determinant
a. drift
a. modulation
a. shift
a. variation
antigenicity
antigen-induced arthritis (AIA)
antigen-nonspecific immune complex
assay
antigen-presenting cell (APC)
antigen-recognition
antigen-sensitive cell

A

antigen-specific immune response

antigenuria
  pneumococcal a.

antigliadin
  a. antibody
  a. IgG, IgA test

antiglobulin-enhanced complement-dependent cytotoxicity (AHG-CDC)

antiglobulin test

antiglomerular basement membrane (anti-GMB)

anti-GMB
  antiglomerular basement membrane

anti-HA antibody

anti-HAV antibody

anti-HB$_s$ antibody

anti-HB$_e$ antibody

anti-HB$_c$ antibody

anti-HCV seropositive

anti-*Helicobacter*

antihelminthic

antihemagglutinin

antihemolysin

antihemolytic

antihepatitis
  a. A virus
  a. C virus seropositive

antihidrotic

Antihist-1

antihistamine
  H$_1$, H$_2$ a.
  nonsedating a.
  oral a.

antihistaminic

Antihist-D

antihistone antibody

antihistone-(H2A-H2B)/deoxyribonucleic acid complex antibody

anti-HLA class I antibody

anti-hnRNP

antihormone

antihost reactivity

antihuman
  a. globulin
  a. globulin crossmatch (AHGXM)
  a. globulin test
  a. parvovirus immunoglobulin G

antihyaluronidase

antihydriotic

antihypertensive agent

antihyperuricemic agent

antiidiotype
  a. antibody
  a. autoantibody
  a. vaccine

anti-IgA antibody (IgE class)

anti-IgE humanized monoclonal antibody

anti-IIb-IIIA mAB therapy

antiimmune body

antiinflammatory
  a.-i. cytokine
  nonsteroidal a.-i.
  a.-i. therapy

anti-Jo-1 antibody

anti-Jp-1 antibody

antikeratin
  a. antibody
  a. autoantibody

antikidney serum nephritis

anti-Ku antibody

anti-La antibody

antilactoferrin antibody

anti-La/SSB antibody

antileukocidin

antileukoproteinase (ALP)

antileukotoxin

anti-Lewisite

Anti-LFA-1

antiluetic

antilymphocyte
  a. antibody (ALA)
  a. globulin (ALG)
  a. induction
  a. serum (ALS)

antilysin

antimalarial
  a. agent
  a. drug

antimelanocyte antibody

antimeningococcus serum

antimetabolite

anti-Mi-2 nuclear antibody

antimicrobial
  A. MPM wound cleanser
  a. spectrum

antimicrobiology susceptibility testing

Antiminth

antimitochondrial antibody

antimonial drug therapy for leishmaniasis

antimony spot

NOTES

anti-MPO
   antimyeloperoxidase
      anti-MPO antibody
antimuscarinic acetylcholine receptor
antimycobacterial
antimycotic
antimyeloperoxidase (anti-MPO)
      a.-m. antibody (anti-MPO antibody)
antimyosin antibody
antinative DNA
antinauseant
antineoplastic
antineuronal antibody
antineurotoxin
antineutrophil
      a. cytoplasmic antibody (ANCA)
      a. cytoplasmic autoantibody
antineutrophilic cytoplasmic antibody (ANCA)
antinuclear
      a. antibody (ANA)
      a. antibody immunodiffusion
      a. antibody immunofluorescence
      a. antibody screening by enzyme immunoassay
      a. antibody screening test
      a. antibody titer
      a. autoantibody
      a. factor (ANF)
      a. matrix antibody
antinucleosomal antibody
antinucleosome autoantibody
antioxidant vitamin
anti-P antibody
antiparallel B-sheet conformation
antiparasitic
antiparvovirus 19 antibody
anti-PCAM
   antiplatelet endothelial cell adhesion molecule
Anti-Pelliculaire
   Shampooing A.-P.
antipeptide antibody
antiperinuclear
      a. autoantibody
      a. factor (APF)
antiperiodic
antiperspirant
antiphagocytic
antiphlogistic
antiphospholipid
      a. antibody (APA, APLA)
      a. antibody syndrome (APS)
antipill finish
antiplatelet endothelial cell adhesion molecule (anti-PCAM)
anti-PM-Scl antibody

antpneumococcal antibody
antipneumococcic
antipneumococcus serum
anti-Pr cold autoagglutinin
antiprecipitin
antiproliferative effect
antiproteasomal
antiprotein S
antipruritic
      a. agent
      a. therapy
      topical a.
antipsoriatic
antipsoric
antipyretic
antipyrine and benzocaine
antipyrotic
antirabies
      a. serum
      a. serum, equine origin
antiresorptive
antireticular cytotoxic serum
antiretroviral
antirheumatic
      a. agent
      a. drug
anti-Ri antibody
antiribonucleoprotein antibody
antiribosomal antibody
antiribosomal-P antibody
antiribosome antibody
antiricin
anti-RNA pol I antibody
anti-RNP antibody
anti-Ro antibody
anti-Ro/SSA
      a.-R. antibody
antirotavirus IgA titer
antirubella antibody
anti-S antibody
antiscabetic
antiscabietic
anti-Scl-70
   antiscleroderma-70 antibody
      anti-Scl-70 antibody
antiscleroderma-70 antibody (anti-Scl-70)
antiseborrheic
antisense
      a. compound
      a. drug
      a. nucleotide
      a. oligodeoxynucleotide
      a. phosphorothioate oligonucleotide
      a. RNA
antisepsis
Anti-Sept bactericidal scrub solution
antiseptic

antiseptic-impregnated central venous catheter
antiserum, pl. **antisera**
   a. anaphylaxis
   blood group a.
   heterologous a.
   homologous a.
   monospecific a.
   monovalent a.
   multivalent a.
   nerve growth factor a.
   NGF a.
   polyvalent a.
   Reenstierna a.
   specific a.
antisignal recognition particle antibody
anti-Sjögren
   a.-S. syndrome A, B antibody
anti-Sm
   a.-S. antibody
anti-Smith antibody
antismooth muscle antibody
antisnakebite serum
antisperm antibody
anti-SRP antibody
anti-SS-A antibody
anti-SS-B antibody
antistaphylococcic
antistaphylolysin
antisteapsin
antistreptococcic
antistreptokinase
antistreptolysin-O (ASLO, ASO)
   antistreptolysin-O test
   antistreptolysin-O titer
antisubstance
antisudorific
antisynthetase
   a. antibody
   a. syndrome
antitac
antitetanus toxin
anti-Th antibody
antithrombin III
antithymocyte
   a. antibody
   a. gamma globulin (ATG, ATGAM)
antithyroid microsomal antibody
antitopoisomerase I antibody
antitoxic
   a. serum

antitoxigen
antitoxin
   bivalent gas gangrene a.
   bothropic a.
   Bothrops a.
   botulinum a.
   botulism a.
   bovine a.
   Crotalus a.
   despeciated a.
   diphtheria a.
   dysentery a.
   gas gangrene a.
   normal a.
   pentavalent gas gangrene a.
   plant a.
   a. rash
   scarlet fever a.
   Staphylococcus a.
   tetanus a.
   tetanus-perfringens a.
   a. unit
antitoxinogen
antitrypsin
anti-tTG antibody
antituberculosis
antituberculous therapy
antitumorigenesis
antitussive
antitype II, IX collagen autoantibody
antityphoid
antityrosinase antibody
anti-U1, -U3 RNP antibody
anti-VEGF antibody
antivenene
   a. unit
antivenin
   anti-Centruroides a.
   black widow spider a.
   a. (*Crotalidae*) polyvalent
antivenom
   Latrodectus mactans a.
   Lyovac a.
   tiger snake a.
Antivert
antiviral
   a. drug
   a. immunity
   a. protein (AVP)
   a. therapy
anti-Yo antibody
Antrizine

NOTES

antrostomy
Anturan
Anturane
Anucort HC suppository
ANUG
    acute necrotizing ulcerative gingivitis
Anuprep HC suppository
Anusol
    A. HC-1 Topical
    A. HC-2.5% Topical
Anusol-HC suppository
Anxanil Oral
AOM
    acute otitis media
aortic arch syndrome
aortitis
    idiopathic a.
AP
    accelerated phase
    CML AP
        chronic
            myelocytic/myelogenous/myeloid
            leukemia accelerated phase
AP1
    activator protein 1
APA
    antiphospholipid antibody
Apacet
APACHE
    acute physiology and chronic health
    evaluation
    APACHE II score
    APACHE II system
apatite
A-P-C
    adenoidal-pharyngeal-conjunctival
    A-P-C virus
APC
    antigen-presenting cell
APEC
    asymmetric periflexural exanthem of
    childhood
APECED
    autoimmune polyendocrinopathy-
    candidiasis-ectodermal dysplasia
    autoimmune polyendocrinopathy-
    candidiasis-ectodermal dystrophy
    APECED syndrome
Apert
    A. hirsutism
    A. syndrome
APF
    antiperinuclear factor
apheresis
APHLT
    auxiliary partial heterotopic liver
    transplantation
aphtha, pl. aphthae

    Bednar a.
    Behçet a.
    cachectic a.
    a. febriles
    herpetiform a.
    aphthae major
    Mikulicz a.
    aphthae minor
    a. tropicae
Aphthasol
aphthoid
aphthosis
    Touraine a.
aphthous
    a. genital ulcer
    a. oral ulcer
    a. stomatitis
Aphthovirus
aphylactic
aphylaxis
apical lobe fibrosis
apicoposterior segment
apiculus
apiospermum
    Monosporium a.
    Scedosporium a.
Apis
    A. mellifera
    A. mellifera sting
apis
    Spiroplasma a.
APL
    acquired progressive lymphangioma
APLA
    antiphospholipid antibody
aplasia
    a. cutis congenita
    gold-induced a.
    pure red cell a. (PRCA)
Apley maneuver
Apligraf
    A. skin substitute
    A. tissue-engineered skin
Aplisol
apnea
    obstructive sleep a. (OSA)
    sleep a.
apneustic breathing
ApoA, ApoB
apo AI
Apo-Allopurinol
Apo-Amoxil
Apo-Ampi
Apo-ASA
ApoB
    ApoA, A.
Apo-Beclomethasone
Apo-Cetirizine

Apo-Cimetidine
apocrine
    a. acne
    a. adenoma
    a. bromhidrosis
    a. carcinoma
    a. chromhidrosis
    a. cystadenoma
    a. epithelioma
    a. hidrocystoma
    a. malaria
    a. miliaria
    a. poroma
    a. retention cyst
    a. sweat gland
apocrinitis
Apodemus
    A. *agrarius*
    A. *flavicollis*
Apo-Diclo
Apo-Diflunisal
Apo-Doxy Tabs
Apo-Erythro E-C
Apo-Famotidine
Apo-Fluconazole
Apo-Flurbiprofen
Apo-Gain
Apo-Hydroxyzine
Apo-Ibuprofen
Apo-Indomethacin
Apo-Ipravent
Apo-Keto
Apo-Keto-E
apolipoprotein
    a. AI (apo AI)
APOLT
    auxiliary partial orthotopic liver
      transplant
    auxiliary partial orthotopic liver
      transplantation
Apo-Metronidazole
Apo-Minocycline
Apo-Nabumetone
Apo-Napro-Na
Apo-Naproxen
aponeurosis
    palmar a.
aponeurotic fibroma
Apo-Pen VK
apophylaxis
apophyseal joint
Apo-Piroxicam

apoplexy
    cutaneous a.
Apo-Prednisone
apoptosis
    cellular inhibitors of a. (cIAPs)
    crypt epithelial cell a.
    dysregulated lymphocytic a.
    lymphocytic a.
apoptosis-associated molecule
apoptotic
    a. bleb
    a. body
    a. cell
    a. index
    a. keratinocyte
Apo-Ranitidine
apostematosa
    cheilitis glandularis a.
Apo-Sulfinpyraz
Apo-Sulin
Apo-Tetra
Apo-Zidovudine
apparatus
    Golgi a.
    internal hair a.
    Kidde a.
    pilosebaceous a.
    spark-gap a.
    vacuum tube a.
apparent leukonychia
AP-PCR
    arbitrary primed PCR
appearance
    ball-in-claw a.
    cluster-of-grapes a.
    coral-head a.
    enamel paint spot a.
    finger-in-glove a.
    ground-glass a.
    hair-on-end a.
    hair-standing-on-end a.
    hidebound a.
    orange peel a.
    plucked chicken papules a.
    safety-pin a.
    slapped-cheek a.
    slapped-face a.
    stuck-on a.
    Swiss cheese a.
    tire-patch a.
    toxic a.

NOTES

appendage
    epidermal a.
appendageal cord
appendicular
    a. disease
    a. tuberculosis
apple
    a. jelly nodule
    a. jelly papule of lupus vulgaris
appliance
    TheraSnore oral a.
applied kinesiology
approach
    CLIP replacement a.
appropriate culture
approximation
    zigzag a.
APR
    acute phase reactant
apraxia
    speech a.
Aprodine
    A. Syrup
    A. Tablet
apron pattern
aprotinin
APRV
    airway pressure release ventilation
APS
    antiphospholipid antibody syndrome
    autoimmune polyglandular syndrome
    APS type 1, 2
APSGN
    acute poststreptococcal
      glomerulonephritis
APT
    atopy patch test
APTT
    activated partial thromboplastin time
APUD
    amine precursor uptake and
      decarboxylation
apurpuric
APV
    ANCA-positive vasculitis
AQ
    Nasacort AQ
Aqua Care moisturizer
Aquacare topical
Aquacel
    A. Hydrofiber dressing
    A. wound packing and dressing
Aquacort
aquagenic
    a. pruritus
    a. urticaria
AquaMEPHYTON injection

Aquanil
    A. lotion
Aquaphor
    A. Antibiotic topical
    A. gauze
aquaphorin
    a. 1, 2
Aquaphyllin
aquarium granuloma
AquaSite Ophthalmic solution
Aquasol
    A. A
    A. A & D
    A. E
    A. E Oral
Aquasorb
    A. hydrogel sheet
    A. transparent hydrogel dressing
aquaspera
    Acrotheca a.
    Rhinocladiella a.
AquaTar
aqueous
    a. epinephrine
    a. extract
    penicillin a.
    a. solution
    a. vaccine
AR
    acoustic rhinometry
    amphiregulin
ARA
    American Rheumatism Association
    ARA criteria
arabic acid
arabicum
    elephantiasis a.
arabinoside
    adenine a.
    cytosine a.
Arabum
    elephantiasis A.
    lepra A.
ara-C
arachidonic
    a. acid (AA)
    a. acid cascade
    a. acid metabolism
    a. acid metabolite
    a. acid pathway
arachnidism
    necrotic a.
arachnodactylia
arachnodactyly
    congenital contractural a.
    contractural a.
arachnoideus
    nevus a.

A

Aralen phosphate with primaquine
   phosphate
Aramine
araneidism
araneosus
     nevus a.
araneus
     nevus a.
A-range
     dihydroxyacetone-psoralen
        ultraviolet A.-r. (DHA-PUVA)
     psoralen ultraviolet A.-r. (PUVA)
aranodactylia
Arava
arbitrary primed PCR (AP-PCR)
arbor
     a. vitae
     a. vitae tree
arborescens
     lipoma a.
arborize
arbovirus, arborvirus
ARC
     acquired immunodeficiency syndrome-
       related complex
     AIDS-related complex
arc
     mercury a.
arcade
     fibrous a.
     vascular a.
arcanobacterial pharyngitis
Archeaopsylla erinacei
arch-loop-whorl system (ALW)
arciform distribution of lesion
arcuate
arcuatus
     Chortoglyphus a.
ARDS
     adult respiratory distress syndrome
area
     butterfly a.
     Celsus a.
     dermatomic a.
     flush a.
     Hof a.
     intertriginous a.
     Jonston a.
     periocular a.
     perioral a.
     periorbital a.

     total body surface a. (TBSA)
     a. under the curve (AUC)
areata
     alopecia universal a.
     ophiasic alopecia a.
     pseudoalopecia a.
areate
areatus
areflexic paraparesis
aregenerative anemia
arenaceous
Arenaviridae
     A. virus
Arenavirus
areola, pl. areolae
     Chaussier a.
     nevoid hyperkeratosis of nipple
      and a.
     primary a.
     vaccinal a.
areolar
areolate
ARF
     acute respiratory failure
     acute rheumatic fever
ArF
     argon fluoride
Argasidae
Arg^{519}-Cys mutation in type II collagen
Argentine
     A. hemorrhagic fever
     A. hemorrhagic fever virus
Argentinean hemorrhagic fever
Argesic-SA
arginine codon
argininosuccinate synthetase deficiency
argininosuccinicaciduria
argon
     a. fluoride (ArF)
     a. laser
argon-pumped tunable-dye laser
Argostideae
Argyll Robertson pupil
argyria
argyriasis
argyric
argyrism
Argyrol S.S.
argyrosis
Aria CPAP system
ARI Group I–IV filter

NOTES

Aristocort
    A. A
    A. A Topical
    A. Forte
    A. Forte Injection
    A. Intralesional Injection
    A. Intralesional Suspension
    A. Oral
    Syrup of A.
    A. Tablet
Aristospan
    A. Intraarticular
    A. Intraarticular Injection
    A. Intralesional
    A. Intralesional Injection
Arizona
    A. ash
    A. ash tree
    A. coral snake
    A. cypress
    A. cypress tree
arizonae
    Salmonella a.
Arizona/Fremont
    A. cottonwood
    A. cottonwood tree
arm
    a. duration maneuver
    a. raises maneuver
    a. straighten maneuver
Arm-a-Med
    A.-a.-M. isoetharine
    A.-a.-M. Isoproterenol
    A.-a.-M. Metaproterenol
armamentarium
    cytotoxic a.
Armed
    A. Forces Institutes of Pathology
    (AFIP)
armed macrophage
ARN
    acute retinal necrosis
Arndt-Gottron
    A.-G. disease
    A.-G. syndrome
Arning tincture
AROA
    autosomal recessive ocular albinism
aromatic hydrocarbon
**around-the-clock oral maintenance
  bronchodilator therapy**
arrangement
    chromosome a.
    corymbose a.
    lesion a.
    V-D-J gene a.

array
    reticulate a.
arrector, pl. **arrectores**
    a. pili muscle
    arrectores pilorum
    arrectores pilorum muscle
    a. pilus
arrest
    cardiorespiratory a.
arresting
    high-efficiency particulate a.
    (HEPA)
Arrhenius-Madsen theory
arrhizus
    Rhizopus a.
arrhythmia
Arrow pneumothorax kit
arrowroot
Arroyo
    Whitewater A.
arsenic
    Mapharsen organic a.
    neoarsphenamine organic a.
    a. pigmentation
    a. trioxide
    tryparsamide organic a.
arsenical
    a. contact dermatitis
    a. keratosis
arsphenamine dermatitis
ArtAssist
    A. compression dressing/wrap
    A. leg compression dressing
artefact (*var. of* artifact)
artefacta
    dermatitis a.
Artemisia
    A. salina
artemisiifolia
    Ambrosia a.
Artemis vulgaris
Arteparon
arterial
    a. blood gas (ABG)
    a. hypoxemia
    a. spider
    a. ulcer
**arterial-ecchymotic type Ehlers-Danlos
  syndrome**
arterioles
    afferent a.
arteriopathy
    Takayasu a.
arteriosclerosis
    fibrotic a.
    a. obliterans
arteriosclerotic gangrene
arteriovenous (AV)

a. block
a. fistula
a. malformation (AVM)
a. shunt
arteritis
    allergic granulomatous a.
    cranial a.
    equine viral a.
    giant cell a. (GCA)
    granulomatous a.
    intimal a.
    Takayasu a.
    temporal giant cell a.
Arterivirus
artery
    interlobularly a.
    nutrient a.
Artha-G
arthralgia
Arthrisin
arthrites pseudoseptiques et bacterides d'Andrews
arthritic tuberculosis
arthriticum
    erythema a.
arthritidis
    Mycoplasma a.
arthritis, pl. **arthritides**
    acne a.
    acute rheumatic a.
    acute rheumatoid a.
    additive a.
    adult-type rheumatoid a.
    anaerobic bacterial a.
    antigen-induced a. (AIA)
    atypical mycobacterial a.
    axial psoriatic a.
    bacterial a.
    Borrelia-associated a.
    brucella a.
    burnt-out rheumatoid a.
    Candida a.
    candidal a.
    carrageenan a.
    chronic postrheumatic fever a.
    collagen-induced a. (CIA)
    crystal a.
    crystal-induced a.
    degenerative a.
    dislocation a.
    dysenteric a.
    enterogenic reactive a.

enteropathic a.
enthesitis-related a.
erosive a.
familial recurrent a.
A. Foundation ibuprofen
A. Foundation Nighttime
A. Foundation Pain Reliever
fungal a.
glenohumeral a.
gonococcal a.
Gram-negative bacilli a.
granulomatous idiopathic a.
hemochromatotic a.
hemorrhagic a.
hepatitis A, B a.
herpes simplex virus a.
idiopathic destructive a. (IDA)
a. impact measurement scale (AIMS)
infectious a.
inflammatory a.
intestinal bypass a.
juvenile chronic a.
juvenile idiopathic a. (JIA)
juvenile rheumatoid a. (JRA)
large-joint inflammatory a.
leukemic a.
lipopolysaccharide-induced a. (LPS-induced arthritis)
LPS-induced a.
    lipopolysaccharide-induced arthritis
Lyme a.
meningococcal a.
monoarticular antigen-induced a.
mutilans a.
a. mutilans
neuropathic a.
nongonococcal bacterial a.
noninflammatory a.
ochronotic a.
oligoarticular seronegative rheumatoid a.
ovalbumin-induced a.
patellofemoral a.
pauciarticular juvenile chronic a.
pauciarticular juvenile rheumatoid a.
peripheral a.
phase I, II rheumatoid a.
polyarticular gonococcal a.
polyarticular juvenile rheumatoid a.
polyarticular septic a.

NOTES

arthritis *(continued)*
    polymicrobial a.
    poststreptococcal reactive a. (PSRA)
    posttraumatic a.
    postvenereal reactive a.
    pseudocystic rheumatoid a.
    pseudoseptic a.
    psoriatic a.
    purulent a.
    pyogenic a.
    reactive a. (ReA)
    retinyl acetate-induced a.
    rheumatoid a. (RA)
    a. robustus
    rubella a.
    Salmonella a.
    sarcoid a.
    senescent a.
    septic a.
    seronegative rheumatoid a.
    seropositive rheumatoid a.
    sexually acquired reactive a.
      (SARA)
    Staphylococcus aureus a.
    suppurative a.
    systemic juvenile rheumatoid a.
    traumatic a.
    tuberculous a.
    unicondylar a.
    venereal-associated a.
    viral a.
    a. without deformity
    Yersinia a.
arthritis-pseudogout
    pyrophosphate a.-p. (PPA)
arthritogenic
    a. peptide
    a. protein
arthritogenicity
Arthro-BST arthroscopic probe
arthrocentesis
arthrochalasia-type Ehlers-Danlos syndrome
arthrochalasis multiplex congenita
arthrodesis
arthrography
    double-contrast a.
arthrogryposis
    a. congenita, distal, type I, II syndrome
    distal a.
arthroophthalmopathy
    hereditary a.
Arthropan
arthropathia psoriatica
arthropathica
    psoriasis a.

arthropathy
    acromegalic a.
    cuff tear a.
    cystic fibrosis a. (CFA)
    enteropathic a.
    facet joint a.
    gonococcal a.
    hemophilic a.
    Jaccoud a.
    myxedematous a.
    neuropathic a.
    ochronotic a.
    primary amyloidotic a.
    psoriatic a.
    pyrophosphate a.
    resorptive a.
    seronegativity, enthesopathy, a. (SEA)
arthropica
    psoriasis a.
arthropism
arthroplasty
    hybrid total a.
    Mayo modified total elbow a.
arthropod
    a. bite
    a. dermatosis
    a. sting
arthropod-borne virus
arthroscope
    Citoscope-16 a.
    30-degree oblique a.
    Medical Dynamics 5990 needle a.
    Stryker a.
arthroscopy
    needle a.
arthrosia
    exanthesis a.
arthrosis
    uncovertebral a.
arthrospore
arthrosteitis
    pustulotic a.
Arthrotec
arthrotomy
Arthus
    A. phenomenon
    A. reaction
Arthus-type reaction
articular
    a. amyloid
    a. chondrocyte
    chronic infantile neurological, cutaneous, and a. (CINCA)
    a. disease
    a. joint tissue catabolism
    a. leprosy

articulation
    acromioclavicular a.
    scapulothoracic a.
    sternoclavicular a.
articulorum
    eczema a.
Articulose-50 injection
artifact, artefact
    buffer a.
    crush a.
artificial
    a. active immunity
    a. passive immunity
    a. skin
    a. tears
artificialis
    acne a.
Artria
art/trs gene
arum plant
ARV
    acquired immunodeficiency syndrome-related virus
    AIDS-related virus
aryepiglottic
arylalcoanoic acid
AS
    aerosol sensitization
    angiosarcoma
    ankylosing spondylitis
A.S.
    Crysticillin A.S.
ASA
    acetylsalicylic acid
    MSD Enteric-Coated ASA
asaccharolyticus
    Peptostreptococcus a.
Asacol Oral
Asadrine
Asaphen
asbestos
    a. corn
    a. wart
Asboe-Hansen
    A.-H. disease
    A.-H. sign
ascariasis
ascaris
Ascaris lumbricoides
ascending lymphangitis
Ascher syndrome
asci (*pl. of* ascus)

ascites
    North American Study of Treatment for Refractory A. (NASTRA)
Ascoli
    A. reaction
    A. test
    A. treatment
Ascomycetes
ascospore
Ascriptin
ascus, pl. **asci**
ASD
    adult/adolescent spectrum of HIV disease
asepsis
aseptic
    a. necrosis
    a. technique
Asepticator unit
ASFV
    African swine fever virus
ash
    Arizona a.
    green a.
    a. leaf spot
    Oregon a.
    a. tree
    a. tree pollen
    white a.
ashgray
    a. blister beetle
    a. blister beetle sting
ash-leaf macule
ashsphere
ashy
    a. dermatitis
    a. dermatosis
    a. dermatosis of Ramirez
ASI
    active specific immunotherapy
Asiatic
    A. cholera
    A. pill
asimadoline
Askin biopsy
Aslera
ASLO
    antistreptolysin-O
    ASLO titer
ASM
    airway smooth muscle
Asmalix

NOTES

ASO
> antistreptolysin-O
> ASO test
> ASO titer

asparagine-linked oligosaccharide
asparagus
aspartic proteinase
aspen
> a. tree

aspergilloma
aspergillosis
> allergic bronchopulmonary a.
> (ABPA)
> disseminated a.
> invasive a.
> primary cutaneous a.
> pulmonary a.
> rhinocerebral a. (RA)

Aspergillus
> A. *amstelodami*
> A. *avenaceus*
> A. *caesiellus*
> A. *candidus*
> A. *carneus*
> A. *clavatus*
> A. *deltoidea*
> A. *flavus*
> A. *fumigatus*
> A. *nidulans*
> A. *niger*
> A. *oryzae*
> A. osteomyelitis
> A. *restrictus*
> A. *sydowi*
> A. *terreus*
> A. *ustus*
> A. *versicolor*

aspergillustoxicosis
aspirate
> nasopharyngeal a. (NPA)

aspiration
> a. biopsy
> fine-needle a. (FNA)
> myringotomy with a.
> recurrent a.

Aspirator
> Cavitron Ultrasonic Surgical A.
> (CUSA)

aspirin
> Bayer Buffered A.
> enteric-coated a.
> Extra Strength Bayer Enteric
> 500 A.
> A. Free Anacin Maximum Strength
> A. Plus Stomach Guard
> a. sensitivity
> St. Joseph Adult Chewable A.
> a. triad

Aspirin-Free Bayer Select Allergy Sinus Caplets
aspirin-induced papillary necrosis
aspirin-intolerant asthma (AIA)
aspirin-sensitive
> a.-s. asthma
> a.-s. respiratory disease (ASRD)

Asprimox
ASRD
> aspirin-sensitive respiratory disease

assassin
> a. bug
> a. bug bite

assay
> adherence a.
> agar diffusion a.
> AH50 a.
> AlaSTAT a.
> alpha-glutathione S-transferase a.
> amplification a.
> antibody blocking a.
> anti-C3 a.
> anti-D enzyme-linked
> immunosorbent a.
> antigen-nonspecific immune
> complex a.
> *Borrelia burgdorferi* DNA a.
> CH50 a.
> chemiluminescence a.
> Colorimeti A.
> competitive binding a.
> complement binding a.
> conglutinin a.
> Cotinine a.
> C1q a.
> *Crithidia luciliae*
> immunofluorescence a.
> 21-Day Cumulative Irritancy A.
> double antibody sandwich a.
> EAC rosette a.
> Ehrlich ascites carcinoma rosette a.
> electrophoretic mobility shift a.
> (EMSA)
> enzyme-linked immunosorbent a.
> (ELISA)
> enzyme-linked immunospot a.
> (ELISPOT)
> Farr a.
> FlowPRA a.
> fluid-phase C1q-binding a.
> fluorescent antinuclear antibody a.
> (FANA)
> food immune complex a. (FICA)
> frozen section a. (FSA)
> glycoprotein-based enzyme-linked
> immunosorbent a. (ggELISA)
> hemolytic plaque a.
> hepatitis B viral DNA a.

HIV DNA amplification a.
human androgen receptor a.
  (HUMARA)
human immunodeficiency virus
  deoxyribonucleic acid
  amplification a.
hybrid capture a. (HCA)
immune adherence
  immunosorbent a. (IAHIA)
immune complex a.
immunobead a.
immunochemical a.
immunoprecipitation a.
immunoradiometric a. (IRMA)
indirect a.
Jerne plaque a.
leukocyte attachment a.
Limulus lysate a.
local lymph-node a. (LLNA)
lymphocyte function a.
murex hybrid capture a.
PCR a.
polyethylene glycol precipitation a.
polymerase chain reaction a.
precipitin a.
Premier H. pylori a.
QPCR a.
quantitative complement a.
quantitative polymerase chain
  reaction a.
Quickscreen a.
radioimmunoprecipitation a. (RIPA)
radioligand a.
radioreceptor a.
Raji cell radioimmune a.
RCR a.
recombinant immunoblot a. (RIBA)
replication-competent retrovirus a.
ribonuclease protection a. (RPA)
Roche Amplicor CMV DNA a.
sandwich a.
skin-based a.
solid-phase C1q-binding a.
staphylococcal-binding a.
staphylococcal protein A binding a.
TaqMan a.
TIL cell a.
two-site immunoradiometric a.
in vitro cytotoxic a.
Assessment Measure for Atopic
  Dermatitis (AMAD)
Assess peak flow meter

Assmann tuberculous infiltrate
associated macrophage
associates
  microbial a.
association
  American Rheumatism A. (ARA)
  a. constant
  Cosmetic, Toiletries, and
    Fragrance A.
associative reaction
astacoid rash
asteatode
asteatosis cutis
asteatotic
  a. dermatitis
  a. eczema
Astech peak flow meter
Astelin Nasal Spray
astemizole
Asteraceae
asteroid body
asteroides
  Nocardia a.
asthenia
  neurocirculatory a.
  tropical anhidrotic a.
asthma
  allergen-induced a.
  allergic a.
  aspirin-intolerant a. (AIA)
  aspirin-sensitive a.
  atopic a.
  baker's a.
  brittle a.
  bronchial a.
  catechol-*O*-methyl transferase a.
  chronic a.
  COMT a.
  cough-variant a.
  Crocodile Bile Pill for A.
  exercise-induced a. (EIA)
  extrinsic a.
  fatal a.
  food a.
  functional abnormality in a.
  hay a.
  intrinsic a.
  malignant potentially fatal a.
  Millar a.
  miller's a.
  mixed a.
  near-fatal a.

NOTES

asthma *(continued)*
> nocturnal a.
> nonallergic a.
> occupationally induced a. (OA)
> occupational non-IgE-dependent a.
> poorly reversible a.
> potentially fatal a.
> premenstrual exacerbation of a. (PMA)
> steroid-dependent a.
> subclinical a.
> summer a.
> *Trichophyton*-induced a.
> variant a.
> virus-induced a.
> wine-induced a.

AsthmaHaler Mist
asthma-like symptom
AsthmaMentor Peak Flow Meter
AsthmaNefrin
asthmatic
> a. bronchitis
> tight a.

asthmatica
> Tylophora a.

asthmaticus
> status a.

asthmogenic
AstraZeneca LP
astringent
> Clean & Clear Deep Cleaning a.

astrocyte
astrocytoma cell
astronyxis
> *Acanthamoeba a.*

Astroviridae virus
ASTS
> American Society of Transplant Surgeons

Asturian leprosy
asturiensis
> elephantiasis a.

asymmetric
> a. distribution
> a. oligoarthritis
> a. oligoarthropathy
> a. periflexural exanthem of childhood (APEC)
> a. peripheral sensory neuropathy
> a. polyarthritis

asymptomatic cricoarytenoid synovitis
asystolia
AT
> amegakaryocytic thrombocytopenia

ATA
> acquired tufted angioma

Atabrine
Atarax Oral

atavism
> phylogenetic a.

ataxia
> cerebellar a.
> locomotor a.
> a. telangiectasia
> a. telangiectasia syndrome

ataxia-telangiectasia
ATCC
> American Type Culture Collection

ATD
> autoimmune thyroid disease

A/Texas/36/91-like influenza
ATG
> antithymocyte gamma globulin
> Enbrel plus ATG

ATGAM
> antithymocyte gamma globulin
> 5 ATGAM antilymphocyte therapy

Atgam
Athabascan type of severe combined immunodeficiency disease (SCIDA)
atheroembolic disease
atheroembolus, pl. atheroemboli
atherogenicity
atheroma
atheromatosis cutis
atheromatous embolus
atherosclerosis
> accelerated graft a. (AGAS)

athlete's
> a. foot
> a. nodule

athletic nail
Athos laser
athrepsia
ATL
> adult T-cell leukemia

atlantoaxial
> a. joint
> a. subluxation

atlantodental dislocation
ATLL
> adult T-cell leukemia/lymphoma

atmoknesis
Atolone Oral
atonic ulcer
atopen
atopic
> a. allergy
> a. asthma
> a. dermatitis (AD)
> A. Dermatitis Area and Severity Index (ADASI)
> a. dermatitis rash
> A. Dermatitis Severity Index (ADSI)
> a. diathesis

a. eczema
a. hypersensitivity
a. keratoconjunctivitis
a. reagin
a. sensitivity
atopy patch test (APT)
atovaquone
Atozine Oral
ATP
adenosine triphosphate
ATPase
adenosine triphosphatase
ATPase activity
atra
Stachybotrys a.
Atra-Tain
atrepsy
atresia
biliary a.
junctional epidermolysis bullosa
with pyloric a.
atretic meningocele
atria (*pl. of* atrium)
atrial conduction disturbance
atrichia
atrichosis
atrichous
atrioventricular (AV)
a. block
Atrisone
atrium, pl. **atria**
a. of infection
Atrohist
Atropair Ophthalmic
atrophedema
atrophia
a. maculosa varioliformis cutis
a. pilorum propria
atrophic
a. candidiasis
a. glossitis
a. hyperkeratotic lesion
a. lichen planus
a. macule
a. papulosis
a. plaque
a. rhinitis of swine
a. stria
a. white scar
atrophica
acne a.
hyperkeratosis figurata centrifuga a.

macula a.
morphea a.
stria a.
atrophicae
lineae striae a.
atrophicans
acrodermatitis chronica a. (ACA)
dermatitis cruris pustulosa et a.
epidermolysis bullosa a.
folliculitis cruris a.
keratosis pilaris a.
lichen planus et acuminatus a.
lichen sclerosus et a.
pityriasis alba a.
poikiloderma vasculare a.
poikiloderma vascularis a.
atrophicus
lichen sclerosus et a. (LS&A)
atrophie
a. blanche
a. blanche lesion
a. noire
atrophoderma
a. albidum
a. biotripticum
a. diffusum
follicular a.
idiopathic a.
neuritic a.
a. neuriticum
a. of Pasini and Pierini
Pasini-Pierini idiopathic a.
progressive idiopathic a.
a. reticulatum
a. reticulatum symmetricum faciei
a. scleroatrophy
senile a.
a. striatum
a. striatum et maculatum
a. ulerythematosa
a. vermicularis
vermiculate a.
a. vermiculatum
atrophodermatosis
atrophy
blue a.
Buchwald a.
central papillary a.
cigarette-paper a.
diffuse a.
a. of fat
fat-replacement a.

NOTES

atrophy *(continued)*
    honeycomb a.
    intrinsic muscle a.
    linear a.
    macular a.
    optic a.
    papillary a.
    primary idiopathic macular a.
    skin a.
    syphilitic spinal muscular a.
    traction a.
    villous a.
    wucher a.
Atropine-Care Ophthalmic
atropine sulfate
Atropisol Ophthalmic
Atrovent
    A. Aerosol Inhalation
    A. Inhalation Solution
A/T/S
    A. lotion
    A. topical
attachment plaque
attack
    acute asthma a.
    drop a.
    syncopal a.
attenuant
attenuate
    a. vaccinia virus
attenuated
    a. live mumps virus vaccine
    a. poxvirus vector
    rickettsia vaccine, a.
    a. tuberculosis
    a. virus
attenuation
attenuator
Attenuvax
atypical
    a. erythema multiforme
    a. fibroxanthoma (AFX)
    a. histiocytosis
    a. ichthyosiform erythroderma
    a. Kawasaki disease (AKD)
    a. lipoma
    a. measles
    a. mole
    a. mole syndrome
    a. mycobacterial arthritis
    a. mycobacterial colonization
    a. mycobacterial infection
    a. pityriasis rosea
    a. pneumonia
AU
    allergy unit
Au antigen

AUC
    area under the curve
Auchmeromyia
audiometry
    screening a.
    threshold a.
audiovestibular dysfunction
audouinii
    Microsporum a.
Audouin microsporon
augmentation
    paraffin breast a.
    silicone breast a.
    a. therapy
augmented histamine test
augmenti
    stadium a.
Augmentin
Aujeszky
    A. disease
    A. disease virus
Aura
    A. Laser
    A. Laser system
aural
    a. fistula
    a. keratosis
Auralate
Auralgan
auranofin
aurantiasis cutis
Aureobasidium pullulans
aureotherapy
aureus
    Staphylococcus a.
auriasis
auricle
    accessory a.
auricular
    a. chondritis
    a. perichondritis
auriculotemporal syndrome
aurid
aurochromoderma
Aurolate
aurothioglucose
    sodium a.
aurothiomalate
    sodium a.
Auroto
Aus antigen
Auspitz
    A. dermatosis
    A. sign
Australia antigen
Australian
    A. parrot droppings
    A. parrot feather

A. parrot protein
A. pine
A. pine tree
A. punch
A. X disease
A. X disease virus
A. X encephalitis
australis
Rickettsia a.
autacoid
autoagglutination
autoagglutinin
anti-Pr cold a.
cold a.
autoaggression
systemic a.
autoallergen
autoallergic
autoallergization
autoallergy
autoamputate
autoanaphylaxis
autoantibody
antibasement membrane zone a.
anti-BMZ a.
anticalpastatin a.
anticardiolipin a.
antiendothelial cell a. (AECA)
antiidiotype a.
antikeratin a.
antineutrophil cytoplasmic a.
antinuclear a.
antinucleosome a.
antiperinuclear a.
antitype II, IX collagen a.
brain-reactive a.
cold a.
Donath-Landsteiner cold a.
hemagglutinating cold a.
idiotype a.
monoclonal a.
muscarinic receptor a.
myositis-associated a.
myositis-specific a. (MSA)
PARP a.
poly(ADP-ribose)polymerase
autoantibody
plasma protein a.
poly(ADP-ribose)polymerase a.
(PARP autoantibody)
warm a.
autoanticomplement

autoantigen
a. collagen
48-kd La a.
52-kd Ro a.
60-kd Ro a.
auto-antiidiotypic antibody
autochemotherapy
autoclasis
autocrine hormone
autocytolysin
autocytolysis
autocytotoxin
autodermic
autodigestion of connective tissue
autoeczematization
autoerythrocyte
a. sensitivity
a. sensitization
a. sensitization syndrome
autogeneic graft
autogenous vaccine
autograft
autografting
cultured epithelial a.
autogram
autographism
Autohaler
Maxair A.
autohemagglutination
autohemolysin
autohemolysis
autoimmune
a. atrophic gastritis
a. blistering mucocutaneous disease
a. chronic hepatitis
a. disorder
a. encephalomyelitis
a. exocrinopathy
a. hemolysis
a. hemolytic anemia (AIHA)
a. hepatitis (AIH)
a. lymphoproliferative syndrome
(ALPS)
a. neonatal thrombocytopenia
a. neutropenia
a. panhypopituitarism
a. paraneoplastic syndrome
a. phenomenon
a. pituitary disease
a. polyendocrinopathy-candidiasis-
ectodermal dysplasia (APECED)

NOTES

autoimmune *(continued)*
- a. polyendocrinopathy-candidiasis-ectodermal dystrophy (APECED)
- a. polyglandular syndrome (APS)
- a. progenitor cell
- a. progesterone dermatitis
- a. purpura
- a. response
- a. thrombocytopenia (AITP)
- a. thrombocytopenic purpura
- a. thyroid disease (ATD)
- a. type of reaction

autoimmunity
- cell-mediated a.

autoimmunization
autoimmunocytopenia
autoinfection
Autoinjector
autoinoculable
autoinoculation
autoisolysin
AuTolo Cure Process wound treatment
autologous
- a. antibody
- a. antigen
- a. bone marrow transplant
- a. cultured epithelium
- a. graft
- a. mixed leukocyte reaction
- a. transplantation

autolyse
autolysin
autolysis
autolytic
autolyze
automated
- A. Cellular Imaging System (ACIS)
- A. Cellular Imaging System immunohistochemical stain
- a. cytochemical system

Automeris
automobile exhaust
autonomic
- a. epilepsy flush
- a. imbalance syndrome
- a. nervous system
- a. urticaria

autonomous
autophagia
autophagic
autophagy
autophytica
- dermatitis a.

autoplast
autoplastic graft
autoplasty
autoradiography

autoreactive B cell
autoreinfection
autoreproduction
autosensitivity
- deoxyribonucleic acid a.
- DNA a.

autosensitization dermatitis
autosensitize
autosepticemia
autoserotherapy
autoserum therapy
autosomal
- a. codominant
- a. dominant
- a. dominant lamellar ichthyosis
- a. dominant oculocutaneous albinism
- a. recessive
- a. recessive ichthyosis
- a. recessive ocular albinism (AROA)
- a. recessive severe combined immunodeficiency disorder
- a. recessive trait

autosomal-dominant periodic fever syndrome
autosplenectomy
Auto Suture SFS stapler
autotherapy
autotoxicans
- horror a.

autotoxicus
- horror a.

autotransplant
autotransplantation
autovaccination
auxiliary
- a. partial heterotopic liver transplantation (APHLT)
- a. partial orthotopic liver transplant (APOLT)
- a. partial orthotopic liver transplantation (APOLT)

auxilytic
AV
- arteriovenous
- atrioventricular
- AV block

Avanta implant
Avant Garde Shampoo
avascularity
avascular necrosis (AVN)
avasculosus
- nevus a.

AVC
- AVC Cream
- AVC suppository

Aveeno
>A. Cleansing Bar
>A. Moisture Cream
>A. oatmeal bath
>Oilated A.
>regular A.

Aveeno/colloidal oatmeal bath
avellana
>*Corylus a.*

avenaceus
>*Aspergillus a.*

Aventyl
Aviadenovirus
avian
>a. diphtheria
>a. encephalomyelitis virus
>a. erythroblastosis virus
>a. infectious encephalomyelitis
>a. infectious laryngotracheitis
>a. infectious laryngotracheitis virus
>a. influenza
>a. influenza virus
>a. leukosis
>a. leukosis-sarcoma complex
>a. leukosis-sarcoma virus
>a. lymphomatosis
>a. lymphomatosis virus
>a. mite dermatitis
>a. monocytosis
>a. myeloblastosis
>a. myeloblastosis virus
>a. neurolymphomatosis virus
>a. pneumoencephalitis virus
>a. reticuloendotheliosis
>a. sarcoma
>a. sarcoma virus
>a. viral arthritis virus

Avicine vaccine
avidin-biotin-horseradish peroxidase complex (ABC)
avidin-biotin-peroxidase
>a.-b.-p. complex method
>a.-b.-p. staining

avidity
>a. antibody
>high a.
>low a.

Avipoxvirus
Avirax
avirulent
Avita acne cream
avitaminosis

avium
>*Mycobacterium a.*

avium-intracellulare
>*Mycobacterium a.-i.* (MAC, MAI)

Avlosulfon
AVM
>arteriovenous malformation

AVN
>avascular necrosis

avobenzone
avocational intervention
avoidance
Avon Skin-So-Soft
AVP
>antiviral protein

AVXR
>acute vascular xenograft rejection

A-Wuhan/359/95-like influenza
axenic
AX-HSA
>amoxicilloyl-human serum albumin

axial
>a. disease
>a. psoriatic arthritis
>a. type

axilla
>ringworm of a.

axillaris
>hidradenitis a.
>tinea a.
>trichomycosis a.
>trichonocardiosis a.

axillary
>a. freckling
>a. hair
>a. nerve palsy
>a. venom gland

axiltraction
axis
>HPA a.
>hypothalamic-pituitary a. (HPA)
>psycho-neuro-immuno-endocrine a.
>a. of symmetry

Axsain
Ayercillin
Ayndet moisturizing soap
AZA
>azathioprine

Azactam
azalide
azapropazone

NOTES

azar
  kala a.
azatadine maleate
azathioprine (AZA)
azathioprine-induced myelosuppression
azelaic
  a. acid
  a. acid cream
azelastine
  a. hydrochloride nasal spray
  a. hydrochloride ophthalmic solution
Azelex
azidothymidine (AZT)
azithromycin
Azlocillin
Azmacort
azobenzene dye

azodicarbonamide
azo dye
azole compound
azoprotein
azotemia
  progressive a.
AZT
  azidothymidine
aztreonam
azul
Azulfidine EN-tabs
azure lunula of nail
azurocidin
azurophil
  a. granule
  a. granule protein
Azzopardi phenomenon

Z. Bigatti

B
    amphotericin B
    blood group-specific substances A
      and B
    B cell
    B cell fibroblast
    B fraction serum
    B lymphocyte
    Prevex B
    B virus
B1
    B1 cell
    nuclear lamin B1
B4
    B4 blocked ricin
    leukotriene B4 (LTB$_4$)
B5
    B5 solution
B$_6$
    vitamin B$_6$
B7
    B7 costimulatory molecule
    B7 protein
B19
    parvovirus B19
    B19 virus
B60
    HLA B60
b$_{558}$
    membrane-bound cytochrome b.
BA
  betamethasone acetate
B&A
  before and after
Babesia
    B. bigemina
    B. bovis
    B. canis
    B. divergens
    B. equi
    B. felis
    B. major
    B. microti
    B. rodhaini
babesiosis
Babies
    Water B.
Babinski
    B. sign
    B. syndrome
Babinski-Vaquez syndrome
baboon syndrome
baby
    Baby's Own Ointment
    blueberry muffin b.

    carbon b.
    collodion b.
    B. Magic soap
BABYbird respirator
bacampicillin hydrochloride
Baccharus
Baciguent topical
bacillary angiomatosis
bacillary-barren tuberculids
Bacille bilié de Calmette-Guérin (BCG)
bacille Calmette-Guérin vaccine
bacilli (*pl. of* bacillus)
bacilliformis
    Bartonella b.
bacillogenic sycosis
bacillosis
Bacillus
    B. abortus
    B. acnes
    B. alvei
    B. anthracis
    B. anthracis toxin
    B. cereus
    B. circulans
    B. laterosporus
    B. licheniformis
    B. megaterium
    B. polymyxa
    B. pseudodiphtheriticum
    B. pumilus
    B. sphaericus
    B. stearothermophilus
    B. subtilis
bacillus, pl. **bacilli**
    acid-fast b. (AFB)
    acne b.
    Calmette-Guérin b.
    b. Calmette-Guérin (BCG)
    b. Calmette-Guérin Live
    b. Calmette-Guérin vaccine
    cholera b.
    comma b.
    Frish b.
    fusiform b.
    Gram-negative b. (GNB)
    Gram-positive b. (GPB)
    Hansen b.
    Koch b.
    lepra b.
    Park-Williams b.
    vole b.
    Warthin-Starry-staining b.
    Whipple b.
bacitracin
    b., neomycin, and polymyxin b

bacitracin *(continued)*
    b., neomycin, polymyxin b, and hydrocortisone
    b., neomycin, polymyxin b, and lidocaine
    b. and polymyxin b
Back-Ese M
Backhaus towel clip
back mice
backtitration
baclofen
bacoti
    Liponyssus b.
BacT/Alert Microbial Detection System
BACTEC
    B. 550
    B. 16B-17D
    B. radiometry
    B. system
bacteremia
    coagulase-negative staph b. (CNSB)
    Gram-negative b. (GNB)
    Gram-positive b. (GPB)
    MAI b.
    Mycobacterium avium-intracellulare b.
    polymicrobial b.
    Pseudomonas aeruginosa b.
    puerperal b.
    vancomycin-resistant *Enterococcus faecium* b.
    VREF b.
bacteria (*pl. of* bacterium)
bacteria-free stage of bacterial endocarditis
bacterial
    b. allergy
    b. antagonism
    b. antigen
    b. arthritis
    b. conjunctivitis
    b. contamination
    b. disease
    b. endocarditis
    b. exotoxin
    b. hemolysin
    b. infection
    b. interference
    b. intertrigo
    b. macromolecule
    b. meningitis (BM)
    b. paronychia
    b. peptidoglycan
    b. phagocytosis test
    b. plaque
    b. pneumococcal pneumonia
    b. septicemia
    b. synergistic gangrene

    b. toxin
    b. translocation
    b. vaccine
    b. virus
bacterial-induced vascular damage
bacterially induced hemostatic disorder
bactericidal-permeability-increasing protein (BPI protein)
bactericide
    specific b.
bacterid
    pustular b.
bacterioagglutinin
bacteriocide
bacteriocidin
bacteriocin factor
bacteriocinogen
bacteriocinogenic plasmid
bacteriogenic agglutination
bacteriolysin
bacteriolysis
    immune b.
bacteriolytic serum
bacteriolyze
bacteriopexy
bacteriophage
    defective b.
    filamentous b.
    b. immunity
    lambda b.
    mature b.
    b. phi-X174
    b. resistance
    temperate b.
    typhoid b.
    b. typing
    vegetative b.
    virulent b.
bacteriophagia
bacteriophagic
bacteriophagology
bacteriopsonin
bacteriosis
bacteriostasis
bacteriostat
bacteriostatic
bacteriotic
bacteriotoxic
bacteriotropic substance
bacteriotropin
bacterium, pl. bacteria
    Bordetella pertussis b.
    commensal bacteria
    coryneform b.
    facultative b.
    heterotopic plate count bacteria (HPC bacteria)
    HPC bacteria

heterotopic plate count bacteria
lysogenic b.
pyogenic b.
resistant b.
bacteriuria
Bacteroides fragilis
Bacticort Otic
Bactine Hydrocortisone
Bactocill
B. injection
B. Oral
Bactolysins
BactoShield topical
Bactrim DS
Bactroban topical
Baculoviridae
baculovirus
Baelz disease
Baerensprung (*var. of* Barensprung)
Bäfverstedt syndrome
bag
B. Balm lubricant/emollient
2-L rubber b.
bagassosis
Baghdad
B. boil
bouton de B.
Bahia grass
Bairnsdale ulcer
baked tongue
Baker-Cummings punch
Baker cyst
baker's
b. asthma
b. dermatitis
b. eczema
b. itch
B. P&S liquid
baking soda paste
BAL
bioartificial liver
bronchoalveolar lavage
BAL therapy
Balamuthia mandrillaris
balanitis, pl. **balanitides**
Candida b.
b. circinata
circinate b.
b. circumscripta
erosive *Candida* b.
Follmann b.
fusospirochetal b.

plasma cell b.
b. plasmacellularis
pseudoepitheliomatous keratotic and micaceous b.
b. xerotica obliterans
b. of Zoon
balanoposthitis
streptococcal b.
balantidial
b. colitis
b. dysentery
Balantidium coli
balatus
Acarus b.
bald
b. cypress
b. cypress tree
Baldex
baldness
common b.
congenital b.
male pattern b.
moth-eaten b.
pubic b.
BALF
bronchoalveolar lavage fluid
ball
fungus b.
b.'s of mucus
red b.'s
ball-in-claw
b.-i.-c. appearance
b.-i.-c. pattern
Ballingall disease
ballistospore
balloon
b. cell
b. cell nevus
ballooning degeneration
balm
Extra-Strength B.
b. of Gilead
Balminil Decongestant
balnea
pruritus b.
balnei
Mycobacterium b.
Balneol lotio
balneotherapy
Balnetar
Baló
B. concentric encephalitis

NOTES

63

Baló (*continued*)
    B. concentric sclerosis
    B. concentric syndrome
Balpred
balsam
    Mecca b.
    b. of Peru
    b. of tolu
balsamic
BALT
    bronchus-associated lymphoid tissue
Baltic amber
bamboo
    b. hair
    b. spine
banal bacterial infection
banana roll
banana-shaped body
Bancroft filariasis
bancrofti
    Filaria b.
    Wuchereria b.
Bancroftian filariasis
band
    b. keratopathy
    longitudinal hyperpigmented b.
    marginal b.
    Muehrcke b.
bandage
    Ace b.
    Coban cohesive medium stretch b.
    Coplus cohesive medium stretch b.
    Crepe short stretch b.
    Elastomull elastic gauze b.
    Elset long stretch b.
    Gelocast b.
    Hamilton b.
    Hollister medial adhesive b.
    Isoelast adhesive short stretch b.
    Isoplast adhesive short stretch b.
    4-layer b. (FLB)
    3M Clean Seals b.
    Nylexogrip cohesive long stretch b.
    Profore 4-layer b.
    b. sign
    Stegman-Tromovitch b.
    Tricoplast adhesive elastic b.
    TubiFast b.
    Ulcosan Unna boot with inelastic zinc plaster b.
Band-Aid composite dressing
banding
Banff rejection grade 1, 2, 3
Bang disease
Banishing cream
bank
    gene b.
    New England Organ B. (NEOB)

Banker type dermatomyositis
bankokerend
Bannayan-Riley-Ruvalcaba syndrome
Bannister disease
Bannwarth syndrome
Banophen
    B. Decongestant Capsule
    B. Oral
BANS
    budesonide aqueous nasal spray
Banti syndrome
bar
    Acne Aid cleansing b.
    Aveeno Cleansing B.
    Fostex B.
    Olay Sensitive Skin b.
    PanOxyl B.
    Steel Bars high protein nutrition b.
    ZNP b.
barba, pl. **barbae**
    folliculitis barbae
    pseudofolliculitis barbae (PFB)
    sycosis barbae
    tinea barbae
    trichophytosis barbae
Barbados leg
barbed
    b. hypostome
    b. stinger
barber
    b. itch
    b. pilonidal sinus
    B. psoriasis
    pustular psoriasis of the palms and soles of B.
Barbour-Stoenner-Kelly (BSK)
    B.-S.-K. broth
barbula hirci
Barc Liquid
Barcoo
    B. disease
    B. rot
Bard Absorption dressing
Bardet-Biedl 1–5 syndrome
Bard-Parker blade
bare lymphocyte syndrome
Barensprung, Baerensprung
    B. erythrasma
barium sulfide
bark
    b. scorpion
    b. scorpion sting
barking cough
barley
Barmah Forest virus

barn
 b. dust
 b. itch
Barnett classification
Barraquer forceps
Barraquer-Simons syndrome
barrier
 blood-aqueous b.
 blood-ocular b.
 blood-retinal b.
 blood-urine b.
 b. layer
 physical b.
 b. protective cream
 b. zone
Barriere-HC
Bart
 B. syndrome
 B. thalassemia
Bartholin adenitis
bartholinitis
Barth syndrome
Bartonella
 B. bacilliformis
 B. elizabethan
 B. henselae
 B. henselae detection
 B. quintana
bartonellosis
Bart-Pumphrey syndrome
basal
 b. cell
 b. cell carcinoma (BCC)
 b. cell epithelioma (BCE)
 b. cell layer
 b. cell membrane
 b. cell nevus
 b. cell nevus syndrome
 b. cell papilloma
 b. lamina
 b. meningitis
 b. transalveolar fluid
basale
 stratum b.
basalis
 decidua b.
basaloid
 b. cell
 b. folliculolymphoid hyperplasia
Basan syndrome
base
 meningitis of the b.

basedoid
Basedow disease
basement
 b. membrane
 b. membrane zone (BMZ)
 b. membrane zone antibody
basic
 b. calcium phosphate (BCP)
 b. calcium phosphate crystal
 B. Clinical Scoring System (BCSS)
 b. fibroblast growth factor (bFGF)
 b. multicellular unit (BMU)
 b. red 46
basidiobolae
 entomophthoramycosis b.
basidiobolomycosis
Basidiomycetes
basidiospore
basilar
 b. meningitis
 b. vasculopathy
basiliximab
basiloma terebrans
basis
 nonimmunologic b.
 B. soap
basket-weave vacuolization
basolateral transport
basophil
 b. degranulation test
 b. kallikrein
basophilic degeneration
basosquamous carcinoma
basosquamous-cell acanthoma
BASOTEST
bastard measles
Bateman
 B. disease
 B. purpura
 B. syndrome
bath
 B. AS Functional Index
 Aveeno/colloidal oatmeal b.
 Aveeno oatmeal b.
 coal tar b.
 colloidal oatmeal b.
 b. itch
 oil b.
 potassium permanganate b.
 b. pruritus
 starch b.

B

NOTES

bath *(continued)*
    stop b.
    tar b.
bathing-trunk nevus
bathtub refinisher's lung
battery
    b. acid
    b. patch testing
BAU
    biological allergic unit
Baumgartner needle holder
bax gene
bayberry tree
Bayer
    B. Buffered Aspirin
    B. Low Adult Strength
    B. Select Pain Relief Formula
Bayle disease
bayonet hair
bay sore
Bazex syndrome
Bazin
    B. disease
    B. ulcer
B1–B5
    Coxsackievirus B1–B5
Bb
    Borrelia burgdorferi
B/Beijing/184/93-like influenza
BBP
    butylbenzyl phthalate
BC
    blast crisis
    CML BC
        chronic
            myelocytic/myelogenous/myeloid
            leukemia blast crisis
B-Caro-T
BCC
    basal cell carcinoma
BCE
    basal cell epithelioma
B-cell
    B.-c. antigen receptor
    B.-c. chronic lymphocytic leukemia
    (B-CLL)
    B.-c. differentiation/growth factor
    B.-c. epitope
    B.-c. growth factor-1, -2
    B.-c. lymphocytic leukemia
    B.-c. lymphocytoma cutis
    B.-c. lymphoma
    B.-c. malignancy
    B.-c. memory
    B.-c. pseudolymphoma
BCG
    Bacille bilié de Calmette-Guérin

bacillus Calmette-Guérin
    Pacis BCG
    TICE BCG
        TICE Bacillus Calmette-Guérin
        live
    BCG vaccine
BCH
    benign cephalic histiocytosis
bcl-2, -6 gene
B-CLL
    B-cell chronic lymphocytic leukemia
BCNU
    bischloroethylnitrosourea
    topical BCNU
B7:counterreceptor interaction
BCP
    basic calcium phosphate
bcr-abl chimeric transcript
BCR/abl gene re-arrangement test
BCSS
    Basic Clinical Scoring System
BCYE
    buffered charcoal yeast extract
    BCYE agar
16B-17D
    BACTEC 16B-17D
Bdellovibrio
BDI
    Beck Depression Inventory
bDNA
    branched chain deoxyribonucleic acid
bead
    Bio-Enza B.
    Sephadex B.
beaded hair
beading
beam
    electron b.
    Gaussian b.
    total skin electron b. (TSEB)
bean
    broad b.
    castor b.
    coffee b.
    green coffee b.
    kidney b.
    lava b.
    lima b.
    navy b.
    string b.
Be^a antigen
beard
    ringworm of b.
Bearn-Kunkel-Slater syndrome
Bearn-Kunkel syndrome
Beau line
beauty mark

Beaver
>B. blade
>B. ES miniblade

Beben

becaplermin

Bechterew syndrome

Beck
>B. Depression Inventory (BDI)
>B. Depression Inventory score

Becker
>B. antigen
>B. hairy hamartoma
>B. muscular dystrophy
>B. nevus

Beclodisk

Becloforte

beclomethasone dipropionate

Beclovent Oral Inhaler

Beconase AQ Nasal Inhaler

bed
>air-fluidized b.
>Biologics Airlift b.
>low air-loss b.
>powder b.
>b. sore
>tanning b.

bedbug
>b. bite
>b. disease transmission

Bednar
>B. aphtha
>B. tumor

bedsore

bee
>b. glue
>honey b.
>b. sting
>sweat b.
>b. venom

beech tree

beefsteak fungus

beefwood

Beepen-VK Oral

beet
>sugar b.

beetle
>ashgray blister b.
>blister b.
>piper b.
>striped blister b.

before and after (B&A)

Behçet
>B. aphtha
>B. disease
>B. syndrome

Behring
>B. law
>B. serum

Beigel disease

beigelii
>*Trichosporon b.*

bejel
>b. treponematosis

Bekhterev-Strümpell spondylitis

Belix Oral

Bell
>B. international unit
>B. palsy

belladonna, phenobarbital, and ergotamine tartrate

Bellergal-S

belli
>*Isospora b.*

belly
>crix b.

Bel-Phen-Ergot S

Belzer solution

Bena-D injection

Benadryl
>B. Allergy/Cold Fastmelt
>B. Decongestant Allergy Tablet
>B. Injection
>B. Oral
>B. topical

Benahist injection

Ben-Allergin-50 Injection

Ben-Aqua

Bence
>B. Jones albumin
>B. Jones protein

Benefin

BeneJoint cream

Benemid

Ben-Gay

benign
>b. cephalic histiocytosis (BCH)
>b. dry pleurisy
>b. dyskeratosis
>b. familial chronic pemphigus
>b. giant cell synovioma
>b. hemangiopericytoma
>b. hyperplasia
>b. inoculation lymphoreticulosis

NOTES

benign *(continued)*
  b. inoculation reticulosis
  b. intracranial hypertension
  b. juvenile melanoma
  b. lichenoid keratosis
  b. lipoblastomatosis
  b. lymphadenosis
  b. lymphangioendothelioma
  b. lymphocytic infiltrate of Jessner-Kanof
  b. lymphocytoma cutis
  b. migratory glossitis
  b. monoclonal gammopathy
  b. mucosal pemphigoid
  b. papular acantholytic dermatosis
  b. paroxysmal peritonitis
  b. pemphigus vegetans
  b. recurrent endothelioleukocytic meningitis
  b. symmetric lipomatosis
  b. systemic mastocytosis
  b. trichilemmoma
  b. tumor
benigna
  lymphadenosis cutis b.
  lymphogranulomatosis b.
  variola b.
benignum
  lymphogranuloma b.
Benisone
Benoject injection
Benoquin
benoxaprofen
Benoxyl
benserazide
bent-fork deformity
bentonite
  b. flocculation test
  quaternium-18 b.
bentoquatam
Benuryl
Benylin
  B. for Allergies
  B. Cold
  B. Cough Syrup
  B. Decongestant
Benzac
  B. AC Gel
  B. AC Wash
  B. W
  B. W Gel
  B. W Wash
BenzaClin gel
Benzagel
5-Benzagel
10-Benzagel
benzalkonium chloride

Benzamycin Pak
Benzashave Cream
benzathine
  penicillin g b.
benzbromarone
benzene
benzethonium chloride
benzimidazole
benziodarone
benznidazole
benzoate
  benzyl b.
  betamethasone b.
  b. preservative
benzocaine
  antipyrine and b.
  b. butyl aminobenzoate, tetracaine, and benzalkonium chloride
  b. gelatin, pectin, and sodium carboxymethylcellulose
  Orabase with b.
Benzodent
benzodiazepine midazolam
benzoic acid and salicylic acid
benzoin
benzophenone
benzoyl
  b. peroxide
  b. peroxide and hydrocortisone
benzphetamine hydrochloride
benzyl
  b. alcohol
  b. benzoate
benzylamine
benzylpenicilloyl-polylysine
Beradinelli-Seip syndrome
bergamot
  oil of b.
Berger IgA nephropathy
Bergh forceps
beriberi
Berkeley scarifier
Berkow formula
berlock, berloque
  b. dermatitis
Bermuda
  B. grass
  B. grass pollen
  B. smut
Bernard-Soulier syndrome
Bernese periacetabular osteotomy
Berotec
berylliosis
beryllium
  b. dermatitis
  b. disease
  b. granuloma

B

Besnier
  B. disease
  B. lupus pernio
  B. protoporphyria
  B. prurigo
  prurigo gestationis of B.
Besnier-Boeck disease
Besnier-Boeck-Schaumann disease
Beta-2
beta
  b. adrenergic stimulation
  b. carotene
  b. corynebacteriophage
  b. hemolysin
  b. hemolysis
  interferon b. (IFN-beta)
  b. lactoglobulin
  b. phage
  b. thalassemia trait
beta-adrenergic agonist
beta-carotene
beta-cell destruction
betacellulin (BTC)
Betachron E-R
Betacort
Betaderm
**Betadine First Aid Antibiotics +
  Moisturizer**
betae
  Phoma b.
Betagel
beta-$_{1C}$ globulin
beta-$_{1E}$ globulin
beta-$_{1F}$ globulin
betaglycan
beta-glycoprotein
  glycine-rich b.-g.
beta-glycoproteinase
  glycine-rich b.-g.
beta$_2$-glycoprotein I (beta$_2$-GPI)
beta$_2$-glycoprotein II
beta$_2$-GPI
  beta$_2$-glycoprotein I
beta-HCH
  beta-hexachlorocyclohexane
**17-beta-hydroxysteroid dehydrogenase
  (17β-HSD)**
beta-heavy-chain disease

beta-hemolytic
  b.-h. streptococcus
  b.-h. streptococcus infection
beta-hexachlorocyclohexane (beta-HCH)
**3-beta-hydroxysteroid dehydrogenase (3β-
  HSD)**
beta-interferon
beta-lactam
beta-lactamase
  CAZ b.-l.
  ceftizoxime b.-l.
beta-lactoglobulin
Betalene Topical
beta-mannosidase deficiency
beta-melanocyte-stimulating hormone
betamethasone
  b. acetate (BA)
  b. benzoate
  b. and clotrimazole
  b. dipropionate
  b. mousse
  b. sodium phosphate and acetate
    suspension
  b. valerate
beta-2-microglobulin
beta$_2$-microglobulin
  beta$_2$-microglobulin level
Betapen-VK Oral
beta-pleated sheet
Betaseron
beta-thalassemia intermedia
Betatrex Topical
Beta-Val Topical
betel
  b. pepper
Bethesda
  B. Conference on Cardiac
    Transplantation
  B. unit (BU)
Betimol Ophthalmic
Betnesol
Betnovate
Betulaceae
Betula verrucosa
betulus
  Carpinus b.
bexarotene
**Bexxar radiolabeled monoclonal
  antibody**
bFGF
  basic fibroblast growth factor

NOTES

BFP
  biologic false positive
BGC
  B. Matrix collagen
  B. Matrix hydrocolloid
  B. Matrix hydrocolloid dressing
BHAP
  bisheteroarylpiperazine
BHD
  Birt-Hogg-Dubé syndrome
bhiwanol dermatitis
BHR
  bronchial hyperresponsiveness
BIA
  bioelectrical impedance analysis
Biafine
  B. RE
  B. WDE
biallelic polymorphism
Bi antigen
Biavax II
Biaxin
  B. Filmtab
  B. XL
bicarbonate (HCO_3)
  sodium b.
bichloracetic acid
bicho dos pes
Bicillin
  B. C-R
  B. C-R 900/300 injection
  B. L-A injection
bicipital
  b. syndrome
  b. tendinitis
Bicitra
biclonal
  b. gammopathy
  b. peak
BIDS
  brittle hair, intellectual impairment,
    decreased fertility, short stature
    ichthyosis plus BIDS (IBIDS)
    BIDS syndrome
Biederman sign
bieneusi
  Enterocytozoon b.
Biernacki sign
Bier spot
Biet
  collarette of B.
Biett collar
Bifidobacterium
  anaerobic *B.*
Bi-Flex
  Osteo B.-F.
bifonazole shampoo
bifurcati

bifurcatus
  pilus b.
bigemina
  Babesia b.
biglycan
Big V
Biken-CAM vaccine
BILAG
  British Isles Lupus Assessment Group
  index
bilateral sensorineural deafness
Bile antigen
bilevel positive airway pressure (BiPAP)
bilharzial granuloma
bilharziasis
bilharzioma
biliaire
  masque b.
biliary
  b. atresia
  b. pruritus
bili light
biliostasis
bilious cholera
bilirubinemia
Billingham Classification of Rejection,
  grade 0, 1A, 1B, 2, 3A, 3B, 4
Biltricide
bi-luer lock adaptor
bimodal immunofluorescent pattern
binary nomenclature
binding
  b. constant
  deoxyribonucleic acid b.
  DNA b.
binomial theorem
bioactive lipid derivative
bioartificial liver (BAL)
bioassay
bioavailability
Biobrane
  B. adhesive
  B. glove
  B. synthetic dressing
  B. synthetic skin substitute
Biobrane/HF skin substitute
Biocef
biochemical
  b. abnormality
  b. biopsy
  b. metastasis
biocidal
Bioclot test
Bioclusive
  B. MVP transparent film
  B. synthetic dressing
bioelectrical impedance analysis (BIA)
Bio-Enza Bead

B

biogenic amine
Biohist-LA
bioinformatics
Biolex
    B. hydrogel dressing
    B. impregnated gauze
    B. wound cleanser
biologic
    b. false positive (BFP)
    b. hemolysis
    b. unit (BU)
biological
    b. allergic unit (BAU)
    b. immunotherapy
    b. standard unit
    b. vector
    b. warfare (BW)
Biologics Airlift bed
biomagnetic therapy
Biomox
Bionaire Air Cleaner
Bionicare 1000 stimulator system
Bion Tears solution
Biopatch
    B. antimicrobial dressing
    B. foam dressing
biophylactic
biophylaxis
BioPress plate
biopsy, pl. biopsies
    Askin b.
    aspiration b.
    biochemical b.
    donor b.
    elliptical b.
    endomyocardial b. (EMB)
    excisional b.
    incisional b.
    International Society for Heart and
      Lung Transplant b.
    intestinal b.
    ISHLT b.
    lymph node b.
    muscle b.
    nasopharyngeal b.
    needle b.
    needle-core b. (NCB)
    open lung b.
    peroral intestinal b.
    punch b.
    renal b.

    scissors b.
    shave b.
    synovial b.
    tangential b.
    temporal artery b. (TAB)
    total b.
    transjugular hepatic b.
    wedge renal b.
biopsy-negative graft dysfunction
  (BNGD)
bioreactor
    magnetic-resonance imaging-
      compatible hollow-fiber b.
    MRI-compatible hollow-fiber b.
BioSpan tissue expander
Bio-Tab Oral
Biotene
Biothrax
biotin deficiency
biotinidase
    b. deficiency
    b. enzyme
biotinylated antihuman IgG
biotoxin
biotripticum
    atrophoderma b.
Biotropine
biotropism
Biozyme-C
BiPAP
    bilevel positive airway pressure
biphasic response
biphosphonate
bipolar electrosurgery
bipolymer
Birbeck granule
birch
    red b.
    river b.
    b. tree
    b. tree pollen
bird
    b. egg syndrome
    b. fancier lung
    b. nest anaphylaxis
bird-breeder's
    b.-b. disease
    b.-b. lung
birdshot retinochoroidopathy
birefringent collagen bundle
Birex

NOTES

birminghamensis
    Legionella b.
Birmingham Vasculitis Activity Score (BVAS)
Birnaviridae
Birnavirus
Birtcher hyfrecator
birthmark
    hemangioma b.
    strawberry b.
    vascular malformation b.
Birt-Hogg-Dubé syndrome (BHD)
bischloroethylnitrosourea (BCNU)
bisheteroarylpiperazine (BHAP)
Bishop-Harmon ophthalmic forceps
Biskra
    bouton de B.
    B. button
Bismatrol
bismuth
    b. granule
    b. subgallate
    b. subsalicylate
Bisolvon
bispecific antibody
bisphosphonate
bitartrate
    hydrocodone b.
    levarterenol b.
    metaraminol b.
    norepinephrine b.
bite
    ant b.
    arthropod b.
    assassin bug b.
    bedbug b.
    black fly b.
    black widow spider b.
    brown recluse spider b.
    cat flea b.
    centipede b.
    chigger b.
    conenose bug b.
    Congo floor maggot b.
    copperhead snake b.
    coral snake b.
    cottonmouth snake b.
    Ctenocephalides canis b.
    Ctenocephalides felis b.
    deer fly b.
    dog flea b.
    Eastern coral snake b.
    fiddle-back spider b.
    fly b.
    giant desert centipede b.
    Gila monster b.
    Glossina b.
    gnat b.
    harvest mite b.
    Heloderma suspectum b.
    horsefly b.
    insect b.
    kissing bug b.
    Latrodectus mactans b.
    Loxosceles reclusa b.
    midge b.
    mite b.
    moccasin snake b.
    mosquito b.
    northern rat flea b.
    Nosopsyllus fasciatus b.
    Oriental rat flea b.
    b. pathology
    pit viper b.
    rat flea b.
    rattlesnake b.
    red bug b.
    sand flea b.
    sandfly b.
    Scolopendra heres b.
    sea snake b.
    snake b.
    spider b.
    stable fly b.
    Stomoxys b.
    Texas coral snake b.
    tick b.
    Triatoma gerstaeckeri b.
    Triatoma sanguisuga b.
    tsetse fly b.
    Tunga penetrans b.
    violin-back spider b.
    Xenopsylla cheopis b.
    Yersinia pestis b.
biterminal coagulation
biting
    b. insect
    nail b.
    b. reef worm
bitolterol mesylate
Bitot spot
bitter dock
Bittner
    B. agent
    B. milk factor
    B. virus
biundulant meningoencephalitis
bivalency
    monogamous b.
bivalent
    b. antibody
    b. antigen
    b. gas gangrene antitoxin
BIWB2
Bizzozero node
Björnstad syndrome

BK
>BK viruria
>BK virus

black
>b. ant
>b. currant rash
>b. dermatographia
>b. dermogram
>b. dot hair
>b. dot tinea
>b. dot tinea capitis
>b. eschar
>b. eye
>b. fever
>b. fly
>b. fly bite
>b. hairy tongue
>b. heel
>B. Lagoon virus
>b. light fluorescent lamp
>b. locust
>b. locust tree
>b. measles
>b. mulberry
>b. palm
>b. pepper
>b. piedra
>b. ray lamp
>b. rubber mix
>b. seeds in wart
>Sudan b.
>b. sweat
>b. toe
>b. walnut
>b. walnut tree pollen
>b. widow spider
>b. widow spider antivenin
>b. widow spider bite

blackberry
black-dot ringworm
Blackfan-Diamond
>B.-D. anemia
>B.-D. Langerhans cell histiocytosis

blackhead
blackjack disease
black-legged tick
blade
>Bard-Parker b.
>Beaver b.
>CLM articulating laryngoscope b.
>Derma b.
>Gillette Blue B.

blain
blanch
blanchable red lesion
blanche
>atrophie b.

blanched cutaneous elevation
blanching
>delayed b.

Blancophor, blankophore
bland
>b. aerosolized liquid
>b. occlusive disorder

blank
>b. allele
>b. antigen

blanket
>cooling b.

blankophore (*var. of* Blancophor)
Blaschko
>B. line
>B. linear dermatosis
>lines of B.

blast
>b. cell
>b. crisis (BC)
>refractory anemia with excess b.'s (RAEB)
>b. transformation

blastema
blastoconidia
>*Candida* b.

blastogenesis
blastogenetic
Blastomyces
>B. brasiliensis
>B. dermatitidis

blastomycetes
>pathogenic b.

blastomycetica
>erosio interdigitalis b.

blastomycetic dermatitis
blastomycosis
>cutaneous b.
>European b.
>keloidal b.
>North American b.
>primary cutaneous b.
>South American b.

blastomycosis-like pyoderma
blastomycotica
>dermatitis b.

blastomycotic osteomyelitis

B

NOTES

73

Blatin
>B. sign
>B. syndrome

bleached rubber syndrome

bleb
>apoptotic b.
>b. stapling

bleeding
>punctate b.

BlemErase Lotion

blemish
>B. Control

Blenderm patch technique

blennorrhagia

blennorrhagic

blennorrhagica
>keratoderma b.
>keratosis b.

blennorrhagicum
>keratoderma b.

blennorrhea
>b. neonatorum

blennorrheal conjunctivitis

Blenoxane

bleomycin
>b. sulfate

Bleph-10 Ophthalmic

Blephamide Ophthalmic

blepharitis
>mixed seborrheic-staphylococcal b.
>seborrheic b.
>staphylococcal b.

blepharochalasia

blepharochalasis

blepharochromidrosis

blepharoconjunctivitis

blepharoplasty scissors

blepharoptosis adiposa

bleuâtres
>tache b.

blind
>b. boil
>b. loop syndrome
>b. passage

blinding disease

blindness
>night b.
>river b.

blister
>b. beetle
>b. beetle dermatitis
>b. beetle sting
>blood b.
>central b.
>diabetic b.
>fever b.
>fly b.
>flying b.

>friction b.
>pressure b.
>b. serum
>subcorneal b.
>sucking b.
>water b.

BlisterFilm transparent film

blistering
>b. collodion
>b. dermatitis
>b. distal dactylitis
>b. lesion
>b. skin

Blis-To-Sol

Blizzard syndrome

Blocadren Oral

Bloch reaction

Bloch-Siemens-Sulzberger syndrome

Bloch-Sulzberger
>B.-S. disease
>B.-S. syndrome

block
>arteriovenous b.
>atrioventricular b.
>AV b.
>congenital complete heart b. (CCHB)
>stellate ganglion b.
>Sun Defense Lip B.

blockade
>costimulatory b.
>reticuloendothelial b.
>stellate ganglion b.
>virus b.

blockage
>mechanical vessel b.
>vessel b.

blocker
>H2 b.

blocking
>b. antibody
>b. vagal afferent fiber
>b. vagal efferent fiber

Blomia tropicalis

blood
>b. blister
>b. chemistry
>b. coagulation
>b. coagulation test
>cord b. (CB)
>b. eosinophilia
>b. fluke
>b. gas
>b. group
>b. group agglutinin
>b. group agglutinogen
>b. group antibody
>b. group antigen

B

b. group antiserum
b. grouping
b. group-specific substances A and B
b. group substance
b. group system
occult b.
b. pH
b. pressure
b. progenitor cell
b. serum
b. transfusion
b. transfusion therapy
b. type
umbilical cord b. (UCB)
whole b.
b. worm
blood-aqueous barrier
bloodborne
blood-filled slit-like space
blood-ocular barrier
blood-retinal barrier
bloodstream infection (BSI)
bloodsucking
blood-urine barrier
Bloom syndrome
Bloom-Torre-Machacek syndrome
blossom
orange b.
blot
Southern b.
Western b.
blotch
palpebral b.
blousing garter dermatitis
blubber finger
blubbery lips
Bluboro solution
blue
b. atrophy
Bonney's b.
b. bottle sting
b. grass
b. grass pollen
methylene b.
b. mussel
b. nail
B. Peel skin health product
b. rubber-bleb nevus
b. rubber-bleb nevus syndrome
Selsun B.

B. + Spitz nevus
b. spot
trypan b.
blueberry
b. muffin baby
b. muffin child
b. muffin lesion
bluecomb
b. disease of turkey
b. virus
bluegrass
annual b.
Kentucky b.
blue-gray
b.-g. lesion
b.-g. pigmentation
blue-toe syndrome
bluetongue virus
Bluettes cotton knit-lined glove
blunt dissection
blunted villus
blush
blushing
BLU-U blue light photodynamic therapy illuminator
BLV
bovine leukemia virus
BM
bacterial meningitis
BMC
bone marrow cell
bone mineral content
BMCMC
bone marrow-derived cultured mast cell
BMD
bone mineral density
BMI
body mass index
B-mode ultrasound
BMT
bone marrow transplant
bone marrow transplantation
BMU
basic multicellular unit
BMZ
basement membrane zone
BMZ antibody
BNGD
biopsy-negative graft dysfunction
BNLF-1 oncogene

NOTES

board
Data Safety Monitoring B.
(DSMB)
institutional review b. (IRB)
Bockenheimer syndrome
Bockhart
B. folliculitis
B. impetigo
BOD
burden of disease
Bodechtel-Guttmann disease
Bodian stain
body
antiimmune b.
apoptotic b.
asteroid b.
banana-shaped b.
Bollinger b.
Borrel b.
caterpillar b.
b. cavity-based B-cell lymphoma
cigar b.
ciliary b.
Civatte b.
colloid b.
Cowdry intranuclear inclusion b.
Cowdry intranuclear inclusion b.
type A, B
Cowdry type A, B inclusion b.
Creola b.
cytoid b.
cytomegalic inclusion b.
cytoplasmic inclusion b.
Dohle inclusion b.
Donovan b.
b. dysmorphic disorder
elementary b. (EB)
Farber b.
foreign b. (FB)
fuchsin b.
glass b.
glomus b.
Guarnieri b.
Halberstaedter-Prowazek b.
Heinz b.
Henderson-Paterson b.
Howell-Jolly b.
inclusion b.
Joest b.
lamellar b. (LB)
Leishman-Donovan b.
Lindner b.
Lipschütz b.
loose b.
b. louse
b. mass
b. mass index (BMI)
Medlar b.

Miyagawa b.
b. moisturizer
molluscum b.
Negri b.
nuclear inclusion b.
Odland b.
Paschen b.
polyhedral b.
Prowazek b.
Prowazek-Greeff b.
psittacosis inclusion b.
reticulate b.
rice b.
ringworm of b.
round b.
Russell b.
Schaumann b.
sclerotic b.
b. somatotype
tingible b.
trachoma b.
vitreous b.
zebra b.
Boeck
B. itch
B. sarcoid
B. sarcoidosis
B. scabies
Boerhaave sweat gland
boggy swelling
Bohn nodule
boil
Aleppo b.
Baghdad b.
blind b.
botfly b.
date b.
Delhi b.
Madura b.
Oriental b.
salt water b.
sea water b.
tropical b.
bois
pian b.
Bolivian hemorrhagic fever
Bollinger
B. body
B. granule
bolster finger
Bombay phenotype
Bombus sting
bone
b. culture
b. decay
b. densitometry
b. erosion
b. felon

b. formation marker
b. fragility
b. marrow cell (BMC)
b. marrow-derived cultured mast cell (BMCMC)
b. marrow examination
b. marrow reserve
b. marrow transplant (BMT)
b. marrow transplantation (BMT)
b. mineral content (BMC)
b. mineral density (BMD)
b. morphogenetic protein receptor
b. resorption marker
b. sialoprotein (BSP)
b. turnover marker
bone-seeking substance
Bonferroni
B. correction
Bonine
Bonney's blue
Bonviva
bony
b. ankylosis
b. erosion
b. spur
Böök syndrome
BOOP
bronchiolitis obliterans with organizing pneumonia
booster
b. dose
b. phenomenon
b. response
boot
Dome-Paste b.
gelatin compression b.
Unna b.
borax
Borda
melanotic prurigo of B.
border
coast of Maine b.
indurated b.
irregular b.
raised b.
vermilion b.
volcanic b.
borderline
b. lepromatous leprosy
b. malignant hemangiopericytoma
b. tuberculoid leprosy

Bordetella
B. parapertussis
B. pertussis
B. pertussis bacterium
Bordet-Gengou phenomenon
Borg
B. scale
B. score
boric acid
Borna
B. disease
B. disease virus
Bornholm
B. disease
B. disease virus
Borofax Topical
Borrel body
Borrelia
B. afzelii
B. burgdorferi (Bb)
B. burgdorferi DNA assay
B. garinii
B. lymphocytoma
B. recurrentis
Borrelia-associated arthritis
borreliacidal
borreliosis, pl. borrelioses
Lyme b.
BORSA strain
Borsieri
B. line
B. sign
Borst-Jadassohn type intraepidermal epithelioma
BOS
bronchiolitis obliterans syndrome
bosch yaw
bosentan
bossing
frontal b.
Bostock disease
Boston exanthema
botfly
b. boil
b. facultative myiasis
b. obligate myiasis
bothropic antitoxin
Bothrops antitoxin
Botox
Botryomyces caespitosus
botryomycosis

NOTES

botryosum
>*Stemphylium b.*

Botrytis cinerea

Bottle
>ENTsol Refillable B.

botulin

botulinum antitoxin

botulinus toxin

botulism
>b. antitoxin
>food-borne b.
>wound b.

botulismotoxin

boubas

Bouchard node

Bouffardi
>B. black mycetoma
>B. white mycetoma

bougie

bougienage

Bouin solution

bound
>total counts b. (TCB)

boundary
>intron-exon b.

bouquet fever

Bourneville
>B. disease
>B. syndrome

Bourneville-Brissaud disease

Bourneville-Pringle
>B.-P. disease
>B.-P. syndrome

bouton
>b. de Baghdad
>b. de Biskra
>b. d'Orient

boutonneuse fever

boutonnière deformity

bovine
>b. antitoxin
>b. collagen dermal implant
>b. colloid
>b. colostrum
>b. ephemeral fever
>b. herpes mammillitis
>b. leukemia virus (BLV)
>b. leukosis virus
>b. mastitis
>b. papular stomatitis
>b. papular stomatitis virus
>pegademase b.
>b. rhinovirus
>b. rotavirus stain
>b. spongiform encephalopathy
>b. superoxide dismutase
>b. ulcerative mammillitis
>b. vaccinia mammillitis

>b. virus diarrhea
>b. virus diarrhea virus
>b. whey protein concentrate

bovis
>*Actinomyces b.*
>*Babesia b.*
>*Mycobacterium b.*

bowed finger

bowel bypass syndrome

Bowen
>B. disease
>B. disease of the glans penis
>B. precancerous dermatosis

Bowenoid
>b. cell
>b. papulosis

Bowins suction

Bowman layer

box
>b. elder maple
>b. elder maple tree
>b. elder tree pollen
>b. jellyfish
>b. jellyfish sting

Box-Cox transformation

Boyden
>B. chamber
>B. chamber technique

boydii
>*Allescheria b.*
>*Petriellidium b.*
>*Pseudallescheria b.*

Boyd surgical light

bozemanii
>*Legionella b.*

BP
>bullous pemphigoid
>Acnomel BP 5

BPA
>bullous pemphigoid antigen

BPI protein

BQ Tablet

BR
>breathing reserve

BR96-doxorubicin monoclonal antibody

brace
>Knight-Taylor b.

bracelet
>identification b.

brachial neuritis of Lyme disease

brachio-oto-renal syndrome

brachioradial pruritus

brachydactyly
>b., mental retardation syndrome
>b., type B1, C, E syndrome

brachymetaphalangism

brachyonychia

B

brachytherapy
    endobronchial b.
bracket fungus
Braden score for skin integrity
bradykinin
braiding
    corn-row b.
brain
    b. abscess
    b. PGD$_2$ synthase
Brainerd diarrhea
brain-reactive autoantibody
branched
    b. chain deoxyribonucleic acid
    (bDNA)
    b. DNA signal amplification assay
    for hepatitis B
branchial
    b. cleft
    b. cyst
    b. plexus
Brandy flap
B-range
    ultraviolet B.-r. (UVB)
Branhamella catarrhalis
branny
    b. desquamation
    b. scale
    b. tetter
Brasfield
    B. chest radiograph score
    B. scoring system
brasiliensis
    Blastomyces b.
    Hevea b.
    Nocardia b.
    Paracoccidioides b.
Brasivol
brawny
    b. edema
    b. induration
    b. tetter
Brazilian
    B. pemphigus
    B. rubber
    B. rubber tree
braziliense
    Ancylostoma b.
Brazil nut
breadloafing
BreakAway absorptive wound dressing
breakbone fever

breaker
    Castroviejo blade b.
Breathe
    B. Right
    B. Right nasal strip
breathing
    apneustic b.
    intermittent positive pressure b.
    (IPPB)
    Ondine curse, periodic b.
    pursed lips b.
    b. reserve (BR)
    sleep-disordered b.
breathlessness
Breda disease
bredeney
    Salmonella b.
breed
    short-haired b.
breeding
    random b.
Breezee Mist Antifungal
Brehmer
    B. method
    B. treatment
Brequinar sodium
Breslow
    B. thickness
    B. thickness in melanoma staging
Brethaire Inhalation Aerosol
Brethine
    B. injection
    B. Oral
Bretonneau
    B. angina
    B. disease
Brett syndrome
Breuerton view of the hand
Brevibacterium
brevicaulis
    Scopulariopsis b.
Brevicon
brevis
    Demodex b.
Brevoxyl Gel
Bricanyl
    B. injection
    B. Oral
bridge
    intercellular b.
bridou
brief metabolic remission

NOTES

bright erythema
Brill disease
Brill-Zinsser disease
Brion-Kayser disease
bristle-worm dermatitis
British
    B. Anti-Lewisite therapy (BAL therapy)
    B. Isles Lupus Assessment Group index (BILAG)
brittle
    b. asthma
    b. hair, intellectual impairment, decreased fertility, short stature (BIDS)
    b. hair, intellectual impairment, decreased fertility, short stature syndrome
    b. nail
    b. nail syndrome
broad
    b. bean
    b. beta disease
    b. spectrum
broad-based rete ridge
broccoli
Brocq
    B. disease
    B. erythrose peribuccale pigmentaire
    erythrose péribuccale pigmentaire of B.
    B. lupoid sycosis
    pseudopelade of B.
    B. pseudopelade
Brodie abscess
Brofed Elixir
broken vein
Bromaline Elixir
Bromanate Elixir
Bromarest
Bromatapp
Bromavir
Brombay
brome
    b. grass
    b. grass pollen
bromelain
Bromfed
    B. Syrup
    B. Tablet
Bromfed-PD
Bromfenex PD
bromhexine
bromhidrosiphobia
bromhidrosis, bromidrosis
    apocrine b.
    eccrine b.

bromide
    b. acne
    ethidium b.
    b. intoxication
    ipratropium b.
    pancuronium b.
bromidism
    vegetating b.
bromidrosiphobia
bromidrosis (*var. of* bromhidrosis)
bromine
bromism
bromocriptine
bromoderma
bromohyperhidrosis
2-Bromo-2-nitropropane-1,3-diol
bromovinyldeoxyuridine
Bromphen
    B. Elixir
    B. Tablet
brompheniramine
    b. maleate
    b. and phenylephrine
    b. and phenylpropanolamine
    b. and pseudoephedrine
bromsulfophthalein retention
Bronalide
bronchi (*pl. of* bronchus)
bronchial
    b. artery embolization
    b. asthma
    b. candidiasis
    b. epithelial cell
    b. epithelium
    b. hygiene
    b. hyperresponsiveness (BHR)
    b. inhalation challenge test
    b. mucous membrane
    b. provocation
    b. provocation test
    b. smooth muscle
    b. smooth muscle tone
    b. stenosis
    b. toilet
bronchiectasis
    proximal b.
bronchiolitis
    b. obliterans syndrome (BOS)
    b. obliterans with organizing pneumonia (BOOP)
bronchitis
    asthmatic b.
    Castellani b.
    chronic b.
    infectious avian b.
    wheezy b.
bronchoactive agonist

B

bronchoalveolar
  b. cell carcinoma
  b. lavage (BAL)
  b. lavage fluid (BALF)
bronchoconstriction
  exercise-induced b. (EIB)
bronchoconstrictor response
bronchodilatation
bronchodilation
  plateau b.
bronchodilator
  Inhal-Aid b.
  Maxi-Myst b.
  nebulized b.
bronchogenic
  b. carcinoma
  b. cyst
bronchogram
  air b.
bronchomoniliasis
bronchopleural fistula
bronchopneumonia
  eosinophilic b.
bronchoprotective subsensitivity
bronchorrhea
Broncho Saline
bronchoscope
  Dumon-Harrell b.
  fiberoptic b.
bronchoscopy
  fiberoptic b.
  ultrasound-guided b.
bronchospasm
  exercise-induced b. (EIB)
bronchovascular marking
bronchus, pl. **bronchi**
  lobar b.
  subsegmental b.
bronchus-associated lymphoid tissue
  (BALT)
Bronitin Mist
Bronkaid Mist
Bronkephrine injection
Bronkodyl
Bronkometer
Bronkosol
bronopol
Brontex
Bronzage
  Huile Solaire B.

bronze
  b. diabetes
  b. hyperpigmentation
bronzed skin
bronzinum
  chloasma b.
Brooke
  B. disease
  B. tumor
Brooke-Spiegler syndrome
bropirimine
Brotane
broth
  Barbour-Stoenner-Kelly b.
  BSK b.
  Quant b.
  b. test
  Todd-Hewitt b.
brown
  B. and Brenn stain
  b. moth larvae sting
  b. oculocutaneous albinism
  b. recluse spider
  b. recluse spider bite
  b. tumor
Brown-Adson forceps
brown-black lesion
Brown-Brenn stain
brown-spot syndrome
brown-tail
  b.-t. moth dermatitis
  b.-t. moth larva
  b.-t. moth sting
  b.-t. rash
brucei
  Trypanosoma b.
Brucella
  B. canis
  B. card test
brucella
  b. arthritis
  b. dermatitis
  b. strain 19 vaccine
brucellar meningitis
brucellergin
brucellin
brucellosis
  chronic b.
brucellum
  erythema b.
Bruce septicemia
Bruch membrane

NOTES

Bruck syndrome
Brugia
    B. malayi
    B. timori
brugian filariasis
Brugsch syndrome
bruise
brumptii
    Scopulariopsis b.
Brumpt white mycetoma
Brunati sign
Brunner gland
Bruns syndrome
Brunsting-Perry
    localized pemphigoid of B.-P.
    B.-P. pemphigoid
Brunsting-type dermatomyositis
brush
    b. border receptor
    b. burn
    b. burn abrasion
    rotating wire b.
Brussels sprout
Bruton
    B. agammaglobulinemia
    B. disease
    B. tyrosine kinase (BTK, Btk)
    B. tyrosine kinase gene
bruxism
Brymill
    B. CryAc cryosurgical unit
    B. 30 cryosurgical unit
BSI
    bloodstream infection
BSK
    Barbour-Stoenner-Kelly
    BSK broth
BSLE
    bullous systemic lupus erythematosus
BSP
    bone sialoprotein
BTC
    betacellulin
B-thalassemia syndrome
BTI-322
    humanized B.
BTK, Btk
    Bruton tyrosine kinase
BU
    Bethesda unit
    biologic unit
buaki
buba madre
bubas
bubble
    b. gum dermatitis
    b. hair
bubo, pl. buboes

Frei b.
gonorrheal b.
indolent b.
malignant b.
nonvenereal b.
pestilential b.
primary b.
satellite buboes
strumous b.
venereal b.
bubon d'emblée
bubonic plague
bubonulus
Bucast
buccalis
    psoriasis b.
buccarum
    morsicatio b.
Buchscher scleroderma
Buchwald atrophy
bucillamine
Buckley syndrome
buckwheat
Bucladin-S
buclizine
BU/CY
    busulfan and Cytoxan
bud
    farcy b.
Budd-Chiari syndrome
budesonide aqueous nasal spray (BANS)
Buehler method
Buerger disease
buffalo
    b. fly
    b. hump
buffer
    b. artifact
    glucose-gelatin Veronal b. (GGVB)
    HEPES b.
    hybridization b.
    Laemmli sample b.
buffered
    b. charcoal yeast extract (BCYE)
    b. charcoal yeast extract agar
Bufferin
buff puff
bug
    assassin b.
    conenose b.
    kissing b.
Buhler test
Buin
    Piz B.
bulb
    hair b.
bulbar

bulbosa
    myringitis b.
bulge-activation hypothesis of hair cycle
bulge sign
bulla, pl. **bullae**
    coma b.
    friction b.
    hemorrhagic b.
    intraepidermal b.
    pressure b.
    sausage-shaped b.
bullate
bullation
bullectomy
    transaxillary apical b.
bullosa
    cicatricial junctional
      epidermolysis b.
    Cockayne-Touraine epidermolysis b.
    dermatitis striata pratensis b.
    Dowling-Meara epidermolysis b.
    dystrophic epidermolysis b.
    epidermolysis b. (EB)
    generalized atrophic benign
      epidermolysis b. (GABEB)
    Hallopeau-Siemens epidermolysis b.
    Herlitz epidermolysis b.
    impetigo contagiosa b.
    inherited epidermolysis b.
    junctional epidermolysis b. (JEB)
    Köbner epidermolysis b.
    Pasini epidermolysis b.
    purpura b.
    recessive dystrophic
      epidermolysis b. (RDEB)
    urticaria b.
bullosis diabeticorum
bullosum
    erythema multiforme b.
bullosus
    herpes circinatus b.
bullous
    b. amyloidosis
    b. congenital ichthyosiform
      erythroderma
    b. disease
    b. drug reaction
    b. edema
    b. erythema multiforme
    b. fever
    b. hemorrhagic pyoderma
      gangrenosum
    b. hives
    b. impetigo
    b. impetigo of newborn
    b. lichen planus
    b. myringitis
    b. pemphigoid (BP)
    b. pemphigoid antigen (BPA)
    b. pemphigoid-like eruption
    b. skin lesion
    b. syphilid
    b. systemic lupus erythematosus
      (BSLE)
bull's eye lesion
bumblebee sting
bump
    goose b.
bundle
    birefringent collagen b.
bunion bursitis
Bunnell
    B. intrinsic tightness
    B. sign
Bunyamwera
    B. fever
    B. virus
Bunyaviridae
Bunyavirus
bunyavirus
    b. encephalitis
bupivacaine
    b. hydrochloride
Bupleurum
burden of disease (BOD)
burgdorferi
    Borrelia b. (Bb)
buried subcutaneous stitch
Burkard spore trap
Burkholderia
    B. cepacia
    B. pseudomallei
Burkitt lymphoma
burn
    actinic b.
    brush b.
    chemical b.
    b. eschar
    first-degree b.
    flash b.
    full-thickness b.
    mask b.
    mat b.
    partial-thickness b.

NOTES

burn (*continued*)
    radiation b.
    road b.
    rope b.
    second-degree b.
    superficial b.
    thermal b.
    third-degree b.
burnetii
    Coxiella b.
burning
    b. mouth
    b. mouth syndrome
    b. tongue
    b. vulva syndrome
burnt-out rheumatoid arthritis
Burow
    B. solution
    B. triangle
burr
burrobrush
    white b.
burrow
burrowing hair
bursa, pl. **bursae**
    diarthrodial joint bursae
    distended b.
    pes anserinus b.
bursectomy
bursitis
    Achilles b.
    anserine b.
    bunion b.
    fungal b.
    iliopectineal b.
    iliopsoas b.
    infrapatellar b.
    ischial b.
    ischiogluteal b.
    obturator internus b.
    olecranon b.
    prepatellar b.
    subacromial b.
    subdeltoid b.
    tendinitis b.
    traumatic b.
    trochanteric b.
bursography
burst
    oxidative b.
    phagocyte oxidative b.
    prednisone b.
    respiratory b.
    steroid b.
Buruli ulcer
burweed
Bury disease
Busacca nodule

Buschke
    B. disease
    B. scleredema
Buschke-Löwenstein
    B.-L. giant condyloma
    B.-L. tumor
    B.-L. variant of verrucous
      carcinoma
Buschke-Ollendorf
    B.-O. disease
    B.-O. sign
    B.-O. syndrome
bush
    iodine b.
    rabbit b.
    b. yaw
bushy capillary
buski
    Fasciolopsis b.
buspirone
Busse-Buschke disease
busulfan and Cytoxan (BU/CY)
butamben picrate
butanedione monoxime
butcher's tubercle
butenafine
    b. HCl
    b. hydrochloride
Butesin
butoconazole
butopyronoxyl
butorphanol
butoxide
    piperonal b.
    pyrethrins and piperonyl b.
butterfly
    b. area
    b. eruption
    b. lung
    b. patch
    b. rash
    b. sign
buttock
    perinatal gangrene of b.
button
    Amboyna b.
    Biskra b.
    Oriental b.
butylbenzyl phthalate (BBP)
butylethylpropandiol
butyl methacrylate
butyrate
    hydrocortisone b.
butyrophilin
BV-ara-U
BVAS
    Birmingham Vasculitis Activity Score
BvgAS regulon

BvgS protein
BW
    biological warfare
Bwamba
    B. fever
    B. virus

Bydramine Cough Syrup
bypass arthritis-dermatitis syndrome
byssinosis
bystander T cell
by-the-wind sailor dermatitis
Bywaters lesion

NOTES

B

C

calphostin C
C carbohydrate antigen
Dalacin C
C fraction serum
C group virus
C propeptide of type II collagen (CPII)
C protein
C syndrome

C1

C1 esterase
C1 esterase inhibitor

C3

C3 anaphylatoxin (C3a)
complement C3
C3 proactivator
C3 proactivator convertase
serum C3
C3 test

C4

complement C4
C4 deficiency (C4D)
serum C4
C4 test

C7

complement C7
C7 deficiency (C7D)

C8

complement C8

C9

complement C9

C100-3 hepatitis C virus antibody
C2 deficiency (C2D)
2C3 anti-VEGF antibody
C3/C4 receptor
C5b-C8 complex
C5b-C9 complex
CA

condyloma acuminatum
croup-associated
CA virus

C3a

C3 anaphylatoxin

C5a

Alexion anticomplement C5a
C5a complex

cable rash
CAC

cryptogenic autoimmune cirrhosis

cachectica

purpura c.

cachectic aphtha
cachecticorum

acne c.

melanoderma c.
melanosis c.

cachexia

rheumatoid c.
c. syndrome

Cachexon
C5a complex
CAD

cadaver donor
chronic actinic dermatitis
chronic airways disease
coronary artery disease

CADASIL

cerebral autosomal dominant arteriopathy
with subcortical infarcts and
leukoencephalopathy

cadaver

c. donor (CAD)
c. donor transplantation

cadaverous
caddis fly
Cade oil
cadherin
CAE

cefuroxime axetil suspension

caecutiens

Onchocerca c.

Caenorhabditis
caerulea (*var. of* cerulea)
caesiellus

Aspergillus c.

caespitosus

Botryomyces c.

Cafatine
café-au-lait

c.-a.-l. macule (CALM)
c.-a.-l. spot

café coronary syndrome
Cafergot
Cafetrate
CAH

chronic active hepatitis
cryptogenic autoimmune hepatitis

CAHC

chronic active hepatitis with cirrhosis

caine mix
Cairns syndrome
cajennense

Amblyomma c.

Cajuput oil
Calabar swelling
Caladryl

C

Calamatum
calamine lotion
calcaneal
> c. petechia
> c. rudiment
> c. spur

calcar
Calciferol
> C. injection
> C. Oral

calcific
> c. periarthritis
> c. tendinitis

calcification
> metastatic c.
> soft tissue c.
> subcutaneous c.

calcifying
> c. epithelioma
> c. epithelioma of Malherbe

Calcijex
calcineurin
calcinosis
> c. circumscripta
> c. cutis
> c. cutis, osteoma cutis, poikiloderma, and skeletal abnormalities (COPS)
> c. cutis, osteoma cutis, poikiloderma, and skeletal abnormalities syndrome
> c. cutis, Raynaud phenomenon, esophageal motility disorder, sclerodactyly, telangiectasia (CREST)
> c. cutis, Raynaud phenomenon, esophageal motility disorder, sclerodactyly, and telangiectasia syndrome
> dystrophic c.
> iatrogenic c.
> traumatic c.
> tumoral c.
> c. universalis

calciphylaxis
calcipotriene therapy
calcipotriol
calcitonin
> c. gene-related peptide (CGRP)
> oral c.
> salmon c.

calcitonin-origin amyloid deposit
calcitriol
calcium
> c. carbonate crystal
> fenoprofen c.
> c. gluconate

> c. hydroxyapatite crystal deposition disease
> leucovorin c.
> c. oxalate crystal
> c. pentosan polysulfate
> c. phosphate crystal deposition disease
> c. pyrophosphate crystal deposition disease
> c. pyrophosphate dihydrate (CPPD)
> c. pyrophosphate dihydrate deposition disease (CPDD)

calcium-dependent transcription
calcium-signal modulating cyclophilin B ligand (CAML)
calcoaceticus
> *Acinetobacter c.*

calcofluor stain
Calcort
calculated mean organism (CMO)
CaldeCort
> C. Anti-Itch Topical Spray
> C. Topical

Caldesene topical
Caldwell-Luc procedure
Caldwell syndrome
Calgitrol calcium alginate wound dressing with maltodextrin
Caliciviridae virus
Calicivirus
California
> C. black-legged tick
> C. encephalitis (CE)
> C. peppertree
> C. peppertree tree
> C. virus

californica
> *Torpedo c.*

caliper
> Mitutoyo digital c.

CALLA
> common acute lymphocytic leukemia antigen
> CALLA positive

Calliphora
Calliphoridae
callositas
callosity
callous
callus
> C. Salve

CALM
> café-au-lait macule

Calmette-Guérin
> Bacille bilié de C.-G. (BCG)
> bacillus C.-G. (BCG)
> C.-G. bacillus
> C.-G. vaccine

Calmette test
Calmex
calmodulin antagonist
Calmurid
Calm-X Oral
calor
    c. mordax
    c. mordicans
calorica
    dermatitis c.
caloric intake
caloricum
    erythema c.
caloris
    stadium c.
Calpain
Calpastatin
calphostin C
calreticulin
calvities
Calycophora dermatitis
Calymmatobacterium granulomatis
CAM
    cell adhesion molecule
    complementary and alternative medicine
Camcreme ECG paste
camera
    Starcam large field of view
        gamma c.
CAML
    calcium-signal modulating cyclophilin B
    ligand
CAMP
    Childhood Asthma Management Program
cAMP
    cyclic adenosine monophosphate
Campath 1H
Campbell-De Morgan spot
camp fever
Campho-Phenique
camphorated menthol
camphor, menthol and phenol
camptodactyly
    congenital c.
Campylobacter
    C. fetus enteritis
    C. jejuni
    C. pylori
CAN
    chronic allograft nephropathy
Canada blue grass
Canada-Cronkhite syndrome

canal
    external auditory c. (EAC)
    Sucquet-Hoyer c.
Canale-Smith syndrome
canaliculi
    pili triangulati et c.
    pili trianguli et c.
canaliculitis
canary
    c. feather
    c. grass
    c. grass pollen
    reed c.
canarypox virus
C-ANCA, c-ANCA
    cytoplasmic antineutrophil cytoplasmic
    antibody
    C-ANCA titer
cancellous
cancer
    anti-EGF receptor antibody for c.
    antiepidermal growth factor receptor
      antibody for c.
    chimney sweep's c.
    c. en cuirasse
    epidermoid c.
    European Organization for Research
      and Treatment of C. (EROTIC)
    c. immunology
    c. immunotherapy
    kangri c.
    nailbed c.
    nonmelanoma skin c. (NMSC)
    skin c.
    c. vaccination
cancericidal, cancerocidal
cancerophobia, cancerphobia
cancerous
cancer-testis antigen
cancrum oris
Candela laser
Candida
    C. albicans
    C. albicans IgG
    C. arthritis
    C. balanitis
    C. blastoconidia
    C. folliculitis
    C. glabrata
    C. glossitis
    C. glossodynia
    C. granuloma

NOTES

Candida (continued)
  C. *guillermondii*
  C. *inconspicua*
  C. infection
  C. intertrigo
  C. *kefyr*
  C. *krusei*
  C. leukoplakia
  C. *lipolytica*
  C. *lusitaniae*
  C. onychia
  C. osteomyelitis
  C. *parapsilosis*
  C. *parapsilosis* colonization
  C. paronychia
  C. *rugosa*
  C. septicemia
  C. skin test
  C. therapy
  C. *tropicalis*
candidal
  c. angular cheilitis
  c. arthritis
  c. infection
  c. leukoplakia
  c. osteomyelitis
  c. paronychia
candidiasis
  acute atrophic oral c.
  atrophic c.
  bronchial c.
  chronic atrophic c.
  chronic hyperplastic c.
  chronic mucocutaneous c. (CMC)
  congenital c.
  cutaneous c.
  disseminated c.
  invasive c.
  localized mucocutaneous c.
  mucocutaneous c.
  neonatal systemic c.
  oral c.
  oropharyngeal c.
  osteoarticular c.
  systemic c.
  vulvovaginal c. (VVC)
candidid
candidosis
candiduria
candidus
  Aspergillus c.
  strophulus c.
Candistatin
candle dripping
Caner-Decker syndrome
Canesten
canestick deformity

canimorsus
  Capnocytophaga c.
canine
  c. adenovirus 1
  c. distemper virus
  c. herpesvirus
  c. herpetovirus
  c. oral papilloma
caninum
  Ancylostoma c.
  Dipylidium c.
canis
  Babesia c.
  Brucella c.
  Ctenocephalides c.
  Demodex c.
  Ehrlichia c.
  hepatitis contagiosa c.
  Microsporum c.
  Toxocara c.
canities
  rapid c.
  c. segmentata sideropenica
  c. unguium
canium
  Neospora c.
canker
  c. sore
  water c.
Cann-Ease moisturizing nasal gel
cannonball pattern
Cannon curette
cannula
  Accelerator c.
  Cobra c.
  Cook c.
  Illouz c.
  Klein c.
  Lamprey c.
  Narins c.
  Pinto c.
canonical polyadenylylation
cantaloupe
cantharic acid
cantharidal collodion
cantharidin
cantharis, pl. cantharides
Cantharone
canthaxanthin
canthorum
  dystrophia c.
canthus, pl. canthi
  inner c.
  nasal c.
  outer c.
  temporal c.
Cantle line
canyon ragweed

cao gio
CAP
community-acquired pneumonia
cap
cradle c.
capacity
forced vital c. (FVC)
functional residual c. (FRC)
inspiratory c. (IC)
maximum breathing c. (MBC)
slow vital c. (SVC)
total lung c. (TLC)
vital c. (VC)
Caparinia
Capastat sulfate
CAPD
chronic ambulatory peritoneal dialysis
capillariasis
capillaries (*pl. of* capillary)
capillaritis
capillaropathy
capillaroscopy
nail fold c.
capillary, pl. capillaries
alveolar c.
c. angioma
bushy c.
c. fragility test
c. hemangioma
c. hemangioma of infancy
c. malformation
c. nevus
c. resistance test
synovial c.
capilli (*pl. of* capillus)
capillitii
dermatitis papillaris c.
pediculosis c.
capillorum
defluvium c.
defluxio c.
capillus, pl. capilli
Capim virus
capitate
capitatum-multangular-lunatum
capitis
black dot tinea c.
endothelioma c.
epithelioma c.
gray-patch tinea c.
inflammatory tinea c.
pediculosis c.

Pediculus humanus c.
pityriasis c.
pthiriasis c.
seborrhea c.
tinea c.
trichophytosis c.
vitiligo c.
Capitrol
Caplan
C. nodule
C. syndrome
Caplets
Advil Cold & Sinus C.
Aspirin-Free Bayer Select Allergy Sinus C.
Dimetapp Sinus C.
Dristan Sinus C.
Miles Nervine C.
TripTone C.
Capnocytophaga canimorsus
Capoten
capreomycin (CM)
c. sulfate
caprin
caprine
c. herpesvirus
c. herpetovirus
Capripoxvirus
caproate
hydroxyprogesterone c.
Caps
Compoz Gel C.
Drixoral Cough & Congestion Liquid C.
capsaicin oleoresin
Capsicum
capsicum
capsid
Capsin
capsomer
capsular
c. antigen
c. precipitation reaction
capsulatum
Histoplasma c.
capsule
Alka-Seltzer Plus Cold Liqui-Gels C.
Banophen Decongestant C.
Dapacin Cold C.
Dimetapp 4-Hour Liqui-Gel C.
Duadacin C.

NOTES

capsule *(continued)*
    Guaivent PD c.
    Kaletra c.
    lopinavir/ritonavir c.
    Poly-Histine-D C.
    Pseudovent PED c.
    Tenon c.
capsulitis
    adhesive c.
Captia
    C. test
    C. test for syphilis
captopril
Capzasin-P
car allergy
Caraparu virus
carate
carateum
    Treponema c.
carbacephem
carbamazepine
carbamide
    c. body lotion
    c. cream
Carba mix
carbapenem
Carbaryl
carbate
    dimethyl c.
carbenicillin
    Indanyl c.
carbide
    cobalt in tungsten c.
carbinoxamine and pseudoephedrine
Carbiset Tablet
Carbiset-TR Tablet
Carb-N-Sert needle holder
Carbocaine injection
Carbodec
    C. Syrup
    C. TR Tablet
carbohydrate intolerance
carbol-fuchsin solution
carbon
    c. arc lamp
    c. baby
    c. dermatosis
    c. dioxide (CO_2)
    c. dioxide laser
    c. dioxide laser scanner system
    c. monoxide
carbovir
carboxamide
    aminoimidazole c. (AIC)
    imidazole c.
carboxyhemoglobin (HbCO)

carboxymethylcellulose
    benzocaine, gelatin, pectin, and sodium c.
    c. sodium
carboxymethyllysine
carboxypeptidase
carbuncle
carbuncular
carbunculoid
carbunculosis
carcinoembryonic antigen (CEA)
carcinogen
carcinogenesis
carcinoid
    c. flush
    c. syndrome
    c. tumor
carcinoma, pl. **carcinomata**
    acantholytic squamous cell c.
    adenoid cystic c.
    adnexal c.
    apocrine c.
    basal cell c. (BCC)
    basosquamous c.
    bronchoalveolar cell c.
    bronchogenic c.
    Buschke-Löwenstein variant of verrucous c.
    cloacogenic c.
    c. cuniculatum
    cylindromatous c.
    de novo squamous cell c.
    eccrine c.
    Ehrlich ascites c. (EAC)
    c. en cuirasse
    epidermoid c.
    esophageal c.
    fibroepithelioma basal cell c.
    fibrosing basal cell c.
    genital squamous cell c.
    hair-matrix c.
    infiltrative basal cell c.
    intermediate c.
    intraepidermal c.
    invasive squamous cell c.
    keloidal basal cell c.
    Lucké c.
    melanotic c.
    Merkel cell c.
    metatypical c.
    microcystic adnexal c. (MAC)
    morbilliform basal cell c.
    morpheaform basal cell c.
    mucinous eccrine c.
    nasopharyngeal c.
    nevoid basal cell c.
    nodular basal cell c.
    noduloulcerative basal cell c.

pigmented basal cell c.
pilomatrix c.
pilomatrixoma c.
prickle-cell c.
primary cutaneous adenoid cystic c.
primary neuroendocrine c.
pseudoglandular squamous cell c.
reticulum cell c.
sclerosing sweat duct c.
sebaceous c.
c. in situ
in situ squamous cell c.
spindle cell c.
squamous cell c. (SCC)
superficial basal cell c.
sweat gland c.
syringoid c.
trabecular c.
trichilemmal c.
V-2 c.
verrucous c.
carcinomatosa
lymphangitis c.
meningitis c.
carcinomatosis
carcinomatous dermatitis
Cardec-S Syrup
cardiac
c. allograft
c. allograft vascular disease
c. allograft vasculopathy (CAV)
c. allotransplantation
c. complications
c. glycoside
c. pacemaker dermatitis
c. rejection
c. sarcoidosis
C. Transplant Research Database
cardiocutaneous
c. myxoma
c. syndrome
cardio-facio-cutaneous syndrome
cardiolipin
cardiomyocyte transplantation
cardiomyopathy
restrictive c.
cardiopulmonary resuscitation
cardiorespiratory arrest
cardiotrophin 1
cardiovascular
c. collapse
c. involvement

Cardiovirus
Cardiovit AT-10 ECG/spirometry combination system
careless weed
Carey Coombs murmur
carindacillin
carinii
Pneumocystis c.
Carlesta
Carmalt forceps
Carmol
C. 40
C. 10 body lotion
C. 20 cream
C. HC cream
C. scalp treatment kit
C. scalp treatment lotion
C. Shampoo
C. topical
Carmol-HC topical
carmustine
carnauba-wax-like keratoderma
carneus
Aspergillus c.
Carney
C. complex
C. syndrome
carnitine palmitoyltransferase deficiency
carob
Caroguard
Caroli disease
carotene
beta c.
carotenemia
carotenoderma
carotenosis cutis
carotid intima-media wall thickness
carotinemia
carotinosis cutis
carpal
c. to metacarpal ratio
c. tunnel syndrome (CTS)
carpet beetle dermatitis
carpet-tack scale
Carpinus betulus
carpometacarpal (CMC)
c. joint
carprofen
CarraFilm
C. transparent film
C. wound dressing
CarraGauze impregnated gauze

NOTES

carrageenan arthritis
carrageenin-induced footpad inflammation model
CarraSmart foam dressing
CarraSorb
> C. H alginate wound cover
> C. H calcium alginate wound dressing
> C. hydrogel dressing
> C. M

Carrasyn hydrogel wound dressing
Carrel patch
carrier
> active c.
> c. cell
> chronic c.
> contact c.
> convalescent c.
> healthy c.
> incubatory c.
> intermittent c.
> c. state
> c. strain

Carrión disease
carrionii
> *Cladosporium c.*

carrot
Carter black mycetoma
Carticel autologous cultured chondrocyte
cartilage
> cricoid c.
> hyaline articular c.
> c. implant
> c. intermediate layer protein (CILP)
> c. matrix protein
> c. oligomeric matrix protein (COMP)
> c. proteoglycan
> tensile strength of osteoarthritic c.

cartilage-hair hypoplasia
cartilaginous collagen
Cartrofen
carumonam
caruncle, pl. **carunculae**
> trichosis carunculae

Casal
> C. collar
> C. necklace

cascade
> adhesion molecule c.
> alternative pathway of complement c.
> arachidonic acid c.
> caspase c.
> clotting c.
> complement activation c.
> complementary c.
> C. impactor

inflammatory c.
rejection c.
terminal c.
caseating granuloma
caseation necrosis
case control study
casei
> *Lactobacillus c.*

casein
cashew
Casoni
> C. intradermal test
> C. reaction
> C. skin test

caspase
> c. 3, 8
> c. cascade
> c. inhibitor

casseii
> *Penicillium c.*

cassette
> susceptibility c.

CAST
> color allergy screening test

cast
> erythrocyte c.
> hair c.
> Minerva c.
> Night C. R
> spica c.
> total contact c.

Castaneda principle
Castellani
> C. bronchitis
> C. Natural Formula
> C. paint
> C. point
> C. treatment

castellani
> *Acanthamoeba c.*

Castle examination light
Castleman disease
castor bean
Castroviejo
> C. blade breaker
> C. blade holder
> C. forceps
> C. needle holder

casual blood pressure (CBP)
CAT
> chloramphenicol acetyltransferase
> conventional asthma therapy
> CAT enzyme

cat
> c. dander
> c. distemper virus
> c. epithelium
> c. flea

c. flea bite
c. hookworm
panleukopenia virus of c.'s
catabolin isoform
catabolism
articular joint tissue c.
Cataflam Oral
catagen growth phase
catalase-negative
catalysis
catalytic domain
catalyze
catamenial hemothorax
Catapres
cataract
poikiloderma atrophicans and c.
secondary c.
catarrhalis
Branhamella c.
herpes c.
Moraxella c.
catarrhal jaundice
catatrichy
catcher's crouch
catecholamine
catechol-*O*-methyl
c.-m. transferase (COMT)
c.-m. transferase asthma
caterpillar
c. body
c. dermatitis
puss c.
c. rash
saddleback c.
c. sting
stinging c.
catfish
saltwater c.
c. sting
cathepsin
c. D, G, L
c. K mRNA
catheter
antiseptic-impregnated central
venous c.
double-balloon triple lumen c.
P.A.S. Port c.
pheresis c.
**catheter-related bloodstream infection
(CR-BSI)**
catholysis
Cath-Secure tape

cati
Toxocara c.
cationic compound
catkins
cat-scratch disease (CSD)
cattle
ephemeral fever of c.
infectious papilloma of c.
malignant catarrh of c.
papular stomatitis virus of c.
c. plague
c. plague virus
c. wart
winter dysentery of c.
Catu virus
cauda equina syndrome
cauliflower
causalgia
causative
caustic
cauterant
cauterization
cauterize
cautery
chemical c.
gas c.
CAV
cardiac allograft vasculopathy
cavernosum
angioma c.
lymphangioma c.
cavernosus
nevus c.
cavernous
c. angioma
c. hemangioma
c. lymphangioma
c. sinusoid
caviae
Aeromonas c.
Nocardia c.
caviar tongue
Cavilon barrier ointment
cavitary
cavitation
**Cavitron Ultrasonic Surgical Aspirator
(CUSA)**
Cavity
Cutinova C.
cayenne
mal de C.

NOTES

cayenne *(continued)*
    c. pepper-like macule
    c. pepper spot
CAZ beta-lactamase
Cazenave
    C. disease
    C. lupus
    C. vitiligo
CB
  cord blood
C3b
    C3b receptor
C4b
    C4b receptor
C3bBb
    C. receptor
CBDC
  chronic bullous disease of childhood
CBH
  cutaneous basophil hypersensitivity
CBMC
  cord blood mononuclear cell
CBP
  casual blood pressure
C5b-9 receptor
CC49 monoclonal antibody
CCA
  chimpanzee coryza agent
CCHB
  congenital complete heart block
CCHF
  Congo-Crimean hemorrhagic fever
CCLE
  chronic cutaneous lupus erythematosus
CCMM
  conventional cutaneous malignant
    melanoma
C3-coated
    C.-c. cell
    C.-c. erythrocyte
CCP
  complement control protein
CCR2
    chemokine receptor C.
CCR5
    chemokine receptor C.
CCS
  composite cultured skin
CCSA
  central centrifugal scarring alopecia
CCTAT
  Cooperative Clinical Trials in Adult
    Transplantation
CCTPT
  Cooperative Clinical Trials in Pediatric
    Transplantation
C2D
  C2 deficiency

CD2–72
  cluster of differentiation 2–72
C4D
  C4 deficiency
C7D
  C7 deficiency
CD28
    C. antibody
    C. protein
C&D
  curettage and desiccation
CD1a antibody
CD3 monoclonal antibody
CD4+
    C. helper/inducer cell
    C. Measure
    C. T cell subset
CD4
    CD4 cell
    CD4 count
    CD4, human recombinant soluble
      rCD4
    CD4, human truncated-365 AA
      polypeptide
    CD4, immunoglobulin G,
      recombinant human
    CD4 monoclonal antibody
    CD4 T cell subset
    CD4 T-lymphocyte count
CD4/CD8 ratio
CD5
    CD5 antibody
    CD5 cell
CD5+ antibody
CD8
    CD38 on CD8
    CD8 cell
    CD8 monoclonal antibody
    CD8 T cell subset
CD8+ T cell
CD10 antibody
CD11a antibody
CD11b antibody
CD11c antibody
CD14 antibody
CD15 antibody
CD16 monoclonal antibody
CD18 antibody
CD19 antibody
CD20 antibody
CD21 antibody
CD22 antibody
CD24 antibody
CD25 monoclonal antibody
CD26/vitronectin receptor
CD29 antibody

CD38
>C. antibody
>C. on CD8

CD40
>C. ligand gene
>C. soluble protein

CD43 antibody

CD44
>C. antibody
>C. Hyaluronic acid receptor

CD49a antibody
CD49b antibody
CD49c antibody
CD49e antibody
CD49f antibody
CD54 antibody
CD57
>DAKO CD57

CD69 monoclonal antibody
CD71 monoclonal antibody
CD106 antibody
CDC
>Centers for Disease Control
>Centers for Disease Control and
> Prevention
>complement-dependent cytotoxicity

CDE
>chlordiazepoxide
>CDE antigen

C3dg receptor
CDI
>Children's Depression Inventory

CDM
>childhood dermatomyositis

CD56 monoclonal antibody
cDNA
>complementary deoxyribonucleic acid
>complementary DNA
> PGHS-1, -2 cDNA
> cDNA probe

CDP 870
CDR
>complementarity-determining region
> CDR grafting

CE
>California encephalitis
>coefficient of error
>curettage and electrodesiccation

CEA
>carcinoembryonic antigen

Ceclor

cedar
>Japanese c.
>mountain c.
>red c.
>salt c.
>Western red c.

CeeNU Oral
cefaclor
cefadroxil monohydrate
Cefadyl
cefamandole nafate
Cefanex
cefazolin sodium
cefditoren pivoxil
cefepime
cefixime
Cefizox
cefmenoxime
cefmetazole sodium
Cefobid
cefodizime
cefonicid sodium
cefoperazone sodium
ceforanide
cefotaxime sodium
cefotetan
cefoxitin sodium
cefpiramide
cefpodoxime proxetil
cefprozil
ceftazidime
ceftibuten
Ceftin Oral
ceftizoxime
>c. beta-lactamase
>c. sodium

ceftriaxone sodium
cefuroxime axetil suspension (CAE)
Cefzil
CEL
>Celsior

Celebrex
celecoxib cell
celery
Celestoderm
Celestone
>C. Oral
>C. Phosphate Injection
>C. Soluspan

celiac
>c. disease
>c. sprue

NOTES

cell

acid-secreting gastric parietal c.
acinar c.
adenovirus-reactive T c.
c. adhesion molecule (CAM)
c. adhesion protein
allogenic dendritic c.
alloreactive c.
alpha c.
anergic T c.
antibody-forming c. (AFC)
antigen-presenting c. (APC)
antigen-sensitive c.
apoptotic c.
astrocytoma c.
autoimmune progenitor c.
autoreactive B c.
B c.
B1 c.
balloon c.
basal c.
basaloid c.
blast c.
blood progenitor c.
bone marrow c. (BMC)
bone marrow-derived cultured
  mast c. (BMCMC)
Bowenoid c.
bronchial epithelial c.
bystander T c.
carrier c.
C3-coated c.
CD4 c.
CD5 c.
CD8 c.
CD4+ helper/inducer c.
CD8+ T c.
celecoxib c.
chronic inflammatory c.
ciliated epithelial c.
circulating B c.
Clara c.
clear c.
cleaved giant c.
common lymphoid progenitor c.
conjunctival goblet c.
contrasuppressor c.
cord blood mononuclear c.
  (CBMC)
corneal epithelial c.
cuboidal c.
cytolytic effector c.
cytomegalic c.
cytoplasmic islet c.
cytotoxic T c.
Daudi lymphoma c.
daughter c.
dendritic epidermal c.

c. deposition
disorder of phagocytic c.
Dorothy Reed-Sternberg c.
c. dose
double negative   c.
Downey c.
effector c.
end c.
endomysial mononuclear c.
endothelial c.
enterochromaffin c.
Epicel autologous skin c.
epidermal Langerhans c.
epithelioid c.
extravillous cytotrophoblast c.
fibroblast-like spindle c.
foam c.
foreign body giant c.
Friend erythroleukemia c.
frozen-thawed red c.
germinative c.
giant c.
goblet c.
granular c.
grape c.
hairy c. (HC)
HeLa c.
helper T c.
hematopoietic stem c.
high endothelial venule c.
homozygous typing c.
horny c.
HPC c.
human skin nurse c. (HSNC)
human umbilical vein endothelial c.
  (HUVEC)
hybrid c.
hyperplastic mucus-secreting
  goblet c.
I c.
IgE-sensitized c.
IgM-coated c.
immunoblastic sarcoma of B, T c.
immunocompetent c.
immunoglobulin E-sensitized c.
immunoglobulin M-coated c.
immunoglobulin-secreting c.
immunologically activated c.
immunologically competent c.
inclusion c.
inducer c.
inflammatory c.
innocent bystander c.
c. interaction (CI)
c. interaction gene
intestinal epithelial c. (IEC)
intracytoplasmic inclusion c.
intraepithelial mast c.

islet alpha c.
JKA c.
Jurkat c.
K c.
  killer cell
keratinized c.
killer c. (K cell)
Kulchitsky c.
Kupffer c.
LAK c.
c. lamina
lamina propria immune c.
Langerhans c.
Langhans c.
lazy NK c.
LE c.
lepra c.
Leroy I c.
Leu-3+ helper T c.
leuko-poor red blood c.
limiting precursor c. (LPC)
c. line
linker for activation of T c.
  (LAT)
Lipschütz c.
lupus erythematosus c.
lymph c.
lymphoid c.
lymphokine-activated killer c.
lymphoplasmacytoid lymphoma c.
lymphoreticular c.
M c.
Madin-Darby bovine kidney c.
mast c.
maturation B c.
MDBK c.
mediator c.
Merkel c.
mesenchymal progenitor c.
mesothelial c.
metaplastic mucus-secreting c.
microchimeric c.
mononuclear c.
morula c.
Mott c.
mucosal mast c.
multifocal Langerhans c.
multinucleated giant c. (MGC)
multipotent hematopoietic c.
myeloid stem c.
naive B c.
natural killer c.

neoplastic c.
nests of nevus c.'s
nevus c.
nevus c., A-, B-, C-type
NK c.
nonadherent c.
non-B c.
nonlymphocytic c.
nuclear factor of activated T c.
  (NFAT)
nucleated endothelial c.
null c.
nurse c.
OKT c.
Ortho-Kung T c.
osteoblast-lineage c.
Paget c.
pagetoid c.
palisade c.
pannus c.
pepsinogen-secreting zymogenic c.
peripheral blood mononuclear c.
  (PBMC)
peripheral blood progenitor c.
  (PBPC)
peripheral blood stem c. (PBSC)
pig aortic endothelial c. (PAEC)
pigmented spindle c. (PSC)
plasma c.
pluripotential c.
polyclonal B c.
polymorphonuclear c.
pre-B c.
preformed granule-associated
  mast c.
prickle c.
Primed c.
progenitor lymphoid c.
proliferative c.
pull c.
pyknotic c.
quantitation of B c.
Raji c.
red blood c. (RBC)
Reed-Sternberg c.
regulatory CD4+ T c.
responder T c.
reticuloendothelial c.
retinal pigment epithelial c. (RPE)
rheumatoid synovial macrophage-
  like/dendritic c.
rosette-forming c.

NOTES

cell *(continued)*
    rosettes of c.
    satellite c.
    scavenger c.
    Schwann c.
    sensitized c.
    Sézary c.
    sheath c.
    sheets of nevus c.'s
    sinusoidal c.
    small noncleaved c. (SNC)
    spindle c.
    spindle-shaped c.
    squamous c.
    stem c.
    c. strain
    stromal c.
    suicide c.
    suppressor c.
    c. surface expression
    surface Ig-expressing B c.
    c. surface marker
    syngeneic c.
    synovial lining c. (SLC)
    synovia T c.
    T c.
    tanned red c.
    target c.
    Tart c.
    tartrate-resistant acid phosphatase positive c.
    Tc1, Tc2 c.
    T cytotoxic c. (Tc)
    TDTH c.
    Tg c.
    Th1 c.
    Th2 c.
    T-helper c. (Th)
    T-helper type 2 c. (Th2)
    T-helper type 3 c. (Th3)
    thymic epithelial c.
    thymus nurse c.
    TIL c.
    Tm c.
    Touton giant c.
    c. transformation
    transiently amplifying c. (TAC)
    TRAP-positive c.
    T-suppressor c.
    tumor-infiltrating lymphocyte c.
    type II alveolar c.
    unifocal Langerhans c.
    Unna c.
    veiled c.
    Vero c.
    virus-infected c.
    virus-transformed c.
    Warthin-Finkeldey c.
    white blood c. (WBC)

cell-bound antibody

cell-cell
    c.-c. adhesion
    c.-c. interaction

CellCept

Cellex-C

cell-mediated
    c.-m. autoimmunity
    c.-m. hypersensitivity
    c.-m. immunity (CMI)
    c.-m. immunologic drug reaction

Cellufresh

cellular
    c. adoptive immunotherapy
    c. blue nevus
    c. casts in urine
    c. diapedesis
    c. immune deficiency syndrome (CIDS)
    c. immune panel
    c. immune theory
    c. immunity deficiency syndrome
    c. immunodeficiency with abnormal immunoglobulin synthesis
    c. inhibitors of apoptosis (cIAPs)
    c. pannus
    c. xenograft rejection
    c. xenotransplantation

cellularis
    plasma c.

cellulite

cellulitis
    acute scalp c.
    anaerobic c.
    demarcated c.
    dissecting c.
    eosinophilic c.
    epizootic c.
    gaseous c.
    perianal streptococcal c.
    phlegmonous c.
    streptococcal c.

cellulose
    hydroxypropyl c.
    oxidized c.

cellulosic/cuprophan

Celluvisc

CELO
    chicken embryo lethal orphan
    CELO virus

celonychia

Celovirus

celsi
    kerion c.

Celsior (CEL)

Celsus
- C. alopecia
- C. area
- C. kerion
- C. papule
- C. vitiligo

Cel-U-Jec
- C.-U.-J. Injection

cement
- c. dermatitis
- c. line

cemented
- finger-packing doughy c.

cementoma
Cenafed Plus Tablet
CENP-B
- scleroderma autoantigen C.-B.

center
- C.'s for Disease Control (CDC)
- C.'s for Disease Control and Prevention (CDC)
- microtubule organizing c.
- necrotic c.

center-edge angle
centimorgan (cM)
centipede
- c. bite
- giant desert c.

central
- c. blister
- c. centrifugal scarring alopecia (CCSA)
- c. clearing
- C. European tick-borne encephalitis virus
- c. fibrinoid necrosis
- c. nervous system (CNS)
- c. papillary atrophy
- c. pruritus
- c. Recklinghausen disease type II
- c. stratum
- c. type neurofibromatosis

centrifugal lipoatrophy
centrifugation
- density gradient c.
- discontinuous plasma-Percoll gradient c.

centrifugum
- erythema annulare c. (EAC)
- leukoderma acquisitum c.
- ulerythema c.

centrilobar necrosis (CLN)

centroblast
centrofacial
- c. lentiginosis
- c. plaque

centromere antigen
Centruroides
- C. exilicauda
- C. exilicauda sting
- C. sculpturatus
- C. sculpturatus sting
- C. vittatus
- C. vittatus sting

Centurion
- C. SiteGuard MVP transparent film
- C. SorbaView composite dressing

CEP
- chronic eosinophilic pneumonia
- congenital erythropoietic porphyria

cepacia
- *Burkholderia* c.

cephalexin monohydrate
cephalhematoma
cephalic
- c. brainlike heterotopia
- c. histiocytosis

cephalocele
- rudimentary c.

cephalooculocutaneous telangiectasia
cephalosporin
- third-generation c.

Cephalosporium
cephalothin sodium
cephamycin
cephapirin sodium
cephradine
Ceptaz
ceramidase deficiency
ceramide-S1P rheostat
ceramide trihexoside (CTH)
Ceratopogonidae
cercaria, pl. **cercariae**
cercarial dermatitis
cerea
- seborrhea c.

cerebellar ataxia
cerebelliformis
- nevus c.

cerebral
- c. allergy
- c. amyloidosis

NOTES

C

cerebral *(continued)*
    c. autosomal dominant arteriopathy with subcortical infarcts and leukoencephalopathy (CADASIL)
    c. macula
    c. malaria
    c. venous sinus thrombosis (CVST)
cérébrale
    tache c.
cerebri
    pseudotumor c.
cerebritis
    lupus c.
cerebrospinal
    c. fever
    c. fluid immunofixation electrophoresis (CSF-IFE)
    c. meningitis
    c. rhinorrhea
cerebrotendinous xanthomatosis
Ceredase injection
cereolysin
cereus
    Bacillus c.
cerevisiae
    Saccharomyces c.
Cerezyme
Cerose-DM
Certican
Certified decongestant
Cerubidine
cerulea, caerulea, pl. **ceruleae**
    macula c.
ceruloplasmin
cerumen
Cerumenex ear drops
ceruminal
ceruminoma
ceruminous gland
cervical
    c. acceleration-deceleration syndrome
    c. actinomycosis
    c. lymph node swelling
    c. patagium
cervicitis
cervicofacial
    c. actinomycosis
    c. rhytidectomy
cervicothoracic kyphosis
cervicothymic remnant
cestodic tuberculosis
Cetacaine
Cetacort Topical
Cetamide Ophthalmic
Cetaphil
Cetapred Ophthalmic
cetirizine

cetyl
    c. alcohol-coal tar distillate
    c. palmitate
cevimeline HCl
CF
    complement fixation
    complement-fixing
    cystic fibrosis
       CF antibody
       CF test
CFA
    cryptogenic fibrosing alveolitis
    cystic fibrosis arthropathy
CFIDS
    chronic fatigue immune deficiency syndrome
    chronic fatigue and immune dysfunction syndrome
c-fos protein
CFR
    coronary flow reserve
CFTR
    cystic fibrosis-transmembrane conductance regulator
CFU
    colony-forming unit
CGD
    chronic granulomatous disease
CGRP
    calcitonin gene-related peptide
CH50 assay
Chaetomium globosum
chafe
chaffeensis
    Ehrlichia c.
Chagas disease
chagasic
chagoma
Chagres virus
chagrin
    peau de c.
chain
    acyl c.
    alpha c.
    glycosaminoglycan c.
    heavy c.
    hemolytic c.
    homology of c.
    IgG heavy c.
    immunoglobulin delta c.
    immunoglobulin epsilon c.
    immunoglobulin G heavy c.
    immunoglobulin heavy c.
    immunoglobulin mu c.
    invariant c.
    J c.
    kappa light c.
    lambda light c.

light c.
myosin light c.
polypeptide c.
chair-rise maneuver
chalazion, pl. **chalazia**
c. clamp
c. knife
chalazodermia
chalk
steroid c.
challenge
allergen specific nasal c.
c. diet
dinitrochlorobenzene c.
direct c.
double-blind placebo-controlled
food c. (DBPCFC)
food c.
histamine c.
methacholine bronchoprovocation c.
nasal allergen c. (NAC)
open food c. (OFC)
oral c.
c. test
chalones
chamber
aluminum Finn c.
Boyden c.
Finn c.
Van der Bend c.
chamber-scarification test
Chanarin-Dorfman syndrome
chancre
erosive c.
fungating c.
hard c.
hunterian c.
indurated c.
mixed c.
monorecidive c.
c. recidive
c. redux
Ricord c.
Rollet c.
soft c.
sporotrichositic c.
sporotrichotic c.
sulcus c.
syphilis c.
tuberculous c.
tularemic c.

chancriform
c. pyoderma
c. syndrome
chancroid
chancroidal
chancrous
change
clinical c.
environmental c.
fibrinoid c.
formula c.
histologic c.
hormonal c.
mitral valve prolapse, aortic
anomalies, skeletal changes, and
skin c.'s (MASS)
nail c.
nonspecific climatic c.
oil drop c.
perigranulomatous fibrotic c.
pigment c.
polyneuropathy, organomegaly,
endocrinopathy, monoclonal
gammopathy, and skin c.'s
(POEMS)
respiratory c.
symmetric reticulonodular x-ray c.
synovial fluid c.
tinctorial c.
vacuolar c.
channel
voltage-gated potassium c.
Chantemesse reaction
Chaoul tube
chappa
chapped
chapping
CHAQ
Childhood Health Assessment
Questionnaire
characteristic
lesion surface c.
charcoal
activated c.
Charcot joint
Charcot-Leyden crystal
chard
Swiss c.
Charlin syndrome
Charlouis disease
Chase-Sulzberger phenomenon

NOTES

C

chat
    langue au c.
Chauffard-Still syndrome
Chauffard syndrome
Chaussier areola
cheat grass pollen
Chediak-Higashi syndrome (CHS)
cheek
    c. chewing
    c. cosmetic
    c. phenomenon
cheese washer's lung
cheesy abscess
cheilectomy procedure
cheilitis, chilitis
    actinic c.
    c. actinica
    allergic apostematous c.
    angular c.
    candidal angular c.
    commissural c.
    contact c.
    c. exfoliativa
    c. glandularis
    c. glandularis apostematosa
    c. granulomatosa
    c. granulomatosa impetiginous
    granulomatous c.
    impetiginous c.
    Miescher granulomatous c.
    migrating c.
    c. mycotic venenata
    solar c.
    Volkmann c.
cheilosis
cheiroarthropathy
    diabetic c.
cheiropompholyx (*var. of*
  chiropompholyx)
chelating agent
chelator
    intracellular calcium c.
chelerythrine chloride
chelicera, pl. **chelicerae**
cheloid
cheloidalis
    acne c.
    acné chéloïdique
    folliculitis c.
chelonae
    Mycobacterium c.
chemabrasion
chemes
chemexfoliation
chemical
    c. agent
    c. burn
    c. cautery

    c. depilatory
    c. dermatitis
    c. grouping
    c. hemostasis
    c. hypersensitivity syndrome
    c. leukoderma
    c. meningitis
    c. panniculitis
    c. peel
    c. peeling
    c. prophylaxis
    c. stimulus
    c. sunscreen
chemicocautery
chemiluminescence assay
chemiluminescent
    c. DNA
    c. in situ hybridization for
      detection of CMV DNA
    c. in situ hybridization for
      detection of cytomegalovirus
      deoxyribonucleic acid
chemistry
    blood c.
chemoattract
chemoattractant
chemocautery
chemoembolization
    transarterial c. (TACE)
chemoimmunology
chemokine
    cutaneous T-cell attracting c.
      (CTACK)
    macrophage-derived c. (MDC)
    c. receptor CCR2
    c. receptor CCR5
    thymus and activation-regulated c.
      (TARC)
chemokinetic factor
chemonucleolysis
chemonucleosis
    chymopapain c.
chemoprophylaxis
chemoresistance
chemorrhexis
chemosis
chemosurgery
    Mohs c.
chemotactic
    c. factor
    c. peptide
chemotaxis
    eosinophilic c.
    impaired neutrophil c.
    leukocyte c.
    neutrophil c.
chemotechnique
chemotherapeutic index

chemotherapy
    c. agent
    combination c.
    interleukin-2 adjunctive c.
chenodeoxycholic acid
Chenopodiaceae
Chenopodium
cheopis
    Xenopsylla c.
cherry
    c. angioma
    c. hemangioma
    c. spot
chest
    c. cold
    c. percussion and vibration
    "silent" c.
Chevron nail
Chewables
    Dimetapp C.
chewing
    cheek c.
Cheyletiella **infestation**
Cheyne-Stokes respiration
CHF
    congestive heart failure
chicken
    c. embryo lethal orphan (CELO)
    c. embryo lethal orphan virus
    c. feather
    c. ovalbumin (OVA)
    c. pox
chickenpox
    c. immune globulin (human)
    c. immunoglobulin
    c. vaccine
    c. virus
chiclero ulcer
Chido-Rodgers antigen
chief agglutinin
Chiesi powder inhaler
chigga
chigger
    c. bite
    c. dermatitis
    c. flea
chigoe
chikungunya virus
chilblain
    c. lupus

    c. lupus erythematosus
    c. lupus erythematosus of
      Hutchinson
    necrotized c.
chilblain-like erythema
CHILD
    congenital hemidysplasia with
    ichthyosiform erythroderma and limb
    defects
    CHILD syndrome
child
    blueberry muffin c.
    Cuna moon c.
childbed fever
childhood
    C. Asthma Management Program
    (CAMP)
    asymmetric periflexural exanthem
    of c. (APEC)
    c. bullous dermatosis
    chronic bullous dermatosis of c.
    chronic bullous disease of c.
    (CBDC)
    c. dermatomyositis (CDM)
    c. eczema
    C. Health Assessment Questionnaire
    (CHAQ)
    c. myositis
    C. Myositis Assessment Scale
    (CMAS)
    papular acrodermatitis of c. (PAC)
    polyarteritis in c.
childhood-type tuberculosis
Child-Pugh score
children
    chronic granulomatous disease of c.
    linear IgA bullous disease in c.
    Self-Perception Profile for c.
Children's
    C. Advil
    C. Advil Suspension
    C. Depression Inventory (CDI)
    C. Motion Sickness liquid
    C. Motrin Suspension
    C. Silfedrine
    C. Vaccine Initiative (CVI)
Child-Turcotte-Pugh
    C.-T.-P. classification
    C.-T.-P. score
chilitis (*var. of* cheilitis)

C

NOTES

CHIME
coloboma of the eye, heart defect, ichthyosiform dermatosis, mental retardation, and ear defect
CHIME syndrome
chimera
chimeric antibody
chimerism
hematopoietic c.
hepatocellular c.
leukocyte c.
mixed hematopoietic c.
chimney sweep's cancer
chimpanzee coryza agent (CCA)
Chinese
C. elm
C. elm tree
C. restaurant syndrome
Chiou equation
chip
protein c.
Chiron bDNA viral load test
Chironex
C. fleckeri
C. fleckeri sting
chiropompholyx, cheiropompholyx
chirp-pulse amplification
chi sequence
Chisolm scale
chi-square test
chitin
chitinases
chive
CHL
chloramphenicol
Chlamydia
C. disease
C. pneumoniae
C. psittaci
C. trachomatis
chlamydial
c. inclusion conjunctivitis
c. infection
c. urethritis
Chlamydiazyme II
chlamydospore
chlamydosporum
Fusarium c.
Chlo-Amine Oral
chloasma
c. bronzinum
c. faciei
c. gravidarum
c. hepaticum
melanoderma c.
c. periorale virginium
c. phthisicorum
c. traumaticum

chloracne
chloracnegens
Chlorafed Liquid
chloral hydrate
chlorambucil
chloramine
c. T
taurine c.
chloramphenicol (CHL)
c. acetyltransferase (CAT)
c. acetyltransferase enzyme
c., polymyxin b, and hydrocortisone
c. and prednisolone
Chloraprep
Chloraseptic
Chlorate Oral
chlorcyclizine
chlordiazepoxide (CDE)
c. antigen
Chloresium Soln wound cleanser
chlorhexidine gluconate
chloride
Adrenalin C.
aluminum c.
benzalkonium c.
benzethonium c.
benzocaine, butyl aminobenzoate, tetracaine, and benzalkonium c.
chelerythrine c.
ethyl c.
ferric c.
Gebauer ethyl c.
liquid ethyl c.
methacholine c.
methylbenzethonium c.
methylrosaniline c.
polyvinyl c. (PVC)
stearalkonium ammonium c.
sweat c.
c. sweat test
vinyl c.
chlorine acne
chlorocarbons
2-chlorodeoxyadenosine
chlorofluorocarbon
chloroform
chloroguanide hydrochloride
chlorohydrate
aluminum c.
chloroma
Chloromycetin
(chlorophenothane)
dichlorodiphenyltrichloroethane (chlorophenothane) (DDT)
chloroprocaine hydrochloride
Chloroptic Ophthalmic
Chloroptic-P Ophthalmic

6-chloropurine
chloroquine
    c. phosphate
    c. and primaquine
    c. therapy
chloroquine-mepacrine (CM)
chloroquine-quinine (CQ)
chloroquine-resistant *Plasmodium*
  falciparum **(CRPF)**
chlorosis
chlorothiazide diuretic
chloroxine
Chlorphed
Chlorphed-LA Nasal Solution
chlorpheniramine
    Efidac/24 c.
    c. maleate
    c., phenylephrine, and codeine
    c., phenylephrine, and
      dextromethorphan
    c., phenylephrine, and
      phenylpropanolamine
    c., phenylephrine, and
      phenyltoloxamine
    c., phenylpropanolamine, and
      acetaminophen
    c., phenyltoloxamine,
      phenylpropanolamine, and
      phenylephrine
    c. and pseudoephedrine
    c., pyrilamine, phenylephrine, and
      phenylpropanolamine
chlorpromazine hydrochloride
chlorpropamide flush
chlorprothixene
chlortetracycline hydrochloride
Chlor-Trimeton (CTM)
    C.-T. 4 Hour Relief Tablet
    C.-T. Injection
    C.-T. Oral
Chlor-Tripolon
    C.-T. Decongestant
    C.-T. N.D.
chocolate
cholangiocarcinoma
cholangiohepatoma
cholangiolitic hepatitis
cholangitis
    primary sclerosing c. (PSC)
    sclerosing c.
Choledyl

cholera
    Asiatic c.
    c. bacillus
    bilious c.
    European c.
    hog c.
    c. infantum
    c. morbus
    c. nostras
    c. sicca
    c. toxin
    typhoid c.
    c. vaccine
cholerae
    Vibrio c.
choleraesuis
    Salmonella c.
choleragen
choleraic
cholera-red reaction
cholerica
    vox c.
Cholesky model
cholestatic hepatitis
cholesterinic molluscum
cholesterinized antigen
cholesteroderma
cholesterol
    c. crystal
    c. embolus
    low-density lipoprotein c. (LDL-C)
    very-low-density lipoprotein c.
cholesterolosis
    c. cutis
    extracellular c.
cholestyramine
cholic acid
choline
    c. magnesium trisalicylate
    c. salicylate
cholinergic
    c. agent
    c. response
    c. urticaria
cholinogenic dermatosis
chondrification
chondrin pellet
chondritis
    auricular c.
chondroadherin
chondrocalcinosis
    hydroxyapatite c.

NOTES

chondrocyte
    articular c.
    Carticel autologous cultured c.
    c. cytoskeletal actin polymerization
    c. mitochondrial oxidative
      phosphorylation
    c. proteoglycan synthesis
    c. sponge
chondrocytic chondrolysis
chondrodermatitis
    c. helicis nodularis
    nodular c.
    c. nodularis chronica helicis
chondrodysplasia
    lethal c.
    c. punctata
    c. punctata dysplasia
    c. punctata syndrome
    thanatophoric diastrophic c.
    twisted c.
chondrogenesis
chondroid syringoma
chondroitin
    c. sulfate
    c. sulfate B
    c. sulfate/dermatan sulfate (CS/DS)
chondrolysis
    chondrocytic c.
chondroma
chondromalacia patellae
chondromatosis
chondroprogenitor
chondroprotective drug
chondrosarcoma
chorda tympani syndrome
chorea
    Sydenham c.
choreal
choriomeningitis
chorionic human recombinant
    gonadotropin
Chorioptes
chorioretinitis
choristoma
    phakomatous c.
choroidal angiitis
choroiditis
Chortoglyphus arcuatus
CHP
    histiocytic cytophagic panniculitis
Chr^a antigen
Christmas
    C. tree pattern
    C. tree test
Christopher spot
Christ-Siemens-Touraine syndrome
chromate dermatitis

chromatica
    trichomycosis c.
chromatin antibody
chromatism
chromatogenous
chromatography
    gas c.
    high-performance liquid c. (HPLC)
chromatophore nevus of Naegeli
chromatophorotropic
chromatosis
chrome
    c. holes on the hand
    c. patch test
    c. sore
    c. ulcer
chromhidrosis, chromidrosis
    apocrine c.
    eccrine c.
chromic gut suture
chromidroses plantaire
chromidrosis (*var. of* chromhidrosis)
chromobacteriosis
chromoblastomycosis
chromogenic
chromomycosis
chromonychia
chromophage
chromophore
chromophototherapy
chromosomal translocation
chromosome
    c. arrangement
    c. 6, class III MHC
    c. number
    Philadelphia c. (Ph)
    c. 6q
    c. walking
    X c.
    yeast artificial c. (YAC)
chromotherapy
chromotrichia
chromotrichial
chronic
    c. acral dermatitis
    c. actinic dermatitis (CAD)
    c. active hepatitis (CAH)
    c. active hepatitis with cirrhosis
      (CAHC)
    c. airways disease (CAD)
    c. allograft nephropathy (CAN)
    c. allograft rejection
    c. ambulatory peritoneal dialysis
      (CAPD)
    c. anaphylaxis
    c. anterior poliomyelitis
    c. asthma
    c. atrophic candidiasis

c. atrophic vulvitis
c. autoimmune thyroiditis
c. blood loss
c. bronchitis
c. brucellosis
c. bullous dermatosis of childhood
c. bullous disease of childhood (CBDC)
c. carrier
c. cold agglutinin disease
c. conjunctivitis
c. cutaneous leishmaniasis
c. cutaneous lupus erythematosus (CCLE)
c. cyclosporine nephropathy
c. diarrhea
c. discoid lupus erythematosus
c. eczema
c. eosinophilic pneumonia (CEP)
c. Epstein-Barr virus infection
c. erythema multiforme
c. familial giant urticaria
c. fatigue immune deficiency syndrome (CFIDS)
c. fatigue and immune dysfunction syndrome (CFIDS)
c. fatigue syndrome
c. fibroid tuberculosis
c. graft dysfunction
c. graft-versus-host disease
c. granulomatous disease (CGD)
c. granulomatous disease of children
c. hemolytic anemia
c. hemosideric dermatosis
c. hereditary lymphedema
c. histiocytosis
c. hyperplastic candidiasis
c. hyperplastic sinusitis with nasal polyposis (CHS/NP)
c. hypersensitivity pneumonitis
c. idiopathic thrombocytopenic purpura
c. idiopathic urticaria (CIU)
c. infantile neurological, cutaneous, and articular (CINCA)
c. infantile neurological cutaneous and auricular syndrome
c. inflammatory cell
c. inflammatory demyelinating polyradiculoneuropathy (CIDP)
c. inflammatory disease

c. interstitial lung disease
c. intestinal pseudoobstruction (CIPO)
c. ITP
c. jejunal inflammation
c. lymphocytic leukemia (CLL)
c. monoarthritis
c. mucocutaneous candidiasis (CMC)
c. mucocutaneous candidiasis syndrome
c. multifocal osteomyelitis
c. myelocytic/myelogenous/myeloid leukemia accelerated phase (CML AP)
c. myelocytic/myelogenous/myeloid leukemia blast crisis (CML BC)
c. myelocytic/myelogenous/myeloid leukemia chronic phase (CML CP)
c. myeloid leukemia (CML)
c. nephrotoxicity
c. obstructive pulmonary disease (COPD)
c. otitis media
c. pain syndrome
c. papular dermatitis
c. paranasal sinusitis
c. paronychia
c. phase shoulder impairment
c. posterior basic meningitis
c. postrheumatic fever arthritis
c. radiodermatitis
c. recurrent multifocal osteitis (CRMO)
c. T-cell leukemia
c. thromboembolic pulmonary hypertension (CTEPH)
c. tophaceous gout
c. transplant nephropathy (CTN)
c. undermining burrowing ulcer
c. undermining ulcer of Meleney
c. widespread pain

chronica
acrodermatitis c.
keratosis lichenoides c.
mycosis cutis c.
c. parapsoriasis lichenoid
pityriasis lichenoides c. (PLC)
purpura pigmentosa c.
urticaria c.

chronicum
erythema c.

NOTES

C

chronicus
> genital lichen simplex c.
> lichen simplex c. (LSC)

chrysanthemum
chrysarobin
chrysiasis
chrysoderma
Chrysomyia
chrysorrhoea
> *Euproctis c.*

Chrysosporium pruinosum
chrysotherapy
CHS
> Chediak-Higashi syndrome

CHS/NP
> chronic hyperplastic sinusitis with nasal polyposis

CHUK
> conserved helix-loop-helix ubiquitous kinase

church spire pattern
Churg-Strauss
> C.-S. angiitis
> C.-S. granulomatosis
> C.-S. syndrome (CSS)
> C.-S. vasculitis
> C.-S. vasculopathy

chylidrosis
chyloderma
chylomicronemia
chylomicron metabolism
chylous
chyluria
chymase
chymopapain chemonucleosis
chytide
CI
> cell interaction
> CI gene

CI-1004
CIA
> collagen-induced arthritis

cIAPs
> cellular inhibitors of apoptosis

Ciarrocchi disease
CIC
> circulating immune complex

Cica-Care topical gel sheeting
cicatrices (*pl. of* cicatrix)
cicatricial
> c. alopecia
> c. horn
> c. junctional epidermolysis bullosa
> c. pemphigoid (CP)
> c. pemphigoid antigen
> c. pemphigoid disease
> c. stenosis

cicatrisata
> alopecia c.

cicatrix, pl. **cicatrices**
> hypertrophic c.
> vicious c.

cicatrization
> exuberant c.

cicatrizing alopecia
ciclopirox
> c. olamine
> c. topical solution

CID
> combined immunodeficiency disease
> cytomegalic inclusion disease

cidal effect
Cidecin
cidofovir
CIDP
> chronic inflammatory demyelinating polyradiculoneuropathy

CIDS
> cellular immune deficiency syndrome

CIE
> congenital ichthyosiform erythroderma
> counterimmunoelectrophoresis
> crossed immunoelectrophoresis

cigar body
cigarette-paper
> c.-p. atrophy
> c.-p. scar
> c.-p. scarring
> c.-p. wrinkling

cigarette smoke
ciguatera poisoning
cilastatin
> imipenem and c.

ciliaris
> acne c.
> tylosis c.

ciliary
> c. beat frequency
> c. body
> c. disorder
> c. neurotrophic factor

ciliated epithelial cell
ciliate dysentery
ciliorum
> defluxio c.
> tinea c.

Ciloxan Ophthalmic
CILP
> cartilage intermediate layer protein

cimetidine
Cimex
> *C. hemipterus*
> *C. lectularius*

Cimicidae
cimicosis

CINCA
    chronic infantile neurological, cutaneous, and articular
    CINCA syndrome
cincinnatiensis
    Legionella c.
cinecienta
    dermatosis c.
cine computed tomography
cinerea
    Botrytis c.
C1INH
    first component of complement
cinnabar red spot
cinnamate
cinnamic
    c. alcohol
    c. aldehyde
cinnamon
Cinobac Pulvules
cinoxacin
cinoxate
CIPO
    chronic intestinal pseudoobstruction
Cipro
    C. injection
    C. Oral
ciprofloxacin hydrochloride
circadian
    c. cortisol
    c. function
circinata
    balanitis c.
    impetigo c.
    pityriasis c.
    psoriasis c.
    tinea c.
circinate
    c. balanitis
    c. psoriasis
    c. syphilitic erythema
circinatum
    erythema c.
circinatus
    favus c.
CircPlus leg compression dressing
circuit
    heart-lung c.
    immunoregulatory c.
Circulaire aerosol drug delivery system
circulans
    Bacillus c.

circular plasmid DNA
circulating
    c. anticoagulant
    c. antiepidermal BMZ IgG
    c. B cell
    c. immune complex (CIC)
Circulon
    C. leg compression dressing
    C. System Step 1, 2 venous ulcer kit
circumflexa
    ichthyosis linearis c. (ILC)
circumscribed
    c. albinism
    c. myxedema
    c. neurodermatitis
    c. precancerous melanosis of Dubreuilh
circumscripta
    allotrichia c.
    alopecia c.
    balanitis c.
    calcinosis c.
    osteoporosis c.
    poliosis c.
circumscriptum
    c. angiokeratoma
    lymphangioma c.
circumscriptus
    albinismus c.
cirrhosis
    chronic active hepatitis with c. (CAHC)
    cryptogenic autoimmune c. (CAC)
    HCV-related c.
    hepatitis C virus-related c.
    primary biliary c. (PBC)
    xanthomatous biliary c.
cirrhotic lacrimal gland
cisplatin
13-*cis*-retinoic acid
cistern
    Pecquet c.
cisternae
    lymphatic c.
Citanest
    C. Forte
    C. Plain
Citoscope-16 arthroscope
citrate
    daunorubicin c.
    piperazine c.

NOTES

111

citrate *(continued)*
    saline sodium c. (SSC)
    c. synthase
citric acid
citrine skin
Citrobacter
    C. diversus
    C. freundii
citronellal
citronella oil
citrullination
citrullinemia
    neonatal c.
Citrus Red dermatitis
CIU
    chronic idiopathic urticaria
Civatte
    C. body
    C. disease
    poikiloderma of C.
    C. poikiloderma
CJD
    Creutzfeldt-Jakob disease
c-jun
    c.-j. N-terminal kinase
    c.-j. protein
c-kit
    soluble c.-k. (sc-kit)
CKR5 mutation
CL
    cutaneous leishmaniasis
CLA
    cutaneous lymphocyte antigen
cladiosis
cladosporioides
    Cladosporium c.
cladosporiosis
Cladosporium
    C. carrionii
    C. cladosporioides
    C. herbarum fungus
    C. mansonii
    C. werneckii
Claforan
clamdigger's itch
clamp
    chalazion c.
    Crile c.
    Dardik c.
    Desmarres c.
    Hirsch mucosal c.
    Providence c.
    Serrefine c.
Clara cell
clarifier
clarithromycin
Claritin
    C. D-24

    C. Extra
    C. RediTab
Claritin-D
    C.-D. 24-Hour
Clark
    C. level (I–V)
    C. malignant melanoma
    classification
Clark-Elder malignant melanoma
    classification
CLAS
    congenital absence of skin
clasmatocyte
class
    functional c. II–IV
    HLA c. 1
    Ig c.
    c. I, II, III antigen
    c. II invariant chain-derived peptide
    (CLIP)
    immunoglobulin c.
    MHC c. I, II
        major histocompatibility complex
            class I
    c. switch
classic
    c. allergy symptom
    c. neurofibromatosis
    c. type Ehlers-Danlos syndrome
classical pathway (CP)
classification
    Acorn c.
    Barnett c.
    Child-Turcotte-Pugh c.
    Clark-Elder malignant melanoma c.
    Clark malignant melanoma c.
    Durie and Salmon multiple
       myeloma c.
    Elder c.
    European-American Lymphoma c.
    FAB c.
    French-American-British c.
    Gell and Coombs c.
    ILO pneumoconiosis c.
    Jopling c.
    Lancefield c.
    Lever and Schamberg-Lever c.
    Loesche c.
    Lukes-Collins non-Hodgkin
       lymphoma c.
    Lund-Browder c.
    morphologic c.
    Nalebuff c.
    Rappaport c.
    REAL c.
    Revised European-American
       Lymphoma c.
    Ridley c.

Runyon c.
Rye c.
Steinbrocker c.
transplant rejection c.
Walter Reed c.
clastothrix
claudication
jaw c.
c. of tongue
clavatus
Aspergillus c.
clavi (*pl. of* clavus)
clavicular sign
clavulanate
clavulanic acid
clavus, pl. **clavi**
c. syphiliticus
clawing
c. deformity
rheumatoid c.
claw nail
Clay-Adams stain
CLE
clean
C. & Clear Deep Cleaning
astringent
C. & Clear Invisible Clearasil
Clearstick
Dey-Wash skin wound c.
cleaner
air c.
Bionaire Air C.
unclassified air c.
Cleanmix DNA purification kit
cleanser
Antimicrobial MPM wound c.
Biolex wound c.
Chloresium Soln wound c.
Clinical Care wound c.
Clinswound wound c.
Contant-Clens wound c.
Curaklense wound c.
Curasol wound c.
Debrisan wound c.
Dermagran wound c.
DermaMend wound c.
DiaB Klenz wound c.
Elta Dermal wound c.
Gentell wound c.
Hyperion wound c.
Iamin Wound C.
lipid-free c.

Lobana wound c.
MicroKlenz wound c.
MPM Antimicrobial wound c.
Optipore Sponge wound c.
Perineal Skin C.
Puri-Clens wound c.
Purpose c.
Restore wound c.
SAF-Clens wound c.
Sea-Clens wound c.
SeptiCare wound c.
Shur-Clens wound c.
SkinTegrity wound c.
Techni-Care wound c.
UltraKlenz wound c.
cleansing
c. cream
Fostex Medicated C.
clear
C. Away Disc
C. By Design
C. By Design Gel
C. Caladryl Spray
c. cell
c. cell acanthoma
c. cell hidradenoma
c. cells scattered in a buckshot
fashion
c. cell syringoma
C. Confident antifungal topical
lotion
Dimetapp C.
C. Pore Treatment
clearance
alveolar fluid c.
creatinine c.
immune complex c.
measure mucociliary c. (MCC)
mucociliary c.
Clearasil
C. B.P. plus
C. Maximum Strength
C. Pads
clear-cell papulosis
clear-cut granuloma
clearing
central c.
ClearLight treatment for acne
ClearSite
C. hydrogel sheet
C. impregnated gauze

NOTES

Clearstick
Clean & Clear Invisible
Clearasil C.
cleavage
collagenase-mediated c.
granzyme B-mediated c.
lines of c.
metal-catalyzed oxidative c.
cleaved giant cell
cleft
branchial c.
lucent c.
clefting
ectrodactyly, ectodermal, c. (EEC)
suprabasal c.
cleidocranial dysplasia
clemastine
c. fumarate
c. and phenylpropanolamine
Cleocin
C. HCl Oral
C. hydrochloride
C. Pediatric
C. Pediatric Oral
C. Phosphate Injection
C. T
C. T Topical
C. Vaginal
CLH
cutaneous lymphoid hyperplasia
Clickhaler
clicking
palatal c.
CLIFT
Crithidia luciliae indirect
immunofluorescence test
climacterica
keratoderma c.
climactericum
keratoderma c.
keratosis c.
climatotherapy
Clinda-Derm Topical
clindamycin
clindamycin/benzoyl peroxide gel
Clindoxyl
CLINHAQ
Clinical Health Assessment Questionnaire
clinic
Systemic Lupus International
Collaborating C.'s (SLICC)
clinical
C. Care wound cleanser
c. change
C. Health Assessment Questionnaire
(CLINHAQ)
c. hyperthyroidism
c. judgment

c. manifestation
c. myocarditis
c. transplant coordinator (CTC)
Clinicel silicon gel-filled cushion
Clinique
C. Antiacne Soap
C. Continuous Coverage
Clinoril
Clinswound wound cleanser
clioquinol and hydrocortisone
CLIP
class II invariant chain-derived peptide
CLIP replacement approach
clip
Backhaus towel c.
ClipTip reusable sensor
CLL
chronic lymphocytic leukemia
CLM articulating laryngoscope blade
CLN
centrilobar necrosis
cloacae
Enterobacter c.
cloacogenic carcinoma
Clobetasol
C. E Cream
clobetasol
c. dipropionate
c. propionate
c. propionate foam
clock-face pattern
Clocort Maximum Strength
clocortolone pivalate
Cloderm topical
clodronate-containing liposome
clofazimine palmitate
clofibrate
clomipramine
Clomycin
clonal
c. deletion theory
c. expansion
c. ignorance
c. selection theory
clonazepam
Cloncorchis sinensis
clone
vector-transfected cell c.
clonidine hydrochloride
clonorchiasis
clonospecific oligoprobe hybridization
clonotype
clopidogrel
clorazepate
Clorpactin WCS-90
closed
c. accordion sign
c. comedo

C

c. patch test
c. wet dressing
closed-space infection
clostridia
clostridial myonecrosis
Clostridium
 Clostridium difficile
 Clostridium difficile test (CLOtest)
closure
 lazy-S c.
 S-shaped c.
 Velcro c.
CLOtest
 Clostridium difficile test
clothes louse
clothing
 c. dermatitis
 FrogWear sunscreen c.
 Solumbra sunscreen c.
 sunscreen c.
Clotrimaderm
clotrimazole
 betamethasone and c.
 c. buccal troche
clotrimazole/betamethasone dipropionate lotion
Clot Stop drain
clotting cascade
Cloudman melanoma
Clouston syndrome
clove oil
clover
 sweet c.
cloxacillin sodium
Cloxapen
Clr deficiency
clubbed finger
clubbing
 idiopathic c.
 nail c.
 c. of nail
club hair
cluster
 aggressive cell c.
 c. of differentiation 2–72 (CD2–72)
cluster-of-grapes appearance
Clutton joint
CM
 capreomycin
 chloroquine-mepacrine
cM
 centimorgan

CMA
 cow's milk allergy
CMAS
 Childhood Myositis Assessment Scale
CMC
 carpometacarpal
 chronic mucocutaneous candidiasis
 CMC syndrome
CMI
 cell-mediated immunity
 Multitest CMI
CMI-392
CML
 chronic myeloid leukemia
 CML AP
 CML BC
 CML CP
CMO
 calculated mean organism
CMP-NANA
 cytidine monophospho-*N*-acetyl neuraminic acid
CMS AccuProbe 450 system
CMV
 cytomegalovirus
 Copalis ToRC automated antibody assay for CMV
CMV-IGIV
 cytomegalovirus immune globulin intravenous
c-myc
 c.-m. gene
 c.-m. protooncogene
cnidoblast
cnidosis
CNS
 central nervous system
CNSB
 coagulase-negative staph bacteremia
CO$_2$
 carbon dioxide
 CO$_2$ laser
coadministration
coagglutinin
coagulase-negative staph bacteremia (CNSB)
coagulase-positive micrococci
coagulation
 biterminal c.
 blood c.
 disseminated intravascular c. (DIC)
 c. factor Va

NOTES

codes E/M CPT ICD-9

coagulation *(continued)*
    c. meshwork
    sepsis-induced disseminated
      intravascular c.
coagulopathy
    consumption c.
coal
    c. tar
    c. tar bath
    c. tar, lanolin, and mineral oil
    c. tar and salicylic acid
coalescence
coalescing
Coamatic protein C test
co-amoxiclav
coarse
    c. breath sound
    c. facies
    c. rale
    c. texture
coast
    Ebola Ivory C.
    c. erysipelas
    c. of Maine border
    c. sage
coated tongue
cobalamin deficiency
cobalt
    c. dermatitis
    c. dichloride
    c. in tungsten carbide
cobalt-chrome head
Coban
    C. cohesive medium stretch
      bandage
    C. dressing
    C. wrap
Cobas Amplicor CMV Monitor test
cobblestoning
Cobb syndrome
cobra
    C. auto-gamma counter
    C. cannula
    c. hemotoxin
    c. venom cofactor
    c. venom factor (CVF)
cocarde reaction
cocardiform
cocci (*pl. of* coccus)
coccidioidal
    c. granuloma
    c. osteomyelitis
Coccidioides immitis
coccidioidin
    c. skin test
coccidioidomycosis
    cutaneous c.
    disseminated c.

coccidiosis
coccogenic sycosis
coccus, pl. **cocci**
    Gram-negative cocci
    Gram-positive cocci
Cochin sore
Cochran-Mantel-Haenszel test
cockade pattern
cockatiel feather
Cockayne syndrome
Cockayne-Touraine epidermolysis bullosa
cocklebur weed pollen
cockroach
    American c.
    German c.
cockscomb ulcer
cocktail
    immunosuppressant c.
cock-up deformity
cocoa
coconut
codeine
    chlorpheniramine, phenylephrine,
      and c.
codfish vertebrae
Codiclear
coding joint
codominant
    autosomal c.
codon
    arginine c.
coefficient
    diffusion c.
    c. of error (CE)
    intraclass correlation c. (ICC)
    Kendall correlation c.
    c. of variation (CV)
coelenterate sting
coenzyme
    3-hydroxy-3-methylglutaryl c. A
      (HMG-CoA)
Coe virus
cofactor
    cobra venom c.
coffee bean
Coffin-Lowry syndrome
Coffin-Siris syndrome
Coflex flexible wrap
Cogan syndrome
Cogentin
cognate
    c. interaction
    c. recognition
cognitive-behavioral technique
coherence therapy
Coherent UltraPulse CO$_2$ laser
Co-Hist

cohort
- Hopkins lupus c.
- c. study

coil
- air c.
- c. gland
- secretory c.

coimmunoprecipitate

Coinage Act

coincidental symptom

coin-rubbing dermatitis

coin-sized lesion

COL1A1 gene

COL2A1 (type II procollagen gene COL2A1)
- type II procollagen gene C. COL2A1
- C. type II procollagen gene

ColBENEMID

colchicine
- c. and probenecid

cold
- c. abscess
- c. agglutination
- c. agglutinin
- c. allergy
- C. & Allergy Elixir
- c. antibody
- c. autoagglutinin
- c. autoantibody
- Benylin C.
- chest c.
- c. cream
- c. exposure
- c. gangrene
- c. hemagglutinin disease
- c. hemolysin
- c. ischemia
- c. ischemia time
- Ornex C.
- c. panniculitis
- c. quartz lamp
- c. quartz radiation
- c. reflex urticaria
- rose c.
- c. sore
- c. stage
- c. steel debulking
- c. storage (CS)
- c. ulcer
- c. virus
- c. water immersion foot (CWIF)

cold-dependent
- c.-d. dermographism
- c.-d. disorder

Cold-Eezer Plus

cold-induced
- c.-i. cell injury
- c.-i. necrosis
- c.-i. skin antigen
- c.-i. urticaria
- c.-i. vasospasm

Coldloc-LA

cold-reactive antibody

Coleman microinfiltration system

Coleoptera

Coley toxin

coli
- *Balantidium c.*
- *Escherichia c.*
- c. granuloma

colic
- infantile c.

colicin

colicinogeny

coliphage

colistimethate sodium

colistin
- c., neomycin, and hydrocortisone
- c. sulfate

colitis
- antibiotic-associated c.
- balantidial c.
- collagenous c.
- dietary protein-induced c.
- milk-induced c.
- pseudomembranous c.
- ulcerative c.

colitose

collaboration
- T cell-B cell c.
- C. Transplant Study

collacin

collagen
- Arg^{519}-Cys mutation in type II c.
- autoantigen c.
- BGC Matrix c.
- cartilaginous c.
- conformational kinks in c.
- C propeptide of type II c. (CPII)
- c. CS
- Cys-containing type II c.
- c. denaturation
- Fibracol c.

NOTES

collagen *(continued)*
    c. fibril
    fibrillar c.
    hydroxylysine content of c.
    c. implant
    c. implantation
    injectable c.
    c. injection
    intimal c.
    Matrix c.
    Medifil c.
    c. polymer
    short-chain type X c.
    Skin Temp c.
    type I–XI, XIV c.
    c. vascular disease
    c. vascular serologic test
    Woun'Dres c.
    Zyderm II c.
    Zyplast c.
collagenase
    c. inhibitor
    polymorphonuclear leukocyte c.
    type IV c.
    type V c.
collagenase-mediated cleavage
collagen-induced arthritis (CIA)
collagenization
collagenolysis
collagenolytic enzyme
collagenoma
collagenosis
    reactive perforating c. (RPC)
collagenous
    c. colitis
    c. fibroma
collapse
    cardiovascular c.
collar
    Biett c.
    Casal c.
    c. of pearls
    c. of Venus
collarette of Biet
collastin
CollaTape
collateral damage
collectins
collection
    American Type Culture C. (ATCC)
    gravitational particle c.
    isokinetic c.
Colles fracture
colli
    erythromelanosis follicularis faciei
      et c.
    fibromatosis c.
    leukoderma c.

    melanoleukoderma c.
    pterygium c.
Collier needle holder
collimated bema handpiece (CBH-1) for laser surgery
collimator
    fan-beam c.
Collins
    C. dynamometer
    C. solution
colliquativa
    tuberculosis cutis c.
colliquative
    c. degeneration
    c. sweat
collodion
    c. baby
    blistering c.
    cantharidal c.
    flexible c.
    hemostatic c.
    iodized c.
    c. membrane
    salicylic acid c.
    styptic c.
colloid
    c. acne
    c. body
    bovine c.
    c. cyst
    c. degeneration
    c. milium
    c. pseudomilium
colloidal
    c. oatmeal
    c. oatmeal bath
colloidalis conglomerata
Collyrium Fresh Ophthalmic
coloboma
    c. of the eye, heart defect,
      ichthyosiform dermatosis, mental
      retardation, and ear defect
      (CHIME)
    c., heart anomaly, ichthyosis,
      mental retardation, and ear
      abnormality syndrome
colocalization
cologne
colonic adenocarcinoma
colonization
    airway bacterial c.
    atypical mycobacterial c.
    Candida parapsilosis c.
colony
    myeloid c.
colony-forming unit (CFU)
colony-stimulating
    c.-s. factor (CSF)

c.-s. factor developed by Venereal Disease Research Laboratory (CSF-VDRL)

c.-s. factor fluorescent treponemal antibody-absorption test (CSF-FTA-ABS)

c.-s. factor microhemagglutination-*Treponema pallidum* test (CSF-MHA-TP)

colophony

color

c. allergy screening test (CAST)
constitutive skin c.
facultative skin c.
inducible skin c.
lesion c.
pale c.

Colorado

C. microdissection needle
C. tick fever
C. tick fever virus (CTF virus)

coloration

colored alcoholic shake lotion

Colorimeti Assay

coloring agent

Colorists

American Association of Textile Chemicals & C.

ColorZone tape

colostrum

bovine c.

colpate

colporate

Columbia S. K. virus

columnar

c. epithelium

Coly-Mycin

C.-M. M Parenteral
C.-M. S Oral
C.-M. S Otic drops

coma bulla

Combantrin

CombiDERM

C. ACD hydrocolloid
C. ACD hydrocolloid dressing

combi-effect

combination

c. chemotherapy
c. retinoid and PUVA therapy (Re-PUVA)
c. skin

combined

c. antibody and cellular deficiency
c. immunodeficiency disease (CID)
c. immunodeficiency syndrome
measles, mumps and rubella vaccines, c.
c. nevi
penicillin g, benzathine and procaine, c.
rubella and mumps vaccines, c.

combining site

combining-site antibody

combion test

Combi test

Combivir

Combo

FP/Salm C.
flucatisone propionate/salmeterol

combustionis

dermatitis c.

Comby sign

comedo, pl. **comedones, comedos**

c. acne
closed c.
comedones epidermal nevus
c. extraction
c. extractor
c. nevus
open c.
solar c.

comedocarcinoma

comedogenic

comedolytic agent

comedone extractor

comedones (*pl. of* comedo)

comedonicus

nevus c.
c. nevus
nevus unilateralis c.

comedos (*pl. of* comedo)

Comfeel

C. hydrocolloid
C. hydrocolloid dressing
C. synthetic dressing
C. Ulcus dressing

Comfort Tears solution

Comhist

C. LA

comma bacillus

commensal bacteria

commercial antigen

commissural cheilitis

NOTES

Committee

National Vaccine Advisory C.
(NVAC)

common

c. acne
c. acute lymphocytic leukemia
antigen (CALLA)
c. acute lymphocytic leukemia
antigen positive
c. baldness
c. blue nevus
c. cold virus
c. lymphoid progenitor cell
c. opsonin
c. peroneal nerve
c. reed
c. reed grass
c. striped scorpion
c. striped scorpion sting
c. variable immune deficiency
(CVID)
c. variable immunodeficiency (CVI,
CVID)
c. variable unclassifiable
immunodeficiency
c. wart

commune

integumentum c.

communicable disease

community-acquired pneumonia (CAP)

COMP

cartilage oligomeric matrix protein

compacta Jeanselmei pedrosoi

compactum

Fonsecaea c.
Hormodendron c.
stratum c.

Companion 314 nasal CPAP system

compartment load distribution

compatibility

compatible

Compeed Skinprotector dressing

competence

immunological c.

competition

antigenic c.

competitive binding assay

competitor DNA

complement

c. activation
c. activation cascade
c. activity
c. binding assay
c. C3
c. C4
c. C7
c. C8
c. C9

c. chemotactic factor
component of c.
c. control protein (CCP)
c. deficiency
c. deviation
erythrocytes, antibody, c. (EAC)
first component of c. (C1INH)
c. fixation (CF)
c. protein (C protein)
c. receptor 1–4 (CR (1–4))
c. sequence
serum c. C1–C9
c. system
c. test
total hemolytic c.
c. unit

complement-activating antigen-antibody

complementarity

**complementarity-determining region
(CDR)**

complementary

c. and alternative medicine (CAM)
c. and alternative medicine
treatment
c. cascade
c. deoxyribonucleic acid (cDNA)
c. DNA (cDNA)
c. strand

complementation

**complement-dependent cytotoxicity
(CDC)**

complement-fixation

c.-f. reaction
c.-f. test

complement-fixing (CF)

c.-f. antibody

complement-mediated

c.-m. anaphylaxis
c.-m. host defense process
c.-m. tumor cell immunopurging

complete

c. antibody
c. antigen
c. blood count
c. imperfect albinism
c. perfect albinism
c. transduction

complex

*Acinetobacter calcoaceticus-
baumannii* c.
acne-seborrhea c.
acquired immunodeficiency
syndrome-related c. (ARC)
AIDS-related c. (ARC)
Allovectin-7 DNA/lipid c.
amphotericin B cholesteryl
sulfate c.
amphotericin B lipid c.

antigen-antibody c.
antigenic c.
avian leukosis-sarcoma c.
avidin-biotin-horseradish
  peroxidase c. (ABC)
C5a c.
Carney c.
C5b-C8 c.
C5b-C9 c.
circulating immune c. (CIC)
cytolytic macromolecular c.
death-inducing signaling c. (DISC)
desmosome-tonofilament c.
DNA-carrier c.
EAHF c.
    eczema, asthma, hay fever
      complex
eczema, asthma, hay fever c.
  (EAHF complex)
elastomeric c.
feline leukemia-sarcoma virus c.
gene c.
Ghon c.
Golgi c.
GP ib-IX c.
H-2 c.
heterodimeric c.
heterooligomeric c.
HLA c.
hyaluronate-polylysine c.
IgG c.
immune c. (IC)
insulin-like growth factor BP3 c.
killer inhibitor receptors-human
  leukocyte antigen c.
KIR-HLA c.
C. 15 lotion
major histocompatibility c. (MHC)
major histocompatibility c. class I
  (MHC class I)
major histocompatibility c. class II
  (MHC class II)
membrane attack c. (MAC)
membranolytic attack c. (MAC)
Merkel-cell-neurite c.
Mycobacterium avium c. (MAC)
peptidoglycan-polysaccharide c.
phosphatidylserine-prothrombin c.
popliteal-arcuate c.
primary c.
c. regional pain syndrome (CRPS)
semimembranosus c.

triangular fibrocartilage c. (TFCC)
tuberous sclerosis c. (TSC)
complexion
  T zone c.
complication
  cardiac c.'s
  delayed c.
  immunologic c.
  nonimmunologic c.
component
  absent dermal c.
  amyloid P c.
  c. of complement
  glenoid c.
  leuko-poor blood c.
  matrix c.
  secretory c.
  serum amyloid A, P c.
  spliceosomal c.
  ultrastructural c.
composite
  c. cultured skin (CCS)
  c. graft
compound
  amide c.
  antisense c.
  azole c.
  cationic c.
  c. cyst
  c. nevus
  psoralen c.
  saligenin c.
  sulfhydryl c.
  C. W
  C. W plus
Compoz
  C. Gel Caps
  C. Nighttime Sleep Aid
compress
  cool c.
  ice c.
compression
  suprascapular nerve c. (SSC)
Comprilan wrap
computed tomography (CT)
computer-assisted arthritis detection
computerized tomodensitometry
COMT
  catechol-*O*-methyl transferase
  COMT asthma
Comtrex
concanamycin A

NOTES

concanavalin A-stimulated T^H cell line supernatant
concentrate
> bovine whey protein c.
> E-Toxa-Clean C.
> hyperimmune bovine colostrum IgC c.
> leukocyte c.
> parvum bovine Ig c.
> platelet c.

concentration
> femtomolar c.
> geometric mean c. (GMC)
> grass pollen c.
> intradermal test c.
> median effective c. (EC$_{50}$)
> minimal bactericidal c. (MBC)
> minimal inhibitory c. (MIC)
> minimum inhibitory c. (MIC)
> prick test c.

concentricum
> *Trichophyton c.*

concomitant
> c. condition
> c. immunity

concrete seborrhea
condition
> concomitant c.
> Fordyce c.
> isocapnic c.
> nondenaturing c.
> seborrheic dermatitis-like c.
> severe chronic allergic c.

conditional-lethal mutant
conditionally lethal mutant
conditioned hemolysis
conditioning
> air c.
> myeloablative c.

condom dermatitis
condyloma, pl. condylomata
> c. acuminatum (CA)
> Buschke-Löwenstein giant c.
> flat c.
> giant c.
> c. lata
> c. latum
> c. planus
> pointed c.

condylomatosis
condylomatous
Condylox
cone
> keratosic c.

conenose, cone-nose
> c. bug
> c. bug bite

Conex

conferta
> urticaria c.

confetti macule
Confide HIV test
configuration
> lesion c.
> string of pearls c.

confirmation
> tissue c.

confluent
> c. measles
> c. and reticulate papillomatosis

confocal laser scanning microscopy
Conformant
> C. contact layer sheet
> C. wound dressing

conformation
> antiparallel B-sheet c.

conformational
> c. determinant
> c. kinks in collagen

congelation
> c. urticaria

congelationis
> dermatitis c.

congeneric
congenita
> adermia c.
> aplasia cutis c.
> arthrochalasis multiplex c.
> cutis marmorata telangiectasia c.
> cutis marmorata telangiectatica c.
> dyskeratosis c.
> hyperkeratosis universalis c.
> keratosis universalis c.
> melanosis diffusa c.
> pachyonychia c.
> type II pachyonychia c.

congenital
> c. absence of skin (CLAS)
> c. anemia
> c. aplasia of thymus
> c. baldness
> c. camptodactyly
> c. candidiasis
> c. circumscribed hypomelanosis
> c. complete heart block (CCHB)
> c. contractural arachnodactyly
> c. cytomegalovirus
> c. depigmentation
> c. disorder
> c. dysphagocytosis
> c. ectodermal defect
> c. ectodermal dysplasia
> c. elephantiasis
> c. erythrodermic ichthyosis
> c. erythropoietic porphyria (CEP)
> c. fascial dystrophy

c. generalized fibromatosis
c. generalized phlebectasia
c. giant pigmented nevus
c. hemidysplasia
c. hemidysplasia with ichthyosiform erythroderma and limb defects (CHILD)
c. hemidysplasia with ichthyosiform erythroderma and limb defects syndrome
c. HIV infection
c. human immunodeficiency virus infection
c. hypomelanotic macule
c. ichthyosiform erythroderma (CIE)
c. Lyme disease
c. rubella
c. rubella syndrome
c. sebaceous gland hyperplasia
c. self-healing reticulohistiocytosis
c. sutural alopecia
c. syphilis
c. telangiectatic erythema
c. total lipodystrophy
c. toxoplasmosis
c. triangular alopecia
c. varicella

congenitale
hemangioma c.
keratoma malignum c.
poikiloderma c.
Thomson poikiloderma c.

congenitalis
alopecia triangularis c.
erythroderma ichthyosiformis c.

Congess
C. Jr
C. Sr

Congestac ND
Congest Aid
Congestant D
Congest-Eze
congestion
nasal c.
Vicks 44D Cough & Head C.

congestive heart failure (CHF)
congestivum
erythema c.

conglobata
acne c.

conglobate
c. abscess
c. acne

conglomerata
colloidalis c.
elastosis colloidalis c.

conglutination
conglutinin assay
Congo
C. floor maggot
C. floor maggot bite
C. red stain

Congo-Crimean hemorrhagic fever (CCHF)
congolensis
Dermatophilus c.

congruence
joint c.

conidium, pl. **conidia**
conjugated
c. antigen
c. estrogen
c. hapten

conjugation
conjugative plasmid
conjunctiva, pl. **conjunctivae**
lepra conjunctivae
limbi c.

conjunctival
c. goblet cell
c. injection
c. provocation test (CPT)
c. testing

conjunctivitis
acute contagious c.
acute epidemic c.
acute follicular c.
allergic c.
angular c.
bacterial c.
blennorrheal c.
chlamydial inclusion c.
chronic c.
giant papillary c. (GPC)
gonococcal c.
herpes simplex c.
infantile purulent c.
Lymphogranuloma venereum c.
Moraxella c.
seasonal allergic c. (SAC)
toxicogenic c.

NOTES

C

conjunctivitis *(continued)*
    vernal c.
    viral c.
Connaught flu
connective
    c. tissue
    c. tissue-activating peptide (CTAP)
    c. tissue disease (CTD)
    c. tissue nevus
    c. tissue panniculitis
    c. tissue proteinase
connector
    transmembrane c.
connexin hemichannel
conniventes
    valvulae c.
connori
    Nosema c.
conorii
    Rickettsia c.
Conradi disease
Conradi-Hünermann syndrome
consciousness
    disturbance of c.
conscriptus
    albinismus c.
consecutive achromia
consensus sequence
conserved helix-loop-helix ubiquitous kinase (CHUK)
consistency
    lesion c.
consolidation
    airspace c.
    patchy airspace c.
    progressive acinar c.
constant
    association c.
    binding c.
    diffusion c.
    dissociation c.
    intrinsic association c.
    c. region
constitutional
    c. hirsutism
    c. reaction
    c. ulcer
constitutive skin color
consumption
    c. coagulopathy
    maximal oxygen c. (VO_2 max)
Contac
    C. Allergy Formula
    C. Cold Non-Drowsy
contact
    allergen c.
    c. allergy
    c. carrier

    c. cheilitis
    c. dermatitis
    C. Dermatitis Research Group
    c. eczema
    c. hypersensitivity
    c. leukoderma
    c. metastasis
    c. photodermatitis
    c. photosensitization
    c. poison
    c. urticaria
contactant
contact-layer wound dressing
contact-type dermatitis
contagion
    immediate c.
    mediate c.
contagiosa
    impetigo c.
    keratosis follicularis c.
    sycosis c.
contagiosum
    ecthyma c.
    epithelioma c.
    erythema c.
    molluscum c.
contagiosus
    pemphigus c.
contagious
    c. disease
    c. ecthyma
    c. ecthyma (pustular dermatitis) virus of sheep
    c. pustular dermatitis
    c. pustular stomatitis virus
contagiousness
contagium
contaminant
contaminate
contamination
    bacterial c.
Contant-Clens wound cleanser
content
    bone mineral c. (BMC)
    high liquid c.
    total body bone mineral c.
Contergan
contig
continua
    acrodermatitis c.
continued fever
continuous
    c. low-flow oxygen
    c. passive motion (CPM)
    c. positive airway pressure (CPAP)
    c. subcutaneous insulin infusion (CSII)

c. subcutaneous insulin infusion pump (CSIIP)
c. venovenous hemodialysis (CVVHD)

continuous-wave
c.-w. dye laser surgery
c.-w. laser

contortus
Haemonchus c.

contraceptive dermatitis

contraction
epitope c.
wound c.

contractural arachnodactyly

contracture
Dupuytren c.
flexion c.

contralateral sign

contransfection

contrast effect

contrasuppression

contrasuppressor cell

control
air pollution c.
c. animal
Blemish C.
c. of emotional factor
Lamis PressureFuse automatic pressure c.
Lander Dandruff C.
mite c.
mold c.
odor c.
Oxy C.
c. protein
Shaklee Dandruff C.

controlled
c. anaphylaxis
c. cough

Controller
Maalox H2 Acid C.
Pepcid AC Acid C.

contusiforme
erythema c.

contusiformis
dermatitis c.
erythema c.

contusion

Contuss
C. XT

conus
tinea c.

convalescence serum

convalescent
c. carrier
c. serum
c. stage

conventional
c. animal
c. asthma therapy (CAT)
c. cutaneous malignant melanoma (CCMM)

conversion
index of marrow c. (IMC)

convertase
C3 proactivator c.
furin c.

convex nail

convoluted foam mattress

convulsion
theophylline-induced c.

ConXn

COOH-terminal peptide

Cook cannula

cookei
Ixodes c.

cool compress

Cooley anemia

coolie itch

cooling
c. agent
c. blanket
rapid c.

CoolSpot skin-cooling device

Coombs
C. serum
C. test

Cooperative
C. Clinical Trials in Adult Transplantation (CCTAT)
C. Clinical Trials in Pediatric Transplantation (CCTPT)
C. Systematic Studies of the Rheumatic Disease (CSSRD)

coordinator
clinical transplant c. (CTC)

CO-Oximeter module

Copalis ToRC automated antibody assay for CMV

Copaxone

COPD
chronic obstructive pulmonary disease

Cophene-B
C.-B. injection

NOTES

copious sputum
Coplus cohesive medium stretch
bandage
copper
    c. bromide laser
    c. deficiency
    c. deposition
    c. dermatitis
    c. itch
    c. metabolism
    c. vapor laser
copperhead
    c. snake
    c. snake bite
Coppertone
    C. Lipkote
    C. Oil-Free
    C. Skin Selects
    C. Sport
    C. Sunscreen
    C. Waterproof Sunblock
copra
    c. itch
    c. mite dermatitis
coprecipitation
coproantibodies
coproporphyria
    erythropoietic c. (ECP)
    hereditary c. (HCP)
coproporphyrin
coproporphyrinogen
COPS
    calcinosis cutis, osteoma cutis,
    poikiloderma, and skeletal
    abnormalities
    COPS syndrome
Co-Pyronil 2 Pulvules
coral
    c. cut
    c. dermatitis
    fire c.
    c. snake
    c. snake bite
coral-head appearance
Corbus disease
cord
    appendageal c.
    c. blood (CB)
    c. blood mononuclear cell (CBMC)
    C. Blood Registry
    umbilical c.
Cordran
    C. SP
    C. SP topical
    C. tape
Cordyceps
Cordylobia anthropophaga
core window

Corgard
Coricidin D
corii
    sclerosis c.
corium
    superficial c.
corkscrew
    c. hair
    c. spirochete
Corlett pyosis
Cormax Ointment
corn
    asbestos c.
    hard c.
    c. meal agar
    seed c.
    c. smut
    soft c.
cornea, pl. corneae
    herpes c.
    ichthyosis sebacea corneae
corneal
    c. epithelial cell
    c. opacification
    c. transplantation
    c. ulcer
corneocyte
    c. adhesion
    c. desquamation
corneous
corner stitch
corneum
    Nosema c.
    stratum c. (SC)
corneus
    c. hypertrophicus
    lichen obtusus c.
cornification
    disorder of c. (DOC)
    c. disorder
    normal c.
    type 1-24 c.
cornified
    c. cell envelope
    c. layer
cornmeal
cornoid lamella
corn-row braiding
cornual
cornuate
cornu cutaneum
corona
    c. phlebectasia
    c. seborrheica
    c. veneris
    zona c.
coronal view

coronary
>c. artery disease (CAD)
>c. fistula
>c. flow reserve (CFR)
>c. vasculitis

Coronaviridae
>C. virus

coronavirus
coronoid fossa
corporis
>pediculosis c.
>*Pediculus c.*
>pthiriasis c.
>seborrhea c.
>tinea c.
>trichophytosis c.

corps ronds
cor pulmonale
corpuscle
>Hassall c.
>Hayem c.
>Meissner c.
>molluscum c.
>Negri c.
>Vater-Pacini c.
>Wagner-Meissner tactile c.

Corque topical
correction
>Bonferroni c.
>Frechet three-flap slot c.
>Tukey post-hoc c.

corrosive
>c. poison
>c. ulcer

corset
Cort
>S-T C.

Cortacet
CortaGel Topical
Cortaid
>C. Maximum Strength
>C. Maximum Strength Topical
>C. with Aloe
>C. with Aloe Topical

Cortate
Cortatrigen Otic
Cort-Dome Topical
Cortef
>C. Feminine Itch
>C. Feminine Itch Topical

Cortenema
cortex of hair

Corticaine cream
corticale
>*Cryptostroma c.*

cortical fusi
corticosteroid
>fluorinated c.
>inhaled c. (ICS)
>parenteral c.
>c. rosacea
>synthetic depot c.
>systemic c.
>topical c.

corticotrope
corticotropin
corticotropin-releasing hormone (CRH)
Corticoviridae
Cortifoam
Cortin topical
cortisol
>circadian c.
>urinary free c. (UCF)

cortisone acetate
Cortisporin
>C. Ophthalmic Ointment
>C. Ophthalmic Suspension
>C. Otic
>C. Topical Cream
>C. Topical Ointment

cortivazol
Cortizone-5 Topical
Cortizone-10 Topical
Cortoderm
Cortone
>C. Acetate
>C. Acetate injection
>C. Acetate Oral

Corylus avellana
corymbiform
corymbose
>c. arrangement
>c. syphilid

corynebacteria
corynebacteriophage
>beta c.

Corynebacterium
>*C. acnes*
>*C. diphtheriae*
>*C. minutissimum*

corynebacterium acne
coryneform bacterium
Coryphen

NOTES

coryza
   allergic c.
Coryzavirus
CO Sleuth
Cosmederm-7
Cosmegen
cosmesis
cosmetic
   c. allergy test
   cheek c.
   c. dermatitis
   eyelash c.
   eyelid c.
   c. intolerance syndrome
   lip c.
   c. skin resurfacing (CSR)
   C., Toiletries, and Fragrance
      Association
   undercover c.
cosmetica
   acne c.
cosmetician
cosmeticus
   status c.
cosmetologist
cosmetology
cosmid
costa
   erysipelas de la c.
costal fringe
costaricensis
   Angiostrongylus c.
Costa's Simple Scoring System
Costello syndrome
costimulation
costimulatory
   c. blockade
   c. molecule
   c. receptor
costovertebral-girdle joint
Cotinine assay
cotriggering hypothesis
Cotrim DS
cotrimoxazole
cotton
   defoliating of c.
   defoliation of c.
   c. linter
   c. roll stomatitis
cottonmouth
   c. snake
   c. snake bite
cottonseed
cottonwood
   Arizona/Fremont c.
   c. tree
   c. tree pollen

cotton-wool
   c.-w. patch
   c.-w. spot
cough
   barking c.
   controlled c.
   Diphen C.
   dry c.
   huff c.
   nonproductive c.
   reflex c.
   Silphen C.
   whooping c.
coughing
   paroxysm of c.
cough-variant asthma
Coulter
   C. counter
   C. ICD-Prep test
coumarin
   c. necrosis
Council
   Medical Research C. (MRC)
count
   absolute blood eosinophil c. (AEC)
   CD4 c.
   CD4 T-lymphocyte c.
   complete blood c.
   hemolysis, elevated liver enzymes,
      low platelet c.
   lymphocyte subset c.
   peripheral blood c.
   reticulocyte c.
   WBC c.
   white blood cell c.
countenance
   Hippocratic c.
counter
   Cobra auto-gamma c.
   Coulter c.
   scintillation c.
   Top-Count microplate
      scintillation c.
counterimmunoelectrophoresis (CIE)
counterirritant
counterirritation
counterregulatory effect
countervailing
coup
   c. de sabre
   c. d'ongle
coupling
   rhodopsin-type c.
Covaderm composite dressing
covariate
cover
   AgiSite alginate wound c.
   AlgiDerm alginate wound c.

alginate wound c.
Algosteril alginate wound c.
CarraSorb H alginate wound c.
Curasorb Zinc alginate wound c.
Dermacea alginate wound c.
FyBron alginate wound c.
Gentell alginate wound c.
Kalginate alginate wound c.
Maxorb alginate wound c.
PolyMem alginate wound c.
Restore alginate wound c.
SeaSorb alginate wound c.
Sorbsan alginate wound c.
Tegagen HG, HI alginate
  wound c.
Coverage
Clinique Continuous C.
Coverlet composite dressing
Covermark corrective makeup
Cover-Roll gauze
coverslip
Cover-Strip wound closure strip
Covertell composite dressing
cow
c. dander
c. milk
c. milk allergy (CMA)
Cowden disease
Cowdria ruminantium
Cowdry
C. intranuclear inclusion body
C. intranuclear inclusion body type
  A, B
C. type A, B inclusion body
cowl
monk's c.
cow-milk protein intolerance
cowpox virus
COX
cyclooxygenase
COX enzyme
COX-1
cyclooxygenase-1
COX-1 enzyme
COX-1 inhibitor
COX-2
cyclooxygenase-2
COX-2 inhibitor
Cox
C. organism
C. regression
coxarthrosis

Coxiella burnetii
Cox-Mantel test
Coxsackie
C. B virus
C. encephalitis
Coxsackievirus
C. B1–B5
Cox-Spjotvoll method
CP
cicatricial pemphigoid
classical pathway
  CML CP
    chronic
      myelocytic/myelogenous/myeloid
      leukemia chronic phase
CP disease
CP-336
CPAP
continuous positive airway pressure
  NightBird nasal CPAP
CPDD
calcium pyrophosphate dihydrate
  deposition disease
CPE
cytopathic effect
C-peptide secretion
CPII
C propeptide of type II collagen
CPM
continuous passive motion
  CPM machine
C-polysaccharide
pneumococcal C.-p. (CPS)
CPPD
calcium pyrophosphate dihydrate
CPS
pneumococcal C-polysaccharide
CPT
conjunctival provocation test
CQ
chloroquine-quinine
C1q
C. assay
C. deficiency
C. immune complex detection
C. receptor
C1qR radioassay
C-R
Bicillin C.-R.
CR (1–4)
complement receptor 1–4
C1r

C

NOTES

129

crab
- c. grass
- c. hand
- c. larvae irritation
- c. louse
- c. yaw

crabro
- *Vespula c.*

cracked
- c. heel
- c. lips

crackle
- end-inspiratory c.
- inspiratory "Velcro" c.
- "Velcro" c.

crackled hair
cradle cap
Crandall syndrome
cranial arteritis
cranialis
- hyperostosis c.

craniocarpotarsal syndrome
craniosynostosis
- c. Adelaide type syndrome
- c. type 1, 2 syndrome

craquelé
- eczema c.
- erythema c.
- onychia c.

crateriform ulcer
craw-craw, kra-kra
crazy paving dermatosis
CR-BSI
- catheter-related bloodstream infection

C-reactive protein (CRP)
cream
- Acnomel c.
- Acticin C.
- adapalene c.
- Akrinol C.
- Aldara c.
- AVC C.
- Aveeno Moisture C.
- Avita acne c.
- azelaic acid c.
- Banishing c.
- barrier protective c.
- BeneJoint c.
- Benzashave C.
- carbamide c.
- Carmol 20 c.
- Carmol HC c.
- cleansing c.
- Clobetasol E C.
- cold c.
- Corticaine c.
- Cortisporin Topical C.
- Cutivate c.
- Cytolex c.
- Differin c.
- diflorasone diacetate c./ointment USP
- docosanol c.
- doxepin hydrochloride c.
- ELA-Max c.
- Eldopaque Forte c.
- Elimite C.
- EMLA c.
- Eucerin c.
- Exact C.
- facial undercover c.
- fluorouracil c.
- Glyquin c.
- hydrocortisone acetate c.
- hydroquinone c.
- Kinerase N6-furfuryladenine skin c.
- Kwell C.
- Lamisil topical c.
- Lasan c.
- Lidakol c.
- LipoTECA c.
- Locilex pexiganan acetate c.
- Locilex topical c.
- Lotrimin AF C.
- Lustra c.
- masoprocol c.
- Maximum Strength Desenex Antifungal C.
- Mentax c.
- Micanol c.
- Naftin c.
- Neosporin C.
- Neutrogena Hand c.
- nonoxynol-9 c.
- Noritate c.
- Pramosone c.
- Prevex Diaper Rash c.
- Prudoxin c.
- Psorion C.
- Renova c.
- Solaquin Forte c.
- SSD C.
- Stokoguard outdoor c.
- Sween C.
- terbinafine hydrochloride c.
- tretinoin c.
- triamcinolone c. (TAC)
- Unibase c.
- Vaniqa c.
- water-washable c.
- Zanfel c.
- Zetone c.
- Zonalon Topical c.

crease
- allergic c.

earlobe c.
palmar c.
creatinine
c. clearance
c. kinase
creatininemia
CREB protein
creeping
c. eruption
c. myiasis
c. ulcer
c. vesiculation
CREG
cross-reactive antigen group
CREG mismatch
Creme
Acid Mantle C.
Fungoid HC C.
Gormel C.
Vite E C.
Creola body
creosote
Crepe short stretch bandage
crepey poikiloderma
crepitans
peritendinitis c.
crepitant
crepitation
crepitus
crescentic glomerulonephritis
CREST
calcinosis cutis, Raynaud phenomenon,
esophageal motility disorder,
sclerodactyly, telangiectasia
CREST syndrome
Cresylate
Creutzfeldt-Jakob disease (CJD)
CRH
corticotropin-releasing hormone
Cricket recording pulse oximeter
cricoarytenoid joint
cricoid cartilage
Crigler-Najjar syndrome
Crile clamp
Crile-Wood needle holder
Crimean-Congo
C.-C. hemorrhagic fever
C.-C. hemorrhagic fever virus
crinis, pl. **crines**

crinium
fragilitas c.
nodositas c.
crisis, pl. **crises**
anaphylactic c.
anaphylactoid c.
blast c. (BC)
chronic
myelocytic/myelogenous/myeloid
leukemia blast c. (CML BC)
scleroderma renal c. (SRC)
criteria
ACR c.
ARA c.
Jones c.
O'Duffy c.
Paulus c.
Sapporo c.
Steinbrocker c.
WHO c.
World Health Organization c.
Crithidia
C. luciliae
C. luciliae immunofluorescence
assay
C. luciliae indirect
immunofluorescence test (CLIFT)
criticus
status c.
crix belly
Crixivan
CRMO
chronic recurrent multifocal osteitis
crocodile
C. Bile Pill for Asthma
c. skin
Crohn disease
Crolom Ophthalmic solution
cromoglycate
disodium c. (DSC)
PMS-Sodium C.
sodium c.
cromolyn sodium
Cronkhite-Canada syndrome
cross
c. agglutination
c. infection
Maltese c.
c. reaction
c. sensitization
cross-antigenicity
cross-desensitization

NOTES

crossectomy
crossed immunoelectrophoresis (CIE)
crosslink
    pyridinoline c.
    urine pyridinoline collagen c.
crosslink hydroxylysylpyridinoline
crosslinking
    abnormal loricrin c.
crossmatch
    antihuman globulin c. (AHGXM)
    flow cytometric c.
    flow cytometry c. (FCXM)
    negative c.
crossmatching
crossmatch-positive recipient
Cross-McKusick-Breen syndrome
cross-presentation
cross-priming pathway
cross-reacting
    c.-r. agglutinin
    c.-r. antibody
    c.-r. material
cross-reaction
cross-reactive
    c.-r. antigen group (CREG)
    c.-r. antigen group mismatch
    c.-r. idiotype
cross-reactivity
cross-sensitivity
cross-sensitization
cross-tachyphylaxis
cross-talk
Cross Top replacement oxygen sensor
Crotalidae
Crotalus antitoxin
crotamiton
crouch
    catcher's c.
croup
croup-associated (CA)
    c.-a. virus
croupous membrane
Crouzon
    C. disease
    C. syndrome
Crowe-Dickermann syndrome
Crowe sign
Crow-Fukase syndrome
crowned dens syndrome
crown of Venus
CRP
    C-reactive protein
CRPF
    chloroquine-resistant *Plasmodium*
      falciparum
CRPS
    complex regional pain syndrome

cruenta
    ephidrosis c.
Cruex topical
crural fold
cruris
    epidermophytosis c.
    tinea c.
    trichophytosis c.
crurum
    erythrocyanosis c.
crush artifact
crust
    amiantaceous c.
    milk c.
    oyster-shell c.
crustacean
crustaceous eruption
crusta lactea
crusted
    c. excoriation
    c. ringworm
    c. scabies
    c. tetter
crustosum
    eczema c.
cruzi
    Trypanosoma c.
Cryac
crymophilic
crymophylactic
cryoanesthesia
cryobiology
Cryocrit
Cryocuff
cryofibrinogenemia
cryogen
cryoglobulin
cryoglobulinemia
    essential mixed c.
    familial c.
    mixed c.
    purpura c.
cryolysis
cryopathy
cryophilic
cryophylactic
cryoprecipitable
cryoprecipitagogue
cryoprecipitate
cryoprecipitation
cryoprotein
cryospray
Cryostat
cryosurgery
Cryo-Surg liquid nitrogen spray unit
cryotherapy
cryotolerant

crypt
    c. abscess
    c. epithelial cell apoptosis
    c. epithelial cell dropout
    c. hyperplasia
cryptic epitope
cryptococcal meningoencephalitis
cryptococcica
    folliculitis decalvans c.
cryptococcosis
Cryptococcus neoformans
cryptogenic
    c. autoimmune cirrhosis (CAC)
    c. autoimmune hepatitis (CAH)
    c. fibrosing alveolitis (CFA)
    c. infection
Cryptomeria japonica
cryptoplasmic
cryptopyic
cryptosporidiosis antibody
Cryptosporidium **oocysts**
Cryptostroma corticale
cryptostromosis
cryptotoxic
cryptotrichotillomania
crystal
    c. arthritis
    basic calcium phosphate c.
    calcium carbonate c.
    calcium oxalate c.
    Charcot-Leyden c.
    cholesterol c.
    dehydrate c.
    c. deposition disease
    hematoidin c.
    hemoglobin c.
    lipid liquid c.
    monosodium urate monohydrate c.
    oxalate c.
    plate-like c.
    potassium permanganate c.
    c. rash
    c. violet
    c. violet vaccine
    xanthine c.
crystal-induced arthritis
crystallina
    miliaria c.
    uridrosis c.
    variola c.

Crysticillin
    C. A.S.
    C. A.S. injection
CS
    citrate synthase
    cold storage
        collagen CS
        invariant chain CS
C1s
CSA, CsA
    cyclosporin A
C1s–C3s
CSD
    cat-scratch disease
        CSD skin test
CS/DS
    chondroitin sulfate/dermatan sulfate
        decorin CS/DS
        fibromodulin CS/DS
        seglycin CS/DS
        versican CS/DS
CSF
    colony-stimulating factor
CSF-FTA-ABS
    colony-stimulating factor fluorescent
    treponemal antibody-absorption test
CSF-IFE
    cerebrospinal fluid immunofixation
    electrophoresis
CSF-MHA-TP
    colony-stimulating factor
    microhemagglutination-*Treponema*
    pallidum test
CSF-VDRL
    colony-stimulating factor developed by
    Venereal Disease Research Laboratory
CSII
    continuous subcutaneous insulin infusion
CSIIP
    continuous subcutaneous insulin infusion
    pump
Csillag disease
CS/KS
    aggrecan C.
CSR
    cosmetic skin resurfacing
CSS
    Churg-Strauss syndrome
CSSRD
    Cooperative Systematic Studies of the
    Rheumatic Disease

C

NOTES

CT
computed tomography
thin-section CT
CTACK
cutaneous T-cell attracting chemokine
CTAP
connective tissue-activating peptide
CTC
clinical transplant coordinator
CTCL
cutaneous T-cell lymphoma
CTD
connective tissue disease
Ctenocephalides
C. canis
C. canis bite
C. felis
C. felis bite
CTEPH
chronic thromboembolic pulmonary
hypertension
C-terminal homolog
C-terminus
CTF virus
CTH
ceramide trihexoside
CTL
cytotoxic T lymphocyte
CTLA-4
cytotoxic T lymphocyte antigen-4
CTLA-4 soluble protein
CTM
Chlor-Trimeton
CTN
chronic transplant nephropathy
CTNS gene
CT-1501R
CTS
carpal tunnel syndrome
CTX
cyclophosphamide
ctx
Cytoxan
Cuban itch
cubital tunnel syndrome
cuboidal cell
cucumber
sea c.
cuff
rotator c.
c. tear arthropathy
cuff-tear arthropathy shoulder
cuirasse
cancer en c.
carcinoma en c.
culbertsoni
Acanthamoeba c.
Culex

Culicidae
culicosis
Cullen sign
culprit organism
cultivated
c. barley grass
c. barley smut
c. corn grass
c. corn smut
c. oat grass
c. oat smut
c. rye grass
c. rye smut
c. wheat grass
c. wheat smut
cultivation
culture
appropriate c.
bone c.
elective c.
enrichment c.
fetal thymus organ c. (FTOC)
fungal c.
mixed lymphocyte c. (MLC)
Nicolle-Novy-MacNeal medium c.
(NNN)
organ c.
stool c.
cultured
c. autologous melanocyte
c. epithelial autografting
c. thymic epithelium
cumulative
c. insult dermatitis
c. toxicity
Cuna moon child
cunicular
cuniculatum
carcinoma c.
epithelioma c.
cuniculi
Encephalitozoon c.
cuniculus
Cunninghamella **pathogen**
Cupressaceae pollinosis
Cupressiaceae
Cuprimine
curable serous meningitis
Curaderm
C. hydrocolloid
C. hydrocolloid dressing
Curafil
C. hydrogel dressing
C. impregnated gauze
Curafoam
C. foam dressing
C. wound dressing

Curagel
    C. Hydrogel dressing
    C. Hydrogel sheet
Curaklense wound cleanser
Curasol
    C. hydrogel dressing
    C. impregnated gauze
    C. wound cleanser
Curasorb
    C. calcium alginate dressing
    C. Zinc alginate dressing
    C. Zinc alginate wound cover
curate
curettage
    c. and desiccation (C&D)
    c. and electrodesiccation (CE)
curette, curet
    Cannon c.
    Fox c.
    Heath c.
    Meyhoeffer c.
    Piffard c.
    Reu c.
    Skeele c.
curettement
Curity ABD absorptive dressing
Curling ulcer
curly dock weed pollen
currant
currens
    larva c.
current
    d'Arsonval c.
    direct galvanic c.
    Oudin c.
    vacuum tube cutting c.
Curschmann spiral
Curth-Maklin cornification disorder
Curtinova hydrocolloid dressing
curve
    area under the c. (AUC)
    dose-response c.
    epidemic c.
Curvularia lunata
CUSA
    Cavitron Ultrasonic Surgical Aspirator
Cushing
    C. disease
    C. syndrome
cushingoid facies
cushion
    Clinicel silicon gel-filled c.

    Ficoll c.
    SkareKare silicon gel-filled c.
cut
    coral c.
cutanea
    sclerosis c.
cutaneomeningospinal angiomatosis
cutaneous
    c. abscess
    c. absorption
    c. albinism
    c. amyloid
    c. ancylostomiasis
    c. anergy
    c. anthrax
    c. apoplexy
    c. basophil hypersensitivity (CBH)
    c. B-cell lymphocytic leukemia
    c. B-cell lymphoma
    c. blastomycosis
    c. candidiasis
    c. coccidioidomycosis
    c. diphtheria
    c. drug eruption
    c. dyschromia
    c. ectasia
    c. elastosis
    c. focal mucinosis
    c. gangrene
    c. graft-versus-host reaction
    c. histoplasmosis
    c. horn
    c. hyperpigmentation
    c. larva migrans
    c. leishmaniasis (CL)
    c. leukocytoclastic vasculitis
    c. lupus
    c. lupus erythematosus
    c. lymphocyte antigen (CLA)
    c. lymphoid hyperplasia (CLH)
    c. manifestation
    c. mastocytosis
    c. meningioma
    c. muscle
    c. myelofibrosis
    c. necrotizing vasculitis
    c. necrotizing venulitis
    c. neoplasia
    c. nodule
    c. polyarteritis nodosa
    c. polyarthritis
    c. pseudolymphoma

C

NOTES

Team Cuti Ceuticals (Cutoff-ed group)

cutaneous *(continued)*
    c. purpura
    c. pustular lesion
    c. sarcoidosis
    c. sign
    c. sinus
    c. sporotrichosis
    c. tag
    c. T-cell attracting chemokine
      (CTACK)
    c. T-cell lymphoma (CTCL)
    c. toxoplasmosis
    c. tuberculin test
    c. tuberculosis
    c. tumor
    c. ulcer
cutaneous-subcutaneous nodule
cutaneum
    cornu c.
    sebum c.
cutaneus
    nodulus c.
cutem
cuticle
    c. of hair
    c. of inner root sheath
cuticularization
Cutifilm
    C. Plus
    C. Plus composite dressing
Cutinova
    C. Cavity
    C. Cavity filler
    C. foam dressing
    C. Hydro
    C. Hydro dressing
    C. Thin hydrocolloid
    C. Thin hydrocolloid dressing
cutireaction test
cutis
    amebiasis c.
    amyloidosis c.
    ancylostomiasis c.
    angiolipoma, posttraumatic neuroma,
      glomus tumor, eccrine
      spiradenoma, and leiomyoma c.
      (ANGEL)
    c. anserina
    asteatosis c.
    atheromatosis c.
    atrophia maculosa varioliformis c.
    aurantiasis c.
    B-cell lymphocytoma c.
    benign lymphocytoma c.
    calcinosis c.
    carotenosis c.
    carotinosis c.
    cholesterolosis c.

    cysticercosis c.
    diphtheria c.
    dystrophic calcinosis c.
    endothelioma c.
    hemangioma hypertrophicum c.
    histiocytoma c.
    c. hyperelastica
    hypertrophicum c.
    idiopathic calcinosis c.
    c. laxa
    leiomyoma c.
    leukemia c.
    lymphadenosis benigna c.
    lymphocytoma c.
    c. marmorata
    c. marmorata telangiectasia
      congenita
    c. marmorata telangiectatica
      congenita
    membranous aplasia c.
    metastatic calcinosis c.
    neuroma c.
    osteoma c.
    osteosis c.
    c. pendula
    c. pensilis
    c. rhomboidalis nuchae
    sarcomatosis c.
    sulci c.
    T-cell lymphocytoma c.
    c. testacea
    tuberculosis fungosa c.
    tuberculosis verrucosa c.
    c. unctuosa
    c. vera
    verrucosa c.
    c. verticis gyrata
cutisector
Cutivate
    C. cream
    C. topical
cutter
    C. insect repellent
    motorized c.
cutting
    c. fluid
    c. oil dermatitis
CV
    coefficient of variation
CVF
    cobra venom factor
CVI
    Children's Vaccine Initiative
    common variable immunodeficiency
CVID
    common variable immune deficiency
    common variable immunodeficiency

CVST
  cerebral venous sinus thrombosis
CVVHD
  continuous venovenous hemodialysis
Cw6
    HLA Cw6
CW dye laser
CWIF
  cold water immersion foot
CyA
  cyclosporine
cyanhidrosis
cyaniventris
    Dermatobia c.
cyanoacrylate
cyanocobalamin
  c. deficiency
cyanohidrosis
cyanosis
    pernio c.
cyanotic
cycle
    bulge-activation hypothesis of
      hair c.
    itch-scratch-lichenification c.
    leukapheresis c.
    purine nucleotide c.
cycler
    thermal c.
cyclic
    c. adenosine monophosphate
      (cAMP)
    c. citrullinated peptide
    c. guanosine monophosphate
    c. neutropenia
    c. nucleotide adenosine
      monophosphate
    c. polypeptide
    c. urticaria
cyclizine hydrochloride
Cyclocort topical
cycloheximide
Cyclomen
cyclomethicone
cyclooxygenase (COX)
    c.-1 (COX-1)
    c.-2 (COX-2)
    c. enzyme
    c. pathway
    c. product
cyclophilin A
cyclophosphamide (CTX)

cyclophosphamide-prednisone
cycloplegic
Cycloprox
cycloserine
cyclosporin A (CSA, CsA)
cyclosporine (CyA)
    high c.
    intermediate c.
    low c.
    c. maintenance therapy
    c. microemulsion
cyclosporine-induced neurotoxicity
Cyclotech dosing device
cylindroma
cylindromatous carcinoma
Cymetra micronized AlloDerm
Cynodon dactylon
cynomolgus macaque tissue
cypress
    Arizona c.
    bald c.
    Italian c.
    Monterey c.
cyproheptadine hydrochloride
cyproterone acetate
Cyrano defect
Cys-containing type II collagen
CysLT1
CysLT2
cyst
    adventitious c.
    anogenital epidermal c.
    anogenital pilar c.
    anogenital sebaceous c.
    anogenital vestibular c.
    apocrine retention c.
    Baker c.
    branchial c.
    bronchogenic c.
    colloid c.
    compound c.
    dermoid c.
    desmoid c.
    epidermal c.
    epidermoid cyst
    epithelial c.
    eruptive vellus hair c.
    false c.
    Favre-Racouchot c.
    follicular infundibular c.
    follicular isthmus c.
    hair c.

NOTES

cyst *(continued)*
    implantation c.
    inclusion c.
    jaw c.
    keratinous c.
    milia c.
    mucinous c.
    mucous c.
    multilocular thymic c. (MTC)
    myxoid c.
    parasitic c.
    parvilocular c.
    pheomycotic c.
    pilar c.
    piliferous c.
    pilonidal c.
    popliteal c.
    preauricular c.
    proliferating pilar c.
    proliferating trichilemmal c.
    pseudohorned c.
    renal c.
    retention c.
    sebaceous c.
    sequestration c.
    subchondral c.
    synovial c.
    thyroglossal c.
    trichilemmal c.
    unicameral c.
    unilocular c.
    vanilla-fudge c.
    vestibular c.
cystadenoma
    apocrine c.
cystatin
    c. C
    c. C amyloidosis
    c. C-origin amyloid deposit
cysteamine
cysteine
    c. proteinase
    c. proteinase inhibitor
cysteinyl leukotriene, LTC$_4$
cystic
    c. acne
    c. deformation
    c. fibrosis (CF)
    c. fibrosis arthropathy (CFA)
    c. fibrosis test
    c. fibrosis-transmembrane
      conductance regulator (CFTR)
    c. hidradenoma
    c. hygroma
    c. lymphatic malformation
cystica
    acne c.
cysticercosis cutis

cysticidal
cysticum
    acanthoma adenoides c.
    epithelioma adenoides c.
    lymphangioma c.
cystides
cystis
cystitis
    acrolein-induced c.
    hemorrhagic c.
cystous
Cystoviridae
cytapheresis
cytarabine hydrochloride
cytase
CY/TBI
    Cytoxan and total body irradiation
cytidine monophospho-*N*-acetyl
    neuraminic acid (CMP-NANA)
cytoadhesion
cytochalasin B, D
cytochrome
    c. C
    c. deficiency
    c. P450
cytocidal
cytodiagnosis
CytoGam
cytogenic technique
cytogram
cytoid body
cytoimmunologic monitoring
cytokine
    antiinflammatory c.
    IL-1, -2, -3, -4, -10, -13 c.
    IL-1-beta c.
    monocyte-derived c.
    motif-bearing c.
    pleiotropic c.
    c. production
    proinflammatory c.
    c. synthesis inhibitory factor
    TH1 c.
    TNF mRNA c.
Cytolex cream
cytology
    fine-needle aspiration c. (FNAC)
cytolysin
cytolysis
cytolytic
    c. effector cell
    c. macromolecular complex
cytomegalic
    c. cell
    c. inclusion body
    c. inclusion disease (CID)
cytomegalovirus (CMV)
    c. antigenemia

congenital c.
c. disease
c. immune globulin intravenous (CMV-IGIV)
c. immune globulin intravenous, human
c. retinitis
tissue-invasive c. (TI-CMV)
cytometer
Epics Elite flow c.
FACScan flow c.
cytometric indirect immunofluorescence
cytometry
flow c.
cytopathic effect (CPE)
cytopathogenic virus
cytophagic
c. histiocytic panniculitis
c. lobular panniculitis
cytophagous
cytophagy
cytophil group
cytophilic antibody
cytophylactic
cytophylaxis
cytoplasm
cytoplasmic
c. antineutrophil cytoplasmic antibody (C-ANCA, c-ANCA)
c. inclusion
c. inclusion body
c. islet cell
c. plaque
cytoprotective agent
cytoryctes
Cytosar-U
cytosine arabinoside
cytoskeleton
cytosolic

CytoTAb
CytoTAb polyclonal antibody
cytotoxic
c. agent
c. armamentarium
c. drug
c. immunologic drug reaction
c. immunosuppressive therapy
c. T cell
c. test
c. T lymphocyte (CTL)
c. T lymphocyte antigen-4 (CTLA-4)
cytotoxicity
antibody-dependent cell-mediated c. (ADCC)
antibody-dependent cellular c. (ADCC)
antiglobulin-enhanced complement-dependent c. (AHG-CDC)
complement-dependent c. (CDC)
lymphocyte-mediated c. (LMC)
natural killer-mediated c.
NK cell-mediated c.
cytotoxin
cytotoxin-positive stain
cytotropic
c. antibody
c. antibody test
cytotropism
Cytovene
Cytovene-IV
Cytoxan (ctx)
busulfan and C. (BU/CY)
C. injection
C. Oral
C. and total body irradiation (CY/TBI)

C

NOTES

D
  D antigen
  Congestant D
  Coricidin D
  D deficiency factor
  Nutrol A D
D2
  prostaglandin D2 (PGD2)
D1927
D-24
  Claritin D-24
D$_2$
  prostaglandin D$_2$ (PGD$_2$)
d4T, didehydrothymidine
Daae disease
Dab-o-Matic
Dabska tumor
dacarbazine (DTIC)
dacliximab monoclonal antibody
daclizumab
DaCosta syndrome
dacryoadenitis
dacryocystitis
dacryocystorhinostomy
dactinomycin
dactyledema
Dactylis glomerata
dactylitis
  blistering distal d.
  distal d.
  multidigit d.
  septic d.
  d. strumosa
  syphilitic d.
  d. tuberculosa
  tuberculous d.
dactylolysis spontanea
dactylon
  Cynodon d.
dactyloscopy
daisy
  oxeye d.
Dakar bat virus
DAKO CD57
Dakrina Ophthalmic solution
Dalacin
  D. C
  D. T
  D. Vaginal
Dalalone
  D. D.P.
  D. L.A.
Dale reaction
dalfopristin
Dalmane

damage
  bacterial-induced vascular d.
  collateral d.
  extravillous trophoblastic d.
  immunologic organ d.
  d. index score
  musculotendinous d.
  residual thermal d. (RTD)
  sun and chemical combination d.
  toxic organ d.
damaged joint progression
dammini
  Ixodes d.
danazol
Danbolt-Closs syndrome
dandelion
dander
  animal d.
  cat d.
  cow d.
  dog d.
  inhaled d.
d'Andrews
  arthrites pseudoseptiques et
    bacterides d.
Dandruff Treatment Shampoo
dandy fever
Dane particle
Danex
Dan-Gard
Danielssen-Boeck
  D.-B. disease
  D.-B. sarcoidosis
Danielssen disease
Danocrine
Danysz
  D. effect
  D. phenomenon
Dapa
Dapacin Cold Capsule
DA pregnancy test
dapsone (DDS)
  D. Pharmacokinetics
  d. topical gel
dapsone/pyrimethamine
daptomycin
Daraprim
DAR breathing system
Dardik clamp
Darier
  D. disease (DD)
  morbus D.
  D. sign
Darier-Roussy sarcoid
Darier-White disease

D

dark dot disease
darkfield
>d. examination of tissue smear
>d. microscopy

dark-staining nodule
Darrach procedure
d'Arsonval current
dartos
>tunica d.

D'Assumpeau rhytidoplasty marker
data
>D. Safety Monitoring Board
>(DSMB)
>x-ray crystallographic d.

Database
>Cardiac Transplant Research D.

date
>d. boil
>d. fever

datura plant
Daudi lymphoma cell
daughter cell
daunorubicin
>d. citrate
>d. hydrochloride

DaunoXome
Davidsohn differential test
Davis
>D. and Geck systemic plastic
>reconstruction P3 or PS3 needle
>D. and Geck systemic PR and
>PRE P3 or PS3 needle

Dawbarn sign
Dawson encephalitis
21-Day Cumulative Irritancy Assay
daylight sign
Daypro
DayQuil Sinus with Pain Relief
2-day ultrarush protocol
DBI
>documented bacterial infection

DBPCFC
>double-blind placebo-controlled food
>challenge

D&C dye
DCL
>disseminated cutaneous leishmaniasis

DCTD
>diffuse connective tissue disease

DD
>Darier disease

ddc
>dideoxycytidine

ddC
>zalcitabine

D-Di
>D-dimers

ddi
>didanosine

D-dimers (D-Di)
DDS
>dapsone

DDT
>dichlorodiphenyltrichloroethane
>(chlorophenothane)

DE
>Ru-Tuss DE

D2E7
de
>de facto
>De Morgan spot
>de novo
>de novo pyrimidine synthesis
>de novo squamous cell carcinoma
>de Quervain disease
>de Quervain stenosing tenosynovitis
>de Quervain syndrome
>De Sanctis-Cacchione syndrome

deacylation
dead
>d. finger
>d. space:tidal volume ratio

dead-end host
deafness
>abnormalities of genitalia,
>retardation of growth, and d.
>bilateral sensorineural d.
>keratitis d.
>lentigines, electrocardiographic
>defects, ocular hypertelorism,
>pulmonary stenosis, abnormalities
>of genitalia, retardation of
>growth, d. (LEOPARD)
>nerve d.

deallergize
deamidated
>d. gliadin
>d. gliadin peptide

deaminase
>adenosine d. (ADA)
>myoadenylate d.

death
>activation-induced cell d. (AICD)
>d. domain
>donor brain d.

death-inducing signaling complex (DISC)
DEBRA
>Dystrophic Epidermolysis Bullosa
>Research Association of America

Debré phenomenon
debridement
debrider
>Accuzyme enzymatic d.
>Panafil enzymatic d.

Panafil-White enzymatic d.
Santyl enzymatic d.
debris
phagocytosable d.
Debrisan
D. topical
D. wound cleanser
Debrox drops
debulking
cold steel d.
DEC
diethylcarbamazine
Decadron
D. and Hexadrol
D. Injection
D. Oral
D. Phosphate
D. Phosphate Respihaler
D. Phosphate Turbinaire
Decadron-LA
Decaject-LA
decalvans
acne d.
folliculitis d.
keratosis follicularis spinulosa d.
porrigo d.
tinea d.
decalvant
decamer
decamethonium
decarboxylase
glutamic acid d. (GAD)
d. inhibitor
decarboxylation
amine precursor uptake and d.
(APUD)
Decaspray
decay
bone d.
decidua
d. basalis
d. parietalis
decidual tissue
deciduous skin
Declomycin
Decofed Syrup
decompensation
Decon
Par D.
Deconamine
D. SR

D. Syrup
D. Tablet
deconditioning
motor d.
physical d.
decongestant
Balminil D.
Benylin D.
Certified d.
Chlor-Tripolon D.
D. Nasal Spray
New D.
D. Nose drops
d. tablet
topical d.
Decongestionnant
Vaporisateur Nasal D.
Deconsal II
Decontabs
decorin CS/DS
decoy DNA
decreased
d. fertility, short stature
d. renal function
decrementi
stadium d.
decubation
decubital gangrene
decubitus ulcer
dedifferentiated
DEDLE
distinctive exudative discoid and
lichenoid dermatitis
Deelman effect
deep
d. felon
d. hemangioma
d. mycosis
d. penetrating nevus
deer
d. fly
d. fly bite
d. fly disease
d. fly fever
d. hair
d. tick
DEET
diethyltoluamide
Deet

D

NOTES

143

defect
 coloboma of the eye, heart defect, ichthyosiform dermatosis, mental retardation, and ear d. (CHIME)
 congenital ectodermal d.
 congenital hemidysplasia with ichthyosiform erythroderma and limb d.'s (CHILD)
 Cyrano d.
 host d.
 human host defense d.
 human nude d.
 humoral d.
 immunoregulatory d.
 limb d.
 neuroectodermal d.
 opsonophagocytic d.
 scleral d.
 standing cutaneous cone d.
 T-cell d.
 tricone d.
defective
 d. bacteriophage
 d. interfering (DI)
 d. interfering particle
 d. phage
 d. probacteriophage
 d. prophage
 d. virus
Defen-LA
defense
 immunological d.
 d. mechanism
defensins
defervesce
defervescence
defervescentiae
 stadium d.
defervescent stage
defibrination syndrome
deficiency
 acetylcholinesterase d.
 acquired biotin d.
 acquired C1 inhibitor d.
 ADA d.
 adenosine deaminase d.
 alpha$_1$-antitrypsin d.
 alpha$_1$ proteinase d.
 antibody d.
 argininosuccinate synthetase d.
 beta-mannosidase d.
 biotin d.
 biotinidase d.
 C2 d. (C2D)
 C4 d. (C4D)
 C7 d. (C7D)
 carnitine palmitoyltransferase d.
 ceramidase d.

 C1r d.
 cobalamin d.
 combined antibody and cellular d.
 common variable immune d. (CVID)
 complement d.
 copper d.
 C1q d.
 cyanocobalamin d.
 cytochrome d.
 essential fatty acid d.
 factor D, H, I d.
 familial alpha-lipoprotein d.
 familial apoprotein CII d.
 folic acid d.
 genetic C2 d.
 glucose-6-phosphatase d.
 growth hormone d.
 HGPRT d.
 histamine-releasing factor d.
 HRF d.
 hyaluronidase d.
 hypoxanthine-guanine phosphoribosyltransferase d.
 IgA d.
 IL-12p40 d.
 IL-2 receptor alpha chain (CD25) d.
 immune d. (ID)
 immunity d.
 immunological d.
 interferon gamma receptor d.
 iron d.
 Jak3 d.
 juvenile biotin d.
 leukocyte adhesion d. (LAD)
 leukocyte adhesion d. type 1 (LAD1)
 leukocyte adhesion d. type 2 (LAD2)
 leukocyte adhesion d. type 3 (LAD3)
 leukocyte adhesion d. type 4 (LAD4)
 lipoprotein lipase d.
 mannan-binding lectin d.
 MHC antigen d.
 MHC class I, II d.
 MPO d.
 multiple sulfatase d.
 myeloperoxidase d.
 myoadenylate deaminase d.
 myophosphorylase d.
 neonatal biotin d.
 neutrophil-specific (secondary) granule d.
 niacin d.
 opsonic d.

ornithine transcarbamylase d.
pantothenic acid d.
phagocytic d.
phosphotransferase d.
placental sulfatase d.
p56 Lck d.
primary cell-mediated d.
prolidase d.
properdin d.
protein C d.
purine nucleoside phosphorylase d.
pyridoxine d.
pyridoxol d.
pyruvate kinase d.
riboflavin d.
secondary antibody d.
secretory component d.
selective antipolysaccharide
  antibody d. (SPAD)
selenium d.
severe combined immune d.
  (SCID)
specific antibody d. (SAD)
steroid sulfatase d.
thiamine d.
tocopherol d.
tyrosine aminotransferase d.
vitamin A d.
vitamin B d.
vitamin B_1 d.
vitamin B_5 d.
vitamin B_6 d.
vitamin B_{12} d.
vitamin C d.
vitamin D d.
vitamin E d.
vitamin K d.
ZAP-70 d.
zinc d.
deflazacort
deflexion
hip d.
deflorescence
defluvium
d. capillorum
d. unguium
defluxio
d. capillorum
d. ciliorum
defluxion
defoliating of cotton
defoliation of cotton

deformans
spondylosis d.
deformation
cystic d.
deformity
angel-wing d.
arthritis without d.
bent-fork d.
boutonnière d.
canestick d.
clawing d.
cock-up d.
habit tic d.
opera-glass d.
pencil and cup d.
piano-key d.
postosteotomy d.
saddle nose d.
swan-neck d.
trap-door d.
violin d.
defurfuration
degenerated microfilaria
degeneration
acromioclavicular d.
amyloid d.
ballooning d.
basophilic d.
colliquative d.
colloid d.
elastoid d.
elastotic d.
epithelial d.
fatty d.
fibrinous d.
glenohumeral d.
granular d.
hepatolenticular d.
hyaline d.
liquefaction d.
malignant d.
mucinous d.
mucoid d.
myxomatous d.
paraneoplastic subacute cerebellar d.
reticular d.
sternoclavicular joint d.
unilateral macular d.
degenerativa
melanosis corii d.
degenerative
d. arthritis

NOTES

D

145

degenerative *(continued)*
    d. collagenous plaque
    d. tendinopathy
Degos
    D. acanthoma
    D. disease
    malignant papillomatosis of D.
    D. syndrome
Degos-Delort-Tricot syndrome
degradation
    postmortem core protein d.
degradomics
degranulation
    goblet cell d.
    piecemeal d. (PMD)
30-degree oblique arthroscope
dehaptenation
dehiscence
Dehist injection
dehumidification
dehumidifier
dehydrate crystal
dehydration
dehydroemetine
dehydroepiandrosterone sulfate (DHEAS)
dehydrogenase
    3-beta-hydroxysteroid d. (3β-HSD)
    17-beta-hydroxysteroid d. (17β-HSD)
    glucose-6-phosphate d. (G6PD)
    inosinic acid d.
    lactate d.
    lactic d. (LDH)
    uridine diphosphoglucose d.
DEI
    Disease Extent Index
Deinococcus radiodurans
DEJ
    dermal-epidermal junction
Dejerine-Sottas disease
Deknatel wound tape
Del
    Del Aqua-5 Gel
    Del Aqua-10 Gel
delavirdine
Delaxin
delayed
    d. allergy
    d. anagen release
    d. blanching
    d. complication
    d. graft function (DGF)
    d. hypersensitivity (DH)
    d. hypersensitivity immunologic drug reaction
    d. hypersensitivity skin testing
    d. patch test reading
    d. pressure urticaria

    d. systemic reaction
    d. tanning
    d. telogen release
    d. transfusion reaction
    d. xenograft rejection (DXR)
delayed-type
    d.-t. hypersensitivity (DTH)
    d.-t. hypersensitivity response
Delcort Topical
deletion
    homozygous autosomal recessive d.
    tolerance through d.
Delhi
    D. boil
    D. sore
deliensis
    Trombicula d.
delitescence
delling
Del-Mycin topical
delta
    d. agent
    d. antigen
    d. antigen hepatitis
    Galton d.
    d. sleep
    d. virus
delta-aminolevulinic acid
Delta-Cortef Oral
Deltasone
    D. Dosepak
    D. Oral
Delta-Tritex Topical
deltoidea
    Anthopsis d.
    Aspergillus d.
delusion of parasitosis
demarcated
    d. cellulitis
    d. reaction
demarcation
Demarquay sign
Dematiaceae
dematiaceous fungus
Demazin
d'emblée
    bubon d.
    mycosis fungoides d.
    syphilis d.
demeclocycline hydrochloride
dementia
    transmissible d.
Demerol
demodectic
    d. acariasis
    d. mange
Demodex
    D. brevis

D. canis
D. equi
D. folliculorum
demodice
demodicidosis
demodicosis
DeMorgan hemangioma
Demulen
demyelinating
denaturation
collagen d.
denaturing agent
Denavir ointment
dendritic
d. epidermal cell
d. macrophage
d. morphology
dendriticum
Dicrocoelium d.
dendritiform
dendrocyte
dengue
d. facies
hemorrhagic d.
d. hemorrhagic fever
d. shock syndrome
d. virus
denileukin diftitox
denitrificans
Alcaligenes d.
Dennie
D. infraorbital fold
D. line
D. sign
Dennie-Marfan syndrome
Dennie-Morgan
D.-M. infraorbital fold
D.-M. line
D.-M. sign
Denorex
densa
lamina d.
sublamina d.
dense-deposit disease
densitometry
bone d.
density
bone mineral d. (BMD)
fixed charge d.
d. gradient bone marrow progenitor enrichment
d. gradient centrifugation

dental
d. abnormality
d. amalgam
d. fistula
d. plaque
d. sinus
d. sinus tract
dentatus
Stephanurus d.
denticola
Treponema d.
dentifrice
dentinogenesis imperfecta
dentocariosa
Rothia d.
denture
d. epulis
d. stomatitis
denture-sore-mouth syndrome
denudation
denude
denuded
Denys-Leclef phenomenon
deodorant dermatitis
2′-deoxyadenosine
deoxycholate
2-deoxy-D-glucose
deoxynucleoside
deoxypyridinoline
deoxyribonuclease (DNase)
fibrinolysin and d.
human recombinant d.
deoxyribonucleic
d. acid (DNA)
d. acid amplicon
d. acid aneuploidy
d. acid autosensitivity
d. acid binding
d. acid hybridization
deoxyribose
deoxyspergualin (DSG)
deoxyvirus
Depakene
Depakote
Depen
dependent edema
Dependovirus
dephosphorylation
depigmentation
congenital d.
depigmentosus
nevus d.

D

NOTES

depilate
depilation
depilatory
    chemical d.
depletion
    acetylcholine d.
depMedalone Injection
Depoject Injection
depolymerize
Depo-Medrol Injection
Depopred Injection
deposit
    calcitonin-origin amyloid d.
    cystatin C-origin amyloid d.
    glycosphingolipid d.
    immune d.
    immunoglobulin light chain-origin amyloid d. (AL protein)
    2-microglobulin-origin amyloid d. (A 2M)
    prion protein-origin amyloid d.
    protein origin amyloid d.
    transthyretin-origin amyloid d.
deposition
    cell d.
    copper d.
    fibrin d.
    hemosiderin d.
    hydroxyapatite crystal d.
    nonlinear IgA d.
    silicone d.
    urate d.
depot reaction
depth
    optical penetration d. (OPD)
depulization
Dercum disease
derivative
    bioactive lipid d.
    ergotamine d.
    piperidine d.
    purified protein d. (PPD)
    undecylenic acid and d.'s
    valproic acid and d.'s
derivative-standard
    purified protein d.-s. (PPD-S)
DERM
    Dermatology Education by Recall
Derma
    D. blade
    D. K laser
    D. 20 laser system
    D. Soap
Dermablend makeup
dermabrader
    Iverson d.
    sandpaper d.
dermabrasion

Dermacea
    D. alginate dressing
    D. alginate wound cover
Dermacentor
    D. andersoni
    D. occidentalis
    D. variabilis
Dermacne
Dermacomb topical
Dermacort Topical
Dermaflex
    D. Gel
    D. HC
Derma-Gel hydrogel sheet
Dermagraft
Dermagraft-TC skin substitute
Dermagran
    D. hydrogel dressing
    D. impregnated gauze
    D. ointment/dressing
    D. wound cleanser
dermagraphy
dermahemia
Dermaide
dermal
    d. duct tumor
    d. hypoplasia
    d. leishmanoid
    d. lesion
    d. lymphatics
    d. microvascular unit
    d. muscle
    d. papilla
    D. Regeneration Template
    d. system
    d. tuberculosis
    d. venular hyperpermeability
dermalaxia
dermal-epidermal junction (DEJ)
DermaMend
    D. cavity foam dressing
    D. foam wound dressing
    D. hydrogel dressing
    D. island foam dressing
    D. wound cleanser
dermametropathism
dermamyiasis linearis migrans oestrosa
Dermanail
Dermanet
    D. contact layer sheet
    D. contact layer wound dressing
Dermanyssus gallinae
Dermapor glove
Dermarest
    D. Dricort
    D. Dricort Topical
DermaSeptic device
Derma-Smoothe/FS topical

Derma-Smoothe Oil
DermaSof gel sheeting
Dermasone
DermAssist
    D. filler
    D. Glycerin
    D. Glycerin hydrogel dressing
    D. hydrocolloid
    D. hydrocolloid dressing
    D. impregnated gauze
    D. transparent film
    D. wound filling material
dermatalgia
Dermatell
    D. hydrocolloid
    D. hydrocolloid dressing
dermatic
dermatica
    zona d.
dermatitic
dermatitidis
    Ajellomyces d.
    Blastomyces d.
dermatitis, pl. **dermatitides**
    acneform d.
    actinic d.
    d. actinica
    acupuncture needle d.
    airborne contact d.
    allergic contact d. (ACD)
    allergic eczematous contact-type d.
    allergic gold d.
    d. ambustionis
    ammonia d.
    ancylostoma d.
    arsenical contact d.
    arsphenamine d.
    d. artefacta
    ashy d.
    Assessment Measure for Atopic D. (AMAD)
    asteatotic d.
    atopic d. (AD)
    autoimmune progesterone d.
    d. autophytica
    autosensitization d.
    avian mite d.
    baker's d.
    berlock d.
    beryllium d.
    bhiwanol d.
    blastomycetic d.

    d. blastomycotica
    blister beetle d.
    blistering d.
    blousing garter d.
    bristle-worm d.
    brown-tail moth d.
    brucella d.
    bubble gum d.
    d. bullosa striata pratensis
    by-the-wind sailor d.
    d. calorica
    Calycophora d.
    carcinomatous d.
    cardiac pacemaker d.
    carpet beetle d.
    caterpillar d.
    cement d.
    cercarial d.
    chemical d.
    chigger d.
    chromate d.
    chronic acral d.
    chronic actinic d. (CAD)
    chronic papular d.
    Citrus Red d.
    clothing d.
    cobalt d.
    coin-rubbing d.
    d. combustionis
    condom d.
    d. congelationis
    contact d.
    contact-type d.
    contagious pustular d.
    contraceptive d.
    d. contusiformis
    copper d.
    copra mite d.
    coral d.
    cosmetic d.
    d. cruris pustulosa et atrophicans
    cumulative insult d.
    cutting oil d.
    deodorant d.
    Dermo-Jet nickel d.
    desquamative d.
    dhobie mark d.
    dialysis d.
    diaper d.
    distinctive exudative discoid and lichenoid d. (DEDLE)

D

NOTES

dermatitis *(continued)*

diving suit d.
dried fruit d.
durable-press allergic contact d.
d. dysmenorrhoeica
earlobe allergic d.
eczematoid d.
endogenous d.
Engman d.
eosinophilic d.
epoxy resin d.
Erysipelothrix d.
d. erythematosa
erythematous macular d.
d. escharotica
d. estivalis
ethylenediamine d.
d. excoriativa infantum
d. exfoliativa
d. exfoliativa epidemica
d. exfoliativa infantum
d. exfoliativa neonatorum
exfoliative d.
exudative discoid and lichenoid d.
eyeglass frame d.
d. factitia
factitial d.
factitious d.
familial rosacea-like d.
feather hydroid d.
fiberglass d.
fire coral d.
fire sponge d.
flea-collar d.
Florida seaweed d.
follicular nummular d.
d. gangrenosa
d. gangrenosa infantum
genital atopic d.
gold d.
hearing aid d.
d. hemostatica
d. herpetiformis (DH)
d. hiemalis
housewives' d.
d. hypostatica
indirect coelenterate d.
industrial d.
d. infectiosa eczematoides
infectious eczematoid d.
infectious eczematous d.
infectious labial d.
insect d.
interdigital d.
irritant contact d. (ICD)
irritant hand d.
Jacquet erosive diaper d.
Japanese hot foot d.

juvenile plantar d. (JPD)
karaya gum d.
Korean yellow moth d.
Leiner d.
lichenified d.
lichenoid contact d.
livedoid d.
Lynghya d.
machine worker d.
mango d.
marine d.
meadow d.
meadow-grass d.
d. medicamentosa
metal d.
moth d.
mother d.
d. multiformis
mycotic d.
napkin d.
nasal cannula d.
nasal solar d.
neck d.
nematode d.
neomycin d.
nickel hand d.
d. nodosa
d. nodularis necrotica
nonspecific d.
nose-pad d.
nummular eczematous d.
nutritional deficiency d.
nylon stocking d.
occupational rubber d.
ocular atopic d.
onion mite d.
oozing d.
Paederus d.
paper d.
d. papillaris capillitii
papular d.
papulosquamous d.
paraphenylenediamine d.
parthenium d.
d. pediculoides ventricosus
pellagra-associated d.
pellagroid d.
Pelodera d.
perfume d.
periocular d.
perioral d.
periorbital d.
periorificial d.
permanent-press finish clothing d.
photoallergic contact d.
photocontact d.
photoingestant d.
photosensitive nonscarring d.

photosensitivity d.
phototoxic contact d.
phototoxic textile d.
phytophototoxic d.
pigmentary atopic d.
pigmented purpuric lichenoid d.
plant d.
plantar d.
poison bun sponge d.
poison ivy d.
poison oak d.
poison sumac d.
poppers' d.
popsicle d.
d. pratensis striata
precancerous d.
primary irritant d.
proliferative d.
propylene glycol d.
protein contact d.
Pseudomonas cepacia d.
psoriasiform d.
d. psoriasiformis nodularis
purple sail d.
purpuric pigmented lichenoid d.
radiation d.
ragweed oil d.
rat mite d.
rebound d.
red feed d.
red moss d.
red sponge d.
red tide d.
d. repens
rhabditic d.
rhus d.
Rockwool d.
roentgen-ray d.
rosaceaform d.
rubber additive d.
sandal strap d.
Schamberg d.
schistosomal d.
schistosome cercarial d.
scombroid d.
sea anemone d.
sea cucumber d.
sea louse d.
sea nettle d.
sea urchin d.
seaweed d.
seborrheic d.

d. seborrheica
Severity Scoring of Atopic D.
  (SCORAD)
shoe dye d.
shoe-leather d.
d. simplex
Six-Area, Six-Sign Atopic D.
  (SASSAD)
d. skiagraphica
skin bends d.
soap d.
soapfish d.
solar d.
d. solaris
sponge spicule d.
starfish d.
stasis d.
d. stasis
stethoscope d.
stinging coral d.
stinging water d.
stomal d.
d. striata pratensis bullosa
subcorneal pustular d.
suction-socket prosthetic d.
sweaty sock d.
swimmer's d.
T-cell-mediated delayed type
  hypersensitivity d.
tetramethylthiuram d.
textile d.
tinea d.
Toxicodendron d.
traumatic d.
traumatica d.
trefoil d.
trunk d.
tulip bulb d.
uncinarial d.
urostomy d.
d. vegetans
Velella velella d.
d. venenata
d. verrucosa
verrucose d.
vesicular d.
weeping d.
x-ray d.
dermatitis-arthritis-tenosynovitis
  syndrome
dermatoalloplasty

D

NOTES

dermatoarthritis
    lipoid d.
dermatoautoplasty
Dermatobia
    D. cyaniventris
    D. hominis
dermatobiasis
dermatoblepharitis
dermatocele
dermatocellulitis
dermatochalasia
dermatochalasis
dermatoconiosis
dermatocyst
dermatodynia
dermatodysplasia verruciformis
dermatofibroma protuberans
dermatofibrosarcoma protuberans (DFSP)
dermatofibrosis
    d. lenticularis
    d. lenticularis disseminata
dermatogenic torticollis
dermatoglyph
dermatoglyphic
dermatoglyphics
dermatograph
dermatographia
    black d.
    urticarial d.
    white d.
dermatographic
dermatographism
dermatography
dermatoheliosis
dermatoheteroplasty
dermatohistopathology
dermatohomoplasty
dermatoid
Dermatologic Diagnostic Algorithm
dermatologist
dermatology
    American Academy of D. (AAD)
    D. Education by Recall (DERM)
    D. Index of Disease Severity (DIDS)
    D. Teachers Exchange Group (DTEG)
dermatolysis palpebrarum
dermatoma
dermatomal
    d. distribution
    d. superficial telangiectasia
    d. zoster
dermatome
    Duval disposable d.
    Reese d.
    Tanner-Vandeput mesh d.

dermatomegaly
dermatomic area
dermatomycosis
    d. furfuracea
    d. microsporina
    d. pedis
    d. trichophytina
dermatomyoma
dermatomyositis (DM)
    amyopathic d.
    Banker type d.
    Brunsting-type d.
    childhood d. (CDM)
    juvenile d. (JDMS)
    d. sine myositis
dermatoneurosis
dermatonosology
Dermatop
dermatopathia pigmentosa reticularis
dermatopathic
    d. anemia
    d. lymphadenitis
    d. lymphadenopathy
dermatopathology
dermatopathy
dermatophagia
Dermatophagoides
    D. farinae
    D. microceras
    D. pteronyssinus
dermatophilosis
Dermatophilus congolensis
dermatophone
dermatophylaxis
dermatophyte
    d. fungal infection
    d. test medium (DTM)
dermatophytid
    erysipelas-like d.
    d. reaction
Dermatophytin
Dermatophytin-O
dermatophytosis, pl. **dermatophytoses**
    d. furfuracea
dermatoplastic
dermatoplasty
    Thompson d.
dermatopolymyositis
dermatopolyneuritis
dermatorrhagia
dermatorrhea
dermatorrhexis
dermatosclerosis
dermatoscope
dermatoscopy
    ABCD rule of d.
dermatosis, pl. **dermatoses**
    acantholytic d.

acarine d.
acquired d.
acute febrile neutrophilic d.
adult bullous d.
angioneurotic d.
arthropod d.
ashy d.
Auspitz d.
benign papular acantholytic d.
Blaschko linear d.
Bowen precancerous d.
carbon d.
childhood bullous d.
cholinogenic d.
chronic hemosideric d.
d. cinecienta
crazy paving d.
dermolytic bullous d.
digitate d.
fall d.
flaky paint d.
gonorrheal d.
Gougerot-Blum d.
ichthyosiform d.
IgA d.
industrial d.
inflammatory d.
intraepidermal neutrophilic IgA d.
juvenile plantar d.
lichenoid chronic d.
linear IgA bullous d. (LABD)
meadow-grass d.
d. medicamentosa
menstrual d.
neutrophilic intraepidermal IgA d.
occupational d.
d. papulosa nigra
papulosa nigra d.
persistent acantholytic d.
pigmented purpuric lichenoid d.
progressive pigmentary d.
pruritic d.
pustular d.
radiation d.
rhythmical d.
Schamberg progressive pigmented
  purpuric d.
seborrheic d.
spring d.
subcorneal pustular d.
summer d.
temperature-dependent d.

transient acantholytic d. (TAD)
ulcerative d.
Unna d.
vascular d.
vulvar d.
dermatosparaxis type
dermatotherapy
dermatothlasia
dermatothlasis
dermatotropic
dermatoxenoplasty
dermatozoiasis
dermatozoon, pl. **dermatozoa**
dermatozoonosis
dermatrophia
dermic
Dermicel tape
DermiCort
dermis
adventitial d.
papillary d.
periadnexal d.
reticular d.
upper d.
dermite
dermitis
DermMaster system
dermoepidermal
d. interface
d. junction
d. nevus
dermogram
black d.
geriatric d.
pediatric d.
dermographia
dermographism
cold-dependent d.
white d.
dermohypodermal
dermoid
d. cyst
inclusion d.
sequestration d.
Dermo-Jet nickel dermatitis
Dermolate Topical
dermolysis
dermolytic bullous dermatosis
dermonecrotic
dermoneurosis
dermonosology
dermopanniculosis formans

D

NOTES

dermopathy
> diabetic d.
> restrictive d.

dermophlebitis
dermoplasty
dermostenosis
dermostosis
dermosyphilopathy
dermotoxin
dermotropic
dermotuberculin reaction
Dermovan
Dermovate
Dermoxyl
Dermtex
> D. HC with Aloe
> D. HC with Aloe Topical

Derm-Vi Soap
DES
> diethylstilbestrol

desaturation
descarboethoxyloratadine
Desenex
> Prescription Strength D.

desensitization
> anaphylactic d.
> heterologous d.
> homologous d.
> massive-dose d.
> penicillin d.

desensitize
desert
> d. ragweed
> d. sore

desetope
desiccant
desiccation
> curettage and d. (C&D)
> mucous d.

desiccative
Desiclovir
design
> Clear By D.
> Morrey-Coonrad d.

desipramine
Desitin topical
Desjardins forceps
desloratadine
Desmarres
> D. clamp
> D. retractor

desmin
desmoglein (Dsg)
> recombinant d. (rDsg)

desmoglein-1 (Dsg1)
desmoglein-3 (Dsg3)

desmoid
> d. cyst
> d. tumor

desmolysis
desmon
desmoplastic
> d. malignant melanoma
> d. trichilemmoma
> d. trichoepithelioma

desmorrhexis
desmosome
desmosome-tonofilament complex
Desocort
desonide otic lotion
DesOwen topical
desoximetasone
despeciated
> d. antitoxin
> d. serum

despeciation
desquamans
> herpes d.

desquamate
desquamating
desquamation
> branny d.
> corneocyte d.
> furfuraceous d.
> generalized d.
> lamellar d.
> membranous d.
> peribronchial d.
> plantar d.
> siliquose d.

desquamative
> d. dermatitis
> d. gingivitis
> d. interstitial pneumonia (DIP)
> d. interstitial pneumonitis

desquamativum, pl. **desquamativa**
> erythema d.
> erythroderma d.

Desquam-E gel
Desquam-X
> D.-X. gel
> D.-X. Wash

destruction
> beta-cell d.
> oligodendrocyte d.
> polymorphonuclear leukocyte-
> dependent tissue d.

destructor
> *Lepidoglyphus* d.

desynchronized sleep
detection
> *Bartonella henselae* d.
> computer-assisted arthritis d.
> C1q immune complex d.

hepatitis B DNA d.
hepatitis C RNA d.
hepatitis C virus antibody d.
Ki-67 marker d.
Lyme disease DNA d.
Mycobacterium tuberculosis d.
myelin-associated glycoprotein
  antibody d.
detergens
liquor carbonis d. (LCD)
detergent
anionic d.
superfatted synthetic d.
synthetic d. (syndet)
detergicans
acne d.
determinant
allotypic d.
antigenic d.
conformational d.
genetic d.
d. group
idiotypic antigenic d.
isoallotypic d.
Kern d.
Km allotypic d.
Oz isotypic d.
sequential d.
determination
fecal fat d.
IgG subclass d.
detersive
detoxicate
detoxication
detoxification
detoxified toxin
detoxify
detritus
tissue d.
Deuteromycetes
DEV
duck embryo origin vaccine
development
Treg d.
Devergie disease
deviation
anterior chamber-associated
  immune d. (ACAID)
complement d.
immune d.
standard d. (SD)
ulnar d.

device
AeroEclipse Aerosol Delivery D.
Antense antitension d.
CoolSpot skin-cooling d.
Cyclotech dosing d.
DermaSeptic d.
electrocoagulation biterminal d.
ElectroRegenesis therapy d. (ERTD)
Endopearl bioabsorbable d.
extracorporeal assist d.
Flexi-Trak skin anchoring d.
flutter d.
Handisol phototherapy d.
Hexascan Mark I, II model robotic
  scanning d.
Orion d.
Prosorba column d.
pulse oximetry d.
Skinscan d.
SkinTech medical tattooing d.
SomnoStar apnea testing d.
Tanner mesher d.
Thoratec ventricular assist d.
Tru-Area Determination
  measuring d.
Vacu-Aide portable suction d.
Venture demand oxygen delivery d.
Vitrasert intraocular d.
Devic syndrome
DeVilbiss Pulmon-Aid nebulizer
devil grip
devil's
d. bite lesion
d. pinch
Devrom
dew
d. itch
D. sign
Dewar flask
DEXA, DXA
dual-energy x-ray absorptiometry
Dexacidin Ophthalmic
Dexacort Phosphate Turbinaire
dexamethasone (DXM)
d. acetate
neomycin, polymyxin b, and d.
d. sodium phosphate
d. suppression test (DST)
tobramycin and d.
Dexasone L.A.
Dexasporin Ophthalmic
Dexchlor

D

NOTES

dexchlorpheniramine maleate
Dexone LA
Dexon suture
Dexotic
dextran 1
dextranomer granule
dextromethorphan
  chlorpheniramine, phenylephrine, and d.
  pseudoephedrine and d.
dextrose
  tetracaine with d.
DEY albuterol inhalation aerosol
Dey-Dose
  D.-D. Isoproterenol
  D.-D. Metaproterenol
Dey-Drop
  D.-D. Ophthalmic solution
Dey-Lute isoetharine
Dey-Wash skin wound clean
DF2 septicemia
DFA
  direct fluorescent antibody
  DFA test
DFA-TP
  direct fluorescent antibody test for *Treponema pallidum*
D/Flex
DFSP
  dermatofibrosarcoma protuberans
DFU
  dideoxyfluorouridine
DGF
  delayed graft function
DH
  delayed hypersensitivity
  dermatitis herpetiformis
DHA
  dihydroacetone
  dihydroxyacetone
DHAP
  dihydroxyacetone phosphate
DHA-PUVA
  dihydroxyacetone-psoralen ultraviolet A-range
Dharmendra antigen
DHEAS
  dehydroepiandrosterone sulfate
D.H.E. 45 injection
d'Herelle phenomenon
dhobie
  d. itch
  d. mark
  d. mark dermatitis
DHS
  dihydrostreptomycin
  DHS Tar
  DHS zinc

DHT
  dihydrotestosterone
  domino heart transplantation
DI
  defective interfering
  HAQ DI
  Health Assessment Questionnaire Disability Index
  DI particle
Di
  Di antigen
diabetes
  bronze d.
  lipoatrophic d.
  d. mellitus
  posttransplant d.
  tacrolimus-associated d.
  type 1, 1A, 1B d.
diabetic
  d. blister
  d. cheiroarthropathy
  d. dermopathy
  d. foot ulcer
  d. gangrene
  d. hand syndrome
  d. muscle infarction (DMI)
  D. Skin Therapy
  d. stiff-hand syndrome
diabetica
  neurotabes d.
diabeticorum
  bullosis d.
  eczema d.
  necrobiosis lipoidica d.
  xanthoma d.
  xanthosis d.
diabetogenic
DiabGel hydrogel dressing
DiaB Klenz wound cleanser
diacerein
diacetate
  diflorasone d.
diacylglycerol
diadermic
diagnosis
  differential d.
  EIA d.
  electrodermal d.
  exercise-induced asthma d.
  problem-oriented d.
diagnostic
  d. algorithm
  d. diphtheria toxin
  d. principle
  d. surgical therapy
  d. test
dialkylthioreas
Dial soap

dialysis
  chronic ambulatory peritoneal d. (CAPD)
  d. dermatitis
  equilibrium d.
dialysis-related amyloidosis
diameter
  mass median aerodynamic d. (MMD)
Diamine
  D. T.D.
  D. T.D. Oral
diamond
  d. fraise
  d. fraise dermabrasion instrument
  D. Jaw needle holder
  d. skin
Diamox
Diaparene
diapedesis
  cellular d.
diaper
  d. dermatitis
  d. granuloma
  d. rash
  d. rash intertrigo
diaphoresis
diaphoretic
diaphragmatic
  d. hernia
  d. pleurisy
diaphysis
diapnoic
diarrhea
  bovine virus d.
  Brainerd d.
  chronic d.
  prolonged d.
  weanling d.
diarthrodial joint bursae
diary
  diet d.
diascope
diascopy
Diasonic ultrasound
diastase-resistant
diastrophic dysplasia
diathesis, pl. **diatheses**
  allergic d.
  atopic d.
  hemorrhagic d.

diathsique
  prurigo d.
diazepam
Diazolidinyl urea (DiU)
Diazo paper
Dibenzyline
Dibucaine
dibutylester
  squaric acid d. (SADBE)
dibutylthiourea
DIC
  disseminated intravascular coagulation
  sepsis-induced DIC
dichloride
  cobalt d.
dichloroacetic acid
dichlorodifluoromethane and trichloromonofluoromethane
dichlorodiphenyltrichloroethane (chlorophenothane) (DDT)
dichlorofluoromethane
dichlorotetrafluoroethane
  ethyl chloride and d.
Dick
  D. method
  D. reaction
  D. test
  D. test toxin
diclazuril
diclofenac
  d. sodium
  d. sodium gel
dicloxacillin sodium
Dicrocoelium dendriticum
Dictyocaulus viviparus
dictyospore
didanosine (ddi)
didehydrothymidine
  d4T, d.
2′-3′-dideoxyadenosine
dideoxycytidine (ddc)
  2′-3′ d.
dideoxyfluorouridine (DFU)
dideoxynucleoside
DIDMOS
  drug-induced delayed multiorgan hypersensitivity syndrome
  DIDMOS syndrome of Sontheimer and Houpt
Didrex
Didrocal
Didronel

D

NOTES

DIDS
    Dermatology Index of Disease Severity
didymospore
diet
    challenge d.
    d. diary
    elemental d.
    elimination d.
    Feingold d.
    gluten-free d.
    hypoallergenic d.
    lactovegetarian d.
    low-phenylalanine d.
    low-tyrosine d.
    Sippy d.
    Zen macrobiotic d.
dietary
    d. protein enterocolitis
    d. protein-induced colitis
    d. protein-induced enterocolitis
Dieterle stain
diethylcarbamazine (DEC)
diethyldithiocarbamate
diethylstilbestrol (DES)
diethylthiourea
diethyltoluamide (DEET)
difference
    geographic d.
differential
    d. diagnosis
    d. expression pattern
    d. gene expression
    d. gene subtraction
differentiation
    d. antigen
    cluster of d. 2–72 (CD2–72)
    tricholemmal d.
Differin
    D. cream
    D. gel
DiffGAM bovine anti-*Clostridium difficile* immunoglobulin
difficile
    Clostridium d.
Diffistat-G polyclonal antibody
Diff-Quik stain
diffusa
    leishmaniasis tegumentaria d.
    psoriasis d.
diffuse
    d. atrophy
    d. connective tissue disease (DCTD)
    d. cutaneous leishmaniasis
    d. cutaneous mastocytosis
    d. erythema
    d. fibrosing alveolitis
    d. histiocytic reaction

    d. hyperkeratosis of palms and soles
    d. idiopathic skeletal hyperostosis (DISH)
    d. infantile fibromatosis
    d. infiltrative lymphocytosis
    d. infiltrative lymphocytosis syndrome
    d. inflammation
    d. interstitial fibrosis of the lung
    d. interstitial lung disease (DILD)
    d. lepromatous leprosy
    d. leprosy of Lucio
    d. phlegmon
    d. plane
    d. plane xanthoma
    d. progressive systemic sclerosis
    d. proliferative glomerulonephritis
    d. pulmonary infiltrate
    d. reflectance spectroscopy (DRS)
    d. scleritis
    d. scleroderma
    d. staining
diffusing capacity for carbon monoxide (DLCO)
diffusion
    agar gel d.
    d. coefficient
    d. constant
    gel d.
    d. of the lunula
diffusum
    angiokeratoma corporis d.
    atrophoderma d.
    keratoma d.
    papilloma d.
diflorasone
    d. diacetate
    d. diacetate cream/ointment USP
Diflucan
    D. injection
    D. Oral
diflunisal
diftitox
    denileukin d.
DiGeorge
    D. anomaly
    D. syndrome
digestion
    intracellular d.
digit
    drummer d.
    rudimentary supernumerary d.
    sausage d.
    supernumerary d.
digital
    d. fibrokeratoma
    d. fibromatosis

d. ischemia
d. mucinous pseudocyst
d. sympathectomy
d. whorl
digitalis
herpes d.
digitata
verruca d.
digitate
d. dermatosis
d. wart
Digitrapper MkIII sleep monitor
dihomogamm
dihydrate
calcium pyrophosphate d. (CPPD)
dihydroacetone (DHA)
dihydrocodeine
dihydroergotamine mesylate
dihydrostreptomycin (DHS)
dihydrotestosterone (DHT)
dihydroxyacetone (DHA)
d. phosphate (DHAP)
d. self-tanning lotion
dihydroxyacetone-psoralen ultraviolet A-range (DHA-PUVA)
dihydroxy leukotriene, LTB4
3,4-dihydroxyphenylalanine (DOPA)
dihydroxypropyl theophylline
Dihyrex Injection
Dilantin
dilated
d. pore
d. pore of Winer
d. venule
DILD
diffuse interstitial lung disease
Dilocaine
Dilor
diloxanide furoate
diluent
dilute Russell viper venom time
dilution
Dimaphen
D. Elixir
D. Tablet
Dimedrine
dimeglumine
gadopentetate d. (Gd-DTPA)
dimenhydrinate
dimension
double (gel) diffusion precipitin test in one d.

gel diffusion precipitin test in one d.
single (gel) diffusion precipitin test in one d.
dimer
dimeric
Dimetabs Oral
Dimetane
D. Decongestant Elixir
D. Extentabs
D. Oral
Dimetapp
D. Chewables
D. Clear
D. Extentabs
D. 4-Hour Liqui-Gel Capsule
D. Sinus Caplets
D. Tablet
dimethicone
dimethyl
d. carbate
d. carbate butopyropoxyl insect repellent
d. phthalate insect repellent
d. sulfoxide (DMSO)
dimethylgloxime nickel spot test
dimidiatum
Scytalidium d.
diminished breath sound
dimorphic fungi
dimorphous leprosy
dimple sign
dimpling
Dinate Injection
dinitrochlorobenzene (DNCB)
d. challenge
dinoflagellate toxin
dinucleotide
diode
d. laser
light-emitting d. (LED)
dioecious
Diomycin
Diopred
dioxide
carbon d. (CO_2)
end-tidal carbon d. ($ETCO_2$)
partial pressure of carbon d. (PCO_2)
solid carbon d.
sulfur d. (SO_2)
titanium d.

D

NOTES

159

dioxybenzone
DIP
> desquamative interstitial pneumonia
> distal interphalangeal

Dipentum
Dipetalonema
> *D. perstans*
> *D. streptocerca*

diphasic milk fever
Diphenacen-50 Injection
Diphen Cough
Diphenhist
diphenhydramine
> acetaminophen and d.
> d. hydrochloride
> parenteral d.
> d. and pseudoephedrine

diphenidol hydrochloride
Diphenylan Sodium
diphenylcyclopropenone
diphenylhydantoin
diphosphate
> adenosine d. (ADP)

diphosphonate
> technetium d.

diphtheria
> d. antitoxin
> d. antitoxin unit
> avian d.
> cutaneous d.
> d. cutis
> false d.
> fowl d.
> d. and tetanus toxoid
> d., tetanus toxoid, and acellular pertussis vaccine
> d., tetanus toxoid, and whole-cell pertussis vaccine
> > d., tetanus toxoid, and whole-cell pertussis vaccine and *Haemophilus* b conjugate vaccine
> d. toxin
> d. toxoid, tetanus toxoid, and pertussis vaccine (DTP)

diphtheriae
> *Corynebacterium d.*

diphtheria-pertussis-tetanus (DPT)
diphtheric desert sore
diphtheritic
> d. membrane
> d. ulcer

diphtheroid
diphtherotoxin
Diphyllobothrium latum
diplococcin
diplopia
Diprolene
> D. AF

> D. AF Topical
> D. Glycol

dipropionate
> alclometasone d.
> beclomethasone d.
> betamethasone d.
> clobetasol d.

Diprosone Topical
dipstick
> d. method
> d. technique

Dipylidium caninum
dipyridamole
direct
> d. agglutination test
> d. challenge
> d. Coombs test
> d. fluorescent antibody (DFA)
> d. fluorescent antibody test
> d. fluorescent antibody test for *Treponema pallidum* (DFA-TP)
> d. galvanic current
> d. histamine releaser
> d. immunofluorescence
> *Mycobacterium* Tuberculosis D. (MTD)
> d. sequencing

directly observed therapy short-course (DOTS)
directory
> Haines d.

dirithromycin
Dirofilaria immitis
dirofilariasis
> subcutaneous d.

disability
> hemarthrotic d.

disaccharide intolerance
Disalcid
DISC
> death-inducing signaling complex

disc
> Clear Away D.
> Durapore membrane d.
> EMLA anesthetic d.

disciform thickening
discoid
> distinctive exudative d.
> exudative d.
> d. LE
> d. lupus
> d. lupus erythematosus (DLE)

discoidea
> psoriasis d.

discoides
> lupus erythematosus d.
> psoriasis d.

discoloration
  oil-spot d.
discontinuous
  d. plasma-Percoll gradient centrifugation
  d. sterilization
discordant
  d. cellular xenograft
  d. organ xenograft
discreta
  porokeratosis plantaris d.
discrete
  d. pit
  d. synovitis
  d. umbilicated papule
discrimination
  self-nonself d.
disease
  acute infectious d.
  Addison d.
  Addison-Gull d.
  adult/adolescent spectrum of HIV d. (ASD)
  adult-onset systemic Still d.
  airways d.
  akamushi d.
  Albright d.
  alcohol-related liver d. (ALD)
  Aleutian mink d.
  Alibert d.
  allograft coronary artery d. (ACAD)
  Almeida d.
  alpha chain d.
  alpha-heavy-chain d.
  amyloid d.
  Anderson-Fabry d.
  Andrews d.
  antibody deficiency d.
  appendicular d.
  Arndt-Gottron d.
  articular d.
  Asboe-Hansen d.
  aspirin-sensitive respiratory d. (ASRD)
  Athabascan type of severe combined immunodeficiency d. (SCIDA)
  atheroembolic d.
  atypical Kawasaki d. (AKD)
  Aujeszky d.
  Australian X d.

  autoimmune blistering mucocutaneous d.
  autoimmune pituitary d.
  autoimmune thyroid d. (ATD)
  axial d.
  bacterial d.
  Baelz d.
  Ballingall d.
  Bang d.
  Bannister d.
  Barcoo d.
  Basedow d.
  Bateman d.
  Bayle d.
  Bazin d.
  Behçet d.
  Beigel d.
  beryllium d.
  Besnier d.
  Besnier-Boeck d.
  Besnier-Boeck-Schaumann d.
  beta-heavy-chain d.
  bird-breeder's d.
  blackjack d.
  blinding d.
  Bloch-Sulzberger d.
  Bodechtel-Guttmann d.
  Borna d.
  Bornholm d.
  Bostock d.
  Bourneville d.
  Bourneville-Brissaud d.
  Bourneville-Pringle d.
  Bowen d.
  brachial neuritis of Lyme d.
  Breda d.
  Bretonneau d.
  Brill d.
  Brill-Zinsser d.
  Brion-Kayser d.
  broad beta d.
  Brocq d.
  Brooke d.
  Bruton d.
  Buerger d.
  bullous d.
  burden of d. (BOD)
  Bury d.
  Buschke d.
  Buschke-Ollendorf d.
  Busse-Buschke d.

D

NOTES

disease *(continued)*

calcium hydroxyapatite crystal deposition d.
calcium phosphate crystal deposition d.
calcium pyrophosphate crystal deposition d.
calcium pyrophosphate dihydrate deposition d. (CPDD)
cardiac allograft vascular d.
Caroli d.
Carrión d.
Castleman d.
cat-scratch d. (CSD)
Cazenave d.
celiac d.
central Recklinghausen d. type II
Chagas d.
Charlouis d.
Chlamydia d.
chronic airways d. (CAD)
chronic cold agglutinin d.
chronic graft-versus-host d.
chronic granulomatous d. (CGD)
chronic inflammatory d.
chronic interstitial lung d.
chronic obstructive pulmonary d. (COPD)
Ciarrocchi d.
cicatricial pemphigoid d.
Civatte d.
cold hemagglutinin d.
collagen vascular d.
combined immunodeficiency d. (CID)
communicable d.
congenital Lyme d.
connective tissue d. (CTD)
Conradi d.
contagious d.
Cooperative Systematic Studies of the Rheumatic D. (CSSRD)
Corbus d.
coronary artery d. (CAD)
Cowden d.
CP d.
Creutzfeldt-Jakob d. (CJD)
Crohn d.
Crouzon d.
crystal deposition d.
Csillag d.
Cushing d.
cytomegalic inclusion d. (CID)
cytomegalovirus d.
Daae d.
Danielssen d.
Danielssen-Boeck d.
Darier d. (DD)

Darier-White d.
dark dot d.
deer fly d.
Degos d.
Dejerine-Sottas d.
dense-deposit d.
de Quervain d.
Dercum d.
Devergie d.
diffuse connective tissue d. (DCTD)
diffuse interstitial lung d. (DILD)
DNA probe test for Lyme d.
dog d.
Dohle d.
Dowling-Degos d.
Dubois d.
Duhring d.
Dukes d.
Duncan d.
Dupuytren d.
Durand-Nicholas-Favre d.
Dutton d.
endocrine d.
end-stage organ d.
Engman d.
Epstein d.
exanthematous d.
D. Extent Index (DEI)
extramammary Paget d. (EMPD)
exudative papulosquamous d.
Fabry d.
Fabry-Anderson d.
Farber d.
Favre-Racouchot d.
fifth d.
Filatov-Dukes d.
Finkelstein d.
first d.
Flegel d.
fly-borne d.
food-borne d.
food-induced respiratory d.
foot-and-mouth d. (FMD)
forced air system d.
Fordyce d.
Forestier d.
Fothergill d.
Fournier d.
fourth d.
Fox d.
Fox-Fordyce d.
Francis d.
Freiberg d.
Friend d.
fungal d.
furuncular d.
fusospirochetal d.

gasping d.
Gaucher d.
genetic d.
Gerhardt d.
Gerhardt-Mitchell d.
Gianotti-Crosti d.
Gibert d.
Gilchrist d.
glycogen storage d.
Gorham d.
Gougerot-Blum d.
Gougerot and Blum d.
Gougerot-Sjögren d.
graft-versus-host d. (GVHD)
graft vessel d. (GVD)
granulomatous d.
Graves d.
Greenhow d.
Griesinger d.
Grover d.
Gumboro d.
Günther d.
gut-associated lymphoid d.
GVH d.
Habermann d.
Hailey-Hailey d. (HHD)
Hallopeau d.
hand-foot-and-mouth d.
Hand-Schüller-Christian d.
Hansen d.
hard pad d.
Hartnup d.
Hashimoto d.
Hashimoto-Pritzker d.
heavy-chain d. (HCD)
Hebra d.
helminthic parasitic d.
hemoglobin C, S d.
hemolytic sickle cell d.
hepatobiliary d.
heritable connective tissue d.
Herlitz d.
hidebound d.
Hirschsprung d.
His-Werner d.
HLA class 1 associated d.
Hodgkin d.
hoof-and-mouth d.
Horton d.
Hunermann d.
Hurler d.
Hurst d.

Hyde d.
idiopathic cold agglutinin d.
idiopathic eczematous d.
immune complex d.
immune-mediated d.
immunobullous d.
immunodeficiency d.
immunologic inflammatory d.
immunoproliferative small
    intestinal d. (IPSID)
inclusion body d.
infarctive inflammatory d.
infectious d. (ID)
inflammatory bowel d. (IBD)
inflammatory lung d.
interstitial lung d. (ILD)
intraepidermal blistering d.
iron storage d.
Isambert d.
island d.
isocyanate d.
itchy red bump d.
Jadassohn d.
Jakob-Creutzfeldt d.
Jessner-Kanof d.
jodbasedow d.
Jüngling d.
Kalischer d.
Kanzaki d.
Kaposi d.
Kashin-Beck d.
Kawasaki d. (KD)
Kellgren d.
Ketron-Goodman d.
Kienböck d.
Kikuchi d.
Kimura d.
kinky-hair d.
Kobberling-Duncan d.
Köbner d.
Köhler d.
Krabbe d.
Kyasanur Forest d.
Kyrle d.
Lafora d.
Lancereaux-Mathieu d.
Landouzy d.
Lane d.
large artery d.
Larrey-Weil d.
Legg-Calvé-Perthes d.
Legionnaires d.

D

NOTES

disease *(continued)*

Leicester d.
Leiner d.
Leloir d.
Lemierre d.
Letterer-Siwe d.
Lewandowski-Lutz d.
Leyden d.
Lhermitte-Duclos d.
linear IgA bullous d.
d. linkage disequilibrium (DLD)
lipid storage d.
lipochrome histiocytosis d.
livedo-patterned d.
liver d.
Lobo d.
Lortat-Jacobs d.
Lou Gehrig d.
lumpy skin d.
lung d.
Lutz-Miescher d.
Lutz-Splendore-Almeida d.
Lyell d.
Lyme d. (stage 1–3)
lymphocytic d.
lymphoproliferative d.
MacIsaac d.
Madelung d.
Majocchi d.
malignant neoplastic d.
mammary Paget d.
maple bark d.
maple-bark stripper's d.
Marburg virus d.
Marek d.
margarine d.
Marie-Strümpell d.
market men d.
McArdle d.
mechanobullous d.
Meleda d.
metabolic bone d.
Mibelli d.
Mikulicz d.
Milian d.
Milroy d.
Milton d.
Mitchell d.
mixed connective tissue d.
  (MCTD)
Mkar d.
Mondor d.
Morvan d.
Moschcowitz d.
mosquito-borne d.
Mseleni d.
Mucha d.
Mucha-Habermann d.

mucocutaneous d.
mucosal d.
mu-heavy chain d.
multicentric d.
mycoplasma d.
myeloproliferative d.
Nasu-Hakola d.
National Institute of Arthritis and
  Metabolic D.'s (NIAMD)
neonatal-onset multisystem
  inflammatory d. (NOMID)
neoplastic d.
Nettleship d.
Neumann d.
neurodegenerative d.
neuroectodermal melanolysomonal d.
neuropathic joint d.
neuropsychiatric d.
neutral lipid storage d.
Newcastle d. (ND)
Niemann-Pick d.
nodular sclerosing Hodgkin d.
  (NSHD)
nonneoplastic d.
obliterative airway d.
obstructive liver d.
occupational immunologic lung d.
  (OLD)
Ockelbo d.
ocular immune d.
ocular inflammatory d.
Ofuji d.
Ohara d.
"oid-oid" d.
orbital inflammatory d.
orphan d.
Osler d.
Osler-Weber-Rendu d.
overlap d.
Paget d.
parasitic d.
Parkinson d.
patellofemoral d.
Paxton d.
pelvic inflammatory d. (PID)
perforating d.
perna d.
Pette-Döring d.
Peyronie d.
phytanic acid storage d.
pigeon breeder's d.
pink d.
Plaut-Vincent d.
polycystic ovary d.
polyglandular autoimmune
  endocrine d.
Pompe d.
Poncet d.

porcupine d.
Posada-Wernicke d.
postthrombotic d.
posttransplantation
 lymphoproliferative d. (PTLD)
posttransplant lymphoproliferative d.
 (PTLD)
poultry handler's d.
Preiser d.
primary pulmonary parenchymal d.
Pringle d.
proliferative inflammatory d.
protozoal parasitic d.
psychocutaneous d.
Puente d.
pulmonary venoocclusive d.
 (PVOD)
pulseless d.
Quincke d.
Quinquaud d.
Ranikhet d.
Rayer d.
Raynaud d.
reactive airways d.
Recklinghausen d.
Recklinghausen d. type I
Reclus d.
Refsum d.
Reiter d.
Rendu-Osler-Weber d.
restrictive lung d.
reticulohistiocytosis d.
rheumatoid d.
Ribas-Torres d.
rippling muscle d.
Ritter d.
Robinson d.
Robles d.
Roitter d.
Rosai-Dorfman d.
Rosenbach d.
Roth-Bernhardt d.
Rubarth d.
runt d.
Rust d.
salivary gland virus d.
sandworm d.
saprophytic d.
Schamberg d.
Schenck d.
Scheuermann d.
Schilder d.

Schönlein d.
Scraple d.
secondary d.
Senear-Usher d.
seropositive d.
serum d.
severe combined
 immunodeficiency d. (SCID)
sexually transmitted d. (STD)
shimamushi d.
sickle cell d. (SCD)
silicone particle d.
sinopulmonary d.
sixth venereal d.
Sjögren d.
skinbound d.
slow virus d.
Sneddon-Wilkinson d.
specific d.
spirochetal d.
sponge diver d.
sponge fisherman d.
SS hemoglobin d.
staging classification for
 Hodgkin d.
Stanton d.
startle d.
stellate patterned d.
sternoclavicular d.
Sticker d.
Still d.
Strümpell d.
Sulzberger-Garbe d.
Sutton d.
Sweet d.
Swift d.
swine vesicular d.
Sylvest d.
d. syndrome
systemic autoimmune d.
systemic febrile d.
Takahara d.
Takayasu d.
Tangier d.
Tarui d.
Taylor d.
Tay-Sachs d.
T- and B-cell severe combined
 immunodeficiency d.
T-cell-mediated autoimmune d.
Teschen d.
Theiler d.

D

NOTES

disease *(continued)*
>Thiemann d.
>third d.
>tickborne d.
>TI-CMV d.
>traumatically induced
>   inflammatory d.
>tropical d.
>tsutsugamushi d.
>twentieth century d.
>type I glycogen storage d.
>Underwood d.
>undifferentiated connective tissue d.
>   (UCTD)
>Unna d.
>Unna-Thost d.
>Urbach-Oppenheim d.
>Urbach-Wiethe d.
>vagabond's d.
>vagrant's d.
>valvular d.
>Van Buchem d.
>varicella d.
>vasoocclusive d.
>vector-borne d.
>venereal d.
>venoocclusivc d. (VOD disease)
>vesiculobullous d.
>Vidal d.
>Vincent d.
>vinyl chloride d.
>viral d.
>virus X d.
>VOD d.
>   venoocclusive disease
>Voerner d.
>von Economo d.
>von Gierke glycogen storage d.
>von Recklinghausen d.
>von Willebrand d. (vWD)
>von Zumbusch d.
>Wardrop d.
>Wassilieff d.
>wasting d.
>Weber-Christian d. (WCD)
>Weber-Cockayne d.
>Weil d.
>Well d.
>Werlhof d.
>Werther d.
>Wesselsbron d.
>Whipple d.
>white spot d.
>Whitmore d.
>Whytt d.
>Willan d.
>Wilson d.
>Winkler d.

>winter vomiting d.
>Witkop-Von Sallman d.
>wood-pulp worker's d.
>Woringer-Kolopp d.
>X-linked lymphoproliferative d.
>   (XLP)
>yellow d.
>Zahorsky d.
>Zoon d.
>Zumbusch d.

disease-modifying antirheumatic drug (DMAD, DMARD)

disease-syphilis
>venereal d.-s. (VDS)

disequilibrium
>disease linkage d. (DLD)
>linkage d.

DISH
>diffuse idiopathic skeletal hyperostosis

disinfect

disinfectant
>phenolated d.
>Sactimed-I-Sinald d.

disinfection

disintegrin
>d. proteinase

disjunctum
>stratum d.

disk
>hair d.
>d. sensitivity method

Diskhaler
>Flutide D.
>D. inhaler

Diskus inhaler

dislocation
>d. arthritis
>atlantodental d.

dismutase
>bovine superoxide d.

disodium
>d. cromoglycate (DSC)
>lobenzarit d.
>ticarcillin d.

disorder
>acquired cornification d.
>acquired vascular d.
>adrenal cortex d.
>anogenital d.
>autoimmune d.
>autosomal recessive severe
>   combined immunodeficiency d.
>bacterially induced hemostatic d.
>bland occlusive d.
>body dysmorphic d.
>ciliary d.
>cold-dependent d.
>congenital d.

cornification d.
d. of cornification (DOC)
Curth-Maklin cornification d.
dysesthesia d.
environmentally associated
  rheumatic d. (EARD)
hematologic d.
hemostatic d.
hereditary vascular d.
heritable d.
ICE d.
immune complex d.
immune-mediated coagulation d.
immunodeficiency d.
immunoglobulin-complexed
  enzyme d.
immunologic d.
immunoproliferative d.
keratitis-deafness cornification d.
lymphoreticular d.
metabolic d.
mineral-related nutritional d.
National Institute of Arthritis,
  Musculoskeletal and Skin D.'s
  (NIAMS)
neurologic d.
nutritional d.
ocular inflammatory d.
pancreatic d.
papulosquamous d.
partial combined
  immunodeficiency d.
periarticular d.
d. of phagocytic cell
pituitary d.
posttransplantation
  lymphoproliferative d. (PTLD, PT-
  LPD)
posttransplant lymphoproliferative d.
  (PTLD)
primary immunodeficiency d.
proliferation d.
psychophysiologic d.
secondary psychiatric d.
severe combined
  immunodeficiency d. (SCID)
thyroid d.
unilateral hemidysplasia
  cornification d.
upper airway d. (UAD)
vascular d.

dispar
  Lymantria d.
disperse dye
dispersing agent
dispersion
  amphotericin B colloidal d.
displacement
  d. analysis
  odontoid process d.
display
  antibody-phage d.
Dispos-a-Med Isoproterenol
disruption
  gene d.
  LTA$_4$ hydrolase gene d.
dissecans
  glossitis d.
  osteochondritis d.
dissecting
  d. cellulitis
  d. cellulitis of scalp
  d. perifolliculitis
  d. scissors
dissection
  blunt d.
  d. cellulitis of scalp
  elective lymph node d. (ELND)
  sharp d.
  d. tubercle
dissector
  Luikart d.
disseminata
  acne d.
  alopecia d.
  dermatofibrosis lenticularis d.
  neurodermatitis d.
  osteitis fibrosa cystica d.
  porokeratosis palmaris plantaris
    et d.
  tuberculosis cutis follicularis d.
  tuberculosis cutis miliaris d.
disseminated
  d. aspergillosis
  d. candidiasis
  d. coccidioidomycosis
  d. cutaneous gangrene
  d. cutaneous leishmaniasis (DCL)
  d. encephalomyelitis
  d. gonococcal infection
  d. herpes simplex
  d. herpes zoster
  d. intravascular coagulation (DIC)

D

NOTES

disseminated *(continued)*
    d. Kaposi sarcoma
    d. lupus erythematosus
    d. neurodermatitis
    d. pagetoid reticulosis
    d. pruriginous angiodermatitis
    d. recurrent infundibulofolliculitis
    d. sporotrichosis
    d. strongyloidiasis
    d. superficial actinic porokeratosis
    (DSAP)
    d. tuberculosis
    d. vaccinia
dissemination
    skin d.
    xanthoma d.
disseminatum
    keratoma d.
    xanthoma d. (XD)
disseminatus
    lupus erythematosus d. (LED)
dissemine
    neurodermite d.
disséminées parapsoriasis en plaques
dissociation constant
distal
    d. arthrogryposis
    d. dactylitis
    d. dystrophy
    d. interphalangeal (DIP)
    d. intestinal obstruction syndrome
    d. nail matrix
    d. radicular joint (DRUJ)
    d. splenorenal shunt (DSRS)
Distaval
distemper virus
distended bursa
distensae
    striae cutis d.
distichia
distichiasis
distillate
    cetyl alcohol-coal tar d.
    Tar D.
distinctive
    d. exudative discoid
    d. exudative discoid and lichenoid
    dermatitis (DEDLE)
distortum
    Microsporum canis, var *d.*
distress
    respiratory d.
distribution
    asymmetric d.
    compartment load d.
    dermatomal d.
    fibrosing alopecia in a pattern d.
    (FAPD)

    lesion d.
    linear d.
    pattern of d.
    shawl d.
    Sips d.
districhiasis
distrix
disturbance
    atrial conduction d.
    d. of consciousness
    microcirculatory d.
dithiothreitol (DTT)
Dithranol
ditiocarb
Ditropan XL oxybutynin chloride extended-release tablet
DiU
    Diazolidinyl urea
diubiquitin
diuretic
    chlorothiazide d.
    loop d.
diutinum
    erythema elevatum d. (EED)
    scleredema d.
divergens
    Babesia d.
diversiloba
    Rhus d.
diversilobum
    Toxicodendron d.
diversity
    antigen-binding d.
diversus
    Citrobacter d.
diving suit dermatitis
division (I–IV) lesion
Dizac injection
Dizmiss
dizygotic
DLCO
    diffusing capacity for carbon monoxide
DLD
    disease linkage disequilibrium
DLE
    discoid lupus erythematosus
DLI
    donor leukocyte infusion
    donor lymphocyte infusion
DM
    dermatomyositis
    Guaifenex DM
    Iobid DM
    Iohist DM
DMAD
    disease-modifying antirheumatic drug
DMARD
    disease-modifying antirheumatic drug

DMDM hydantoin
D-Med Injection
DMI
  diabetic muscle infarction
DMSA
  Tc-dimercaptosuccinic acid
DMSO
  dimethyl sulfoxide
DNA
  deoxyribonucleic acid
  DNA amplicon
  DNA aneuploidy
  antidimer DNA
  antidouble-stranded DNA
  antinative DNA
  DNA autosensitivity
  DNA binding
  chemiluminescent DNA
  chemiluminescent in situ
    hybridization for detection of
    CMV DNA
  circular plasmid DNA
  competitor DNA
  complementary DNA (cDNA)
  decoy DNA
  double-stranded DNA (dsDNA)
  episomal DNA
  DNA gyrase
  HBV DNA
  HLA-G DNA
  DNA homology
  human cloned DNA
  DNA hybridization
  DNA hybridization test
  improper repair of DNA
  naked plasmid DNA
  PCR for HIV DNA
  DNA polymerase
  DNA probe test
  DNA probe test for Lyme disease
  DNA repair
  single-stranded DNA
  DNA topoisomerase I (Topo I)
  DNA vaccination
  DNA vaccine
  DNA virus
DNA-anti-DNA system
DNA-binding test
DNA-carrier complex
DNA-chain terminator
DNase
  deoxyribonuclease

DNCB
  dinitrochlorobenzene
Doak
  Tar D.
Doak-Oil
Doan's
  D. Backache Pill
  Extra Strength D.
  D., Original
dobutamine stress echocardiography
  (DSE)
DOC
  disorder of cornification
dock
  bitter d.
  d. plantain
  tall d.
  yellow d.
docosanol cream
documented
  d. bacterial infection (DBI)
  d. viral infection (DVI)
dodecamer
dog
  d. dander
  d. disease
  d. distemper virus
  d. epithelium
  d. fennel
  d. flea
  d. flea bite
  nonshedding d.
  d. tapeworm
dog-ear
Dogger Bank itch
Dohi
  acropigmentation of D.
Dohle
  D. disease
  D. inclusion body
dolastatin
dolens
  phlegmasia alba d.
Dolichorespula **sting**
Dolobid
dolor
Dolorac
dolorimeter scoliosis
dolorosa
  adiposis d.
  neurolipomatosis d.
  tubercula d.

D

NOTES

domain
> catalytic d.
> death d.
> extracellular d. (ECD)
> Fas-associating protein with
>   death d. (FADD)
> immunoglobulin d.
> pleckstrin homology d.
> silencer of death d. (SODD)

Domeboro
> Otic D.

Dome-Paste boot

domesticus
> *Glycyphagus d.*

dominant
> autosomal d.
> lamellar d.
> d. phenotype

domino
> d. heart transplantation (DHT)
> d. procedure

Domiphen

Donath-Landsteiner
> D.-L. antibody
> D.-L. cold autoantibody
> D.-L. syndrome

d'ongle
> coup d.

Donizetti potion

donor
> d. allopeptide
> d. biopsy
> d. brain death
> cadaver d. (CAD)
> extended criteria d. (ECD)
> heart-beating d. (HBD)
> identical twin d.
> d. leukocyte infusion (DLI)
> living d. (LD)
> living-related d. (LRD)
> d. lymphocyte infusion (DLI)
> marginal d.
> matched related d. (MRD)
> matched unrelated d. (MURD)
> nonheart-beating d. (NHBD)
> d. sclera
> universal d.

donor-related warm ischemia

donor-specific
> d.-s. tolerance
> d.-s. transfusion (DST)

donor-transmitted lymphoma

Donovan body

donovani
> *Leishmania d.*

Donovania granulomatis

donovanosis

door-knob probe

doorknob spray tip

DOPA
> 3,4-dihydroxyphenylalanine

dopa
> d. radiation
> d. reaction

dopamine

dopa-oxidase

Doppler
> Laserflo laser D.
> D. ultrasound

d'orange
> peau d.

Dorcol

Dorfman-Chanarin syndrome

d'Orient
> bouton d.

Dormarex 2 Oral

Dormex

Dormin Oral

Dorothy Reed-Sternberg cell

dorsal
> d. surface
> d. wrist tenosynovitis

dorsalis
> acne d.
> tabes d.

dorsi
> elastofibroma d.

dorsoradial subluxation

Dortu phlebectomy hook

dory flop

Doryx Oral

dose
> booster d.
> cell d.
> effective d. (ED)
> erythema d.
> infecting d. (ID)
> L d.
> L+ d.
> lethal d. (LD)
> Lf d.
> Lo d.
> Lr d.
> maintenance d.
> minimal erythema d. (MED)
> minimal infecting d. (MID)
> minimal lethal d. (MLD)
> minimal phototoxic d. (MPD)
> minimal reacting d. (MRD)
> minimum effective d. (MED)
> minimum effective naproxen d.
>   (MEND)
> sensitizing d.
> shocking d.

Dosepak
Deltasone D.
Medrol D.
dose-related effect
dose-response curve
dosimeter
Rosenthal-French d.
dosing
once-daily d. (ODD)
pulse d.
DOTS
directly observed therapy short-course
dots
Trantas d.
double
d. antibody immunoassay
d. antibody method
d. antibody precipitation
d. antibody sandwich assay
d. drug treatment
d. (gel) diffusion precipitin test in
one dimension
d. immunodiffusion
d. immunodiffusion in agarose gels
test
d. negative cell
d. renal allograft
double-balloon triple lumen catheter
double-blind placebo-controlled food
challenge (DBPCFC)
double-contrast arthrography
double-crush syndrome
double-edge nail
double-hook Tyrell skin hook
double-sandwich IgM ELISA
doublestaining
fluorescent treponemal antibody
absorption d. (FTA-ABS-DS)
double-stranded DNA (dsDNA)
Douche
Yeast-Gard Medicated D.
doughnut wart
Douglas
D. fir
D. fir tree
douloureux
tic d.
Dove soap
Dovonex
dowager hump
dowicide
Dowicil 200

Dowling-Degos disease
Dowling-Meara epidermolysis bullosa
down
malignant d.
D. syndrome
Downey cell
down-regulation
downstream mediator
doxepin
d. HCl
d. hydrochloride cream
Doxil
doxofylline
doxorubicin
liposomal d.
Doxy-200
Doxy-Caps
Doxychel
D. injection
D. Oral
Doxycin
doxycycline pleurodesis
Doxy-Tabs
Doxytec
D.P.
Dalalone D.
DPAP interactive airway management
system
d-penicillamine
DPI
dry powder inhaler
DPOC
placebo-controlled oral challenge testing
DPT
diphtheria-pertussis-tetanus
DQB1
major histocompatibility complex
(MHC) class II allele DRB1,
DRB3, DRB4, DRB5, and D.
DQw1
DQw7
allele HLA D.
allele human leukocyte antigen D.
Dr.
Dr. Scholl's Athlete's Foot
Dr. Scholl's Maximum Strength
Tritin
DR1 allele
DR3 allele
DR5 allele
dracontiasis
dracunculiasis

D

NOTES

dracunculosis
Dracunculus medinensis
Dragon
    Minor Blue D.
drain
    Clot Stop d.
drainage
    enteric pancreatic d.
    paranasal sinus d.
    percussion and postural d. (P and PD)
    percutaneous abscess and fluid d. (PAFD)
    postural d.
    thoracic duct d. (TDD)
Draize Repeat Insult patch test
Dramamine
    D. II
    D. Oral
Dramilin Injection
Drechslera
Drenison
DRESS
    drug rash with eosinophil and systemic symptom
        DRESS syndrome of Bocquet and Roujeau
dressing
    AcryDerm border island d.
    Acticel wound d.
    Acticoat burn d.
    Airstrip composite d.
    AlgiDerm alginate d.
    AlgiDerm wound d.
    alginate d.
    AlgiSite alginate d.
    AlgiSite wound d.
    Algisorb wound d.
    Algosteril alginate d.
    Alldress composite d.
    Allevyn adhesive foam d.
    Allevyn cavity foam d.
    Allevyn island foam d.
    Allevyn synthetic d.
    Allevyn tracheostomy foam d.
    Amerigel topical ointment hydrogel d.
    Aquacel Hydrofiber d.
    Aquacel wound packing and d.
    Aquasorb transparent hydrogel d.
    ArtAssist leg compression d.
    Band-Aid composite d.
    Bard Absorption d.
    BGC Matrix hydrocolloid d.
    Biobrane synthetic d.
    Bioclusive synthetic d.
    Biolex hydrogel d.
    Biopatch antimicrobial d.
    Biopatch foam d.
    BreakAway absorptive wound d.
    CarraFilm wound d.
    CarraSmart foam d.
    CarraSorb H calcium alginate wound d.
    CarraSorb hydrogel d.
    Carrasyn hydrogel wound d.
    Centurion SorbaView composite d.
    CircPlus leg compression d.
    Circulon leg compression d.
    closed wet d.
    Coban d.
    CombiDERM ACD hydrocolloid d.
    Comfeel hydrocolloid d.
    Comfeel synthetic d.
    Comfeel Ulcus d.
    Compeed Skinprotector d.
    Conformant wound d.
    contact-layer wound d.
    Covaderm composite d.
    Coverlet composite d.
    Covertell composite d.
    Curaderm hydrocolloid d.
    Curafil hydrogel d.
    Curafoam foam d.
    Curafoam wound d.
    Curagel Hydrogel d.
    Curasol hydrogel d.
    Curasorb calcium alginate d.
    Curasorb Zinc alginate d.
    Curity ABD absorptive d.
    Curtinova hydrocolloid d.
    Cutifilm Plus composite d.
    Cutinova foam d.
    Cutinova Hydro d.
    Cutinova Thin hydrocolloid d.
    Dermacea alginate d.
    Dermagran hydrogel d.
    DermaMend cavity foam d.
    DermaMend foam wound d.
    DermaMend hydrogel d.
    DermaMend island foam d.
    Dermanet contact layer wound d.
    DermAssist Glycerin hydrogel d.
    DermAssist hydrocolloid d.
    Dermatell hydrocolloid d.
    DiabGel hydrogel d.
    DuoDerm CGF hydrocolloid d.
    DuoDerm SCB leg compression d.
    DuoDerm synthetic d.
    Dyna-Flex leg compression d.
    Elastoplast elastic d.
    Elta Dermal hydrogel d.
    Epi-lock wound d.
    ExuDerm hydrocolloid d.
    Exu-Dry absorptive d.
    Fibracol collagen-alginate d.

Flexzan foam wound d.
FyBron alginate wound d.
Gelocast Unna boot leg
  compression d.
gel wound d.
Gentell alginate wound d.
Gentell foam wound d.
Gentell hydrogel d.
GraftCyte gauze wound d.
Handages d.
hyCare G hydrogel d.
hyCure collagen hemostatic
  wound d.
Hydrasorb foam wound d.
Hydrocol hydrocolloid d.
hydrocolloid d.
hydrogel d.
hydrophilic polymer d.
HyFil hydrogel d.
Hypergel hydrogel d.
Hyperion Advanced alginate d.
Hyperion bordered hydrocolloid d.
Hyperion hydrophilic wound gel
  hydrogel d.
Hyperion thin hydrocolloid d.
Iamin gel wound d.
Iamin hydrogel d.
Inerpan d.
Intelligent d.
IntraSite hydrogel d.
Iodoflex absorptive d.
Iodosorb absorptive d.
Kalginate alginate d.
Kaltostat alginate d.
LYOfoam A, C, T foam d.
LYOfoam Extra foam d.
Maxorb alginate wound d.
Medipore Dress-it d.
Mepore absorptive d.
Mesalt debridement d.
Mitraflex Plus foam d.
Mitraflex SC foam d.
Mitraflex wound d.
MPM composite d.
MPM hydrogel d.
MultiPad absorptive d.
nonocclusive d.
Normlgel hydrogel d.
N-Terface contact layer wound d.
Nu-Derm hydrocolloid d.
Nu Gauze d.
Nu-Gel hydrogel wound d.

Nu-Gel synthetic d.
Oasis wound d.
occlusive d.
Omniderm synthetic d.
open wet d.
OpSite Flexigrid adhesive d.
OpSite Plus composite d.
OpSite postop composite d.
OpSite semipermeable d.
OsmoCyte pillow wound d.
Owens Surgical d.
Panoplex hydrogel d.
plastic adhesive d.
Polyderm foam d.
PolyMem alginate d.
PolyMem foam d.
polymer film d.
polymer foam d.
Polyskin II d.
Primaderm d.
Primapore absorptive wound d.
Primer leg compression d.
Pro-Clude transparent film
  wound d.
ProCyte transparent adhesive
  film d.
Profore leg compression d.
RepliCare hydrocolloid d.
Reston foam wound d.
Reston hydrocolloid d.
Restore alginate d.
Restore hydrocolloid d.
Restore hydrogel d.
Royl-Derm wound hydrogel d.
Saf-Gel hydrogel d.
SeaSorb alginate d.
semipermeable d.
SignaDress Sterile hydrocolloid d.
Silon wound d.
Siloskin d.
SiteGuard MVP transparent
  adhesive film d.
SkinTegrity hydrogel d.
SofSorb absorptive d.
SoftCloth absorptive d.
Sof-Wick d.
SoloSite hydrogel d.
SorbaView wound d.
Sorbsan alginate d.
Sorbsan wound d.
StrataSorb composite wound d.
SurePress leg compression d.

D

NOTES

173

dressing *(continued)*
    Synthaderm wound d.
    Tegaderm semipermeable d.
    Tegaderm transparent d.
    Tegagel hydrogel d.
    Tegagen HG alginate wound d.
    Tegagen HI alginate d.
    Tegapore contact-layer wound d.
    Tegasorb synthetic d.
    Tegasorb Thin hydrocolloid d.
    Telfa composite d.
    Telfamax absorptive d.
    Tendersorb ABD absorptive d.
    Tenderwrap leg compression d.
    Thera-Boot leg compression d.
    d. therapy
    THINSite with BioFilm hydrogel
      topical wound d.
    Tielle absorptive d.
    tie-over bolster d.
    Triad hydrocolloid d.
    Ultec hydrocolloid d.
    Uniflex polyurethane adhesive
      surgical d.
    Unna-Flex leg compression d.
    Unna-Pak leg compression d.
    Vari/Moist wound d.
    Veingard d.
    Ventex composite d.
    Viasorb composite d.
    Vigilon d.
    water-impermeable, nonsilicone-based
      occlusive d.
    wet d.
    Woun'Dres hydrogel d.
    Wound Span Bridge II d.
    Zipzoc Stocking leg compression d.
dressing/sheet
    Tegagel d.
dressing/wrap
    ArtAssist compression d.
Dricort
    Dermarest D.
Dri-Ear Otic
dried
    d. fruit dermatitis
    d. human serum
drift
    antigenic d.
drip
    postnasal d. (PND)
dripping
    candle d.
Drisdol Oral
Dristan
    D. Long Lasting Nasal solution
    D. Sinus Caplets
Drithocreme HP

Dritho-Scalp
drive
    hypoxic ventilatory d. (HVD)
Drixoral
    D. Cough & Congestion Liquid
      Caps
    D. Non-Drowsy
    D. Syrup
DR/MLC cell marker
dronabinol
drop attack
droplet
    d. infection
    d. nucleus
drop-like psoriasis
dropout
    crypt epithelial cell d.
droppings
    Australian parrot d.
    pigeon d.
drops
    Afrin Children's Nose d.
    Allergan Ear d.
    Cerumenex ear d.
    Coly-Mycin S Otic d.
    Debrox d.
    Decongestant Nose d.
    Mallazine Eye d.
    Moisture Ophthalmic d.
    Myapap d.
    Patanol eye d.
    RO-Eye d.
    Rondec d.
    Triaminic Oral Infant d.
    Tri-P Oral Infant d.
dropsy
    epidemic d.
Drotic Otic
drowsiness
Droxia
DRS
    diffuse reflectance spectroscopy
drug
    adrenergic d.
    d. allergy
    d. alopecia
    d. anaphylaxis
    anticholinergic d.
    antimalarial d.
    antirheumatic d.
    antisense d.
    antiviral d.
    chondroprotective d.
    cytotoxic d.
    disease-modifying antirheumatic d.
      (DMAD, DMARD)
    d. eruption
    d. hypersensitivity

immunophilin-binding d.
immunosuppressive d.
d. interaction
d. intolerance
ISAtx247 immunosuppressive d.
large-molecular-weight d.
lysosomotropic antimalarial d.
MR d.
muscle-relaxant d.
myorelaxant d.
noncross-reactive d.
nonsteroidal anti-inflammatory d.
  (NSAID)
orphan d.
d. overdose
d. rash
d. rash with eosinophil and
  systemic symptom (DRESS)
d. rash with eosinophil and
  systemic symptoms of Bocquet
  and Roujeau
rauwolfia d.
d. reaction
second-line d. (SLD)
simple d.
slow-acting antirheumatic d.
  (SAARD)
sulfa d.
uricosuric d.
drug-associated erythema multiforme
drug-fast
drug-induced
d.-i. acanthosis nigricans
d.-i. alopecia
d.-i. bullous photosensitivity
d.-i. delayed multiorgan
  hypersensitivity syndrome
  (DIDMOS)
d.-i. delayed multiorgan
  hypersensitivity syndrome of
  Sontheimer and Houpt
d.-i. depression of immune system
d.-i. erythema
d.-i. lupus
d.-i. lymphadenopathy
d.-i. photodermatitis
d.-i. pneumonia
d.-i. progressive symptom sclerosis
d.-i. purpura
d.-i. SLE syndrome
d.-i. systemic lupus erythematosus
d.-i. thrombocytopenia

drug-related
d.-r. immunohemolytic anemia
d.-r. myopathy
DRUJ
distal radicular joint
drummer digit
DRw53
allele HLA D.
allele human leukocyte antigen D.
dry
d. cough
d. cutaneous leishmaniasis
D. Eyes solution
D. Eye Therapy solution
d. flush
d. gangrene
d. ice
d. leprosy
d. lips
d. mouth
Peri-Strips D.
d. powder inhaler (DPI)
d. skin
d. tetter
dry-ice slush
dryness
excessive d.
Dryox
D. Gel
D. Wash
Drysol
DS
Bactrim DS
Cotrim DS
Septra DS
Sulfatrim DS
Tolectin DS
Uroplus DS
DSAP
disseminated superficial actinic
porokeratosis
DSC
disodium cromoglycate
dsDNA
double-stranded DNA
DSE
dobutamine stress echocardiography
DSG
deoxyspergualin
Dsg
desmoglein

NOTES

D

175

Dsg1
desmoglein-1
Dsg3
desmoglein-3
Dsg3 antigen
DSMB
Data Safety Monitoring Board
DSRS
distal splenorenal shunt
DST
dexamethasone suppression test
donor-specific transfusion
d4T
Zerit
DTaP
acellular pertussis vaccine combined with
diphtheria and tetanus toxoid
DTEG
Dermatology Teachers Exchange Group
DTH
delayed-type hypersensitivity
DTIC
dacarbazine
DTIC-Dome
DTM
dermatophyte test medium
DTP
diphtheria toxoid, tetanus toxoid, and
pertussis vaccine
DTT
dithiothreitol
Duadacin Capsule
dual-beam photon absorptiometry
dual-energy x-ray absorptiometry
(DEXA, DXA)
dual-fluorescence analysis
dual-function enzyme
dual kidney transplant
duazomycin
Dubois
D. abscess
D. disease
D. sign
duboisii
Histoplasma d.
Dubreuilh
circumscribed precancerous
melanosis of D.
D. elastoma
D. precancerous melanosis
precancerous melanosis of D.
Ducas and Kapetanakis pigmented
purpura
Duchenne muscular dystrophy
duck
d. embryo origin vaccine (DEV)
d. feather
d. hepatitis virus

d. influenza virus
d. plague
d. plague virus
ducreyi
Haemophilus d.
Ducrey test
duct
eccrine d.
Pecquet d.
ductopenia
ductopenic rejection
Duffy
D. antigen
D. blood antibody type
D. blood group
Duhring
D. disease
D. pruritus
Dukes disease
Dulbecco medium
dumas
dumdum fever
dumoffii
Legionella d.
Dumon-Harrell bronchoscope
Duncan
D. disease
D. syndrome
d'Unna
Pate d.
Dunnett multiple comparison test
Dunnigan syndrome
duodenale
Ancylostoma d.
DuoDerm
D. CGF hydrocolloid
D. CGF hydrocolloid dressing
D. hydroactive gel
D. SCB
D. SCB leg compression dressing
D. synthetic dressing
DuoFilm
D. Solution
Duoforte
Duo-Medihaler Aerosol
DuoPlant
Duo-Trach
duovirus
Duplex T
duplication
1q d.
Dupuytren
D. contracture
D. disease
durable-press
d.-p. allergic contact dermatitis
d.-p. allergy
Durafedrin

Dura-Gest
Duralone Injection
dural sinus thrombosis
Duralutin injection
Duramist plus
Durand-Nicholas-Favre disease
Duranest injection
Durapore membrane disc
DuraScreen sunscreen
duration
    D. Nasal solution
    d. of treatment
Duratuss
dura twist skin hook
Dura-Vent/DA
Duricef
Durie and Salmon multiple myeloma
  classification
Durrax
durum
    fibroma d.
    heloma d.
    papilloma d.
    ulcus d.
dust
    barn d.
    grain d.
    house d.
    d. mite
    mushroom d.
dustborne
Dutton
    D. disease
    D. relapsing fever
Duval disposable dermatome
Duvenhaga virus
DVI
    documented viral infection
Dwelle Ophthalmic solution
DXA (*var. of* DEXA)
DXM
    dexamethasone
DXR
    delayed xenograft rejection
Dycill
Dyclone
dyclonine hydrochloride
dye
    acid d.
    azo d.
    azobenzene d.

    D&C d.
    disperse d.
    food d.
    injectable d.
    d. laser
Dymenate Injection
dymple
Dynabac
Dyna-Care pressure pad system
Dynacin Oral
Dyna-Flex leg compression dressing
Dyna-Hex topical
dynamometer
    Collins d.
Dynapen
Dy-o-Derm
Dyonics
    D. basket forceps
    D. Dyosite office arthroscopy
    system
    D. InteliJet fluid management
    system
    D. suction punch
dyphylline
dysarthria
dysautonomia
    familial d.
dysbaric
dysbetalipoproteinemia
    familial d.
dyschondroplasia with hemangioma
dyschroia
dyschromatosis symmetrica
dyschromia
    cutaneous d.
dyschromicum
dyscornification
    hypergranulotic d.
dyscrasia
dysenteriae
    Shigella flexneri d.
    viral d.
dysenteric arthritis
dysentery
    d. antitoxin
    balantidial d.
    ciliate d.
    scorbutic d.
    Sonne d.
    spirillar d.
    sporadic d.

D

NOTES

dysesthesia
    d. disorder
    d. pedis
dysfunction
    antibody d.
    audiovestibular d.
    biopsy-negative graft d. (BNGD)
    chronic graft d.
    emotional d.
    erectile d.
    intestinal mucosal d.
    meibomian gland d.
    multiple organ system d. (MOSD)
    myocardial d.
    neuroimmune d.
    phagocyte d.
    sensorineural d.
    small airways d.
    Study of Left Ventricular D.
    temporomandibular d. (TMD)
    vascular d.
dysgammaglobulinemia
dysgenesis
    gonadal d.
    reticular d.
dyshidria
dyshidrosis, dyshydrosis, dysidrosis,
  pl. **dyshidroses**
    lamellar d.
    sole d.
    trichophytic d.
dyshidrotic eczema
dysidria
dysidrosis (*var. of* dyshidrosis)
dyskeratinization
dyskeratoma
    acantholytic d.
    focal acantholytic d.
    warty d.
dyskeratosis, pl. **dyskeratoses**
    acantholytic d.
    benign d.
    d. congenita
    focal acantholytic d.
    malignant d.
    transient acantholytic d.
dyskeratotic keratinocyte
dyskinetic cilia syndrome
dyslipoidosis
dysmenorrhoeica
    dermatitis d.
dysmetabolism
    tryptophan d.
dysmorphobia
dysmorphogenesis
dysmucopolysaccharidosis
    fibrocytic d.

Dysne-Inhal
dysostosis, pl. **dysostoses**
    mandibulofacial d.
dyspareunia
dyspeptic
dysphagia
dysphagocytosis
    congenital d.
dyspigmentation
dysplasia
    acetabular d.
    anhidrotic ectodermal d.
    autoimmune polyendocrinopathy-
      candidiasis-ectodermal d.
      (APECED)
    chondrodysplasia punctata d.
    cleidocranial d.
    congenital ectodermal d.
    diastrophic d.
    ectodermal d.
    familial white folded mucosal d.
    fibrous d.
    hidrotic ectodermal d.
    hypohidrotic ectodermal d. (HED)
    Kniest d.
    late-onset spondyloepiphyseal d.
    lymphopenic thymic d.
    mandibuloacral d.
    mesodermal d.
    metaphyseal d.
    multiple epiphyseal d.
    neutrophil d.
    otospondylometaphyseal d.
      (OSMED)
    polyostotic fibrous d.
    Rapp-Hodgkin ectodermal d.
    sphenoid d.
    spondyloepiphyseal d. (SED)
    thymic d.
dysplastic
    d. nevus
    d. nevus syndrome
dyspnea
dyspneic
dysprosium ferric hydroxide
dysproteinemia
    angioimmunoblastic
      lymphadenopathy with d. (AILD)
dysproteinemic purpura
dysraphism
    spinal d.
dysregulated lymphocytic apoptosis
dysregulation
    immune d.
dyssebacia
dyssynchrony
    thoracoabdominal d.
dysthymia

dystrophia
    d. canthorum
    d. unguium
dystrophic
    d. calcinosis
    d. calcinosis cutis
    d. epidermolysis bullosa
    d. epidermolysis bullosa,
      albopapuloid variant
    D. Epidermolysis Bullosa Research
      Association of America (DEBRA)
    d. palmoplantar hyperkeratosis
dystrophica
    elastosis d.
    epidermolysis bullosa d.
dystrophin
dystrophy
    autoimmune polyendocrinopathy-
      candidiasis-ectodermal d.
      (APECED)

Becker muscular d.
congenital fascial d.
distal d.
Duchenne muscular d.
Emery-Dreifuss d.
epidermolysis bullosa with
  muscular d.
fascioscapulohumeral d.
intermittent hair-follicle d.
lamellar d.
limb-girdle d.
medial canaliform d.
median canaliform d.
median nail d.
merosin deficiency d.
muscular d.
oculopharyngeal d.
reflex sympathetic d. (RSD)
ten-nail d.
twenty-nail d.

NOTES

D

E
- Florone E
- E rosette

E₁
- prostaglandin E_1 (PGE_1)

E₂
- prostaglandin E_2 (PGE_2)
- purine-stimulated prostaglandin E_2 (PGE_2)

E5 monoclonal antibody

EAC
- Ehrlich ascites carcinoma
- erythema annulare centrifugum
- erythrocytes, antibody, complement
- external auditory canal
  - EAC rosette
  - EAC rosette assay

EAE
- experimental allergic encephalitis
- experimental allergic encephalomyelitis

EAG
- experimental autoimmune gastritis

EAHF
- eczema, asthma, hayfever
  - EAHF complex

EAI
- erythema ab igne

ear
- middle e.
- Otocalm E.
- e. pit
- sugarcane e.

EARD
- environmentally associated rheumatic disorder

Earle L fibrosarcoma

earlobe
- e. allergic dermatitis
- e. crease
- e. sign of nickel sensitivity

early
- e. congenital syphilis
- e. latent syphilis
- e. reaction
- e. yaw

early-phase
- e.-p. reaction (EPR)
- e.-p. response

EARTS
- European Anti-ICAM Renal Transplant Study

EASI
- Eczema Area and Severity Index

Easprin

EAST
- enzyme allergosorbent test

eastern
- E. coral snake
- E. coral snake bite
- e. equine encephalomyelitis virus
- E. tick-borne rickettsiosis

easy bruising syndrome

Eaton
- E. agent
- E. agent pneumonia

Eaton-Lambert syndrome

EB
- elementary body
- epidermolysis bullosa
- Epstein-Barr
  - EB nuclear antigen test
  - EB simplex
  - EB viral capsid antigen test
  - EB virus

EBA
- epidermolysis bullosa acquisita

ebastine

EBM
- evidence-based medicine

EBMT
- European Group for Bone Marrow Transplantation

EBNA
- Epstein-Barr nuclear antigen
  - EBNA IgG ELISA test

Ebola
- E. hemorrhagic fever
- E. Ivory Coast
- E. virus

EB-specific IgM test

EBV
- Epstein-Barr virus
  - EBV glycoprotein gp110
  - EBV infection

EC
- Euro-Collins
  - EC solution

E-C
- Apo-Erythro E-C

EC₅₀
- median effective concentration

ECASA
- enteric-coated acetylsalicylic acid

ECBO
- enteric cytopathogenic bovine orphan
  - ECBO virus

E

eccentrica
: hyperkeratosis e.
: keratoderma e.
: poliosis e.

ecchymoma

ecchymosed

ecchymosis, pl. **ecchymoses**
: old e.
: Roederer e.

ecchymotic
: e. mark
: e. rash

ECCL
: encephalocraniocutaneous lipomatosis

eccrine
: e. acrospiroma
: e. adenocarcinoma
: e. angiomatous hamartoma
: e. bromhidrosis
: e. carcinoma
: e. chromhidrosis
: e. duct
: e. epithelioma
: e. hidradenitis
: e. hidrocystoma
: e. poroma
: e. spiradenoma
: e. squamous syringometaplasia
: e. sweat gland
: e. syringofibroadenoma
: e. tumor

ECD
: extended criteria donor
: extracellular domain

ECF-A
: eosinophil chemotactic factor of anaphylaxis

ECG
: electrocardiogram

echidninus
: *Laelaps* e.

echinococcosis

Echinococcus
: *E. granulosus*
: *E. multilocularis*

echinococcus

echinoderm

ECHO
: enteric cytopathogenic human orphan
: ECHO virus

echocardiography
: dobutamine stress e. (DSE)

echo sign

echoviral exanthema

echovirus

eclabium

ECLAM
: European Consensus Lupus Activity Measure

eclipse
: e. period
: e. phase

ECLM
: European Confederation for Laboratory Medicine

ECLP
: extracorporeal liver perfusion

ECM
: erythema chronicum migrans
: extracellular matrix

ECM-degrading proteinase

ECMO
: enteric cytopathogenic monkey orphan
: extracorporeal membrane oxygenation
: ECMO virus

ECN
: epithelioid combined nevi

ECN-BLITZ
: E.-B. nevus

ECN-DPN
: epithelioid combined nevi deep penetrating nevus

EcoCheck oxygen monitor

ecologic alteration

E-Complex-600

EcoNail antifungal

econazole nitrate

Econopred Plus Ophthalmic

Ecostatin

ecotaxis

Ecotrin

ecotropic virus

ECP
: eosinophil cationic protein
: erythropoietic coproporphyria

ecphyma

ECSO
: enteric cytopathogenic swine orphan
: ECSO virus

ectasia
: acral arteriolar e.
: cutaneous e.
: papillary e.
: sacral root sheath e.
: senile e.
: spider e.

Ectasule

ecthyma
: e. contagiosum
: contagious e.
: e. gangrenosum
: e. infectiosum

ecthymatiform

ecthymatous syphilid

ectoantigen
ectoderm
ectodermal
    e. dysplasia
    e. dysplasia, ectrodactyly and cleft
      lip and/or palate (EEC)
ectodermatosis
ectodermogenic neurosyphilis
ectodermosis erosiva pluriorificialis
ectogenous
ectoparasite
ectopic
    e. cutaneous schistosomiasis
    e. keratinization
    e. sebaceous gland
Ectosone
ectothrix infection
ectotoxin
ectozoon
ectrodactyly, ectodermal, clefting (EEC)
ectrodactyly-ectodermal dysplasia-clefting
  syndrome
ectromelia virus
ECU
    extensor carpi ulnaris
eczema
    adolescent e.
    adult e.
    allergic e.
    E. Area and Severity Index
      (EASI)
    e. articulorum
    asteatotic e.
    e., asthma, hayfever (EAHF)
    e., asthma, hay fever complex
      (EAHF complex)
    atopic e.
    baker's e.
    childhood e.
    chronic e.
    contact e.
    e. craquelé
    e. crustosum
    e. diabeticorum
    dyshidrotic e.
    e. epilans
    e. epizootica
    e. erythematosum
    flexural e.
    follicular nummular e.
    hand e.
    e. herpeticum

housewives' e.
e. hypertrophicum
idiopathic late-onset e.
infantile e.
e. intertrigo
intertrigo e.
lichenoid e.
e. madidans
e. marginatum
e. neuriticum
nummular e.
e. nummulare
nutritional deficiency e.
orbicular e.
e. papulosum
e. parasiticum
e. pustulosum
e. rubrum
e. scrofuloderma
seborrheic e.
e. seborrhoeicum
e. siccum
e. solare
e. squamosum
stasis e.
e. stasis
topical e.
tropical e.
e. tyloticum
e. vaccinatum
varicose e.
e. verrucosum
e. vesiculosum
weeping e.
winter e.
xerotic e.
eczematid
    exsiccation e.
eczematization
eczematize
eczematodes
    impetigo e.
eczematogenic
eczematogenous
eczematoid
    e. dermatitis
    e. pruritic plaque
    e. seborrhea
eczematoides
    dermatitis infectiosa e.
eczematous
    e. lesion

E

NOTES

eczematous *(continued)*
  e. patch
  e. PMLE
  e. polymorphous light eruption
  e. reaction
ED
  effective dose
edema
  acute hemorrhagic e. (AHE)
  angioneurotic e.
  brawny e.
  bullous e.
  dependent e.
  e. of feet
  e. of hand
  hemorrhagic e.
  hereditary angioneurotic e. (HAE, HANE)
  hysterical e.
  indolent nonpitting e.
  inflammatory e.
  intercellular e.
  intracellular e.
  laryngeal e.
  massive cerebral e.
  Milton e.
  e. neonatorum
  noninflammatory e.
  palpebral e.
  periodic e.
  persistent e.
  pitting e.
  Quincke e.
  remitting seronegative symmetric synovitis with pitting e. (RS3PE)
  Yangtze e.
edematous
edge effect
Edmonston-Zagreb vaccine
edobacomab
EDRF
  endothelium-derived relaxing factor
EDSS
  expanded disability status scale
EDTA
  ethylenediaminetetraacetic acid
Edwardsiella
EEC
  ectodermal dysplasia, ectrodactyly and cleft lip and/or palate
  ectrodactyly, ectodermal, clefting
  EEC syndrome
EED
  erythema elevatum diutinum
EEE
  EEE virus
E.E.S. Oral

EEU
  environmental exposure unit
EFA
  essential fatty acid
Efalith ointment
efavirenz
Efedron
effect
  allogenic e.
  antiapoptotic e.
  antiproliferative e.
  cidal e.
  contrast e.
  counterregulatory e.
  cytopathic e. (CPE)
  Danysz e.
  Deelman e.
  dose-related e.
  edge e.
  first-pass drug e.
  graft-versus-leukemia e.
  isomorphic e.
  Köbner e.
  Koebner effect
  light-sparing e.
  Lyon e.
  nongenomic glucocorticoid e.
  postanesthetic e.
  postpartum e.
  prepriming e.
  proinflammatory e.
  secondary e.
  side e.
  squeeze e.
  steal e.
  tattooing e.
  tendonesis e.
  Tindall e.
  veto e.
  virostatic e.
effective dose (ED)
effector
  e. cell
  e. molecule
  nephritogenic e.
  e. pathway
Effersyl
efficacy
efficiency
  hair removal e. (HRE)
  sleep e.
effluvium
  anagen e.
  short anagen telogen e.
  telogen e.
effort syndrome

effusion
>joint e.
>parapneumonic e.

Efidac/24 chlorpheniramine

eflornithine hydrochloride

Efodine

Efudex topical

EGF
>epidermal growth factor

egg-passage
>rabies vaccine, Flury strain e.-p.

eggplant

egg shell nail

EGM
>extraglandular manifestation

Ehlers-Danlos
>E.-D. syndrome
>E.-D. syndrome, arthrochalasia type
>E.-D. syndrome, hypermobility type
>E.-D. syndrome, kyphoscoliotic type
>E.-D. syndrome type X
>E.-D. syndrome, vascular type

Ehrlich
>E. ascites carcinoma (EAC)
>E. ascites carcinoma rosette assay
>E. phenomenon
>E. postulate
>E. side-chain theory

Ehrlichia
>*E. canis*
>*E. chaffeensis*
>*E. ewengii*
>*E. sennetsu*

ehrlichiosis
>human granulocytic e.

EI
>erythema infectiosum

EIA
>enzyme immunoassay
>enzyme-linked immunoassay
>exercise-induced anaphylaxis
>exercise-induced asthma
>>EIA diagnosis

EIB
>exercise-induced bronchoconstriction
>exercise-induced bronchospasm

eicosanoid inhibition

eicosapentaenoic acid

Eikenella

EIRDS
>exercise-induced respiratory distress syndrome

EI.U
>ELISA unit

ekiri

elacin

ELAD artificial liver

ELAM
>endothelial-leukocyte adhesion molecule

ELAM-1
>endothelial leukocyte adhesion molecule-1

ELA-Max cream

elapid

Elapidae

Elase-Chloromycetin topical

Elase topical

elastase
>neutrophil e.
>polymorphonuclear leukocyte e.
>*Pseudomonas e.*

elastic
>e. fiber
>e. fibers stain
>e. recoil
>e. skin
>e. tissue
>e. wrap

elastica
>helminthiasis e.

elastic-fiber fragmentation

elasticity
>sputum viscosity and e.

elasticum
>localized acquired cutaneous pseudoxanthoma e.
>periumbilical perforating pseudoxanthoma e.
>pseudoxanthoma e. (PXE)

elasticus
>Lewandowsky nevus e.

Elastikon elastic tape

elastin

elastofibroma dorsi

Elasto-Gel hydrogel sheet

elastoid degeneration

elastolysis
>generalized e.
>middermal e.

elastolytic giant cell granuloma

elastoma
>Dubreuilh e.
>juvenile e.
>Miescher e.

E

NOTES

elastomer
    thermoplastic e. (TPE)
elastomeric
    e. complex
    e. pump
Elastomull elastic gauze bandage
Elastoplast elastic dressing
elastorrhexis
elastosis
    actinic e.
    e. colloidalis conglomerata
    cutaneous e.
    e. dystrophica
    linear focal e.
    nodular e.
    e. perforans serpiginosa (EPS)
    perforating calcific e.
    senile e.
    solar e.
    thermal e.
elastotic
    e. degeneration
    e. nodules of anthelix
    e. stria
Elavil
elbow
    golfer e.
    Little League e.
    Mayo classification of
      rheumatoid e.
    tennis e.
    transplant e.
Eldecort Topical
elder
    E. classification
    marsh e.
    rough marsh e.
    Vitadye makeup by E.
Eldopaque
    E. Forte
    E. Forte cream
Eldoquin
    E. Forte
EleCare medical food
elective
    e. culture
    e. low-risk recipient
    e. lymph node dissection (ELND)
Electra 1000C coagulation analyzer
electroacupuncture
Electro-Acuscope
electrocardiogram (ECG)
    12-lead e.
electrocautery
electrocoagulated
electrocoagulation
    e. biterminal device
    pinpoint e.

electrode
    indifferent e.
    e. siccation
electrodermal
    e. diagnosis
    e. testing
electrodermatome
electrodesiccation
    curettage and e. (CE)
electrofulguration
electroimmunodiffusion
electrolysis
electromagnetic
    e. field
    e. radiation
electromyographic feature
electromyography (EMG)
electron
    e. beam
    e. microscope (EM)
    e. microscopy
electronic filter
electrooculogram
electrophilic
    e. ethylene episulfonium
    e. stress (ES)
electrophoresis
    cerebrospinal fluid
      immunofixation e. (CSF-IFE)
    immunodeficiency e.
    immunofixation e. (IFE)
    polyacrylamide gel e. (PAGE)
    pulsed field gel e. (PFGE)
    serum immunofixation e. (SIFE)
    serum protein e. (SPEP)
    sodium dodecyl sulfate-
      polyacrylamide gel e. (SDS-
      PAGE)
    urinary e.
    urine immunofixation e. (UIFE)
    urine protein e. (UPEP)
electrophoretic mobility shift assay
  (EMSA)
electrophoretogram
    serum protein e. (SPE)
electrophototherapy
ElectroRegenesis therapy device (ERTD)
electrosection
electrosurgery
    bipolar e.
electrosurgical epilation
electrotransfer test
Elejalde syndrome (ES)
element
    kappa-deleting e.
    promotor e.
    Rev-responsive e. (RRE)
    trace e.

elemental diet
elementary
    e. body (EB)
    e. lesion
elephant
    e. leg
    e. skin
elephantiac
elephantiasic
elephantiasis
    e. arabicum
    e. arabum
    e. asturiensis
    congenital e.
    filarial e.
    e. graecorum
    lymphangiectatic e.
    e. neurofibromatosis
    e. neuromatosa
    neuromatosis e.
    nevoid e.
    nostras e.
    e. nostras
    e. nostra verrucosa
    e. telangiectodes
    e. tropica
elephantoid fever
elevation
    blanched cutaneous e.
    rest, ice, compresses, e. (RICE)
elevator
    Freer septum e.
    e. grain dust mite
elevatum
ELF
    epithelial lining fluid
Elgiloy
elicitation
elimination
    e. diet
    food e.
    immune e.
    e. procedure
    sweat chloride e.
Elimite Cream
ELISA
    enzyme-linked immunosorbent assay
    double-sandwich IgM ELISA
    ELISA test
    ELISA unit (EI.U)

ELISPOT
    enzyme-linked immunospot assay
    ELISPOT test
Elixicon
Elixir
    Allergy E.
    Brofed E.
    Bromaline E.
    Bromanate E.
    Bromphen E.
    Cold & Allergy E.
    Dimaphen E.
    Dimetane Decongestant E.
    Genatap E.
Elixophyllin
elizabethan
    Bartonella e.
Elliot sign
Ellipse compact spacer
elliptical
    e. biopsy
    e. incision
elliptocyte
Ellis-van Creveld syndrome
Ellman Surgitron
ELM
    epiluminescence microscopy
elm
    American e.
    Chinese e.
    fall e.
    slippery e.
    e. tree
    e. tree pollen
ELND
    elective lymph node dissection
Elocon topical
elongin
ELP
    extracorporeal liver perfusion
Elset long stretch bandage
Elta
    E. Dermal hydrogel dressing
    E. Dermal impregnated gauze
    E. Dermal wound cleanser
Eltor
eluate
    glomerular e.
EM
    electron microscope
    erythema multiforme
emaculation

NOTES

ematode
EMB
endomyocardial biopsy
ethambutol
emboli (*pl. of* embolus)
embolia cutis medicamentosa
embolic
e. gangrene
e. nodule
embolism
plasmodium e.
pulmonary e.
embolization
bronchial artery e.
renal cholesterol e. (RCE)
embolus, pl. **emboli**
atheromatous e.
cholesterol e.
septal e.
septic e.
embryogenesis
embryology
EMC
encephalomyocarditis
EMC virus
emerging virus
Emery-Dreifuss dystrophy
emetine
EMG
electromyography
Emgel topical
EMIT
enzyme-multiplied immunoassay
technique
EMLA
eutectic mixture of local anesthetics
EMLA anesthetic disc
EMLA cream
EMLA topical
EMMPRIN
extracellular matrix metalloproteinase
inducer
Emo-Cort
emollient
emotional
e. dysfunction
e. flushing
e. hyperhidrosis
e. stress
EMPD
extramammary Paget disease
emperipolesis
emphlysis
emphractic
emphraxis
emphysema
subcutaneous e.
empiric therapy

Empirin
Emplasterium urea **paste**
empty sella syndrome
empyema
empyesis
EMS
eosinophilia-myalgia syndrome
EMSA
electrophoretic mobility shift assay
emulsifiable ointment
emulsifying agent
emulsion
Pusey e.
radiodermatitis e. (RE)
wound dressing e. (WDE)
E-Mycin
E.-M. Oral
E-Mycin-E
EN
erythema nodosum
en
en bloc transplant
en bloc transplantation
en coup de sabre
en coup de sabre scalp lesion
en passant
ENA
extractable nuclear antigen
ENA antigen
enamel
e. paint skin
e. paint spot appearance
enanthem
enanthema
enanthematous
enanthesis
Enbrel plus ATG
Encap
Novo-Rythro E.
encapsulated
e. neuroma
e. organism
encephalitide
encephalitis
acute disseminated e. (ADE)
acute necrotizing e.
Australian X e.
Baló concentric e.
bunyavirus e.
California e. (CE)
Coxsackie e.
Dawson e.
epidemic e.
equine e.
experimental allergic e. (EAE)
Far East Russian e.
fox e.
herpes simplex e.

HHV6 e.
hyperergic e.
Ilhéus e.
inclusion body e.
Japanese B e.
e. japonica
e. lethargica
Mengo e.
Murray Valley e. (MVE)
postvaccinal e.
Powassan e.
Russian autumn e.
Russian spring-summer e.
Russian tick-borne e.
secondary e.
St. Louis e.
subacute inclusion body e.
varicella e.
vernal e.
e. virus
von Economo e.
woodcutter's e.
encephalitogen
encephalitogenic
Encephalitozoon cuniculi
encephalocele
**encephalocraniocutaneous lipomatosis
(ECCL)**
encephalomyelitis
acute disseminated e. (ADEM)
allergic e.
autoimmune e.
avian infectious e.
disseminated e.
enzootic e.
equine e.
experimental allergic e. (EAE)
herpes B e.
infectious porcine e.
Kelly e.
mouse e.
Venezuelan equine e. (VEE)
viral e.
virus e.
western equine e. (WEE)
zoster e.
encephalomyocarditis (EMC)
e. virus
encephalopathy
bovine spongiform e.
HIV e.
subacute spongiform e.

transmissible mink e.
transmissible spongiform e. (TSE)
encoding
naked DNA e.
end
e. cell
E. Lice
E. Lice Liquid
endemia
endemic
e. fogo selvagem
e. fungal infection
e. index
e. nonbacterial infantile
gastroenteritis
e. pemphigus foliaceus
e. syphilis
e. typhus
e. urticaria
endemica
urticaria multiformis e.
endemium
erythema e.
granuloma e.
Treponema e.
endemoepidemic
Endep
endermic
endermism
end-inspiratory crackle
endobronchial brachytherapy
endocardial fibroproliferative
endocarditis
acute bacterial e. (ABE)
bacteria-free stage of bacterial e.
bacterial e.
enterococcal e.
infectious e.
Libman-Sacks e.
subacute bacterial e. (SBE)
endocrine
e. amyloidosis
e. disease
e. hormone imbalance
e. rhinitis
endocrinopathy
endocytosis
reverse e.
endoderm
Endodermophyton
endogenote

E

NOTES

endogenous
    e. antigen
    e. antitumor immunity
    e. dermatitis
    e. factor
    e. immune response
    e. infection
    e. ochronosis
    e. pyrogen
endoluminal
endomophilous
endomyocardial biopsy (EMB)
endomysial mononuclear cell
endonuclease
endoparasitism
Endopearl bioabsorbable device
endopeptidase
    Zn-dependent e.
endoperoxide synthase
endophthalmitis
endoplasmic reticulum
endoprotease
endosclerosis
endoscopy
    intragastral provocation under e. (IPEC)
EndoSheath
endosomal acidification
endosteal
endothelial
    e. cell
    e. cell proliferation
    e. leukocyte adhesion molecule-1 (ELAM-1)
    e. lysis
endothelial-derived nitric oxide
endothelial-leukocyte adhesion molecule (ELAM)
endothelial-relaxing factor
endothelin-1 (ET-1)
endothelioid
endothelioma
    e. capitis
    e. cutis
endothelium-derived
    e.-d. relaxation factor
    e.-d. relaxing factor (EDRF)
endothelium vascular
endothrix infection
endotoxemia
endotoxicosis
endotoxic reaction
endotoxin
    e. shock
    e. signaling pathway
endovascular papillary angioendothelioma

end-product
    advanced glycation e.-p. (AGE)
end-stage organ disease
end-tidal carbon dioxide (ETCO$_2$)
engagement
    immune e.
Engerix-B
English
    E. plantain
    E. plantain weed pollen
    E. walnut tree pollen
englobe
englobement
Engman
    E. dermatitis
    E. disease
engraftment
enhancement
    immunological e.
enhancer
    Aerosol Cloud e. (ACE)
    SEPA dermal absorption e.
enhancing antibody
enisoprost
enolase
    neuron-specific e. (NSE)
Enomine
Enovil
enoxacin
enoxaparin
enrichment
    e. culture
    density gradient bone marrow progenitor e.
Enseals
    potassium iodide e.
EN-tabs
    Azulfidine E.-t.
entactin
Entamoeba histolytica
Entemopoxvirus
enteric
    e. cytopathogenic bovine orphan (ECBO)
    e. cytopathogenic bovine orphan virus
    e. cytopathogenic human orphan (ECHO)
    e. cytopathogenic human orphan virus
    e. cytopathogenic monkey orphan (ECMO)
    e. cytopathogenic monkey orphan virus
    e. cytopathogenic swine orphan (ECSO)
    e. cytopathogenic swine orphan virus

e. fever
e. pancreatic drainage
enteric-coated
e.-c. acetylsalicylic acid (ECASA)
e.-c. aspirin
enteritidis
Salmonella e.
enteritis
e. anaphylactica
Campylobacter fetus e.
feline infectious e.
e. of mink
transmissible e.
enteroadherent
enteroaggregative
Enterobacter cloacae
Enterobacteriaceae
enterobiasis
Enterobius vermicularis
enterochromaffin cell
enterococcal endocarditis
Enterococcus
E. faecalis
E. faecium
vancomycin-resistant *E.* (VRE)
enterocolitica
Yersinia e.
enterocolitis
antibiotic e.
dietary protein e.
dietary protein-induced e.
gold-induced e.
necrotizing e. (NEC)
Enterocytozoon bieneusi
enterogenic reactive arthritis
enterohemorrhagic
enteroinvasive
enteropathic
e. arthritis
e. arthropathy
enteropathica
acrodermatitis e.
enteropathy
food protein-induced e.
gluten e.
gluten-sensitive e. (GSE)
protein-losing e.
enterosepsis
enterotoxigenic
enterotoxin
Escherichia coli e.
staphylococcal e.

enteroviral
e. exanthema
e. infection
Enterovirus
enterovirus (EV)
myelitic e.
nonpolio e.
Entex
E. LA
E. PSE
entheseal ossification
enthesis
enthesitis
enthesitis-related arthritis
enthesopathy
ankylosing e.
ankylosis and ankylosing e.
(ANKENT)
metabolic e.
enthesophyte
enthetic
entire body imaging agent
Entocort
entomophthoramycosis basidiobolae
entomophthoromycosis
entrapment
genitofemoral nerve e.
nerve e.
e. neuropathy
peroneal nerve e.
saphenous nerve e.
sciatic nerve e.
suprascapular nerve e.
sural nerve e.
Entrophen
ENTsol
E. adaptor
E. Mist
E. Packets
E. Refillable Bottle
enucleation
Envacor test
envelope
cornified cell e.
viral e.
envenomation
env gene
environmental
e. allergen

E

NOTES

environmental *(continued)*
  e. change
  e. exposure unit (EEU)
  e. illness
  e. medicine
  e. mite infestation
  e. mycobacterial infection
  e. mycobacteriosis
  e. scabies
  e. scleroderma
  e. survey
environmentally associated rheumatic disorder (EARD)
environment progressive symptom sclerosis
envoplakin
enzootic
  e. bovine leukosis
  e. encephalomyelitis
  e. encephalomyelitis virus
enzymatic saliva
enzyme
  e. allergosorbent test (EAST)
  angiotensin-converting e. (ACE)
  biotinidase e.
  CAT e.
  chloramphenicol acetyltransferase e.
  collagenolytic e.
  COX e.
  COX-1 e.
  cyclooxygenase e.
  dual-function e.
  epoxide hydrolase e.
  fyn kinase e.
  e. heme oxygenase
  e. immunoassay (EIA)
  immunoglobulin-complexed e. (ICE)
  lysosomal e.
  lytic e.
  matrix-degrading e.
  phospholipase e.
  prostanoid biosynthetic e.
  proteolytic e.
  e. replacement
  secretory PLA$_2$ e.
  steroidogenic e.
  ubiquitin-conjugating e.
  upstream e.
  e. worker's lung
enzyme-linked
  e.-l. immunoassay (EIA)
  e.-l. immunosorbent assay (ELISA)
  e.-l. immunosorbent assay test
  e.-l. immunospot assay (ELISPOT)
enzyme-multiplied immunoassay technique (EMIT)
enzyme-related panniculitis

EOA
  erosive osteoarthritis
eosin
  hematoxylin and e. (HE, H&E)
  e. stain
eosinophil
  e. cationic protein (ECP)
  e. chemotactic factor
  e. chemotactic factor of anaphylaxis (ECF-A)
  e. granule cationic protein
  e. peroxidase
  e. protein X
eosinophil-derived neurotoxin
eosinophilia
  airway e.
  angiolymphoid hyperplasia with e. (ALHE)
  blood e.
  peripheral blood e.
  prolonged pulmonary e.
  pulmonary infiltrate with e. (PIE)
  simple pulmonary e.
  tropical e.
eosinophilia-myalgia syndrome (EMS)
eosinophilic
  e. abscess
  e. bronchopneumonia
  e. cellulitis
  e. chemotaxis
  e. dermatitis
  e. fasciitis
  e. fasciitis syndrome
  e. gastroenteritis
  e. granuloma
  e. granulomatosis
  e. myalgia
  e. myalgia syndrome
  e. myositis
  e. panniculitis
  e. pneumonia
  e., polymorphic, and pruritic eruption associated with radiotherapy (EPPER)
  e. pulmonary syndrome
  e. pustular folliculitis
  e. spongiosis
  e. synovitis
eosinophilopoiesis
eosinophiluria
eotaxin
EPAP
  expiratory positive airway pressure
EpDRF
  epithelium-derived relaxation factor
EP1, EP2, EP3, EP4
ephedra

ephedrine
    aminophylline, amobarbital, and e.
    e. sulfate
Ephedsol
ephelis, pl. **ephelides**
    nevi, atrial myxoma, myxoid
    neurofibromas, and ephelides
    (NAME)
    nevi, atrial myxomas, myxomas of
    skin and mammary glands, and
    ephelides (NAME)
ephemeral
    e. fever of cattle
    e. fever virus
ephidrosis cruenta
epicanthus
Epicauta
    E. fabricii
    E. fabricii sting
    E. vitlata
    E. vitlata sting
Epicel
    E. autologous skin cell
    E. skin graft material
Epicoccum purpurascens
epicondylitis
Epics Elite flow cytometer
epicutaneous
    e. reaction
    e. test
epicuticle
epidemic
    e. acne
    e. arthritic erythema
    e. benign dry pleurisy
    e. cerebrospinal meningitis
    e. curve
    e. diaphragmatic pleurisy
    e. dropsy
    e. encephalitis
    e. exanthema
    e. gastroenteritis virus
    e. hemorrhagic fever
    e. hepatitis
    e. keratoconjunctivitis
    e. keratoconjunctivitis virus
    e. myalgia
    e. myalgia virus
    e. myositis
    e. nausea
    e. nonbacterial gastroenteritis
    e. parotiditis

    e. parotitis virus
    e. pleurodynia
    e. pleurodynia virus
    e. polyarthritis
    e. roseola
    e. transient diaphragmatic spasm
    e. tremor
    e. typhus
    e. vomiting
epidemica
    dermatitis exfoliativa e.
    nephropathia e.
    urticaria e.
epidemicity
epidemicum
    erythema arthriticum e.
epidemiography
epidemiologic
epidemiology
epidermal
    e. allergen
    e. appendage
    e. cyst
    e. filaggrin
    e. growth factor (EGF)
    e. Langerhans cell
    e. necrolysis
    e. nevus
    e. stacking
    e. testing
epidermal-dermal separation
epidermal-melanin unit
epidermatoplasty
epidermic-dermic nevus
epidermidalization
epidermides (*pl. of* epidermis)
epidermidis
    Staphylococcus e.
    stratum corneum e.
epidermidosis
epidermis, pl. **epidermides**
    a collarette of e.
    hyperkeratotic e.
    hyperplastic e.
epidermitis
epidermization
epidermodysplasia
    e. verruciformis
    e. verruciformis of Lewandowski-
    Lutz
epidermoid
    e. cancer

E

NOTES

epidermoid *(continued)*
  e. carcinoma
  e. cyst
epidermolysis
  e. bullosa (EB)
  e. bullosa acquisita (EBA)
  e. bullosa acquisita antigen
  e. bullosa atrophicans
  e. bullosa, dermal type
  e. bullosa dystrophica
  e. bullosa, epidermal type
  e. bullosa, Gravis type
  e. bullosa, inverse
  e. bullosa, junctional type
  e. bullosa lethalis
  e. bullosa, localized
  e. bullosa, Mitis type
  e. bullosa simplex
  e. bullosa simplex herpetiformis
  e. bullosa simplex with mottled
    pigmentation
  e. bullosa with muscular dystrophy
  polydysplastic e.
  toxic bullous e.
epidermolytic
  e. acanthoma
  e. hyperkeratosis
  e. keratosis palmaris et plantaris
  e. palmoplantar keratoderma
epidermophytid
Epidermophyton
  E. floccosum
  E. inguinale
epidermophytosis
  e. cruris
  e. interdigitale
epidermosis
epidermotropic
  e. cutaneous toxoplasmosis
  e. reticulosis
epidermotropism
Epi EZ
EpiE-ZPen
Epifoam
Epifrin
epigenetic
epiglottiditis
epiglottitis
  acute e.
epilans
  eczema e.
EpiLaser laser-based hair removal system
epilate
epilation
  electrosurgical e.
  photo e.
  wax e.

epilator
  galvanic e.
epilatory
epilepticus
  status e.
EpiLight
  E. flashlamp
  E. hair removal system
Epi-lock wound dressing
epiloia
epiluminescence microscopy (ELM)
epiluminescent skin surface microscope
Epilyt
epimastical fever
epimerization
epinephrine
  aqueous e.
  e. hydrochloride
  lidocaine and e.
  self-injecting e.
  subcutaneous e.
  Xylocaine with e.
EpiPen Jr
epiphenomenal
epiphora
epiphyseal
epiphysiodesis
epiphysiolysis
epiphysitis
Epiquick
episclera
episcleritis
  nodular e.
  nonrheumatoid e.
  rheumatoid e.
episodic
  e. angioedema
  e. bronchial obstruction
  e. malnutrition
episomal DNA
episome
  resistance-transferring e.
epispastic
EpiStar diode laser system
epistaxis
episulfonium
  electrophilic ethylene e.
epithelial
  e. cyst
  e. degeneration
  e. keratitis
  e. keratopathy
  e. lining fluid (ELF)
  e. nevus
  e. tumor
epitheliale
  molluscum e.
epithelialization

epithelial-mesenchymal
epitheliitis
epithelioid
    e. blue nevus
    e. cell
    e. cell nevus
    e. combined nevi (ECN)
    e. combined nevi deep penetrating
     nevus (ECN-DPN)
    e. granuloma
    e. sarcoma
epithelioma
    e. adenoides cysticum
    apocrine e.
    basal cell e. (BCE)
    Borst-Jadassohn type
     intraepidermal e.
    calcifying e.
    e. capitis
    e. contagiosum
    e. cuniculatum
    eccrine e.
    Ferguson-Smith e.
    Ferguson-Smith-type e.
    Jadassohn e.
    e. of Malherbe
    Malherbe calcifying e.
    multiple benign cystic e.
    prickle-cell e.
    sebaceous e.
    squamous cell e.
    superficial basal cell e.
epitheliomatocylindromatosus
    nevus e.
epitheliomatosis
epitheliomatous
epitheliopathy
epithelioserosa
    zona e.
epitheliotropic
epithelite
epithelium
    autologous cultured e.
    bronchial e.
    cat e.
    columnar e.
    cultured thymic e.
    dog e.
    ferret e.
    goat e.
    monkey e.
    mouse e.
    rabbit e.
    sheep e.
    sloughed bronchial e.
    swine e.
    tegumentary e.
epithelium-derived relaxation factor
  (EpDRF)
epithelization
epithelize
Epitol
epitope
    aGal e.
    allergenic e.
    B-cell e.
    e. contraction
    cryptic e.
    3Gal e.
    Gal$a$1 e.
    e. homozygosity
    J serovar-specific e.
    e. mapping
    ovalbumin-derived e.
    shared e.
epitope-spreading phenomenon
EpiTouch laser
epitoxoid
epitrichium
Epivir
Epivir-HBV
epizootica
    eczema e.
epizootic cellulitis
EPO
    epoetin alfa
epoetin alfa (EPO)
Epogen
eponychia
eponychium
epoprostenol
epoxide hydrolase enzyme
epoxy
    e. resin
    e. resin dermatitis
    e. resin lung
EPP
    erythropoietic porphyria
Eppendorf tube
EPPER
    eosinophilic, polymorphic, and pruritic
     eruption associated with radiotherapy
EPR
    early-phase reaction

E

NOTES

EPS
  elastosis perforans serpiginosa
epsilometric test
epsilon-aminocaproic agent
Epsom salts
Epstein
  E. disease
  E. pearls
Epstein-Barr (EB)
  E.-B. exanthema
  E.-B. glycoprotein gp110
  E.-B. nuclear antigen (EBNA)
  E.-B. nuclear antigen test
  E.-B. simplex
  E.-B. virus (EBV)
  E.-B. virus-induced early antibody
  E.-B. virus infection
  E.-B. virus test
Epstein-Barr-specific immunoglobulin M test
ePTFE
  expanded polytetrafluoroethylene
  ePTFE implant
epulis
  denture e.
  e. fissuratum
  giant cell e.
EQ-5D EuroQol questionnaire
Equagesic
equation
  Chiou e.
equestrian panniculitis
equi
  Babesia e.
  Demodex e.
  Rhodococcus e.
equilibrium
  e. dialysis
  Hardy-Weinberg e.
equine
  e. abortion virus
  e. arteritis virus
  e. coital exanthema virus
  e. encephalitis
  e. encephalomyelitis
  e. infectious anemia
  e. infectious anemia virus
  e. influenza
  e. influenza virus
  e. Morbillivirus
  e. rhinopneumonitis
  e. rhinopneumonitis virus
  e. rhinovirus
  e. serum hepatitis
  e. viral arteritis
equinia
equivalence zone

equivalent
  human skin e. (HSE)
  living skin e. (LSE)
equuli
  Actinobacillus e.
E-R
  Betachron E-R
eradicate
ErbB-2 protein
erbium
  e. laser
  2040 e. SilkLaser
erbium:YAG
erbium:yttrium-aluminum-garnet (Er:YAG)
Ercaf
erectile
  e. dysfunction
  e. nevus
Ergamisol
ergocalciferol
Ergomar
Ergostat
ergosterole
ergotamine
  e. derivative
  Medihaler-Epi E.
ergotism
erinacei
  Archeaopsylla e.
  Trichophyton e.
erosio interdigitalis blastomycetica
erosion
  bone e.
  bony e.
  glenoid e.
  punched-out e.
  radiographic e.
  subchondral e.
  e. volume
erosiva
erosive
  e. arthritis
  e. *Candida* balanitis
  e. chancre
  e. lichen planus
  e. osteoarthritis (EOA)
  e. polyarthritis
EROTIC
  European Organization for Research and Treatment of Cancer
error
  coefficient of e. (CE)
ERT
  estrogen replacement therapy
ERTD
  ElectroRegenesis therapy device
erubescence

erubescent
eruption
    acneform e.
    bullous pemphigoid-like e.
    butterfly e.
    creeping e.
    crustaceous e.
    cutaneous drug e.
    drug e.
    eczematous polymorphous light e.
    erythematous psoriasiform e.
    evanescent e.
    e. evolution
    familial polymorphous light e.
    feigned e.
    fixed drug e. (FDE)
    hypopigmented macular e.
    iodine e.
    juvenile spring e.
    Kaposi varicelliform e.
    lichenoid e.
    light e.
    medicinal e.
    morbilliform e.
    noneczematous persistent papular
      gold e.
    papulosquamous e.
    pemphigus-like e.
    petechial e.
    pityriasis rosea-like e.
    polymorphous light e. (PMLE)
    posttraumatic pustular e.
    psoriasiform e.
    purpuric phototherapy-induced e.
    pustular e.
    Rosen papular e.
    scarlatiniform e.
    scleroderma-like e.
    sea bathers' e.
    serum e.
    skin e.
    summer e.
    tubercular e.
    vesicopustular e.
    vesicular e.
eruptione
    variola sine e.
eruptive
    e. fever
    e. keratoacanthoma
    e. pseudoangiomatosis
    e. syringoma

    e. vellus hair cyst
    e. xanthoma
ERV
    expiratory residual volume
Erwinia
Er:YAG
    erbium:yttrium-aluminum-garnet
Erybid
Eryc
    E. Oral
Erycette topical
EryDerm Topical
Erygel Topical
Erymax Topical
EryPed Oral
erysipelas
    ambulant e.
    coast e.
    e. de la costa
    e. grave internum
    e. internum
    e. migrans
    migrant e.
    e. perstans
    e. perstans faciei
    phlegmonous e.
    e. pustulosum
    surgical e.
    e. verrucosum
    e. vesiculosum
    wandering e.
    zoonotic e.
erysipelas-like
    e.-l. dermatophytid
    e.-l. erythema
    e.-l. skin lesion
erysipelatous
erysipeloid
    Rosenbach e.
    e. of Rosenbach
Erysipelothrix
    E. dermatitis
    E. rhusiopathiae
erysipelotoxin
Ery-Tab Oral
erythema
    e. ab igne (EAI)
    e. acneforme
    acral e.
    acrodynic e.
    annular e.
    e. annulare

E

NOTES

erythema *(continued)*
    e. annulare centrifugum (EAC)
    e. annulare rheumaticum
    e. arthriticum
    e. arthriticum epidemicum
    bright e.
    e. brucellum
    e. caloricum
    chilblain-like e.
    e. chronicum
    e. chronicum figuratum
      melanodermicum
    e. chronicum migrans (ECM)
    circinate syphilitic e.
    e. circinatum
    congenital telangiectatic e.
    e. congestivum
    e. contagiosum
    e. contusiforme
    e. contusiformis
    e. craquelé
    e. desquamativum
    diffuse e.
    e. dose
    drug-induced e.
    e. dyschromicum perstans
    e. elevatum diutinum (EED)
    e. endemium
    epidemic arthritic e.
    erysipelas-like e.
    e. exfoliativa
    facial e.
    e. figuratum
    e. figuratum perstans
    e. fugax
    e. gyratum
    e. gyratum perstans
    e. gyratum repens
    hemorrhagic exudative e.
    e. induratum
    e. infectiosum (EI)
    e. intertrigo
    e. iris
    Jacquet e.
    e. keratodes
    linear extensor e.
    macular e.
    malar e.
    e. marginatum
    Milian e.
    morbilliform e.
    e. multiforme (EM)
    e. multiforme bullosum
    e. multiforme exudativum
    e. multiforme major
    e. multiforme minor
    e. multiforme neonatal
    necrolytic migratory e.

    e. necroticans
    e. neonatorum toxicum
    ninth-day e.
    e. nodosum (EN)
    e. nodosum leprosum
    e. nodosum migrans
    e. nodosum syphiliticum
    e. nuchae
    nummular e.
    palmar e.
    e. palmare
    e. palmare hereditarium
    e. papulatum
    papuloerosive e.
    e. papulosum
    e. paratrimma
    pellagroid e.
    periorbital e.
    periungual e.
    e. pernio
    e. polymorphe
    e. pudicitiae
    e. a pudore
    e. pudoris
    e. punctate
    e. punctatum
    radiation e.
    retiform e.
    rheumatic e.
    e. scarlatiniform
    scarlatiniform e.
    e. scarlatiniforme
    e. simplex
    e. solare
    e. streptogenes
    symptomatic e.
    telangiectatic e.
    e. threshold
    toxic e.
    e. toxicum neonatorum
    e. traumaticum
    e. tuberculatum
    e. urticans
    e. venenatum
    violet-blue e.
erythematic
erythematodes
    lupus e.
erythematosa
    acne e.
    dermatitis e.
erythematosquamous plaque
erythematosum
    eczema e.
erythematosus
    acute cutaneous lupus e. (ACLE)
    bullous systemic lupus e. (BSLE)
    chilblain lupus e.

chronic cutaneous lupus e. (CCLE)
chronic discoid lupus e.
cutaneous lupus e.
discoid lupus e. (DLE)
disseminated lupus e.
drug-induced systemic lupus e.
lupus e. (LE)
neonatal lupus e. (NLE)
neuropsychiatric syndrome of
  systemic lupus e. (NPSLE)
neuropsychiatric systemic lupus e.
  (NPSLE)
pemphigus e.
subacute cutaneous lupus e.
  (SCLE)
systemic lupus e. (SLE)
transient neonatal systemic lupus e.
tumid lupus e.

erythematous
e. macular dermatitis
e. mark
e. plaque
e. psoriasiform eruption
e. syphilid
e. wheal

erythematovesicular
erythemogenic
erythermalgia
erythralgia
erythrasma
Barensprung e.
erythredema
erythrism
erythristic
Erythro-Base
erythroblastosis
fetal e.
e. fetalis
erythroblastotic
erythrocatalysis
Erythrocin Oral
erythrocyanosis
e. crurum
e. crurum puellaris
e. frigida
e. frigida crurum puellarum
e. supramalleolaris
erythrocyte
e. adherence phenomenon
e. adherence test
e. cast
C3-coated e.

IgG-coated e.
e. sedimentation rate (ESR)
e. sheet rosette cell marker
erythrocytes, antibody, complement
  (EAC)
erythrocytolysin
erythrocytolysis
erythrocytosis
posttransplant e.
erythroderma, erythrodermia
atypical ichthyosiform e.
bullous congenital ichthyosiform e.
congenital ichthyosiform e. (CIE)
e. desquamativum
e. exfoliativa
exfoliative e.
ichthyosiform e.
e. ichthyosiformis congenitalis
lamellar congenital ichthyosiform e.
lymphomatous e.
nonbullous congenital
  ichthyosiform e.
e. psoriaticum
Sézary e.
e. squamosum
T-cell e.
Wilson-Brocq e.
erythrodermas
erythrodermatitis
erythrodermia (*var. of* erythroderma)
erythrodermic psoriasis (PsoE)
erythrodysesthesia syndrome
erythrogenic toxin
erythrokeratodermia
e. figurata variabilis
progressive symmetric e. (PSEK)
e. progressive symmetrica
progressive symmetrical
  verrucous e.
erythrokeratolysis hiemalis
erythroleukemia cell line
erythrolysin
erythrolysis
erythromelalgia
erythromelanin
erythromelanosis
e. follicularis faciei
e. follicularis faciei et colli
erythromelia
erythromycin
e. and benzoyl peroxide
e., benzoyl peroxide topical gel

E

NOTES

erythromycin (continued)
 e. and sulfisoxazole
 e. topical
erythromycin-sulfisoxazole
erythrophagia
erythrophagocytosis
erythroplakia
erythroplasia
 e. of Queyrat
 Zoon e.
erythropoietic
 e. coproporphyria (ECP)
 e. porphyria (EPP)
 e. protoporphyria
erythropoietin
erythropolis
 Rhodococcus e.
erythroprosopalgia
erythrose
 e. péribuccale pigmentaire of Brocq
 e. pigmentaire péribuccale
Eryzole Oral
ES
 electrophilic stress
 Elejalde syndrome
 excretory-secretory
eschar
 black e.
 burn e.
 e. separation
escharotic
escharotica
 dermatitis e.
 rupia e.
Escherichia
 E. coli
 E. coli enterotoxin
 E. coli polysaccharide antibody
E-selectin
E-Solve-2 topical
esophageal
 e. carcinoma
 e. hypomotility
esophagitis dissecans superficialis
esophagomycosis
Esoterica
 E. Facial
 E. Regular
 E. Sensitive Skin Formula
 E. Sunscreen
espundia
ESR
 erythrocyte sedimentation rate
ESS
 excited skin syndrome
essential
 e. fatty acid (EFA)
 e. fatty acid deficiency

 e. fever
 e. mixed cryoglobulinemia
 e. pruritus
 e. telangiectasia
 e. thrombocytopenic purpura
established cell line
Estar Gel
ester
 aminobenzoate e.
 fumaric acid e.
 isopropyl e.
 PABA e.
 phorbol e.
esterase
 C1 e.
 lymphocyte serine e.
 nonspecific e. (NSE)
 serine e.
esterified PABA
esthiomene
estivae
estival, aestival
 e. vacciniform
estivale, aestivale
 hydroa e.
estivalis, aestivalis
 acne e.
 dermatitis e.
 protoporphyria e.
 prurigo e.
 pruritus e.
estradiol
estrogen
 conjugated e.
 e. replacement therapy (ERT)
estrone
ET-1
 endothelin-1
et
 keratoderma palmaris e.
etanercept monotherapy
ETCO$_2$
 end-tidal carbon dioxide
E-test
ethambutol (EMB)
 e. hydrochloride
ethanol
 alkyl phenoxyl polyethoxy e.
ethanolamine
 amino ethyl e.
ether
 alkyl aryl e.
Ethicon
 E. P and PS needle
 E. suture
ethidium bromide
Ethilon suture
ethinylestradiol

ethionamide
ethmoidectomy
ethmoid sinusitis
ethyl
  e. alcohol
  e. aminobenzoate
  e. chloride
  e. chloride and
    dichlorotetrafluoroethane
  e. hexanediol
  e. methacrylate
ethyl-2,3-dihydroxybenzoate
ethylenediamine dermatitis
ethylenediaminetetraacetic acid (EDTA)
ethylene oxide (ETO)
ethyleneurea melamine formaldehyde
  resin
ethylnorepinephrine
  e. hydrochloride
ethylsuccinate
  oral erythromycin e.
Etibi
etidocaine hydrochloride
etidronate
  sodium e.
etidronate/calcium
etiolation
etiologic
etiology
  monoarticular arthritis of
    unknown e.
etiopathogenesis
etiopathogenic
ETO
  ethylene oxide
  ETO Sleuth
etodolac
ETOPOPHOS infusion
etoposide phosphate infusion
E-Toxa-Clean Concentrate
Etretin
etretinate treatment
ETS-2% topical
Eubacterium aerofaciens
Eucalyptamint 2000
eucalyptus
  e. oil
  e. saligna
  e. tree
  e. tree pollen

Eucerin
  E. cream
  E. Plus moisturizer
euchromatic
Eudal-SR
eudiaphoresis
EULAR
  European League Against Rheumatism
eumelanin
eumycetoma
eumycotic mycetoma
eupeptic
euphoria
Euproctis
  E. chrysorrhoea
  E. chrysorrhoea sting
Eurax topical
Euro-Collins (EC)
  Euro-Collins solution
Euroglyphus maynei
europa
  Olea e.
europaeus
  Ulex e.
European
  E. Anti-ICAM Renal Transplant
    Study (EARTS)
  E. blastomycosis
  E. blister beetle sting
  E. cholera
  E. Confederation for Laboratory
    Medicine (ECLM)
  E. Consensus Lupus Activity
    Measure (ECLAM)
  E. Group for Bone Marrow
    Transplantation (EBMT)
  E. League Against Rheumatism
    (EULAR)
  E. Organization for Research and
    Treatment of Cancer (EROTIC)
European-American Lymphoma
  classification
eustachian tube
eutectic mixture of local anesthetics
  (EMLA)
euthyroid
  sick e.
  e. sick syndrome
eutrichosis
Euxyl K 400
EV
  enterovirus

E

NOTES

201

evaluation
    acute physiology and chronic
      health e. (APACHE)
evanescent
    e. eruption
    e. macule
Evans blue stain
evening primrose oil
everolimus
evidence-based Medicine (EBM)
evisceration
    total abdominal e. (TAE)
E-Vista
E-Vitamin
EVLW
    extravascular lung water
evolution
    eruption e.
    lesion e.
Evoxac
evulsion
Ewart sign
ewengii
    Ehrlichia e.
Ewing tumor
ex
    ex vivo adenoviral transfection
    ex vivo cell expansion
    ex vivo organ storage
exacerbation
Exact
    E. Cream
    E. skin product
exaggerated bronchoconstrictor response
examination
    bone marrow e.
    full-body cutaneous e.
    immunofluorescent e.
    KOH e.
    Neurobehavioral Cognitive Status e.
    retinal e.
    Wood light e.
exanthem
    unilateral laterothoracic e. (ULE)
    vesicular e.
exanthema, pl. **exanthemas, exanthemata**
    Boston e.
    echoviral e.
    enteroviral e.
    epidemic e.
    Epstein-Barr e.
    keratoid e.
    ordinal designation of the
      exanthemata
    polymorphous e.
    e. subitum
    vesicular e.
    viral e.

exanthematic typhus of São Paulo
exanthematicus
    ichthyismus e.
exanthematique
    typhus e.
exanthematous
    e. disease
    e. fever
    e. typhus
exanthesis arthrosia
excavatum
    pectus e.
Excedrin
    E. IB
    E. P.M.
Excel
    Simplastin E.
excentrica
    hyperkeratosis e.
excess
    antibody e.
    antigen e.
    e. incidence (IDD)
excessive
    e. dryness
    e. hairiness
    e. secretion
    e. sweating
    e. water immersion
exchange
    e. plasmapheresis
    e. transfusion
exchanger
    heat/moisture e. (HME)
excimer lasing medium
excision
    fusiform e.
    surgical e. (SE)
    tangential e.
    tangent-to-circle e.
    wide e.
excisional
    e. biopsy
    e. removal
excited
    e. skin syndrome (ESS)
    e. state
exclamation point hair
exclusion
    allelic e.
excoriate
excoriated
    e. acne
    e. folliculitis
excoriation
    crusted e.
    necrotic e.
    neurotic e.

excrescence
    wart-like e.
excretion
    xanthine stone e.
excretory-secretory (ES)
excursion
Exelderm topical
exercise
    isometric e.
    passive range of motion e.
exercise-induced
    e.-i. anaphylaxis (EIA)
    e.-i. asthma (EIA)
    e.-i. asthma diagnosis
    e.-i. bronchoconstriction (EIB)
    e.-i. bronchospasm (EIB)
    e.-i. cholinergic urticaria
    e.-i. refractoriness
    e.-i. respiratory distress syndrome
    (EIRDS)
exertion
exfoliant
exfoliate
exfoliatio areata lingua
exfoliation
exfoliativa
    cheilitis e.
    dermatitis e.
    erythema e.
    erythroderma e.
    glossitis areata e.
    keratolysis e.
exfoliative
    e. dermatitis
    e. erythroderma
    e. psoriasis
Exgest
exhaust
    automobile e.
exhaustion
    nervous e.
    obvious physical e.
Exidine
    E. Scrub
    E. solution
exilicauda
    Centruroides e.
exine
Exirel
exoantigen
exocrine
exocrinopathic process

exocrinopathy
    autoimmune e.
exocytosis
exogenetic
exogenote
exogenous
    e. antigen
    e. factor
    e. hyperthyroidism
    e. interleukin-12
    e. ochronosis
    e. pigmentation
    e. polyunsaturated fatty acids
    e. substance
exon 5
exonuclease
Exophiala
    E. jeanselmei
    E. werneckii
exophytic
exopolysaccharide
    mucoid e. (MEP)
Exorex
exoserosis
exostosis, pl. exostoses
    subungual e.
exotoxic
exotoxin
    bacterial e.
    streptococcal pyrogenic e. (SPE)
expanded
    e. disability status scale (EDSS)
    e. polytetrafluoroethylene (ePTFE)
    e. polytetrafluoroethylene implant
expander
    BioSpan tissue e.
    Miami STAR tissue e.
expansion
    clonal e.
    ex vivo cell e.
    pre-B cell e.
expectorant
    Fedahist E.
    Genamin E.
    Myminic E.
    Silaminic E.
    Theramin E.
    Triaminic E.
    Tri-Clear E.
    Triphenyl E.
expectorate

E

NOTES

experimental
    e. allergic encephalitis (EAE)
    e. allergic encephalomyelitis (EAE)
    e. autoimmune gastritis (EAG)
experimentally induced Köbner phenomenon (KP-e)
expiration
    prolongation of e.
expiratory
    e. positive airway pressure (EPAP)
    e. prolongation
    e. residual volume (ERV)
explant
explantation
explosive-onset fever
explosive vomiting
exposure
    aerosolized pollutant e.
    allergen e.
    cold e.
    heat e.
    light e.
    limitation of e.
    narrowband UVB therapeutic
      light e.
    occupational e.
    prior drug e.
    repeated e.
    silica dust e.
    sun e.
    vinyl chloride e.
expression
    cell surface e.
    differential gene e.
expressor
    Heilen e.
    Saalfield e.
    Schamberg e.
    Unna e.
    Walton e.
    Zimmerman-Walton e.
exsanguinous metabolic support perfusion
Exsel
    E. Shampoo
Exserohilum
    E. jeanselmei
    E. rostratum
exsiccation eczematid
extended criteria donor (ECD)
extender
    Frechet e.
Extendryl
extensor
    e. carpi ulnaris (ECU)
    e. surface
extensum
    hemangioma planum e.

Extentabs
    Dimetane E.
    Dimetapp E.
exteriorization
externa
    otitis e.
external
    e. absorption
    e. auditory canal (EAC)
    e. meningitis
    e. otitis
Extra
    Claritin E.
    E. Strength Bayer Enteric 500
      Aspirin
    E. Strength Doan's
extraarticular tissue
extracellular
    e. cholesterolosis
    e. crystalloid solution
    e. domain (ECD)
    e. matrix (ECM)
    e. matrix-degrading proteinase
    e. matrix metalloproteinase inducer
      (EMMPRIN)
    e. matrix remodeling
    e. signal-regulated kinase
    e. toxin
extrachromosomal
extracorporeal
    e. assist device
    e. liver perfusion (ECLP, ELP)
    e. membrane oxygenation (ECMO)
    e. photochemotherapy
    e. photophoresis
extract
    allergenic e.
    allergic e.
    alum-precipitated pyridine-extracted
      pollen e.
    aqueous e.
    buffered charcoal yeast e. (BCYE)
    glutaraldehyde-modified-tyrosine-
      absorbed e.
    glycerinated e.
    e. of henna
    inhalant allergen e.
    liver e.
    lyophilized e.
    phenol-preserved e.
    pollen e.
    tobacco leaf e.
    venom e.
    whole-body e.
    whole ragweed e. (WRE)
extractable nuclear antigen (ENA)
extraction
    comedo e.

extractor
>Amico e.
>comedo e.
>comedone e.
>Schamberg comedo e.
>Unna comedo e.
>Walton e.

extraglandular manifestation (EGM)
extralobar
extramammary Paget disease (EMPD)
extraocular sarcoidosis
extrapulmonary
>e. pneumocystosis
>e. sarcoidosis
>e. tuberculosis

Extra-Strength Balm
extrauterine environmental stimulus
extravasation potential
extravascular
>e. granulomatous feature
>e. lung water (EVLW)

extravillous
>e. cytotrophoblast cell
>e. trophoblastic damage

extrinsic
>e. allergic alveolitis
>e. asthma
>e. compression of trachea

exuberant
>e. cicatrization
>e. infectious

exudate
>retinal e.

exudation
exudative
>e. discoid
>e. discoid and lichenoid
>e. discoid and lichenoid dermatitis
>e. neurodermatitis
>e. papulosquamous disease

exudativum
>erythema multiforme e.

exude
ExuDerm
>E. hydrocolloid
>E. hydrocolloid dressing

Exu-Dry absorptive dressing
exulceratio simplex
ex-vivo liver perfusion
eye
>black e.
>e. folliculitis
>raccoon e.'s
>red e.

eyebrow loss
eyeglass frame dermatitis
eyelash
>e. cosmetic
>e. loss

eyelid cosmetic
eyeline tattoo
Eye-Lube-A solution
EZ
>Epi E.

NOTES

E

F

    F agent
    F genote
    F pilus
    F plasmid

F2

    prostaglandin F2 (PGF$_2$)

f

    f factor I, II, IIa, III

F12-MABP fusion protein

FA

    fluorescent antibody stain
    FA virus

FAB

    French-American-British
    FAB classification

Fab

    Fab fragment
    Fab piece

FAB-1 cell marker

Faba vulgaris

Fabc fragment

fabism

fabric

fabrication

    laser-assisted internal f. (LIFT)

fabricii

    Epicauta f.

Fabry

    F. angiokeratoma
    F. disease
    F. syndrome

Fabry-Anderson disease

Facb fragment

faccinia

face

    Hippocratic f.
    F.'s Only
    f. peel
    ringworm of the f.

face-lift

facet

    f. joint arthropathy
    f. joint osteoarthritis

facetal joint

facial

    f. erythema
    Esoterica F.
    f. foundation
    f. moisturizer
    f. nerve palsy
    f. powder
    f. undercover cream
    f. vitiligo

faciale

    granuloma f.
    pyoderma f.

facialis

    herpes f.
    pyodermia f.
    zona f.

faciei

    atrophoderma reticulatum
      symmetricum f.
    chloasma f.
    erysipelas perstans f.
    erythromelanosis follicularis f.
    keratosis pilaris atrophicans f.
    lupus miliaris disseminatus f.
    pityriasis simplex f.
    pyoderma chancriforme f.
    seborrhea f.
    symmetricum f.
    tinea f.

facies

    adenoidal f.
    allergic f.
    coarse f.
    cushingoid f.
    dengue f.
    f. hepatica
    Hippocratic f.
    f. Hippocratica
    hound-dog f.
    leonine f.
    monkey f.
    moon f.
    myxedematous f.
    round f.
    tabetic f.

FACS

    fluorescence-activated cell sorter
    fluorescence-activated cell sorting
    fluorescent-activated cell sorting

FACScan

    F. flow cytometer

F-actin

    subplasmalemmal F.-a.

factitia

    dermatitis f.
    urticaria f.

factitial

    f. dermatitis
    f. panniculitis

factitious

    f. dermatitis
    f. purpura
    f. urticaria

F

facto
    de f.
factor
    f. A, B, C, D, E, H, I
    acidic fibroblast growth f. (a-FGF)
    activated vitamin K-dependent f.
    albumin-autoagglutinating f.
    alloantigen-independent risk f.
    allogenic effect f.
    angiogenesis f.
    anticomplementary f.
    antinuclear f. (ANF)
    antiperinuclear f. (APF)
    bacteriocin f.
    basic fibroblast growth f. (bFGF)
    B-cell differentiation/growth f.
    B-cell growth f.-1, -2
    Bittner milk f.
    chemokinetic f.
    chemotactic f.
    ciliary neurotrophic f.
    cobra venom f. (CVF)
    colony-stimulating f. (CSF)
    complement chemotactic f.
    control of emotional f.
    cytokine synthesis inhibitory f.
    D deficiency f.
    f. D, H, I deficiency
    endogenous f.
    endothelial-relaxing f.
    endothelium-derived relaxation f.
    endothelium-derived relaxing f.
    (EDRF)
    eosinophil chemotactic f.
    epidermal growth f. (EGF)
    epithelium-derived relaxation f.
    (EpDRF)
    exogenous f.
    fertility f.
    fibroblast growth f. (FGF)
    f f. I, II, IIa, III
    genetic f.
    f. Gm
    granulocyte colony-stimulating f.
    (G-CSF)
    granulocyte and macrophage
    colony-stimulating f. (GM-CSF)
    granulocyte-macrophage colony-
    stimulating f. (GM-CSF)
    growth f. (GF)
    Hageman f.
    H deficiency f.
    hemopoietic f.
    heparin-binding epidermal growth
    factor-like growth f. (HB-EGF)
    heparin-binding growth f. (HBGF)
    hepatocyte growth f. (HGF)
    histamine-releasing f. (HRF)

I deficiency f.
IgM rheumatoid f.
    immunoglobulin M rheumatoid
    factor
f. I, II, VII, VIII, IX, X, XI, XII
immunoglobulin G rheumatoid f.
    (IgG RF)
immunoglobulin M rheumatoid f.
    (IgM RF, IgM rheumatoid factor)
inhibition f.
f. Inv
kappa-binding nuclear f.
latent transforming growth f.
LE f.
leucine zipper transcription f.
leukocytosis-promoting f.
leukopenic f.
lymph node permeability f. (LNPF)
macrophage-activating f. (MAF)
macrophage colony-stimulating f.
    (M-CSF)
macrophage-derived tumor
    necrosis f.
migration-inhibitory f. (MIF)
milk f.
monocyte chemotactic f. (MCF)
monocyte-derived neutrophil
    chemotactic f.
multilineage colony-stimulating f.
myeloma growth f.
natural killer cell-stimulating f.
    (NKSF)
nephritic f.
nerve growth f. (NGF)
neutrophil-activating f. (NAF)
neutrophil chemotactant f.
nuclear f.
osteoclast-activating f. (OAF)
osteoclast differentiation f.
platelet f. 4 (PF4)
platelet-activating f. (PAF)
platelet activating/aggregating f.
    (PAF)
platelet-aggregating f. (PAF)
platelet-derived angiogenesis f.
    (PDAF)
platelet-derived epidermal growth f.
    (PDEGF)
platelet-derived growth f. (PDGF)
positive rheumatoid f.
progesterone-induced blocking f.
    (PIBF)
properdin f. A, B, D, E
psychogenic f.
R f.
recognition f.
releasing f. (RF)
f. replacement therapy

resistance f.
resistance-inducing f.
resistance-transfer f.
Rh f.
rhesus f.
Rheumatex test for rheumatoid f.
rheumatoid f. (RF)
Rheumaton test for rheumatoid f.
secretor f.
sex f.
soluble co-stimulatory f.
steel f.
stem cell f. (SCF)
stimulating f. (SF)
streaking leukocyte f.
sun protection f. (SPF)
T-cell growth f. (TCGF)
T-cell replacing f.
thymic lymphopoietic f.
thymus-replacing f.
thyrotoxic complement-fixation f.
tissue f. (TF)
transcription f.
transfer f.
transforming growth f. (TGF)
transforming growth f.-alpha (TGF-alpha)
transforming growth f.-beta (TGFB, TGF-beta)
trigger f.
trypanosome growth f. (TGF)
tumor lysis f.
tumor necrosis f. (TNF)
vascular endothelial growth f. (VEGF)
vascular permeability factor/vascular endothelial cell growth f. (VPF/VEGF)
f. VIIIa
f. VIII:C inhibitor
f. V Leiden
f. V Leiden mutation
von Willebrand f. (vWF)
Willebrand f.
X f.
f. XIII

factor-1
anemia-inducing f.-1 (AIF-1)
heparin-binding growth f.-1 (HBGF-1)
insulin-like growth f.-1 (IGF-1)
stromal-cell-derived f.-1 (SDF-1)
T-cell growth f.-1

factor-2
keratinocyte growth f.-2 (KGF-2)
T-cell growth f.-2
vascular endothelial growth f.-2 (VEGF2)
factor-3
leukocyte antigen f.-3 (LAF-3)
factor-4
factor-alpha
tumor necrosis f.-a. (TNF-alpha)
factor-B
transforming growth f.-B. (TGF-B)
factor-beta
transforming growth f.-b. (TGFB, TGF-beta)
tumor necrosis f.-b.
factor-inducing monocytopoiesis
factor-kappa B
nuclear f. (NF-κB)
facultative
f. anaerobe
f. bacterium
f. myiasis
f. skin color
FADD
Fas-associating protein with death domain
faecalis
Alcaligenes f.
Enterococcus f.
Streptococcus f.
faecium
Enterococcus f.
vancomycin-resistant *Enterococcus f.* (VREF)
faeni
Micropolyspora f.
Faget sign
fagopyrism
failure
acute respiratory f. (ARF)
adrenocortical f.
congestive heart f. (CHF)
fulminant hepatic f. (FHF)
graft f.
impending respiratory f.
late-onset renal f.
multiple organ system f. (MOSF)
premature ovarian f. (POF)
primary adrenocortical f.
renal f.
respiratory f.

F

NOTES

failure *(continued)*
secondary adrenocortical f.
severe respiratory f.
f. to thrive
ventilatory f.
failure-free survival (FFS)
Fairbanks arthritis phenotype
falciparum
Plasmodium f.
fall
f. dermatosis
f. elm
f. elm tree
hair f.
fall-and-rise phenomenon
false
f. agglutination
f. cyst
f. diphtheria
f. membrane
f. ragweed
f. ragweed weed pollen
false-negative
f.-n. patch test
f.-n. reaction
false-positive
f.-p. patch test
f.-p. reaction
f.-p. syphilis test
FAMA
fluorescent antimembrane antibody
famciclovir
familial
f. acanthosis nigrans
f. aggregation
f. alpha-lipoprotein deficiency
f. amyloidosis
f. amyloidotic polyneuropathy (FAP)
f. amyloidotic polyneuropathy syndrome
f. amyloid polyneuropathy
f. apoprotein CII deficiency
f. articular hypermobility syndrome
f. atypical multiple mole melanoma syndrome (FAMMM)
f. benign chronic pemphigus
f. benign pemphigus of Hailey-Hailey
f. cholestasis syndrome
f. cold urticaria
f. combined hyperlipidemia
f. continuous skin peel
f. cryoglobulinemia
f. dysautonomia
f. dysbetalipoproteinemia
f. erythrophagocytic lymphohistiocytosis

f. hemophagocytic lymphohistiocytosis (FHL)
f. Hibernian fever (FHF)
f. hypercholesterolemia
f. hypermobility syndrome
f. hypertriglyceridemia
f. hypocalciuric hypercalcemia
f. juvenile hyperuricemic nephropathy
f. Mediterranean fever
f. myovascular fibroma
f. nephropathic amyloidosis syndrome
f. pancytopenia
f. panmyelophthisis
f. paroxysmal polyserositis
f. PMLE
f. polymorphous light eruption
f. progressive hyperpigmentation (FPH)
f. pulmonary fibroproliferative
f. recurrent arthritis
f. recurrent polyserositis
f. reticuloendotheliosis
f. rosacea-like dermatitis
f. spondyloepiphyseal dysplasia tarda
f. thrombocytopenia
f. urticaria pigmentosa
f. white folded mucosal dysplasia
family
immunoglobulin supergene f.
pentraxin protein f.
FAMMM
familial atypical multiple mole melanoma syndrome
famotidine
Famvir
FANA
fluorescent antinuclear antibody assay
fan-beam collimator
Fanconi
F. anemia
F. syndrome
Fansimef
FAO
Food Agricultural Organization
FAP
familial amyloidotic polyneuropathy
FAPD
fibrosing alopecia in a pattern distribution
Farber
F. body
F. disease
farcinica
Nocardia f.
farcy bud
Far East Russian encephalitis

farinae
  Dermatophagoides *f.*
farinosus
  herpes f.
farmer's
  f. lung
  f. neck
  f. skin
farmyard pox
Farr
  F. assay
  F. law
  F. test
Fas
  F. antigen
  F. ligand (FasL)
  F. ligand gene
  soluble F. (sFas)
Fas-associating protein with death domain (FADD)
Fas-based killing pathway
fascia
  f. lata
  palmar f.
  plantar f.
fasciatus
  Nosopsyllus f.
fascicular lymphosarcoma
fasciculata
  zona f.
fasciitis
  eosinophilic f.
  necrotizing f.
  nodular pseudosarcomatous f.
  proliferative f.
  pseudosarcomatous f.
fasciitis-panniculitis syndrome
fascioliasis
Fasciolopsis buski
fascioscapulohumeral dystrophy
Fas-Fas
  F.-F. ligand
  F.-F. ligand molecule
fashion
  clear cells scattered in a buckshot f.
  ying-yang f.
Fasject
FasL
  Fas ligand
  FasL gene
Fas-L molecule

fastidious
fastigium
Fastmelt
  Benadryl Allergy/Cold F.
fast-twitch morphology of muscle fiber
fat
  atrophy of f.
  hydrous wool f.
  f. malabsorption
  f. necrosis
fatal asthma
fatigue
fat-replacement atrophy
fatty
  f. degeneration
  f. nevus
faucium
  Mycoplasma f.
faun tail nevus
favic alopecia
favid
  f. alopecia
  f. Favre-Racouchot syndrome
favism
favosa
  mycosis f.
  porrigo f.
  tinea f.
  trichomycosis f.
Favre-Racouchot
  F.-R. cyst
  F.-R. disease
  F.-R. skin
  F.-R. syndrome
favus
  f. circinatus
  f. herpeticus
  f. herpetiformis
  f. pilaris
FB
  foreign body
Fb fragment
5-FC
  5-fluorocytosine
Fc
  Fc fragment
  Fc gamma receptor III
  Fc piece
  Fc receptor
FCH
  folliculosebaceous cystic hamartoma

F

NOTES

FCM
fibroblast-conditioned medium
FCP
florid cutaneous papillomatosis
FCXM
flow cytometry crossmatch
FDA
Food and Drug Administration
FDE
fixed drug eruption
FDG-PET
fluorine-18 2-fluoro-2-deoxy-D-glucose-positron emission tomography
feather
Australian parrot f.
canary f.
chicken f.
cockatiel f.
duck f.
goose f.
f. hydroid
f. hydroid dermatitis
mixed f.
parakeet f.
parrot f.
pigeon f.
turkey f.
FeatherTouch CO2 laser
feature
electromyographic f.
extravascular granulomatous f.
immunologic f.
pathologic f.
sicca f.
febricitans
pes f.
febricula
febrile
f. agglutinin
aphtha f.'s
hydroa f.
f. urticaria
febrilis
herpes f.
urticaria f.
febrility
fecal fat determination
Fedahist
F. Expectorant
F. Expectorant pediatric
F. Tablet
feeleii
Legionella f.
feet (*pl. of* foot)
FEF
forced expiratory flow

FEF$_{25-75\%}$
mean forced expiratory flow during the middle of FVC
Fegan technique
Fegeler syndrome
FEH
focal epithelial hyperplasia
FEIA
fluorescent enzyme immunoassay
feigned eruption
Feingold diet
Fekeeh
Feldene
feline
f. agranulocytosis
f. infectious enteritis
f. infectious peritonitis
f. leukemia
f. leukemia-sarcoma virus complex
f. leukemia virus (FeLV)
f. panleukopenia virus (FPV)
f. rhinotracheitis virus
f. viral rhinotracheitis
felineum
Microsporum f.
felis
Afipia f.
Babesia f.
Ctenocephalides f.
felon
bone f.
deep f.
subcutaneous f.
subcuticular f.
subperiosteal f.
thecal f.
Felty syndrome
FeLV
feline leukemia virus
female
f. pattern alopecia
f. pseudo-Turner syndrome
Femizol-M
femoral
f. anteversion
f. nerve
Femstat
femtomolar concentration
fenbufen
Fen-fan-ji
fennel
dog f.
fenoprofen calcium
fenoterol
fentanyl
Fer antigen

Ferguson-Smith
 F.-S. epithelioma
 F.-S. keratoacanthoma
Ferguson-Smith-type epithelioma
fermentans
 Acidaminococcus f.
fermented food
Fernandez reaction
ferox
 protoporphyria f.
 prurigo f.
Ferreira-Marques lipoatrophy
ferret epithelium
ferric
 f. chloride
 f. subsulfate
ferrugineum
 Microsporum f.
fertility
 f. agent
 f. factor
FES
 flame emission spectroscopy
 forced expiratory spirogram
fescue
 meadow f.
FESEM
 field emission scanning electron
 microscopy
fester
festooning
festoons
fetal
 f. alcohol syndrome
 f. erythroblastosis
 f. hydantoin syndrome
 f. liver transplantation
 f. pig cell transplantation
 f. thymus organ culture (FTOC)
 f. thymus transplantation
 f. ventral mesencephalic tissue
 transplantation
fetalis
 erythroblastosis f.
 ichthyosis f.
 keratosis diffusa f.
fetid sweat
fetoplacental unit (FPU)
fetoprotein
 alpha f.
fetor oris

fetus
 harlequin f.
Feuerstein
 ringhook method of F.
FEV
 forced expiratory volume
FEV$_{1\%VC}$
 forced expiratory volume in 1 second as
 percent of FVC
FEV$_1$
 forced expiratory volume in 1 second
fever
 acute rheumatic f. (ARF)
 Aden f.
 African endemic relapsing f.
 African hemorrhagic f.
 African swine f.
 Argentinean hemorrhagic f.
 Argentine hemorrhagic f.
 black f.
 f. blister
 Bolivian hemorrhagic f.
 bouquet f.
 boutonneuse f.
 bovine ephemeral f.
 breakbone f.
 bullous f.
 Bunyamwera f.
 Bwamba f.
 camp f.
 cerebrospinal f.
 childbed f.
 Colorado tick f.
 Congo-Crimean hemorrhagic f.
 (CCHF)
 continued f.
 Crimean-Congo hemorrhagic f.
 dandy f.
 date f.
 deer fly f.
 dengue hemorrhagic f.
 diphasic milk f.
 dumdum f.
 Dutton relapsing f.
 Ebola hemorrhagic f.
 elephantoid f.
 enteric f.
 epidemic hemorrhagic f.
 epimastical f.
 eruptive f.
 essential f.
 exanthematous f.

NOTES

F

fever *(continued)*
   explosive-onset f.
   familial Hibernian f. (FHF)
   familial Mediterranean f.
   flood f.
   food f.
   Fort Bragg f.
   glandular f.
   grain f.
   Haverhill f.
   hay f.
   hemoglobinuric f.
   hemorrhagic f.
   herpetic f.
   hospital f.
   humidifier f.
   Ilhéus f.
   inundation f.
   island f.
   jail f.
   Japanese river f.
   jungle yellow f.
   Katayama f.
   kedani f.
   Korean hemorrhagic f.
   Lassa hemorrhagic f.
   laurel f.
   louse-borne relapsing f.
   low-grade f.
   malignant catarrhal f.
   Malta f.
   Manchurian hemorrhagic f.
   Marseilles f.
   Mediterranean erythematous f.
   Mediterranean exanthematous f.
   Mediterranean spotted f.
   metal fume f.
   miliary f.
   mill f.
   miniature scarlet f.
   monoleptic f.
   mud f.
   nodal f.
   Omsk hemorrhagic f.
   o'nyong-nyong f.
   Oroya f.
   Pahvant Valley f.
   pappataci f.
   papular f.
   paratyphoid f.
   pharyngoconjunctival f.
   Phlebotomus f.
   polka f.
   polyleptic f.
   preicteric f.
   pretibial f.
   protein f.
   puerperal f.

   Pym f.
   pyogenic f.
   Q f.
   quinine f.
   Quotidian f.
   rat-bite f.
   recrudescent typhus f.
   relapsing f.
   rheumatic f.
   Rift Valley f.
   Rocky Mountain spotted f.
   rose f.
   Ross River f.
   saddleback f.
   sandfly f.
   San Joaquin Valley f.
   scarlet f.
   Schamberg f.
   ship f.
   shipping f.
   Sindbis f.
   slow f.
   solar f.
   f. sore
   South African hemorrhagic f.
   South African tick f.
   Southeast Asian f.
   spotted f.
   steroid f.
   streptobacillary f.
   swamp f.
   swine f.
   symptomatic f.
   syphilitic f.
   f. therapy
   three-day f.
   tick f.
   tickborne relapsing f.
   traumatic f.
   trench f.
   tsutsugamushi f.
   typhoid f.
   undifferentiated type f.'s
   undulant f.
   f. of unknown origin (FUO)
   viral hemorrhagic f. (VHF)
   viral sandfly f.
   Wesselsbron f.
   West African f.
   West Nile f.
   Whitmore f.
   wound f.
   yellow f.
   Zika f.

Feverall
fexofenadine
   f. HCl/pseudoephedrine HCl
   f. and pseudoephedrine

FF
    fibrofolliculoma
FFA
    frontal fibrosing alopecia
FFS
    failure-free survival
    five-factor score
FGF
    fibroblast growth factor
FHF
    familial Hibernian fever
    fulminant hepatic failure
FHL
    familial hemophagocytic
       lymphohistiocytosis
FI
    fungal infection
    fusion inhibitor
FIA
    Freund incomplete adjuvant
fiber
    A-alpha nerve f.
    afferent nerve f.
    alpha nerve f.
    blocking vagal afferent f.
    blocking vagal efferent f.
    elastic f.
    fast-twitch morphology of
       muscle f.
    Gomori silver impregnation for
       reticulin f.
    Herxheimer f.
    lattice f.
    parasympathetic nerve f.
    reticulin f.
    reticulum f.
    slow-twitch morphology of
       muscle f.
fiberglass dermatitis
fiber-knob
    Ad f.-k.
fiberoptic
    f. bronchoscope
    f. bronchoscopy
Fibracol
    F. collagen
    F. collagen-alginate dressing
Fibrel gel
fibric acid
fibril
    amyloid f.

    collagen f.
    f. structure
fibrillar collagen
fibrillarin
fibrillation
fibrillin
fibrillin-containing microfibril
fibrillogenesis
    in vitro f.
fibrillogenic *N*-terminal fragment
fibrin
    f. deposition
    f. glue
    f. matrix
    f. sealant
fibrinogen level
fibrinoid
    f. change
    f. necrosis
fibrinolysin and deoxyribonuclease
fibrinolytic purpura
fibrinopeptide
fibrinous degeneration
fibroblast
    B cell f.
    f. growth factor (FGF)
    human embryonic lung f.
    f. interferon
    f. lineage synoviocyte
    macrophage f.
    f. mediation
    rheumatoid synovial f.
    Swiss 3T3 f.
    synovial f.
    T cell f.
    tissue-activated f.
    type B f.
fibroblast-conditioned medium (FCM)
fibroblastic tissue
fibroblast-like
    f.-l. spindle cell
    f.-l. synoviocyte (FLS)
fibroblast-shaped synoviocyte
fibrocartilage
    meniscal f.
fibrocartilage-cell lacunae
fibrocytic dysmucopolysaccharidosis
fibrodysplasia ossification progressiva
fibroepithelial polyp

NOTES

F

fibroepithelioma
  f. basal cell carcinoma
  f. of Pinkus
fibrofolliculoma (FF)
fibrogen-associated amyloidosis
fibrogenesis imperfecta ossium
fibrokeratoma
  acquired digital f.
  acral f.
  digital f.
fibroma
  aponeurotic f.
  collagenous f.
  f. durum
  familial myovascular f.
  infantile digital f.
  irritation f.
  juvenile aponeurotic f.
  f. lipomatodes
  f. molle
  f. molle gravidarum
  pedunculated f.
  f. pendulum
  perifollicular f. (PFF)
  peripheral ossifying f.
  periungual f.
  rabbit f.
  senile f.
  Shope f.
fibromatogenic
fibromatosis
  aggressive infantile f.
  f. colli
  congenital generalized f.
  diffuse infantile f.
  digital f.
  gingival f.
  juvenile hyaline f.
  juvenile palmoplantar f.
  palmoplantar f.
  subcutaneous pseudosarcomatous f.
  f. virus of rabbit
fibromatous
fibromectomy
fibromodulin CS/DS
fibromucinoidosus
  lichen f.
fibromyalgia (FM)
  F. Impact Questionnaire (FIQ)
  f. syndrome (FMS)
  f. trigger point
fibronectin
  large external transformation-
    sensitive f. (LETS)
  plasma f.
  f. receptor
**fibronectin-deficient type Ehlers-Danlos
  syndrome**

fibroplasia
  papular f.
fibroproliferative
  endocardial f.
  familial pulmonary f.
fibrosa
  osteitis f.
fibrosarcoma
  Earle L f.
fibrosing
  f. alopecia in a pattern distribution
    (FAPD)
  f. alveolitis
  f. basal cell carcinoma
  f. syndrome
fibrosis
  apical lobe f.
  cystic f. (CF)
  glomerular f.
  idiopathic pulmonary f. (IPF)
  interstitial f.
  nodular subepidermal f.
  obliterative granulomatous f.
  parenchymal f.
  perifollicular f.
  periglandular f.
  perineural f.
  peripheral f.
  portal tract f.
  progressive interstitial f.
  retroperitoneal f.
  serosal f.
  subepidermal nodular f.
  subepithelial f.
  Symmers pipe-stem f.
fibrositis
fibrosum
  molluscum f.
fibrosus
  annulus f.
  lupus f.
  nevus f.
fibrothorax
fibrotic arteriosclerosis
fibrous
  f. arcade
  f. bacterial virus
  f. dysplasia
  f. hamartoma of infancy
  f. histiocytoma
  f. hyperplasia
  f. intimal thickening (FIT)
  f. pannus
  f. papule
  f. papule fibroxanthoma
  f. sheath
  f. synovium (FS)
  f. xanthoma

fibroxanthoma
  atypical f. (AFX)
  fibrous papule f.
FICA
  food immune complex assay
Ficoll cushion
Ficoll-Hypaque
ficosis
fiddle-back
  f.-b. spider
  f.-b. spider bite
fiddler neck
field
  electromagnetic f.
  f. emission scanning electron
    microscopy (FESEM)
Fiessinger-Leroy-Reiter syndrome
Fiessinger-Leroy syndrome
Fiessinger-Rendu syndrome
fifth disease
fig
  f. wart
  weeping f.
figurata
  keratosis rubra f.
  psoriasis f.
figurate psoriasis
figuratum
  erythema f.
figuratus
figure
  flame f.
filaggrin
  epidermal f.
  protein f.
filament
  intermediate f.
filamentary
  f. keratitides
  f. keratitis
filamentous
  f. actin
  f. bacterial virus
  f. bacteriophage
Filaria
  F. bancrofti
  F. loa
filaria, pl. **filariae**
filarial
  f. abscess
  f. elephantiasis
  f. nematode

filariasis
  Bancroft f.
  Bancroftian f.
  brugian f.
  Loiasis f.
  timorian f.
filaricidal
Filatov-Dukes disease
Filatov spot
filgrastim
filiform
  f. tumor
  f. wart
filiformis
  verruca f.
Filipovitch sign
filler
  AcryDerm Strands f.
  Cutinova Cavity f.
  DermAssist f.
  Humatrix Microclysmic Gel f.
  Multidex f.
  PolyWic f.
filles
  acne excoriée des jeunes f.
film
  Bioclusive MVP transparent f.
  BlisterFilm transparent f.
  CarraFilm transparent f.
  Centurion SiteGuard MVP
    transparent f.
  DermAssist transparent f.
  No Sting barrier f.
  NUVO barrier f.
  Omniderm transparent f.
  OpSite Flexigrid transparent f.
  Polyskin II transparent f.
  Polyskin M.R. transparent f.
  polyurethane f. (PUF)
  Pro-Clude transparent f.
  ProCyte transparent f.
  SureSite transparent f.
  Tegaderm HP transparent f.
  Transeal transparent f.
Filmtab
  Biaxin F.
  Rondec F.
Filoviridae virus
Filovirus
filter
  ARI Group I–IV f.
  electronic f.

F

NOTES

filter *(continued)*
    HEPA f.
    high-efficiency particulate air f.
    membrane f.
    Nuclepore f.
filtrable virus
fimbriatum
    Gliocladium f.
finasteride
finding
    immunofluorescence f.
    serum protein electrophoretic f.
    x-ray f.
fine-needle
    f.-n. aspiration (FNA)
    f.-n. aspiration cytology (FNAC)
finger
    blubber f.
    bolster f.
    bowed f.
    clubbed f.
    dead f.
    Hippocratic f.
    F. Phantom pulse oximeter testing system
    sausage f.
    seal f.
    snapping f.
    spade f.
    speck f.
    trigger f.
    vibration-induced white f. (VWF)
    waxy f.
    whale f.
    white f.
finger-in-glove appearance
fingernail
    half-and-half f.
finger-packing doughy cemented
fingerprints
    Galton system of classification of f.
fingertip unit (FTU)
finish
    antipill f.
Finkelstein
    F. disease
    F. test
Finn chamber
FIO₂
    fraction of inspired oxygen
FIQ
    Fibromyalgia Impact Questionnaire
fir
    Douglas f.
fire
    f. ant
    f. ant anaphylaxis

    f. ant sting
    f. coral
    f. coral dermatitis
    f. coral sting
    Saint Anthony's f.
    f. sponge dermatitis
    St. Anthony f.
firebush
fireweed
firm lesion
first
    F. Check rapid diagnostic test
    f. component of complement (C1INH)
    f. degree frostbite
    f. disease
first-degree burn
first-pass drug effect
first-set rejection
fir-tree-like pattern
Fischer stripper
FISH
    fluorescence in situ hybridization
    FISH protocol in bone marrow transplantation
fish
    f. oil
    scorpion f.
    f. skin
    f. tapeworm anemia
    tuna f.
Fisher
    F. method
    F. syndrome
    F. two-tailed exact test
Fisher-Race theory
fish-mouth
    f.-m. healing
    f.-m. wound
fish-tank granuloma
Fisoneb ultrasonic nebulizer
fissuratum
    acanthoma f.
    epulis f.
    granuloma f.
fissure
    anal f.
    interpalpebral f.
fissured tongue
fissuring
fistula, pl. fistulae, fistulas
    f. in ano
    arteriovenous f.
    aural f.
    bronchopleural f.
    coronary f.
    dental f.

pilonidal f.
postbiopsy f.
FIT
fibrous intimal thickening
FITC
fluorescein isothiocyanate
Fite stain
Fitz-Hugh and Curtis syndrome
Fitzpatrick
F. classification of skin type
F. wrinkle score
five-factor score (FFS)
fixation
complement f. (CF)
f. forceps
Ilizarov external f.
open reduction and internal f.
(ORIF)
f. reaction
fixed
f. airflow obstruction
f. charge density
f. cutaneous sporotrichosis
f. drug eruption (FDE)
f. drug reaction
f. pulmonary infiltrate
f. virus
FK506
tacrolimus
flaccid
flagellar
f. agglutinin
f. antigen
flag sign
Flagyl Oral
flake
sulfur f.
flaky paint dermatosis
Flamazine
flame
f. emission spectroscopy (FES)
f. figure
f. nevus
flammeus
nevus f.
f. nevus
osteohypertrophic nevus f.
Flantadin
FLAP
5-lipoxygenase-activating protein
flap
advancement f.

Brandy f.
interpolation f.
island pedicle f.
Juri f.
Karapandzic f.
Marzola f.
O to T f.
O to Z f. *Peng*
pedicled f.
rhombic f.
rotation f.
sliding-bucket mucosal f.
transposition f.
flare
wheal and f.
Flarex Ophthalmic
flash
f. burn
F. portable spirometer
flashlamp
EpiLight f.
f. photoepilation
**flashlamp-pumped pulsed-dye laser
(FLPD, FPDL)**
flashscanner-enhanced CO_2 laser
flask
Dewar f.
flat
f. condyloma
f. papular syphilid
f. wart
flatworm
flavedo
flavicollis
Apodemus f.
Flavimonas orzihabitans
Flaviviridae
Flavivirus
Flavobacterium meningosepticum
flavus
Aspergillus f.
flaxseed
FLB
4-layer bandage
flea
cat f.
chigger f.
dog f.
northern rat f.
Oriental rat f.
sand f.
f. venom

F

NOTES

flea-borne typhus
flea-collar dermatitis
fleck
fleckeri
    Chironex f.
Flegel disease
Fleischner syndrome
flesh
    goosebump f.
    proud f.
flesh-colored
fleshfly
Flexderm hydrogel sheet
flexed tenosynovitis
Flexercell Strain Unit
flexible
    f. collodion
    f. silicone implant
flexion contracture
Flexi-Trak skin anchoring device
flexneri
    Shigella f.
flexor surface
flexural
    f. eczema
    f. psoriasis
flexure
Flexzan foam wound dressing
flight
    matrix-assisted laser desorption ionization-time of f. (MALDI-TOF)
floating-tooth sign
floccosum
    Epidermophyton f.
flocculation
    f. reaction
    f. test
Flolan
Flonase
flood fever
floor-sit maneuver
flop
    dory f.
flora
    saprophytic f.
Florey unit
florid
    f. cutaneous papillomatosis (FCP)
    f. oral papillomatosis
Florida seaweed dermatitis
Florinef Acetate
floristic zone
Florone
    F. E
    F. E topical

flour
    soybean f.
    wheat f.
Flovent Rotadisk powder
flow
    f. cytometric crossmatch
    f. cytometry
    f. cytometry crossmatch (FCXM)
    forced expiratory f. (FEF)
    peak expiratory f. (PEFR)
    peak nasal inspiratory f. (PNIF)
    sinusoidal blood f.
Flowmeter
    Personal Best Peak F.
flowmetry
    laser Doppler f. (LDF)
FlowPRA assay
Floxin
    F. injection
    F. Oral
FLPD
    flashlamp-pumped pulsed-dye laser vascular FLPD
FLS
    fibroblast-like synoviocyte
flu
    Connaught f.
flucatisone propionate/salmeterol (FP/Salm Combo)
fluconazole
fluctuance
fluctuant
fluctuating
    limes f. (Lf)
fluctuation
5-flucytosine
fludrocortisone acetate
fluence
flufenamic acid
fluffy alveolar infiltrate
fluid
    basal transalveolar f.
    bronchoalveolar lavage f. (BALF)
    cutting f.
    epithelial lining f. (ELF)
    intravenous f.
    middle ear f. (MEF)
    simulated gastric f. (SGF)
    simulated intestinal f. (SIF)
    synovial f. (SF)
    tetanus toxoid, f.
    f. therapy
fluid-filled pressure transducer
fluid-phase C1q-binding assay
Flu-Imune
fluke
    blood f.

intestinal f.
tissue f.
Flumadine Oral
flunisolide nasal solution
fluocinolone acetonide
fluocinonide
Fluoderm
Fluogen
Fluonex topical
Fluonid topical
fluoresce
fluorescein-conjugated monoclonal antibody immunofluorescent test
fluorescein isothiocyanate (FITC)
fluorescein-tagged monoclonal antibody immunofluorescent test
fluorescence
    f. overlay antigen mapping (FOAM)
    f. polarization immunoassay (FPIA)
    f. quenching
    f. in situ hybridization (FISH)
    f. in situ hybridization protocol in bone marrow transplantation
fluorescence-activated
    f.-a. cell sorter (FACS)
    f.-a. cell sorting (FACS)
fluorescent
    f. antibody stain (FA)
    f. antibody technique
    f. antimembrane antibody (FAMA)
    f. antinuclear antibody assay (FANA)
    f. enzyme immunoassay (FEIA)
    f. sun lamp
    f. treponemal antibody absorption (FTA-ABS)
    f. treponemal antibody absorption doublestaining (FTA-ABS-DS)
    f. treponemal antibody-absorption test
fluorescent-activated cell sorting (FACS)
fluorescentiae
    stadium f.
Fluorethyl
fluoride
    argon f. (ArF)
Fluori-Methane Topical Spray
fluorinated
    f. corticosteroid
    f. corticosteroid-occlusive therapy
    f. pyrimidine

fluorine-18 2-fluoro-2-deoxy-D-glucose-positron emission tomography (FDG-PET)
fluorochrome
fluorochroming
5-fluorocytosine (5-FC)
fluorometholone
    sodium sulfacetamide and f.
fluorometric procedure
Fluoroplex topical
Fluor-Op Ophthalmic
fluoroquinolone antibiotic
fluoroscopy
5-fluorouracil (5-FU)
fluorouracil cream
fluoxetine
    f. HCl
    f. hydrochloride
fluphenazine hydrochloride
flurandrenolide
flurazepam
flurbiprofen
Fluro-Ethyl Aerosol
Flurosyn topical
Flury
    F. strain rabies virus
    F. strain vaccine
flush
    f. area
    autonomic epilepsy f.
    carcinoid f.
    chlorpropamide f.
    dry f.
    histamine f.
    idiopathic f.
    medullary carcinoma f.
    wet f.
flushing
    emotional f.
    menopausal f.
    neural-mediated f.
    paroxysmal f.
    pulmonary f.
    thermal f.
flutamide
Flutex Topical
fluticasone propionate (FP)
Flutide Diskhaler
flutter device
flux
    f. allergen
    soldering f.

F

NOTES

Fluzone
fly
    f. bite
    black f.
    f. blister
    buffalo f.
    caddis f.
    deer f.
    horse f.
    house f.
    may f.
    sarcophagi f.
    screw-worm f.
    sewer f.
    Spanish f.
    stable f.
    tsetse f.
    tumbu f.
fly-borne disease
flying blister
Flynn-Aird syndrome
FM
    fibromyalgia
    fragrance mix
FMD
    foot-and-mouth disease
    FMD virus
FML Forte Ophthalmic
FML-S Ophthalmic suspension
FMS
    fibromyalgia syndrome
FNA
    fine-needle aspiration
FNAC
    fine-needle aspiration cytology
FOAM
    fluorescence overlay antigen mapping
foam
    f. cell
    clobetasol propionate f.
    Luxiq ViaFoam betamethasone
     valerate f.
    Olux f.
    Reston f.
foamy
    f. agent
    f. histiocyte
    f. virus
focal
    f. acantholytic dyskeratoma
    f. acantholytic dyskeratosis
    f. acral hyperkeratosis
    f. amyloidosis
    f. anoxia
    f. dermal hypoplasia
    f. embolic glomerulonephritis
    f. epithelial hyperplasia (FEH)
    f. histiocytosis

    f. infection
    f. inflammation
    f. reaction
    f. rupture of basement membrane
    f. segmental glomerulosclerosis
     (FSGS)
focus, pl. **foci**
    granulomatous f.
focusing
    isoelectric f. (IEF)
Foerster forceps
fogo selvagem (FS)
FOII powder inhaler
foil
    f. bath pulsed ultraviolet
     actinotherapy
    f. bath PUVA
fold
    crural f.
    Dennie infraorbital f.
    Dennie-Morgan infraorbital f.
    immunoglobulin f.
    lateral nail f.
    Morgan f.
    nail f.
    nasolabial f. (NLF)
    villous f.
folding
    protein f.
Folex PFS
foliacée
    lame f.
foliaceous pemphigus
foliaceus
    endemic pemphigus f.
    pemphigus f. (PF)
folic
    f. acid
    f. acid deficiency
folinic acid
follicle
    agminated f.
    hair f.
    hypertrophic lymphoid f.
    pilosebaceous f.
    tertiary f.
follicular
    f. abscess
    f. accentuation
    f. alopecia
    f. atrophoderma
    f. degeneration syndrome
    f. ichthyosis
    f. impetigo
    f. infundibular cyst
    f. isthmus cyst
    f. keratosis
    f. lichen planus

f. mange
f. melanin unit
f. mucinosis
f. nummular dermatitis
f. nummular eczema
f. occlusion triad
f. orifice
f. papule
f. plug
f. poroma
f. pustule
f. syphilid
f. vulvitis
follicularis
alopecia f.
ichthyosis f.
isolated dyskeratosis f.
keratosis f.
lichen planus f.
folliculis
folliculitis
agminate f.
f. barbae
Bockhart f.
Candida f.
f. cheloidalis
f. cruris atrophicans
f. decalvans
f. decalvans cryptococcica
f. decalvans et lichen spinulosus
eosinophilic pustular f.
f. et perifolliculitis abscedens et suffodiens
excoriated f.
eye f.
f. gonorrhoeica
hot tub f.
industrial f.
keloidal f.
f. keloidalis
f. nares perforans
oil f.
perforating f.
Pityrosporum f.
pustular f.
scalp f.
superficial f.
f. ulerythema reticulata
f. ulerythematosa reticulata
f. varioliformis
folliculorum
Acarus f.

Demodex f.
pityriasis f.
folliculosebaceous cystic hamartoma (FCH)
folliculosis
traumatic anserine f.
folliculus
Follmann balanitis
fomes
fomite
Fong syndrome
Fonsecaea
F. compactum
F. pedrosoi
food
f. additive
F. Agricultural Organization (FAO)
f. allergy
f. antigen
antigenemically cross-reacting f.
f. asthma
f. challenge
F. and Drug Administration (FDA)
f. dye
EleCare medical f.
f. elimination
fermented f.
f. fever
f. hypersensitivity
f. immune complex assay (FICA)
f. protein-induced enteropathy
Tetramune fish f.
food-associated exercise-induced anaphylaxis
food-borne
f.-b. botulism
f.-b. disease
food-induced respiratory disease
foot, pl. **feet**
athlete's f.
cold water immersion f. (CWIF)
Dr. Scholl's Athlete's F.
edema of feet
fungous f.
Hong Kong f.
immersion f.
Madura f.
moccasin f.
mossy f.
neuropathic f.
perforating ulcer of f.
reddening of soles of feet

NOTES

F

foot (*continued*)
    ringworm of f.
    sea boot f.
    shelter f.
    tennis shoe f.
    f. tetter
    trench f.
    tropical immersion f.
    tropic immersion f. (TIF)
    warm water immersion f. (WWIF)
    f. yaw
foot-and-mouth
    f.-a.-m. disease (FMD)
    f.-a.-m. disease virus
    f.-a.-m. disease virus vaccine
for
    f. skin (FS)
    f. skin reverse cutting needle
Foradil
foramen of Monro
foramina
    neural f.
forbidden-clone theory
force
    f. transducer
    van der Waals f.
forced
    f. air system disease
    f. expiratory flow (FEF)
    f. expiratory spirogram (FES)
    f. expiratory volume (FEV)
    f. expiratory volume in 1 second (FEV$_1$)
    f. expiratory volume in 1 second as percent of FVC (FEV$_{1\%VC}$)
    f. vital capacity (FVC)
forceps
    Adson toothed f.
    Allis f.
    Barraquer f.
    Bergh f.
    Bishop-Harmon ophthalmic f.
    Brown-Adson f.
    Carmalt f.
    Castroviejo f.
    Desjardins f.
    Dyonics basket f.
    fixation f.
    Foerster f.
    Frankel-Adson f.
    Graefe f.
    Hartmann ear f.
    IM Jaws alligator f.
    Iris f.
    Jacobson f.
    jeweler's f.
    Lalonde hook f.
    Mixter f.

    mosquito f.
    Semken f.
    splinter f.
    suction loose body f.
    thumb f.
    Walter splinter f.
Forchheimer
    F. sign
    F. spot
Fordyce
    angiokeratoma of F.
    F. angiokeratoma
    F. condition
    F. disease
    F. granule
    F. spot
forearm ischemic exercise test
forefoot
foreign
    f. body (FB)
    f. body giant cell
    f. body granuloma
    f. body radiation
    f. body rhinitis
    f. protein
    f. protein therapy
    f. serum
foreign-body reaction
forelock
    occipital f.
    white frontal f.
Forestier disease
forest yaw
fork
    tuning f.
form
    hyphal f.
    involution f.
    pentamidine in aerosol f.
    replicative f. (RF)
    yeast f.
formaldehyde-releasing preservative (FRP)
formaldehyde resin
formalin
formalinize
formans
    dermopanniculosis f.
formation
    anterior synechia f.
    antigenic antibody lattice f.
    keloid f.
    lamellipodia f.
    mesangial complex f.
    posterior synechia f.
    scar f.
    spike f.

syndesmophyte f.
web f.
formication
formoterol
Formo-Test test
formula
Alimentum f.
Anti-Acne Control F.
Bayer Select Pain Relief F.
Berkow f.
Castellani Natural F.
f. change
Contac Allergy F.
Esoterica Sensitive Skin F.
Friedewald f.
Grecian F.
Neocate f.
Nursoy f.
Nutramigen f.
Parkland burn resuscitation f.
Poisson-Pearson f.
Triaminic AM Decongestant F.
Vivonex f.
formulary
formulation
amphotericin B liposomal f.
fornix, pl. **fornices**
inferior f.
Forsius-Eriksson-type ocular albinism
Forssman
F. antibody
F. antigen
F. antigen-antibody reaction
Fortaz
Fort Bragg fever
Forte
Aristocort F.
Citanest F.
Eldopaque F.
Eldoquin F.
Robinul F.
Solaquin F.
Stieva-A F.
Triam F.
Forteo
Fortovase
fortuitum
Mycobacterium f.
fos
f. gene
F. protooncogene
Fosamax

foscarnet sodium
Foscavir injection
fosfomycin tromethamine
Foshay test
fossa, pl. **fossae**
antecubital f.
coronoid f.
glenoid f.
olecranon f.
popliteal f.
Foster needle holder
Fostex
F. Bar
F. 10% BPO Gel
F. Medicated Cleansing
F. 10% Wash
Fostril lotion
Fothergill disease
FotoFacial treatment
Fototar
foundation
anhydrous facial f.
facial f.
oil-based facial f.
water-based facial f.
water-free facial f.
fountain-spray splatter
Fournier
F. disease
F. gangrene
F. syphiloma
fourth disease
foveation
foveolate
fowl
f. diphtheria
f. erythroblastosis virus
leukemia of f.'s
f. leukosis
f. lymphomatosis
f. lymphomatosis virus
f. myeloblastosis virus
f. neurolymphomatosis virus
f. paralysis
f. pest
f. plague
f. plague virus
fowleri
Naegleria f.
Fowler solution
fowlpox
f. virus

F

NOTES

fox
 F. curette
 F. disease
 f. encephalitis
 f. encephalitis virus
 F. impetigo
Fox-Fordyce disease
foxtail
 meadow f.
FP
 fluticasone propionate
FPDL
 flashlamp-pumped pulsed-dye laser
FPH
 familial progressive hyperpigmentation
FPIA
 fluorescence polarization immunoassay
FP/Salm Combo
FPU
 fetoplacental unit
FPV
 feline panleukopenia virus
fractional sterilization
fraction of inspired oxygen (FIO₂)
fracture
 Colles f.
 f. fusi
 Segond f.
 stress f.
 transchondral f.
fragarius
 nevus f.
fragilis
 Bacteroides f.
fragilitas
 f. crinium
 f. unguium
fragility
 bone f.
fragment
 Fab f.
 Fabc f.
 Facb f.
 Fb f.
 Fc f.
 fibrillogenic *N*-terminal f.
 Fv f.
 Klenow f.
 Spengler f.
fragmentation
 elastic-fiber f.
fragrance mix (FM)
fraise
 diamond f.
frambesia tropica
frambesiformis
 sycosis f.
frambesiform syphilid

frambesioma
framboesia
 sycosis f.
framboesiaeformis
 sycosis f.
framboesianus
 lichen f.
framboesioides
 mycosis f.
frame-shift
 f.-s. mutagen
 f.-s. mutation
Franceschetti-Jadassohn syndrome
Franceschetti-Klein syndrome
Francis disease
Francisella tularensis
Frankel-Adson forceps
Frankfort horizontal plane
frank virilization
fraterna
 Hymenolepis f.
Frazier-Shepherd skin hook
Frazier skin hook
FRC
 functional residual capacity
FreAmine
Frechet
 F. extender
 F. three-flap slot correction
freckle
 f. of Hutchinson
 Hutchinson f.
 melanotic f.
freckling
 axillary f.
Frederickson type IIa, IIb hyperlipidemia
free
 f. cartilage graft
 f. margin
 f. radical
 f. salicylate level
freeborni
 Anopheles f.
freehand technique
Freeman-Sheldon syndrome
Freer septum elevator
free-tissue xenograft
freeze-dried
 f.-d. protein
 f.-d. skin
freezing
 surface f.
Freezone solution
Frei
 F. antigen
 F. bubo
 F. test

Freiberg disease
Frei-Hoffmann reaction
French-American-British (FAB)
    F.-A.-B. classification
French measles
Freon
frequency
    f. of allergy symptom
    ciliary beat f.
    f. doubled neodymium:yttrium-
      aluminum-garnet laser
freshening peel
fresh frozen plasma
Freund
    F. complete adjuvant
    F. complete adjuvant test
    F. incomplete adjuvant (FIA)
freundii
    Citrobacter f.
Frey
    F. hair
    F. syndrome
friction
    adhesional and glide f.
    f. blister
    f. bulla
Friedewald formula
Friedländer pneumonia
Friend
    F. disease
    F. erythroleukemia cell
    F. leukemia virus
frigida
    erythrocyanosis f.
Frigiderm
frigoris
    stadium f.
fringe
    costal f.
Frish bacillus
Froben
Froben-SINUS RHYTHM
FrogWear sunscreen clothing
frond
    villous f.
frontal
    f. bossing
    f. fibrosing alopecia (FFA)
frontalis
    acne f.
    alopecia liminaris f.

frost
    f. itch
    urea f.
frostbite
    first degree f.
frostnip
frozen
    f. plasma
    f. section assay (FSA)
    f. shoulder
frozen-thawed red cell
FRP
    formaldehyde-releasing preservative
Fruit
    F. of the Earth Moisturizing Aloe
    F. of the Earth Moisturizing Aloe
      Sport
frustrated
    f. phagocyte
    f. phagocytosis
FS
    fibrous synovium
    fogo selvagem
    for skin
      FS reverse cutting needle
      FS Shampoo topical
FSA
    frozen section assay
FSGS
    focal segmental glomerulosclerosis
FSL
    Actin FSL
FTA-ABS
    fluorescent treponemal antibody
      absorption
      FTA-ABS test
FTA-ABS-DS
    fluorescent treponemal antibody
      absorption doublestaining
FTOC
    fetal thymus organ culture
FTU
    fingertip unit
FTY720
5-FU
    5-fluorouracil
fuchsin
    acid f.
    f. body
fucosidosis
fugax
    erythema f.

F

NOTES

fugitive
    f. swelling
    f. wart
fulguration
full-body cutaneous examination
full-coverage facial powder
full-thickness
    f.-t. burn
    f.-t. graft
fulminans
    acne f.
    purpura f.
fulminant hepatic failure (FHF)
fulminating smallpox
Fulvicin P/G
Fulvicin-U/F
fulvum
    Microsporum f.
fumagillin
fumarate
    clemastine f.
fumaric acid ester
fumes
    soldering f.
fumigation
fumigatus
    Aspergillus f.
Fun-boi
function
    circadian f.
    decreased renal f.
    delayed graft f. (DGF)
    gene f.
    International Index of Erectile F. (IIEF)
    phagocytic f.
    poor marrow f.
    pulmonary f. (PF)
    secretory vesicle f.
functional
    f. abnormality in asthma
    f. affinity
    f. C1 esterase inhibitor
    f. class II–IV
    f. impairment
    f. polymorphism
    f. residual capacity (FRC)
funestus
    Anopheles f.
fungal
    f. arthritis
    f. bursitis
    f. culture
    f. disease
    f. id reaction
    f. infection (FI)
    f. scraping
fungate

fungating
    f. chancre
    f. sore
fungemia
fungi (*pl. of* fungus)
fungicidal
fungicide
fungiform
Fungi Imperfecti
Fungi-Nail
fungistasis
fungistat
fungistatic
fungitoxic
Fungizone
    F. intravenous
Fungoid
    F. AF Topical solution
    F. HC Creme
    F. tincture
fungoides
    granuloma f.
    microabscess of mycosis f.
    mycosis f. (MF)
fungosity
fungosus
    nevus vascularis f.
fungous
    f. foot
    f. gonitis
    f. infection
fungus, pl. fungi
    Alternaria alternanta f.
    f. ball
    beefsteak f.
    bracket f.
    Cladosporium herbarum f.
    dematiaceous f.
    dimorphic fungi
    mosaic f.
    nonpathogenic f.
    opportunistic f.
    Phoma f.
    sac f.
    saprophytic fungi
    subcutaneous f.
    Trichophyton tonsurans f.
    umbilical f.
    zoophilic f.
FUO
    fever of unknown origin
Furacin topical
Furadantin
Furalan
Furan
Furanite
furazolidone
furfur, pl. *furfures*

Malassezia f.
Microsporum f.
furfuracea
    alopecia f.
    dermatomycosis f.
    dermatophytosis f.
    impetigo f.
    pityriasis f.
    seborrhea f.
    tinea f.
furfuraceous
    f. desquamation
    f. impetigo
furfurans
    porrigo f.
furfures (*pl. of furfur*)
furin convertase
furoate
    diloxanide f.
    mometasone f.
Furoxone
furrow
    Jadelot f.
    transverse f.
furrowed tongue
furuncle
furuncular disease
furunculitis
    hospital f.
furunculoid
furunculosis orientalis
furunculous
furunculus
Fusarium
    F. chlamydosporum
    F. moniliforme
    F. oxysporum
    F. sacchari
    F. solani

fusca
    lamina f.
fuscoceruleus
    nevus f.
fusi (*pl. of fusus*)
fusidic acid
fusiform
    f. bacillus
    f. excision
fusin
    f. molecule
fusion
    f. inhibitor (FI)
    protoplast f.
    f. toxin
Fusobacterium nucleatum
fusospirochetal
    f. balanitis
    f. disease
    f. stomatitis
fusus, pl. **fusi**
    cortical fusi
    fracture fusi
Futcher line
fuzz
    peach f.
FVC
    forced vital capacity
    forced expiratory volume in 1
        second as percent of FVC
        ($FEV_{1\%VC}$)
    mean forced expiratory flow during
        the middle of FVC ($FEF_{25-75\%}$)
Fv fragment
Fy antigen
FyBron
    F. alginate wound cover
    F. alginate wound dressing
fyn kinase enzyme

NOTES

F

G
>G antigen
>G protein
>G unit of streptomycin

G3139

5G1.1 recombinant C5 complement inhibitor

G5 massage and percussion machine

GA
>granuloma annulare

GABA
>gamma-aminobutyric acid
>>GABA inhibitory neurotransmitter

GABAergic neuron

Gabbromicina

GABEB
>generalized atrophic benign epidermolysis bullosa

GABHS
>group A beta-hemolytic streptococcus

Gaboon ulcer

GAD
>glutamic acid decarboxylase

GAD65

gadolinium

gadopentetate dimeglumine (Gd-DTPA)

GAG
>glycosaminoglycan

gag
>g. gene
>viral protein g.

gait
>g. analysis
>antalgic g.

GAL
>gallus adeno-like
>>GAL virus

Gal
>G. antibody

Gal*a*1 epitope

galactidrosis

galactophlysis

galea

3Gal epitope

gallinae
>*Dermanyssus g.*

gallinarum
>neurolymphomatosis g.
>osteopetrosis g.

Gallipoli sore

gallium-aluminum-arsenide 904-nm laser

gallus
>g. adeno-like (GAL)
>g. adeno-like virus

GALT
>gut-associated lymphoid tissue

Galton
>G. delta
>G. system of classification of fingerprints

galvanic epilator

Gamasidae

gamasoidosis

Gamastan

Gambel
>G. oak
>G. oak tree

gambiae
>*Anopheles g.*

gamekeeper's thumb

gametocytemia

gametophyte

Gamimune N

gamma
>g. globulin
>g. hemolysis
>interferon g.

gamma-aminobutyric acid (GABA)

gamma-1b
>interferon g.-1b

Gammabulin Immuno

gamma-camera

Gammagard S/D

gamma-glutamyltranspeptidase

gamma-linolenic acid

Gammar

Gammar-P I.V.

gammopathy
>benign monoclonal g.
>biclonal g.
>monoclonal g.
>polyclonal g.

ganciclovir

ganglion, pl. **ganglia**
>sensory g.
>trigeminal g.

ganglionectomy
>lumbar g.

ganglioneuroma

gangosa

gangraenescens
>granuloma g.

gangrene
>arteriosclerotic g.
>bacterial synergistic g.
>cold g.
>cutaneous g.
>decubital g.
>diabetic g.

G

gangrene *(continued)*
 disseminated cutaneous g.
 dry g.
 embolic g.
 Fournier g.
 gas g.
 hemorrhagic g.
 hospital g.
 hot g.
 infected vascular g.
 Meleney g.
 moist g.
 nosocomial g.
 peripheral g.
 Pott g.
 presenile spontaneous g.
 pressure g.
 progressive bacterial synergistic g.
 senile g.
 static g.
 symmetrical g.
 synergistic g.
 thrombotic g.
 venous g.
 wet g.
 white g.
gangrenosa
 dermatitis g.
 phagedena g.
 pyodermia g.
 vaccinia g.
 varicella g.
gangrenosum
 bullous hemorrhagic pyoderma g.
 ecthyma g.
 hemorrhagic pyoderma g.
 pyoderma g. (PG)
gangrenosus
 pemphigus g.
gangrenous stomatitis
Gantanol
Gantrisin Oral
Garamycin
 G. injection
 G. Ophthalmic
 G. Topical
Gardner-Diamond
 G.-D. purpura
 G.-D. syndrome
Gardnerella vaginitis
Gardner syndrome
gargoylism
garinii
 Borrelia g.
garlic
garment
 Marena compression g.
 g. nevus

garnet
 neodymium:yttrium-aluminum-g.
 (Nd:YAG)
GART
 genotypic antiretroviral resistance testing
GAS
 group A streptococcus
gas
 g. abscess
 arterial blood g. (ABG)
 blood g.
 g. cautery
 g. chromatography
 g. gangrene
 g. gangrene antitoxin
gaseous cellulitis
gasping disease
Gasterophilus
gastritis
 autoimmune atrophic g.
 experimental autoimmune g. (EAG)
Gastrocrom
 G. Oral
gastroenteritis
 acute infectious nonbacterial g.
 allergic eosinophilic g.
 endemic nonbacterial infantile g.
 eosinophilic g.
 epidemic nonbacterial g.
 infantile g.
 porcine transmissible g.
 rotavirus g.
 viral g.
 g. virus type A, B
gastroenterocolitis
 allergic eosinophilic g.
gastroenteropathy
 protein-losing g.
gastroesophageal (GE)
 g. reflux (GER)
gastrointestinal
 g. anisakiasis (GIA)
 g. symptom
 g. ulceration
gastropathy
 NSAID g.
gastroprotective agent
gastroschisis
gastrotoxin
gatifloxacin
gating
Gaucher disease
gauge
 adjustable-length g.
Gaussian beam
gauze
 Aquaphor g.
 Biolex impregnated g.

CarraGauze impregnated g.
ClearSite impregnated g.
Cover-Roll g.
Curafil impregnated g.
Curasol impregnated g.
Dermagran impregnated g.
DermAssist impregnated g.
Elta Dermal impregnated g.
Gentell impregnated g.
Iodoform g.
MPM GelPad impregnated g.
nonstick g.
N-Terface g.
PanoGauze hydrogel-impregnated g.
PanoGauze impregnated g.
Restore impregnated g.
SkinTegrity impregnated g.
TransiGel impregnated g.
Gaviscon Prevent
GBM
glomerular basement membrane
GBS
group B streptococcus
GC
glucocorticoid
GCA
giant cell arteritis
G-CSF
granulocyte colony-stimulating factor
GCTTS
giant cell tumor of tendon sheath
Gd-DTPA
gadopentetate dimeglumine
GE
gastroesophageal
Ge
Ge antigen
Ge Jie Anti-asthma Pill
Gebauer ethyl chloride
Geiger electrocautery unit
gel
AccuSite injectable g.
adapalene g.
Advanced Formula Oxy
Sensitive G.
agarose g.
Benzac AC G.
BenzaClin g.
Benzac W G.
Brevoxyl G.
Cann-Ease moisturizing nasal g.
Clear By Design G.

clindamycin/benzoyl peroxide g.
dapsone topical g.
Del Aqua-5 G.
Del Aqua-10 G.
Dermaflex G.
Desquam-E g.
Desquam-X g.
diclofenac sodium g.
Differin g.
g. diffusion
g. diffusion precipitin test
g. diffusion precipitin test in one
dimension
g. diffusion reaction
Dryox G.
DuoDerm hydroactive g.
erythromycin, benzoyl peroxide
topical g.
Estar G.
Fibrel g.
Fostex 10% BPO G.
H.P. Acthar G.
Humatrix Microclysmic G.
IntraSite g.
Keralyt G.
NeoStrata g.
Panretin topical g.
Perfectoderm G.
g. phenomenon
polyacrylamide g.
precipitate in g.
PreSun lotion and g.
silicone g.
sodium dodecyl sulfate-
polyacrylamide gradient slab g.
Solarase topical g.
SoloSite wound g.
T g.
tazarotene topical g.
Tisit Blue G.
Triaz g.
Vergogel G.
g. wound dressing
gelatin
g. allergy
g. compression boot
g. zymography
gelatinase
72-kD g.
92-kD g.
Gelfoam

G

NOTES

Gell
- G. and Coombs classification
- G. and Coombs classification system
- G. and Coombs reaction

Gelocast
- G. bandage
- G. Unna boot leg compression dressing

gelsolin amyloidosis

Gem
- Ampliwax PCR G.

gemcitabine HCl

gemellus
- *Paederus* g.

geminata
- *Solenopsis* g.

Gemini automated centrifugal analyzer

Genac Tablet

Genahist Oral

Genamin Expectorant

Gen-Amoxicillin

Genant method

Genapap

Genasense

Genaspor

Genatap Elixir

Gen-Beclo

Gen-Cyproterone

gene
- art/trs g.
- g. bank
- bax g.
- bcl-2, -6 g.
- Bruton tyrosine kinase g.
- CD40 ligand g.
- cell interaction g.
- CI g.
- c-myc g.
- COL1A1 g.
- COL2A1 type II procollagen g.
- g. complex
- CTNS g.
- g. disruption
- env g.
- FasL g.
- Fas ligand g.
- fos g.
- g. function
- gag g.
- germline V g.
- herpes thymidine kinase g.
- HLA-B60 g.
- HLA-DR3 g.
- hormone-related g.
- housekeeping g.
- IL-2 receptor alpha chain g.
- immune response g.
- immune suppressor g.
- immunoglobulin g.
- Ir g.
- Is g.
- J chain g.
- JH g.
- jun g.
- luciferase reporter g.
- manganese superoxide dismutase g.
- g. manipulation
- marker g.
- master regulator g.
- melanoma-associated g. (MAGE)
- 3'orf g.
- g. overexpression
- pol g.
- proapoptotic g.
- P53 tumor suppressor g.
- R g.
- RAG1, RAG2 g.
- recombinase-activating g.
- sor g.
- stealthing g.
- sTNFR g.
- g. structure
- suicide g.
- tat g.
- g. therapy
- TNF receptor II g.
- g. transcription
- transfer g.
- transforming g.
- tumor suppressor g.
- V g.
- vanA, vanH, vanS g.
- V-D-J g.
- VH g.
- von Hippel-Lindau g. (VHL)
- wt g.
- X-encoded immune system g.

gene-based
- g.-b. vaccine
- g.-b. vector

gene-knockout technology

general
- g. immunity
- g. transduction

generalis
- acne g.
- seborrhea g.

generalisata
- alopecia g.

generalisatus
- herpes zoster g.

generalized
- g. anaphylaxis
- g. atrophic benign epidermolysis bullosa (GABEB)

g. desquamation
g. elastolysis
g. epidermolysis bullosa simplex
g. epidermolytic hyperkeratosis
g. eruptive histiocytoma
g. granuloma annulare
g. heat urticaria
g. hyperhidrosis
g. lentiginosis
g. maculopapular rash
g. melanosis
g. morphea
g. morphea variant
g. myxedema
g. plane xanthoma
g. plane xanthomatosis
g. pruritus
g. pustular psoriasis
g. pustular psoriasis of von
   Zumbusch
g. pustular psoriasis of Zambusch
g. Shwartzman phenomenon
g. vaccinia
g. vitiligo
g. weakness
g. xanthelasma
generation time
genetic
g. C2 deficiency
g. depression of immune system
g. determinant
g. disease
g. factor
g. marker
microbial g.'s
g. predisposition
g. recombination
Gengou phenomenon
Gengraf
Gen-Ipratropium
genistein
genistein-inhibited movement
genital
g. aphthous ulcer
g. atopic dermatitis
g. erosive lichen planus
g. hair
g. herpes
g. herpes simplex virus
g. hidradenitis suppurativa
g. lentigo
g. leukoderma

g. lichen sclerosus
g. lichen simplex chronicus
g. neurodermatitis
g. papulosquamous lesion
g. plasma cell mucositis
g. pruritus
g. psoriasis
g. Reiter syndrome
g. squamous cell carcinoma
g. tumor
g. wart
genitalis
herpes g.
genitalium
Mycoplasma g.
genitofemoral nerve entrapment
genitourinary lesion
Gennerich treatment
genodermatology
genodermatosis
neurologic g.
genome
viral g.
genome-side linkage analysis
genomic
g. analysis
g. glucocorticoid mechanism
Genoptic S.O.P. Ophthalmic
genospecies
genote
F g.
genotoxic
genotype
XXYY g.
genotypic antiretroviral resistance testing (GART)
genotyping
Genpril
Gen-Probe rapid tuberculosis test
Gensan
Gentab-LA
Gentacidin Ophthalmic
Gentak Ophthalmic
gentamicin
prednisolone and g.
g. sulfate
Gentell
G. alginate wound cover
G. alginate wound dressing
G. foam wound dressing
G. hydrogel dressing

G

NOTES

Gentell *(continued)*
   G. impregnated gauze
   G. wound cleanser
gentian violet
GentleLASE
   G. laser
   G. Plus laser system
GentlePeel skin exfoliation system
genu valgum
Geocillin
geode
geographic
   g. difference
   g. pattern
   g. stippling of nail
   g. tongue
geographica
   lingua g.
   psoriasis g.
geometric
   g. mean concentration (GMC)
   g. mean titer (GMT)
geophilic
geotrichosis
Geotrichum
GER
   gastroesophageal reflux
geranylgeranyl transferase I
gerbil
Geref
Gerhardt
   G. disease
   G. phenomenon
   G. reaction
   G. test
Gerhardt-Mitchell disease
geriatric
   g. dermogram
   g. psoriasis
Gerimal II
germ
   hair g.
   primary epithelial g.
   g. theory
German
   G. cockroach
   G. measles
   G. measles virus
germicidal
germicide
germinal
germinative
   g. cell
   g. time
germinativum
   stratum g.
Germiston virus

germline
   g. transcription
   g. V gene
geroderma
gerontine
gerstaeckeri
   Triatoma g.
Gerstmann-Straussler-Scheinker
   syndrome
GESICA trial
gestationis
   herpes g. (HG)
   hydroa g.
   impetigo g.
   pemphigoid g.
   protoporphyria g.
   prurigo g.
GF
   growth factor
GFR
   glomerular filtration rate
GG
   Slo-Phyllin GG
ggELISA
   glycoprotein-based enzyme-linked
   immunosorbent assay
GGVB
   glucose-gelatin Veronal buffer
GH
   growth hormone
Ghon complex
ghoul hand
GIA
   gastrointestinal anisakiasis
Gianotti-Crosti
   G.-C. disease
   G.-C. syndrome
giant
   g. cell
   g. cell arteritis (GCA)
   g. cell arteritis syndrome
   g. cell epulis
   g. cell granuloma
   g. cell myocarditis
   g. cell myositis
   g. cell tumor
   g. cell tumor of tendon sheath
   (GCTTS)
   g. condyloma
   g. congenital pigmented nevus
   g. desert centipede
   g. desert centipede bite
   g. eccrine acrospiroma
   g. hives
   g. lichenification
   g. papillary conjunctivitis (GPC)
   g. ragweed
   g. urticaria

giantism
Giardia lamblia
Gibbs-Gradle scissors
Gibert
    G. disease
    G. pityriasis
Giemsa stain
gift spot
gigantea
    lichenificatio g.
    urticaria g.
giganteum
    molluscum g.
Gila
    G. monster
    G. monster bite
Gilbert syndrome
Gilchrist
    G. disease
    G. mycosis
Gilead
    balm of G.
Gillette Blue Blade
Gillies needle holder
ginger
gingiva
gingival
    g. fibromatosis
    g. hyperplasia
    g. lymphoma
gingivitis
    acute necrotizing ulcerative g.
    (ANUG)
    desquamative g.
    gonococcal g.
    ulcerative g.
gingivostomatitis
    acute herpetic g.
    herpetic g.
ginkgo
gio
    cao g.
girdle
    shoulder g.
Girdlestone pseudarthrosis
Giroux-Barbeau syndrome
GL-701
glabella
glabra
    verruca g.

glabrata
    Candida g.
    Torulopsis g.
glabrate
glabrosa
    tinea g.
glabrous skin
gladiatorum
    herpes g.
gland
    apocrine sweat g.
    axillary venom g.
    Boerhaave sweat g.
    Brunner g.
    ceruminous g.
    cirrhotic lacrimal g.
    coil g.
    eccrine sweat g.
    ectopic sebaceous g.
    holocrine g.
    hyperplasia of sebaceous g.
    Krause g.
    lymph g.
    meibomian g.
    merocrine g.
    Moll g.
    oil g.
    paired venom g.
    parotid g.
    Philip g.
    salivary g.
    sebaceous g. (SG)
    stink g.
    sweat g.
    Zeis g.
glanders
glandular fever
glandularis
    cheilitis g.
glans penis
Glanzmann thrombasthenia
glass
    g. body
    Wood g.
Glaucon
glebae
    Acanthamoeba g.
glenohumeral
    g. arthritis
    g. degeneration
    g. joint
    g. ligament

G

NOTES

glenohumeral *(continued)*
    g. osteoarthritis
    g. synovitis
glenoid
    g. component
    g. erosion
    g. fossa
    g. labrum
glenoplasty
gliadin
    deamidated g.
glial nodule
Gliocladium fimbriatum
glioma
    nasal g.
    optic g.
gliomatous proliferation
global rating of pain
globi (*pl. of* globus)
globosum
    Chaetomium g.
globulin
    alpha-2 g.
    antihuman g.
    antilymphocyte g. (ALG)
    antithymocyte gamma g. (ATG, ATGAM)
    beta-$_{1E}$ g.
    beta-$_{1C}$ g.
    beta-$_{1F}$ g.
    gamma g.
    hepatitis B immune g. (H-BIG)
    human gamma g.
    immune serum g.
    intravenous gamma g. (IVGG)
    intravenous immune serum g. (IVIG)
    lymphocyte immune g.
    Minnesota antilymphoblast g.
    pertussis immune g.
    placenta-eluted gamma g.
    rabbit antithymocyte g. (RATG)
    respiratory syncytial virus IV immune g.
    RH$_o$(D) g.
    tetanus immune g.
    vaccinia immune g.
    varicella-zoster immune g.
    zoster immune g.
globus, pl. **globi**
glomangioma
glomangiomatosis
glomera (*pl. of* glomus)
glomerata
    Dactylis g.
glomerular
    g. basement membrane (GBM)
    g. eluate

    g. fibrosis
    g. filtration rate (GFR)
    g. hyperfiltration
glomeruli (*pl. of* glomerulus)
glomerulitis
glomeruloid hemangioma
glomerulonephritis
    acute crescentic g.
    acute hemorrhagic g.
    acute poststreptococcal g. (APSGN)
    antibasement membrane antibody-induced g.
    crescentic g.
    diffuse proliferative g.
    focal embolic g.
    hypocomplementemic g.
    immune complex g.
    lupus g.
    membranoproliferative g.
    membranous g.
    mesangiocapillary g. (MCCN)
    pauciimmune g.
    postinfectious g.
    postpyodermal acute g.
    poststreptococcal g. (PSGN)
    primary pauciimmune necrotizing g.
    proliferative g.
    rapidly progressive necrotizing g. (RPGN)
glomerulosa
    zona g.
glomerulosclerosis
    focal segmental g. (FSGS)
glomerulus, pl. **glomeruli**
glomus, pl. **glomera**
    g. body
    neuromyoarterial g.
    g. tumor
Glossina
    G. bite
glossitis, pl. **glossitides**
    g. areata exfoliativa
    atrophic g.
    benign migratory g.
    Candida g.
    g. dissecans
    Hunter g.
    median rhomboid g. (MRG)
    migratory g.
    Moeller g.
    g. parasitica
    parenchymatous g.
    g. of pellagra
    g. rhombica mediana
    rhomboid g.
    g. rhomboidea mediana
glossodynia
    Candida g.

glossopyrosis
glossy
>g. skin
>g. tongue

glove
>Biobrane g.
>Bluettes cotton knit-lined g.
>Dermapor g.
>invisible g.
>Nimble Fingers g.
>g.'s and socks syndrome (GSS)
>Super Ebonettes flock-lined g.

glove-powder inhalation test
glove-use test
glow
>sunset g.

glowing red lips
glucagon
>gut g.

glucagonoma syndrome
Glucantime
glucocerebrosidase
glucocorticoid (GC)
>intraarticular g.
>g. withdrawal syndrome

glucocorticoid-induced osteoporosis
glucocorticoid-inducible protein
glucocorticoid-mediated stress-induced immune alteration
glucocorticosteroid
gluconate
>calcium g.
>chlorhexidine g.

glucosamine
glucose
glucose-6-phosphatase deficiency
glucose-gelatin Veronal buffer (GGVB)
glucose-6-phosphate dehydrogenase (G6PD)
glucuronate
>trimetrexate g.

glucuronic acid
glucuronidase
glucuronidation salicylate
glue
>bee g.
>fibrin g.
>Loctite 15494 ethyl cyanoacrylate g.

GLUS
>granulomatous lesions of unknown significance
>GLUS syndrome

glutamate
>monosodium g. (MSG)

glutamic acid decarboxylase (GAD)
glutamine-rich polypeptide
glutaraldehyde
glutaraldehyde-modified-tyrosine-absorbed extract
glutathione-dependent, cytosolic isozyme
glutathione S-transferase (GST)
gluten
>g. enteropathy
>g. intolerance

gluten-free diet
gluten-sensitive enteropathy (GSE)
glutinosa
>*Alnus g.*

GLY
>glycerol

glycation
>nonenzymatic g. (NEG)

glycerin
>DermAssist G.

glycerinated extract
glycerol (GLY)
>g. guaiacolate

Glycerol-T
glyceryl monostearate
glycine
glycine-rich
>g.-r. beta-glycoprotein
>g.-r. beta-glycoproteinase

glycobiology
glycocalyx
Glycofed
glycogenolysis
glycogen storage disease
glycol
>Diprolene G.
>propylene g.
>salicylic acid and propylene g.

glycolic acid
glycolipid lipidosis
glycolysis
glycophorin antigen
glycophosphatidylinositol anchor
glycoprotein
>beta$_2$-g. II
>homopentameric g.

G

NOTES

glycoprotein *(continued)*
    human cartilage g. 39
    g. IIa (GPIIa)
    g. IIb (GPIIb)
    g. IIb-IIIa (GPIIbIIIa)
    lysosomal g.
    multifunctional extracellular g.
    myelin-oligodendrocyte g. (MOG)
    pregnancy alpha-2 g. (PAG)
    pregnancy-associated g.
glycoprotein-based enzyme-linked
    immunosorbent assay (ggELISA)
glycoproteinosis
glycopyrrolate
glycosaminoglycan (GAG)
    g. chain
glycoside
    cardiac g.
glycosphingolipid
    g. deposit
    g. metabolism
glycosphingolipidosis
glycosylation
glycosylphosphatidylinositol (GPI)
glycosylphosphatidylinositol-anchored
    protein
glycyl-transfer
    g.-t. ribonucleic acid
    g.-t. ribonucleic acid synthetase
glycyl-tRNA synthetase
Glycyphagus domesticus
Glydant
Glyquin cream
Gm
    Gm allotype
    Gm antigen
    factor Gm
GMC
    geometric mean concentration
GM-CSF
    granulocyte-macrophage colony-
      stimulating factor
    granulocyte and macrophage colony-
      stimulating factor
GMP
    guanosine monophosphate
GMS
    Grocott methenamine silver
GMT
    geometric mean titer
G-myticin topical
gnat bite
Gnathostoma spinigerum
gnathostomiasis
GNB
    Gram-negative bacillus
    Gram-negative bacteremia
gnotobiology

gnotobiota
gnotobiote
gnotobiotic
goat
    g. epithelium
    g. milk
goatpox virus
goat-serum-derived
goblet
    g. cell
    g. cell degranulation
    g. cell hyperplasia
    g. cell metaplasia
Goeckerman
    G. regimen
    G. treatment
Goggia sign
gold
    African G.
    g. 4-amino-2-mercaptobenzoic acid
    g. dermatitis
    parenteral g.
    g. retinoid
    g. salts
    G. Schnapps syndrome
    Selsun G.
    Selsun G. for Women
    g. sodium thioglucose (GSTG)
    g. sodium thiomalate (GSTM)
    g. therapy
    g. thiopropanolsulphonate
    g. thiosulfate
goldenrod
gold-induced
    g.-i. aplasia
    g.-i. enterocolitis
golfer
    g. elbow
    g. skin
golf tee hair
Golgi
    G. apparatus
    G. complex
Goltz-Gorlin syndrome
Goltz syndrome
Gomori silver impregnation for
    reticulin fiber
gonadal dysgenesis
gonadotropin
    chorionic human recombinant g.
gonarthrosis
gondii
    Toxoplasma g.
gonitis
    fungous g.
gonococcal
    g. arthritis
    g. arthropathy

g. conjunctivitis
g. gingivitis
g. septicemia
g. stomatitis
gonococcemia
gonococcic tenosynovitis
gono opsonin
gonophage
gonorrhea
oropharyngeal g.
pharyngeal g.
rectal g.
gonorrheal
g. bubo
g. dermatosis
g. keratosis
g. tenosynovitis
g. urethritis
gonorrhoeae
Neisseria g.
tetracycline-resistant *Neisseria* g.
(TRNG)
gonorrhoeica
folliculitis g.
gonorrhoica
macula g.
gonotoxemia
gonotoxin
Good antigen
goodness-of-fit chi-square test
Goodpasture syndrome
goose
g. bump
g. feather
gooseberry
goosebump flesh
gooseflesh
goosefoot weed pollen
Gopalan syndrome
Gordofilm Liquid
gordonae
Mycobacterium g.
Gordon phenomenon
Gorham disease
Gorlin-Chaudhry-Moss syndrome
Gorlin-Goltz syndrome
Gorlin syndrome
Gorman syndrome
Gormel Creme
Gorney-Freeman straight facelift scissors
Gorney straight facelift scissors
Göthlin test

Gottron
G. papule
G. sign
G. syndrome
Gott shunt
Gougerot
G. and Blum disease
pigmented purpuric lichenoid
dermatitis of G.
G. syndrome
G. triad
Gougerot-Blum
G.-B. dermatosis
G.-B. disease
G.-B. syndrome
Gougerot-Carteaud
papillomatosis of G.-C.
G.-C. syndrome
Gougerot-Sjögren disease
goundou
gout
chronic tophaceous g.
intercritical g.
juvenile g.
saturnine g.
tophaceous g.
underexcretion-type g.
gouttes
parapsoriasis en g.
gouty panniculitis
Gower
G. maneuver
panatrophy of G.
gp110
EBV glycoprotein g.
Epstein-Barr glycoprotein g.
gp120
gp91^{phox} level
GPB
Gram-positive bacillus
Gram-positive bacteremia
GPC
giant papillary conjunctivitis
G6PD
glucose-6-phosphate dehydrogenase
GP47, GP67 protein
GPI
glycosylphosphatidylinositol
GPI-anchored protein
GP ib-IX complex
GPIIa
glycoprotein IIa

G

NOTES

GPIIb
glycoprotein IIb
GPIIbIIIa
glycoprotein IIb-IIIa
GPL unit
GPMT
guinea pig maximization test
G-protein-coupled receptor
grade
Billingham Classification of
Rejection, g. 0, 1A, 1B, 2, 3A,
3B, 4
International Society for Heart and
Lung Transplant g.
ISHLT g.
gradient
alveolar-arterial oxygen g.
grading
wound g. 1-6
Gradle scissors
graecorum
elephantiasis g.
lepra g.
Graefe forceps
Graffi virus
graft
AlloDerm processed tissue g.
AlloDerm universal dermal
tissue g.
allogenic g.
autogeneic g.
autologous g.
autoplastic g.
composite g.
g. failure
free cartilage g.
full-thickness g.
H g.
heterologous g.
heteroplastic g.
heterospecific g.
homologous g.
homoplastic g.
g. injury
interspecific g.
intrahepatic islet g.
islet composite g.
isogeneic g.
isologous g.
isoplastic g.
Papineau g.
pinch g.
g. reinfection
g. rejection
g. septoplasty
split-thickness skin g. (STSG)
g. survival rate
syngeneic g.

Thiersch g.
g. thrombosis
g. vessel disease (GVD)
white g.
XenoDerm g.
xenogeneic g.
GraftCyte gauze wound dressing
grafting
CDR g.
hair g.
Graftskin
graft-to-recipient weight ratio (GRWR)
graft-versus-host (GVH)
g.-v.-h. disease (GVHD)
g.-v.-h. reaction
g.-v.-h. response (GVHR)
graft-versus-leukemia (GVL)
g.-v.-l. effect
Graham-Little-Piccardi-Lasseur syndrome
Graham Little syndrome
grain
g. dust
g. fever
g. itch
grama grass
gramicidin
neomycin, polymyxin b, and g.
Gram-negative
G.-n. bacilli arthritis
G.-n. bacillus (GNB)
G.-n. bacteremia (GNB)
G.-n. cocci
G.-n. organism
G.-n. rod
Gram-positive
G.-p. bacillus (GPB)
G.-p. bacteremia (GPB)
G.-p. cocci
G.-p. organism
G.-p. rod
Gram stain
Gr antigen
granular
g. cell
g. cell layer
g. cell myoblastoma
g. cell schwannoma
g. cell tumor
g. degeneration
g. papulation
g. vaginitis
granulate
granulation
red g.
g. tissue
granule
azurophil g.
Birbeck g.

bismuth g.
Bollinger g.
dextranomer g.
Fordyce g.
keratohyaline g.
lamellar g.
Langerhans cell g.
membrane-coating g.
Much g.
Snaplets-FR G.
sulfur g.
tertiary g.

Granulex
granulocyte
g. colony-stimulating factor (G-CSF)
g. and macrophage colony-stimulating factor (GM-CSF)
g. transfusion
granulocyte-macrophage colony-stimulating factor (GM-CSF)
granulocytic leukemia
granulocytopenia
granuloma
actinic g.
amebic g.
g. annulare (GA)
annular elastolytic giant cell g.
aquarium g.
beryllium g.
bilharzial g.
Candida g.
caseating g.
clear-cut g.
coccidioidal g.
coli g.
diaper g.
elastolytic giant cell g.
g. endemium
eosinophilic g.
epithelioid g.
g. faciale
fish-tank g.
g. fissuratum
foreign body g.
g. fungoides
g. gangraenescens
giant cell g.
g. gluteale infantum
histiocytic g.
Hodgkin g.
infectious g.

g. inguinale
g. inguinale tropicum
lethal midline g.
lipoid g.
lipophagic g.
g. lycopodium
Majocchi g.
g. malignum
mercury g.
metastatic g.
midline lethal g.
Miescher actinic g.
mixed inflammatory g.
monilial g.
g. multiforme
necrobiotic g.
necrotizing g.
noncaseating g.
O'Brien actinic g.
oily g.
orbital g.
palisading g.
paracoccidioidal g.
parasitic g.
perifollicular g.
peripheral giant cell g.
g. pudendi
pyogenic g.
g. pyogenicum
reticulohistiocytic g.
sarcoid g.
schistosome g.
sea urchin g.
silica g.
swimming pool g.
g. telangiectaticum
trichophytic g.
g. trichophyticum
g. venereum
zirconium g.
granulomatis
Calymmatobacterium g.
Donovania g.
granulomatosa
cheilitis g.
Miescher cheilitis g.
granulomatosis
allergic g.
Churg-Strauss g.
g. disciformis et progressiva
eosinophilic g.
lethal midline g.

G

NOTES

granulomatosis *(continued)*
    limited Wegener g.
    lipid g.
    lipophagia g.
    lymphomatoid g.
    midline g.
    Miescher-Leder g.
    necrobiosis g.
    g. rhinitis
    Wegener g. (WG)
granulomatous
    g. angiitis
    g. arteritis
    g. bacterial infection
    g. cheilitis
    g. cutaneous T-cell lymphoma
    g. dermal infiltrate
    g. disease
    g. focus
    g. hepatitis
    g. idiopathic arthritis
    g. inflammatory reaction
    g. lesions of unknown significance
      (GLUS)
    g. pyoderma
    g. rosacea
    g. slack skin
    g. vasculitis
granulosis rubra nasi
granulosity
granulosum
    stratum g. (SG)
granulosus
    Echinococcus g.
granzyme B-mediated cleavage
grape cell
grapefruit
grasper
    nonsuction g.
grass
    alfalfa g.
    Bahia g.
    Bermuda g.
    blue g.
    brome g.
    Canada blue g.
    canary g.
    common reed g.
    crab g.
    cultivated barley g.
    cultivated corn g.
    cultivated oat g.
    cultivated rye g.
    cultivated wheat g.
    grama g.
    Johnson g.
    June g.
    meadow fescue g.

    meadow foxtail g.
    orchard g.
    perennial rye g.
    g. pollen
    g. pollen concentration
    redtop A g.
    salt g.
    sorghum g.
    sweet vernal g.
    timothy g.
    velvet g.
    vernal g.
    wild rye g.
Graves disease
Gravicon VC25
gravidarum
    chloasma g.
    fibroma molle g.
    hydroa g.
    melasma g.
    prurigo g.
    striae g.
gravis
    icterus g.
    junctional epidermolysis bullosa
      atrophicans generalisata g.
    myasthenia g. (MG)
Gravis-type Ehlers-Danlos syndrome
gravitational
    g. particle collection
    g. sampler
    g. ulcer
Gravol
gray-patch
    g.-p. ringworm
    g.-p. tinea capitis
gray-scale intensity
grease
    silicone g.
greasewood
greasy scaly lesion
Grecian Formula
green
    g. amaranth
    g. ash
    g. ash tree
    g. coffee bean
    Guignet g.
    g. hair
    indocyanine g. (ICG)
    malachite g.
    g. monkey virus
    g. nail
    g. nail syndrome
    Paris g.
    g. pepper
    G. soap tincture
    g. tea polyphenol (GTP)

Greenblatt
  groove sign of G.
Greenhow disease
Greenspan scale
green-striped nail
Greither syndrome
grenz
  g. ray
  g. ray therapy
  g. ray treatment
Griesinger disease
Griess analysis
Grifulvin V
grind test
grip, grippe
  devil g.
Grisactin Ultra
Griscelli syndrome (GS)
grisea
  Madurella g.
griseofulvin
  ultramicrosize g.
Grisolle sign
Grisovin-FP
Gris-PEG
grocer's itch
Grocott methenamine silver (GMS)
groin
  ringworm of the g.
  g. ulcer
Grönblad-Strandberg syndrome
groove
  Harrison g.
  nail g.
  g. sign
  g. sign of Greenblatt
  transverse nasal g.
grooved tongue
gross
  g. lesion
  G. leukemia virus
Grossan nasal irrigator
Grotthus-Draper law
ground
  g. itch
  g. substance
ground-glass
  g.-g. appearance
  g.-g. opacification
  g.-g. pattern
grounding pad
groundsel tree

group
  g. A beta-hemolytic streptococcal infection
  g. A beta-hemolytic streptococcus (GABHS)
  g. A carbohydrate antibody
  g. agglutination
  g. agglutinin
  g. antigens
  g. A streptococcus (GAS)
  g. A streptococcus infection
  blood g.
  g. B streptococcus (GBS)
  Contact Dermatitis Research G.
  cross-reactive antigen g. (CREG)
  g. C rotavirus
  cytophil g.
  Dermatology Teachers Exchange G. (DTEG)
  determinant g.
  Duffy blood g.
  g. immunity
  International Contact Dermatitis Research G. (ICDRG)
  g. JK *Corynebacterium* sepsis
  g. JK organism
  Kell-Cellano blood g.
  Kidd blood g.
  Lewis blood g.
  Lutheran blood g.
  MNSs blood g.
  North American Contact Dermatitis G. (NACDG)
  Pigmented Lesion Study G. (PLSG)
  g. reaction
  retrovirus g.
  support g.
  syntenic g.
  g. 5 topical steroid
grouping
  blood g.
  chemical g.
Grover disease
growing season
growth
  g. factor (GF)
  g. hormone (GH)
  g. hormone deficiency
  g. phase
  g. retardation
Gruber reaction

NOTES

G

Gruber-Widal reaction
GRWR
    graft-to-recipient weight ratio
gryphosis
gryphotic
gryposis unguium
GS
    Griscelli syndrome
GSE
    gluten-sensitive enteropathy
GSS
    gloves and socks syndrome
GST
    glutathione S-transferase
GSTG
    gold sodium thioglucose
GSTM
    gold sodium thiomalate
GTP
    green tea polyphenol
    guanosine triphosphate
guaiacolate
    glycerol g.
Guaifed-PD
guaifenesin
    g. and phenylpropanolamine
    g., phenylpropanolamine, and
      phenylephrine
    g. and pseudoephedrine
    theophylline and g.
Guaifenex
    G. DM
    G. LA
    G. PPA 75
    G. PSE
GuaiMAX-D
Guaipax
Guaitab
Guaivent PD capsule
Guaivent/PSE
Guama virus
guanethidine
guanine
guanosine
    g. monophosphate (GMP)
    g. triphosphate (GTP)
guanylic acid
Guard
    Aspirin Plus Stomach G.
guar gum
Guarnieri body
Guaroa virus
Gubler-Robin typhus
Guiatex
Guiatuss PE
Guignet green
Guillain-Barré syndrome

guillermondii
    Candida g.
guinea
    g. corn yaw
    g. pig
    g. pig maximization test (GPMT)
    G. worm
    g. worm infection
Gulf War syndrome (GWS)
gum
    guar g.
    karaya g.
    g. rash
    G. tragacanth
    vegetable g.
Gumboro disease
gumma of tertiary syphilis
gummatous
    g. meningitis
    g. syphilid
    g. syphilis
    g. ulcer
gummosa
    scrofuloderma g.
gummy
Günther
    G. disease
    G. syndrome
gustatory
    g. hyperhidrosis
    g. rhinitis
gut
    g. glucagon
    g. homeostasis
gut-associated
    g.-a. lymphoid disease
    g.-a. lymphoid tissue (GALT)
Guthrie skin hook
gutless adenovirus
guttata
    morphea g.
    parapsoriasis g.
    psoriasis g.
guttate
    g. hypomelanosis
    g. parapsoriasis
    g. psoriasis
guttering
    limbal g.
Guyon
    tunnel of G.
GV
    Healon GV
GVD
    graft vessel disease
GVH
    graft-versus-host
    GVH disease

GVHD
> graft-versus-host disease

GVHR
> graft-versus-host response

GVL
> graft-versus-leukemia

G-well
> G.-w. Lotion
> G.-w. Shampoo

GWS
> Gulf War syndrome

gymnosperm

Gynecort Topical

Gyne-Lotrimin

gypseum
> *Microsporum* g.
> *Trichophyton* g.

gypsy
> g. moth larva
> g. moth larva sting

gyrase
> DNA g.

gyrata
> cutis verticis g.
> psoriasis g.

gyrate psoriasis

gyratum
> erythema g.

gyrose

NOTES

H
   H agglutinin
   H antigen
   H deficiency factor
   H graft
1H
   Campath 1H
H-2
   H-2 antigen
   H-2 complex
H2
   H2 blocker
   prostaglandin H2 (PGH2)
0157-H7 strain
HA
   hepatitis A
   hydroxyapatite
Ha-1A monoclonal antibody
HAA
   hepatitis A antigen
   hepatitis-associated antigen
Haake rheometer
haarscheibe tumor
HAART
   highly active antiretroviral therapy
Habermann disease
Haber syndrome
Haber-Weiss reaction
habit
   h. tic deformity
   wolf-biter h.
habitus
   marfanoid h.
habumatone
hackberry tree
HAE
   hereditary angioneurotic edema
HAEM
   herpes-associated erythema multiforme
   herpes simplex-associated erythema
      multiforme
haematobium
   Schistosoma h.
Haemonchus contortus
haemophilum
   Mycobacterium h.
Haemophilus
   H. ducreyi
   H. influenzae meningitis
   H. influenzae type b (HIB)
   H. parahaemolyticus
   H. parainfluenzae
   H. suis
haemorrhagica
   angina bullosa h. (ABH)

Haenel symptom
Haffkine vaccine
Hafnia alvei
Hagedorn needle
Hageman factor
HA1, HA2 virus
Hailey-Hailey
   H.-H. disease (HHD)
   familial benign pemphigus of H.-H.
Haines directory
hair
   animal h.
   axillary h.
   bamboo h.
   bayonet h.
   beaded h.
   black dot h.
   bubble h.
   h. bulb
   burrowing h.
   h. cast
   club h.
   h. collar sign
   corkscrew h.
   cortex of h.
   crackled h.
   cuticle of h.
   h. cyst
   deer h.
   h. disk
   H. dressing screening tray test
   exclamation point h.
   h. fall
   h. follicle
   h. follicle mite
   h. follicle mite scabies
   h. follicle nevus
   Frey h.
   genital h.
   h. germ
   golf tee h.
   h. grafting
   green h.
   horse h.
   ingrowing h.
   ingrown h.
   kinky h.
   knotted h.
   lanugo h.
   h. loss
   h. matrix
   h. melanin
   moniliform h.
   nettling h.
   h. removal efficiency (HRE)

H

hair *(continued)*
ringed h.
h. rudiment
h. and scalp
Schridde cancer h.
h. shaft
spun-glass h.
stellate h.
telogen h.
terminal h.
h. transplant
tuft of h.
twisted h.
vellus h.
woolly h.

HAIR-AN
hyperandrogenism, insulin resistance, and
acanthosis nigricans
HAIR-AN syndrome

hairiness
excessive h.

hair-like structure
hair-matrix carcinoma
hair-on-end appearance
hair-standing-on-end appearance
hairy
h. cell (HC)
h. cell leukemia (HCL)
h. hamartoma
h. leukoplakia
h. mole
h. nevus

Halberstaedter-Prowazek body
halcinonide
Halcion
Haldrone
Halfan
half-and-half
h.-a.-h. fingernail
h.-a.-h. nail

half-buried mattress stitch
half-moon
red h.-m.

Halfprin
halitosis
Hallermann-Streiff syndrome
Hallopeau
H. acrodermatitis
acrodermatitis continua of H.
H. disease

Hallopeau-Siemens
H.-S. epidermolysis bullosa
H.-S. syndrome

hallux
h. valgus
h. varus

halo
anemic h.

h. melanoma
h. nevus
purpuric h.
red h.
h. vest

halobetasol propionate
haloderma, halodermia
halodes
Helminthosporium h.
halofantrine hydrochloride
halofuginone
halogen acne
halogenated salicylanilides
halogenoderma
halogenosis
vegetating h.

Halog-E topical
Halog topical
haloprogin
Halotex topical
Halothane
Halotussin PE
HALS
Health and Activity Limitation Survey

Halsey needle holder
Halsted
H. law
H. mosquito hemostat

Haltone
Haltran
hamartoma, pl. **hamartomata**
Becker hairy h.
eccrine angiomatous h.
folliculosebaceous cystic h. (FCH)
hairy h.
neurocristic h.
pilar neurocristic h.
smooth muscle h.

Hamilton
H. bandage
H. pseudophlegmon
H. test

Hamman-Rich syndrome
Hamman sign
hammer toe
hamster
Ham test
HAM/TSP
HTLV-1-associated myelopathy or
tropical spastic paraparesis

Hanalux Oslo light
hand
accordion h.
Breuerton view of the h.
chrome holes on the h.
crab h.
h. eczema
edema of h.

ghoul h.
Hunstad h.
Marinesco succulent h.
mechanic h.
pulling boat h.
ringworm of the h.
trench h.
Handages dressing
hand-and-foot syndrome
hand-foot-and-mouth
h.-f.-a.-m. disease
h.-f.-a.-m. disease virus
Handisol phototherapy device
Hand-Schüller-Christian disease
HANE
hereditary angioneurotic edema
hanging skin
hangnail
Hanks balanced salt solution (HBSS)
Hansen
H. bacillus
H. disease
Hantaan virus
Hantavirus **infection**
hapalonychia
haploidentical
haplotype
haplotype-shared transfusion
Happle syndrome
hapten
conjugated h.
h. inhibition of precipitation
h. mechanism of hemolytic anemia
haptenated protein
haptene
Hapten-type reaction
haptoglobin
HAQ
Health Assessment Questionnaire
Stanford Health Assessment
Questionnaire
HAQ DI
Harada syndrome
hard
h. chancre
h. corn
h. keratin
h. nevus
h. pad disease
h. pad virus
h. palate
h. papilloma

h. sore
h. tick
h. ulcer
hardening
harderoporphyrin
hard-milled soap
Hardy-Weinberg equilibrium
harlequin
h. fetus
h. ichthyosis
ichthyosis h.
Harrison groove
Harris pressure mat
Harter syndrome
Hartmann
H. ear forceps
H. hemostat
Hartnup disease
harvest
h. mite
h. mite bite
Harvey murine sarcoma virus
harzianum
Trichoderma h.
Hashimoto
H. disease
H. thyroiditis
Hashimoto-Pritzker disease
Hassall corpuscle
HAT
hypoxanthine, aminopterin and thymidine
HAT medium
Hata phenomenon
Hatchcock sign
hatchetti
Acanthamoeba h.
Hauch
ohne H.
HAV
hepatitis A virus
HAV RNA
Haverhill fever
Haversian system
Havrix vaccine
Hawaiian Tropic Herbal
Hawes-Pallister-Landor syndrome
hay
h. asthma
h. fever
Hayek oscillator
Hayem corpuscle
Hayfebrol Liquid

NOTES

H

hayfever
> eczema, asthma, h. (EAHF)

Hay-Wells syndrome

hazel
> witch h.

hazelnut
> h. tree
> h. tree pollen

HB
> hepatitis B
> Recombivax HB

HB$_c$
> hepatitis B$_c$

HB$_e$
> hepatitis B$_e$

HB$_e$, HBe
> hepatitis B$_e$

HB$_s$
> hepatitis B surface

HB$_e$Ab, HBeAb
> antibody to hepatitis B e antigen

HB$_c$Ab, HBcAb
> antibody to hepatitis B core antigen

HB$_s$Ab, HBsAb
> antibody to hepatitis B surface antigen

HB$_s$Ag, HBsAg
> hepatitis B surface antigen

HB$_c$Ag, HBcAg
> hepatitis B core antigen

HBcAb (*var. of* HB$_c$Ab)
> antibody to hepatitis B core antigen

HbCO
> carboxyhemoglobin

HBD
> heart-beating donor

HBe (*var. of* HB$_e$)

HBeAb (*var. of* HB$_e$Ab)
> antibody to hepatitis B e antigen

HB-EGF
> heparin-binding epidermal growth factor-like growth factor

HBGF
> heparin-binding growth factor

HBGF-1
> heparin-binding growth factor-1

H-BIG
> hepatitis B immune globulin
> hepatitis B immunoglobulin

HBO
> hyperbaric oxygen

HbO$_2$
> oxyhemoglobin

HbOC/DTP vaccine

HbOC vaccine

HBsAb (*var. of* HB$_s$Ab)
> antibody to hepatitis B surface antigen

HBsAg (*var. of* HB$_s$Ag)

HBSS
> Hanks balanced salt solution

HBT
> home-based telemetry
> HBT Sleuth

HBV
> hepatitis B virus
> HBV bDNA signal amplification
> HBV DNA
> HBV DNA probe test

HC
> hairy cell
> hepatitis C
> Dermaflex HC
> Prevex HC
> Sarna HC
> Ti-U-Lac HC

HCA
> hybrid capture assay
> Orabase HCA

HCB
> hexachlorobenzene

HCD
> heavy-chain disease

HCL
> hairy cell leukemia

HCl
> hydrochloride
> amiprilose HCl
> butenafine HCl
> cevimeline HCl
> doxepin HCl
> fexofenadine HCl/pseudoephedrine HCl
> fluoxetine HCl
> gemcitabine HCl
> hydroxyzine HCl
> moxifloxacin HCl
> paroxetine HCl
> pioglitazone HCl
> pramoxine HCl
> promethazine HCl
> pseudoephedrine HCl
> sertraline HCl
> valacyclovir HCl

HCO$_3$
> bicarbonate

HCP
> hereditary coproporphyria

HCQ
> hydroxychloroquine

HCT
> hematopoietic stem cell transplantation

HCV
> hepatitis C virus
> RIBA HCV
> HCV by RIBA
> HCV RNA

HCV-related cirrhosis
HD
　　hemodialysis
　　hepatitis D
HDCV
　　human diploid cell rabies vaccine
　　human diploid cell vaccine
HDI
　　isocyanate HDI
HDIT
　　high-dose immunosuppressive therapy
HDM
　　house dust mite
HDV
　　hepatitis D virus
HE
　　hematoxylin and eosin
　　hepatitis E
H&E
　　hematoxylin and eosin
　　hematoxylin and eosin stain
head
　　cobalt-chrome h.
　　h. compression test
　　h. distraction test
　　h. louse
　　H. & Shoulders
　　H. & Shoulders Shampoo
　　H. zone
headache tablet
headlight sign
Heaf test
healed ulcer
healing
　　fish-mouth h.
　　Pressure Ulcer Scale for H.
　　(PUSH)
　　wound h.
Healon GV
health
　　H. and Activity Limitation Survey
　　(HALS)
　　H. Assessment Questionnaire
　　(HAQ)
　　H. Assessment Questionnaire
　　Disability Index (HAQ DI)
　　h. maintenance organization (HMO)
　　National Institutes of H. (NIH)
health-related quality of life
healthy
　　h. carrier
　　h. years of life lost (HYLL)

He antigen
hearing
　　h. aid dermatitis
　　h. loss
heart
　　AbioCor implantable replacement h.
　　h. allograft
　　h. antigen
　　h. rate reserve (HRR)
　　h. transplantation (HTX)
heart-beating donor (HBD)
heart-lung
　　h.-l. circuit
　　h.-l. transplantation (HLT)
heartworm
heat
　　h. exposure
　　h. lamp
　　prickly h.
　　h. rash
　　h. therapy
　　h. urticaria
Heath curette
heat/moisture exchanger (HME)
heat-phenol inactivated vaccine
heat-shock
　　h.-s. protein (HSP)
　　h.-s. protein 70 (HSP-70)
heavy chain
heavy-chain disease (HCD)
Heberden node
Hebra
　　H. disease
　　H. erythema multiforme
　　melanotic prurigo of H.
　　H. ointment
　　H. pityriasis
　　protoporphyria of H.
　　H. prurigo
hebraeum
　　Amblyomma h.
Hecht
　　H. phenomenon
　　H. pneumonia
Heck syndrome
HED
　　hypohidrotic ectodermal dysplasia
heel
　　black h.
　　cracked h.
　　h. spur
Heelbo decubitus protector

NOTES

H

Heerfordt syndrome
Heilen expressor
Heiner syndrome
Heinz body
Hektoen phenomenon
HEL
    hen egg lysozyme
    HEL protein
HeLa cell
Helanthus
helical
helicis
    chondrodermatitis nodularis
    chronica h.
Helicobacter
    ImmunoCard used for diagnosis of
    H. pylori
    H. mustelae
    H. pylori
heliopathy
heliotherapy
heliotrope rash
Helisal rapid blood test
Helistat collagen matrix sponge
helix
    triple h.
HELLP
    hemolysis, elevated liver enzymes, low
    platelet
    HELLP syndrome
helminth
    multicellular h.
helminthiasis elastica
helminthic parasitic disease
Helminthosporium
    H. halodes
    H. savitum
Heloderma
    H. suspectum
    H. suspectum bite
heloma
    h. durum
    h. molle
helosis
helotomy
helper
    h. T cell
    h. virus
helper-suppressor cell ratio
helplessness
    learned h.
Helweg-Larssen syndrome
hemacytometer
hemadsorption
    h. virus test
    h. virus type 1, 2

hemagglutinating
    h. antibody
    h. cold autoantibody
hemagglutination
    h. inhibition
    passive h. (PHA)
    reverse passive h.
    h. test
    viral h.
hemagglutinin
    influenza virus h.
hemalum
    Mayer h.
hemangioendothelioma
    kaposiform h. (KHE)
    malignant h.
    retiform h.
    spindle cell h.
hemangioma, pl. hemangiomata
    h. birthmark
    capillary h.
    cavernous h.
    cherry h.
    h. congenitale
    deep h.
    DeMorgan h.
    dyschondroplasia with h.
    glomeruloid h.
    h. hypertrophicum cutis
    involuting flat h.
    microvenular h.
    mixed h.
    nuchal h.
    h. planum extensum
    port-wine h.
    sclerosing h.
    senile h.
    spider h.
    strawberry h.
    superficial h.
    synovial h.
    targetoid hemosiderotic h. (THH)
    verrucous h.
hemangioma-thrombocytopenia syndrome
hemangiomatosis
    Osler h.
    Parkes-Weber h.
    pulmonary capillary h.
    thrombocytopenic h.
    unilateral h.
hemangiomatous tissue
hemangiopericytoma (HPC)
    benign h.
    borderline malignant h.
    malignant h.
hemarthrosis
hemarthrotic disability
hematid

hematidrosis
hematogenous metastasis
hematoidin crystal
hematologic
    h. disorder
    h. reaction
hematolysis
hematoma
    paroxysmal hand h.
    spontaneous spinal epidural h.
    (SSEH)
    subungual h.
hematopoiesis
hematopoietic
    h. chimerism
    h. failure syndrome
    h. PGD_2 synthase
    h. reconstitution
    h. stem cell
    h. stem cell transplant
    h. stem cell transplantation (HCT, HSCT)
    h. system
hematotoxin
hematotropic
hematoxin
hematoxylin
    h. and eosin (HE, H&E)
    h. and eosin stain (H&E)
hematoxylin-eosin
hematoxyphilic inclusion
hematuria
hemiarthroplasty
    McKeever and MacIntosh h.
hemiatrophy
    progressive facial h.
    Romberg h.
hemiballismus
hemicallotasis procedure
hemichannel
    connexin h.
hemidesmosome
hemidiaphoresis
hemidiaphragm
hemidrosis
hemidysplasia
    congenital h.
    unilateral h.
hemihepatectomy
hemihidrosis
hemihyperhidrosis

hemihypertrophy
hemijoint
Hemiptera
hemipterus
    Cimex h.
hemithorax
hemoagglutination
hemoagglutinin
hemoantitoxin
hemochromatosis
hemochromatotic arthritis
hemocyanin
    keyhole limpet h.
hemocytoblast
hemocytometer
hemodialysis (HD)
    continuous venovenous h.
    (CVVHD)
    perforating disease of h.
hemodialysis-associated amyloidosis
hemoglobin
    h. crystal
    h. C, S disease
hemoglobinopathy
hemoglobinophilic
hemoglobinuria
    nocturnal h.
    paroxysmal cold h.
    paroxysmal nocturnal h. (PNH)
hemoglobinuric
    h. fever
    h. nephrosis
hemolysate
hemolysin
    alpha h.
    bacterial h.
    beta h.
    cold h.
    heterophil h.
    immune h.
    natural h.
    specific h.
    h. unit
    warm-cold h.
hemolysinogen
hemolysis
    acute intravascular h.
    autoimmune h.
    beta h.
    biologic h.
    conditioned h.

NOTES

H

hemolysis *(continued)*
    h., elevated liver enzymes, low platelet (HELLP)
    h., elevated liver enzymes, low platelet count
    h., elevated liver enzymes, and low platelet syndrome
    gamma h.
    immune h.
    venom h.
    viridans h.
hemolytic
    h. anemia of newborn
    h. chain
    h. disease of newborn
    h. plaque assay
    h. sickle cell disease
    h. streptococcus
    h. uremic syndrome (HUS)
hemolyzation
hemolyze
hemopexin
hemophagocytic syndrome
hemophagocytosis
hemophil
hemophilia
    acquired h.
hemophiliac patient
hemophilic arthropathy
hemopoietic factor
hemoprecipitin
hemoptysis
    Manson h.
hemorrhage
    iliopsoas h.
    intraalveolar h.
    intraosseous h.
    intraventricular h.
    petechial h.
    pulmonary h.
    punctate h.
    retinal h.
    splinter h.
    subaponeurotic h.
hemorrhagic
    h. arthritis
    h. bulla
    h. cystitis
    h. dengue
    h. diathesis
    h. edema
    h. exudative erythema
    h. fever
    h. fever with renal syndrome (HFRS)
    h. gangrene
    h. lesion
    h. pian

    h. pyoderma gangrenosum
    h. rash
    h. smallpox
    h. telangiectasia
hemorrhagica
    purpura h.
    scarlatina h.
    urticaria h.
    variola h.
hemorrhagicus
    lichen h.
    pemphigus h.
hemorrhagins
hemosiderin
    h. deposition
    h. hyperpigmentation
hemosiderin-laden macrophage
hemosiderosis
    idiopathic pulmonary h.
    pulmonary h.
    synovial h.
hemostasis
    chemical h.
hemostat
    Halsted mosquito h.
    Hartmann h.
hemostatic
    h. agent
    h. collodion
    h. disorder
hemostatica
    dermatitis h.
hemothorax, pl. **hemothoraces**
    catamenial h.
hemotoxic
hemotoxin
    cobra h.
hemotropic
hemp
    western water h.
Hemril-HC Uniserts
hen
    h. egg lysozyme (HEL)
    h. egg lysozyme protein
Henderson-Paterson body
Hendersonula toruloidea
Hendra virus
He-Ne lasing medium
Henle-Koch pustulate
Henle layer
henna
    extract of h.
Henoch purpura
Henoch-Schönlein
    H.-S. purpura (HSP)
    H.-S. syndrome (HSS)
    H.-S. vasculitis

henselae
    Bartonella h.
    Rochalimaea h.
HEP
    hepatoerythrocytic porphyria
HEPA
    high-efficiency particulate air
    high-efficiency particulate arresting
       HEPA filter
Hepadnaviridae
hepadnavirus
Hepandrin
heparinase 2
heparin-binding
    h.-b. epidermal growth factor-like
       growth factor (HB-EGF)
    h.-b. growth factor (HBGF)
    h.-b. growth factor-1 (HBGF-1)
heparinization
heparinoid therapy
heparin sulfate
hepatic
    h. ischemia and reperfusion (HIR)
    h. ischemia and reperfusion injury
    h. nevus
    h. porphyria
    h. portoenterostomy
    h. sickling
hepatica
    facies h.
hepaticojejunostomy
    Roux-en-Y h.
hepaticum
    chloasma h.
hepatitic
hepatitis
    h. A (HA)
    h. A antigen (HAA)
    h. A, B arthritis
    aggressive h.
    anicteric virus h.
    autoimmune h. (AIH)
    autoimmune chronic h.
    h. A vaccine
    h. A virus (HAV)
    h. B (HB)
    h. B$_e$ (HBe, HB$_e$)
    h. B$_c$ (HB$_c$)
    h. B core antigen (HB$_c$Ag, HBcAg)
    h. B DNA detection
    h. B e antigen

    h. B immune globulin (H-BIG)
    h. B immunoglobulin (H-BIG)
    branched DNA signal amplification assay for h. B
    h. B surface (HB$_s$)
    h. B surface antigen (HB$_s$Ag, HBsAg)
    h. B vaccine
    h. B viral DNA assay
    h. B virus (HBV)
    h. B virus branched chain deoxyribonucleic acid signal amplification
    h. C (HC)
    cholangiolitic h.
    cholestatic h.
    chronic active h. (CAH)
    h. contagiosa canis
    h. C RNA detection
    cryptogenic autoimmune h. (CAH)
    h. C virus (HCV)
    h. C virus antibody detection
    h. C virus-related cirrhosis
    h. D (HD)
    delta antigen h.
    h. D virus (HDV)
    h. E (HE)
    epidemic h.
    equine serum h.
    h. E virus (HEV)
    h. G
    granulomatous h.
    h. G virus (HGV)
    infectious h. (IH)
    infectious canine h.
    isoniazid-induced h.
    long incubation h.
    lupoid h.
    mouse h.
    murine h.
    NANB h.
    non-A-E h.
    non-A non-B h.
    peliosis h.
    posttransfusion h. (PST)
    serum h. (SH)
    short incubation h.
    transfusion h.
    viral h. (VH)
    h. virus
    virus A h.

NOTES

H

hepatitis-associated
 h.-a. antigen (HAA)
 h.-a. lichen planus
hepatobiliary disease
hepatocellular chimerism
hepatocyte
 h. growth factor (HGF)
 immortalized human h.
hepatoerythrocytic porphyria (HEP)
hepatoerythropoietic porphyria
hepatolenticular degeneration
hepatolysin
hepatomegaly
hepatopulmonary syndrome (HPS)
hepatosplenic
 h. schistosomiasis
 h. tuberculosis
hepatosplenomegaly
hepatotoxic
hepatotoxicity
hepatotoxin
hepatotrophic
Hep-B-Gammagee
HEPES buffer
heptacarboxylporphyrin I
Heptavax immunization
Heptovir
herald patch
Herbal
 H. Answer
 Hawaiian Tropic H.
herbimycin-inhibited movement
Herbogesic
herd immunity
hereditaria
 alopecia h.
hereditarium
 erythema palmare h.
hereditary
 h. allergy
 h. angioneurotic edema (HAE, HANE)
 h. arthroophthalmopathy
 h. cardiopathic amyloidosis
 h. coproporphyria (HCP)
 h. hemorrhagic angioma
 h. hemorrhagic telangiectasia (HHT)
 h. hemorrhagic telangiectasis
 h. hypomelanosis
 h. lymphedema
 h. multiple trichoepithelioma
 h. osteoonychodysplasia (HOOD)
 h. periodic fever syndrome
 h. sclerosing poikiloderma (HSP)
 h. sensory radicular neuropathy
 h. spherocytosis
 h. vascular disorder
 h. vibratory angioedema

heredofamilial
 h. amyloidosis
 h. urticaria
heredolues
heredoluetic
heredopathia atactica polyneuritiformis
heredosyphilis
heredosyphilitic
heres
 Scolopendra h.
Herisan
heritable
 h. connective tissue disease
 h. disorder
Herlitz
 H. disease
 H. epidermolysis bullosa
 H. syndrome
Hermal kit
Hermansky-Pudlak
 H.-P. syndrome
 H.-P. syndrome type IV, VI
hernia
 diaphragmatic h.
herniated presacral fat pad
herpangina pharyngitis
herpes
 h. B encephalomyelitis
 h. catarrhalis
 h. circinatus bullosus
 h. cornea
 h. desquamans
 h. digitalis
 h. facialis
 h. farinosus
 h. febrilis
 genital h.
 h. genitalis
 h. gestationis (HG)
 h. gladiatorum
 inoculation h.
 h. iridis
 h. iris
 h. labialis
 h. menstrualis
 h. mentalis
 nasal h.
 neonatal h.
 h. neonatalis
 h. odeus
 orolabial h.
 h. pharyngitis
 h. phlyctaenodes
 h. praepuffalis
 h. progenitalis
 h. simplex
 h. simplex-associated erythema multiforme (HAEM)

[handwritten annotation: extragenital herpes simplex]

h. simplex conjunctivitis
h. simplex encephalitis
h. simplex infection
h. simplex recurrens
h. simplex virus (HSV)
h. simplex virus arthritis
h. simplex virus thymidine kinase (HSVTK)
h. simplex virus type I, II
h. thymidine kinase gene
h. tonsurans
h. tonsurans maculosus
toxoplasmosis, other, rubella, cytomegalovirus, and h.
traumatic h.
h. vegetans
h. whitlow
wrestler h.
h. zoster (HZ)
h. zoster generalisatus
h. zoster infection
h. zoster ophthalmicus
h. zoster oticus
h. zoster varicellosus
h. zoster virus
herpes-associated erythema multiforme (HAEM)
Herpesviridae
herpesvirus
h. 8
canine h.
caprine h.
h. hominis
human h. 1–7 (HHV)
human h. 6 (HHV-6)
human h. 8 (HHV-8)
human h. 6A (HHV-6A)
human h. 6B (HHV-6B)
McKrae h.
h. saimiri (HVS)
h. simiae
suid h.
h. type 1
Herpesvirus saimiri
herpetic
h. angina
h. fever
h. gingivostomatitis
h. infection
h. keratoconjunctivitis
h. meningoencephalitis
h. paronychia

h. stromal keratitis (HSK)
h. sycosis
h. ulcer
h. vulvovaginitis
h. whitlow
zoster sine h.
herpeticum
eczema h.
herpeticus
favus h.
herpetiform
h. aphtha
h. distribution of lesion
h. pemphigus (HP)
herpetiforme
hydroa h.
herpetiformis
dermatitis h. (DH)
epidermolysis bullosa simplex h.
favus h.
impetigo h.
morphea h.
herpetoid
Herpetoviridae
Herpetovirus
herpetovirus
canine h.
caprine h.
Herplex Ophthalmic
herringbone
h. nail
h. pattern
Hertoghe sign
Herxheimer
H. fiber
H. reaction
H. spiral
HES
hypereosinophilic syndrome
Hess test
HETE
hydroxyeicosatetraenoic acid
heteroagglutinin
heteroantibody
heteroantiserum
heterochromia irides
heteroclitic, heteroclytic
h. antibody
heterocyclic antidepressant
heterocytotropic
h. anaphylaxis
h. antibody

NOTES

H

heterodermic
heterodimer
heterodimeric complex
heterodimerization
heteroduplexing method
heterogenetic
    h. antibody
    h. antigen
heterogenic, heterogeneic
    h. enterobacterial antigen
heterogenote
heterogenous vaccine
heterograft
heterokeratoplasty
heterologous
    h. antiserum
    h. desensitization
    h. graft
    h. protein
    h. serotype
    h. serum
heterology
heterolysin
heterolysis
heterolytic
heteromerization
heterooligomeric complex
heteroosteoplasty
heteropathy
heterophil
    h. antibody
    h. antigen
    h. hemolysin
heterophile
    h. antibody
    h. antigen
heteroplasia
    osseous h.
heteroplastic graft
heteroplastid
heteroplasty
heterospecific graft
heterotopia
    cephalic brainlike h.
heterotopic
    h. heart transplantation (HHT)
    h. plate count bacteria (HPC bacteria)
heterotransplantation
heterotrichosis superciliorum
heterotrimer
heterotrimeric cell-membrane-bound molecule
heterovaccine therapy
heterozygous
heuristic

HEV
    hepatitis E virus
    high endothelial venule
Hevea
    H. brasiliensis
    H. brasiliensis latex
HEVI
    hibernal epidemic viral infection
hexacetonide
    triamcinolone h.
hexachloride
hexachlorobenzene (HCB)
hexachlorophene
Hexadenovirus
Hexadrol
    Decadron and H.
    H. phosphate
hexagonus
    Ixodes h.
hexahydrate
    aluminum chloride h.
hexamer
hexamethylmelamine
hexamethyl violet
hexanediol
    ethyl h.
hexasaccharides
    hyaluronan h.
Hexascan Mark I, II model robotic scanning device
Hexit
hexon antigen
hexosaminidase
hexose monophosphate shunt (HMS)
HFA
    Proventil HFA
H-F Antidote
HFRS
    hemorrhagic fever with renal syndrome
HG
    herpes gestationis
HGA
    homogentisic acid
HGF
    hepatocyte growth factor
HGH
    human growth hormone
HGP-30W vaccine
HGPRT
    hypoxanthine-guanine phosphoribosyltransferase
    HGPRT deficiency
HGV
    hepatitis G virus
H$_1$, H$_2$ antihistamine
HHD
    Hailey-Hailey disease

HHT
> hereditary hemorrhagic telangiectasia
> heterotopic heart transplantation

HHV
> human herpesvirus 1–7

HHV-6
> human herpesvirus 6

HHV-8
> human herpesvirus 8

HHV6 encephalitis

HHV-6A
> human herpesvirus 6A

HHV-6B
> human herpesvirus 6B

HIB
> *Haemophilus influenzae* type b

hibernal epidemic viral infection (HEVI)

hibernoma

Hibiclens topical

Hibistat topical

Hibitane

HibTITER

Hib-TT vaccine

hiccup, hiccough

hickey
> stingray h.

hickory
> shagbark h.
> h. tree

Hi-Cor-1.0 Topical

Hi-Cor-2.5 Topical

HID
> hyperimmunoglobulinemia syndrome

hidden
> h. margin
> h. nail skin

hidebound
> h. appearance
> h. disease

hidradenitis
> h. axillaris
> h. axillaris of Verneuil
> eccrine h.
> idiopathic recurrent palmoplantar h.
> neutrophilic eccrine h. (NEH)
> palmoplantar eccrine h. (PEH)
> recurrent palmoplantar h.
> h. suppurativa

hidradenoma
> clear cell h.
> cystic h.

> malignant nodular h.
> nodular h.
> papillary h.
> h. papilliferum
> poroid h.
> solid h.

hidroa

hidroacanthoma simplex

hidrocystoma
> apocrine h.
> eccrine h.

hidromeiosis

hidropoiesis

hidropoietic

hidrorrhea

hidrosadenitis

hidroschesis

hidrosis

hidrotic ectodermal dysplasia

HIE
> hyper-IgE

hiemalis
> acrodermatitis h.
> dermatitis h.
> erythrokeratolysis h.
> prurigo h.
> pruritus h.

hierarchical clustering discrimination logic

high
> h. avidity
> h. cyclosporine
> h. dose tolerance
> h. endothelial venule (HEV)
> h. endothelial venule cell
> h. frequency oscillation
> H. Frequency Oscillatory ventilator
> h. frequency of recombination
> h. frequency transduction
> h. liquid content
> h. lung volume
> h. molecular weight (HMW)
> h. molecular weight-melanoma-associated antigen (HMW-MAA)

high-arched palate

high-dose immunosuppressive therapy (HDIT)

high-efficiency
> h.-e. particulate air (HEPA)
> h.-e. particulate air filter
> h.-e. particulate arresting (HEPA)

high-egg-passage vaccine

NOTES

H

high-energy, pulse-doublet waveform
high-frequency
 h.-f. jet ventilation
 h.-f. positive pressure ventilation
high-grade small noncleaved cell
 malignant lymphoma
highly
 h. active antiretroviral therapy
  (HAART)
 h. polymorphic microsatellite
  marker
high-performance liquid chromatography
 (HPLC)
high-resolution
 h.-r. computed tomography (HRCT)
 h.-r. computed tomography scan
high-risk recipient (HRR)
Higouménaki sign
hilar
 h. adenopathy
 h. lymphadenopathy
Hildenbrand typhus
hilus tuberculosis
HIM
 hyper-IgM syndrome
hindfoot splint
Hind III polymorphism
hinge region
Hinton test
hip
 h. deflexion
 snapping h.
Hippocratic
 H. countenance
 H. face
 H. facies
 H. finger
 H. look
 H. nail
 H. visage
 H. wreath
Hippocratica
 facies H.
HIR
 hepatic ischemia and reperfusion
 HIR injury
hirci
 barbula h.
Hirsch mucosal clamp
Hirschowitz syndrome
Hirschsprung disease
Hirst spore trap
hirsute
hirsuties
hirsutism
 Apert h.
 constitutional h.
 idiopathic h.

hirtellous
hirudiniasis
Hirudin-sensitive protease
Hismanal
HISS
 human immune status survey
Histadyl
Histaject injection
Histalet
 H. Forte Tablet
 H. Syrup
 H. X
Histalon
histaminase
histamine
 h. challenge
 h. flush
 h. H$_1$ agonist
 h. liberator
 h. phosphate
 h. shock
histamine-releasing
 h.-r. factor (HRF)
 h.-r. factor deficiency
histaminergic
Histantil
Histatrol
Hista-Vadrin Tablet
histidinemia
histidyl-tRNA synthetase
histiocyte
 alveolar infiltration by h.
 foamy h.
 interstitial infiltration by h.
 palisading h.
histiocytic
 h. cytophagic panniculitis (CHP)
 h. granuloma
 h. lymphoma
 h. medullary reticulosis
 h. response
histiocytoma
 h. cutis
 fibrous h.
 generalized eruptive h.
 malignant fibrous h. (MFH)
histiocytosis
 acute disseminated h.
 atypical h.
 benign cephalic h. (BCH)
 Blackfan-Diamond Langerhans
  cell h.
 cephalic h.
 chronic h.
 focal h.
 indeterminate cell h.
 juvenile xanthogranuloma h.
 Langerhans cell h. (LCH)

malignant h.
multifocal h.
nodular non-X h.
regressing atypical h.
sea-blue h.
sinus h. (SH)
skin-limited h.
h. X
h. Y
histoblot method
histochemical
histocompatibility
h. antigen
h. antigen class I
h. locus (HL)
major h.
h. testing
Histofreezer
H. cryosurgical wart remover
H. cryosurgical wart treatment
histoid leprosy
histoincompatibility
histoincompatible
histologic
h. change
h. lesion
histological
histology
joint h.
Histolyn-CYL
histolytica
Ameba h.
Entamoeba h.
histone antibody
histone-DNA antibody
Histopaque
Histoplasma
H. capsulatum
H. duboisii
histoplasmin
histoplasmin-latex test
histoplasmosis
African h.
cutaneous h.
primary pulmonary h.
progressive disseminated h.
history
Köbner phenomenon by h. (KP-h)
relevant sting h.
histotope
histotoxic
His-Werner disease

Hitzig syndrome
HIV
human immunodeficiency virus
HIV DNA amplification assay
HIV DNA PCR test
HIV encephalopathy
HIV neutralizing antibody
HIV protease inhibitor
HIV-1
human immunodeficiency virus-1
HIV-2
human immunodeficiency virus-2
HIV-associated
hives
bullous h.
giant h.
Hivid
HIVIG
human immunodeficiency virus
immunoglobulin
HL
histocompatibility locus
HLA
human leukocyte antibody
human leukocyte antigen
human lymphocyte antigen
HLA allele
HLA B60
HLA class 1
HLA class 1 associated disease
HLA complex
HLA Cw6
HLA intercellular interaction
HLA typing
HLA-129
HLA-A
HLA-A11
HLA antigen
HLA-B
HLA-B8
HLA-B13
HLA-B17
HLA-B27
HLA-B60 gene
HLA-B27 gene product
HLA-C
HLA-Cw6
HLA-DP
HLA-DQ
HLA-DR
HLA-DR2

NOTES

H

HLA-DR4
  allele H.-D.
HLA-DR7
  allele H.-D.
HLA-DRB1 allele
HLA-DRB and HLA-DRQ DNA typing
HLA-DR3 gene
HLA-DRw4
HLA-DRw52
HLA-E
HLA-F
HLA-G DNA
HLT
  heart-lung transplantation
HM-175
HME
  heat/moisture exchanger
    Tracheolife HME
HMG-CoA
  3-hydroxy-3-methylglutaryl coenzyme A
    HMG-CoA reductase inhibitor
HMO
  health maintenance organization
HMPAO-SPECT
  technetium-99m hexamethylpropylene
    amine oxime-single-photon-emission
    computed tomography
HMR-3480
HMS
  hexose monophosphate shunt
  hypothetical mean strain
    HMS Liquifilm
    HMS Liquifilm Ophthalmic
HMW
  high molecular weight
HMW-MAA
  high molecular weight-melanoma-
    associated antigen
Ho antigen
hobnail tongue
Hodgkin
  H. disease
  H. granuloma
  H. lymphoma
Hoechst staining
Hof area
Hoffman-Clayton procedure
Hoffman sign
Hofmann violet
hog
  h. cholera
  h. cholera vaccine
  h. cholera virus
holder
  Baumgartner needle h.
  Carb-N-Sert needle h.
  Castroviejo blade h.
  Castroviejo needle h.

  Collier needle h.
  Crile-Wood needle h.
  Diamond Jaw needle h.
  Foster needle h.
  Gillies needle h.
  Halsey needle h.
  Neuro-smooth needle h.
  neurosurgery needle h.
  Olsen-Hegar needle h.
  smooth jawed needle h.
  Webster needle h.
Hollister medial adhesive bandage
Hollister-Stier Laboratory
Holmes-Adie syndrome
holmium ethylenediamine tetramethylene
  phosphonic acid
holocrine gland
holoenzyme
Hologic
holothurin
Holt-Oram syndrome
homatropine hydrobromide
home-based telemetry (HBT)
home cleaning product
homeobox protein
homeopathy
homeoplasia
homeoplastic
homeostasis
  gut h.
homeostasis-driven proliferation
homeotherapy
homing receptor
hominis
  Actinobacillus h.
  Actinomyces h.
  Dermatobia h.
  herpesvirus h.
  Mycoplasma h.
  Pentatrichomonas h.
  poliovirus h.
  Sarcoptes h.
  Staphylococcus h.
homme rouge
homocystinuria
homocytotropic
  h. anaphylaxis
  h. antibody
  h. reaction
homodimer
homodimeric
homodimerization
homogenates
homogeneous
homogenous
homogentisic acid (HGA)
homograft reaction
homoioplasia

homolog
    C-terminal h.
    murine h.
homologous
    h. antigen
    h. antiserum
    h. desensitization
    h. graft
    h. to lymphotoxin, shows inducible
    expression and competes with
    herpes simplex virus glycoprotein
    D for herpes virus entry
    mediator, a receptor expressed by
    T lymphocyte (LIGHT)
    h. serotype
    h. serum
    h. serum jaundice
homology
    h. of chain
    DNA h.
    h. of strand
homolysin
homolysis
homopentameric glycoprotein
homophil
homophilic cell-cell adhesion
homoplastic graft
homotransplantation
homotrimeric
homozygosity
    epitope h.
homozygous
    h. autosomal recessive deletion
    h. typing cell
homunculus
honeybee, honey bee
    African h.
    h. sting
honeycomb
    h. atrophy
    h. hyperkeratosis
    h. lung
    h. nevus
    h. plaque
    h. ringworm
    h. staining pattern
    h. tetter
honeymoon period
Hong
    H. Kong foot
    H. Kong influenza
    H. Kong toe

HOOD
    hereditary osteoonychodysplasia
hoof-and-mouth disease
hook
    Dortu phlebectomy h.
    double-hook Tyrell skin h.
    dura twist skin h.
    Frazier-Shepherd skin h.
    Frazier skin h.
    Guthrie skin h.
    Joseph skin h.
    Millet phlebectomy h.
    Muller phlebectomy h.
    Oesch phlebectomy h.
    Ramelet phlebectomy h.
    single-hook Frazier skin h.
    skin h.
    Tyrell skin h.
    Varady phlebectomy h.
hookworm
    cat h.
Hoover sign
Hopf
    acrokeratosis verruciformis of H.
Hopkins lupus cohort
hops
hordeolum
Horder spot
horizontal
    h. growth phase
    h. mattress stitch
    h. section
    h. transmission
Hormodendron
    H. compactum
    H. pedrosoi
Hormodendrum
hormonal change
hormone
    adrenocorticotropic h. (ACTH)
    alpha-melanocyte-stimulating h.
    (alpha-MSH, alpha-MSH)
    autocrine h.
    beta-melanocyte-stimulating h.
    corticotropin-releasing h. (CRH)
    growth h. (GH)
    human growth h. (HGH)
    immunoreactive h.
    melanocyte-stimulating h. (MSH)
    polypeptide h.
    syndrome of inappropriate excretion
    of antidiuretic h. (SIADH)

NOTES

H

hormone *(continued)*
    thymic h.
    thyroid-stimulating h. (TSH)
hormone-related gene
horn
    cicatricial h.
    cutaneous h.
    nail h.
    sebaceous h.
    warty h.
hornbeam
Horner syndrome
hornet
    h. sting
    white-faced h.
    yellow h.
hornification
horny
    h. cell
    h. cell layer
    h. spine
horripilation
horror
    h. autotoxicans
    h. autotoxicus
horse
    h. fly
    h. hair
    h. serum
horsefly bite
horsepox virus
horses
    infectious arteritis virus of h.
hortae
    Piedraia h.
Horton disease
hose
    Medi-Strumpf support h.
hospital
    h. fever
    h. furunculitis
    h. gangrene
hospital-acquired infection
host
    accidental h.
    amplifier h.
    dead-end h.
    h. defect
    humoral h.
    h. immunity
    immunocompromised h.
    reservoir h.
    h. response
host-cell lysis
host-generated neutrophils recruitment
host-immune process
hot
    h. comb alopecia

    h. gangrene
    h. quartz vapor lamp
    h. tub folliculitis
Hotchkiss-McManus
    H.-M. stain
    H.-M. technique
hot-cross-bun skull
hotfoot
hound-dog facies
Houpt
    DIDMOS syndrome of Sontheimer and H.
    drug-induced delayed multiorgan hypersensitivity syndrome of Sontheimer and H.
24-Hour
    Claritin-D 24-H.
hour
    Actifed 12 H.
    Sudafed 12 H.
hourglass
house
    h. dust
    h. dust mite (HDM)
    h. dust mite F, P
    h. fly
housefly
housekeeping gene
housemaid knee
housewives'
    h. dermatitis
    h. eczema
Houssay animal
Howell-Evans
    H.-E. keratoderma
    H.-E. syndrome
Howell-Jolly body
H2Oxyl
Hoyne sign
HP
    herpetiform pemphigus
    hypersensitivity pneumonitis
HPA
    hypothalamic-pituitary-adrenal
    hypothalamic-pituitary axis
    hypothalamo-pituitary adrenal
    HPA axis
H.P. Acthar Gel
HPC
    hemangiopericytoma
    HPC bacteria
    HPC cell
HPLC
    high-performance liquid chromatography
HPS
    hepatopulmonary syndrome

HPV
    human papillomavirus
    human parvovirus
HQ
      NeoStrata HQ
HRCT
    high-resolution computed tomography
      HRCT scan
HRE
    hair removal efficiency
HRF
    histamine-releasing factor
      HRF deficiency
HRR
    heart rate reserve
    high-risk recipient
HS
    hyperplastic synovium
HSCT
    hematopoietic stem cell transplantation
      nonmyeloablative HSCT
3β-HSD
    3-beta-hydroxysteroid dehydrogenase
17β-HSD
    17-beta-hydroxysteroid dehydrogenase
HSE
    human skin equivalent
HSK
    herpetic stromal keratitis
H-SLAP
    human stromelysin aggregated
      proteoglycan
      H-SLAP test
HSNC
    human skin nurse cell
HSP
    heat-shock protein
    Henoch-Schönlein purpura
    hereditary sclerosing poikiloderma
      mycobacteria HSP
HSP-70
    heat-shock protein 70
HSS
    Henoch-Schönlein syndrome
HSV
    herpes simplex virus
      Mollaret HSV
HSV-thymidine kinase ex-vivo cell therapy
HSVTK
    herpes simplex virus thymidine kinase
H-tetanase

HTLV
    human T-cell leukemia/lymphoma virus
    human T-cell leukemia virus
    human T-cell lymphotrophic virus
HTLV-1-associated myelopathy or tropical spastic paraparesis (HAM/TSP)
HTLV-I
    human T-cell lymphotrophic virus type I
HTLV I
    human T-cell leukemia virus I
HTLV-II
    human T-cell lymphotrophic virus type II
HTLV III
    human T-cell leukemia virus III
HTLV-III
    human T-cell lymphotrophic virus type
      III
HTX
    heart transplantation
Hu-901
hu1124
Hu antigen
huff cough
Huile Solaire Bronzage
human
    h. alpha-1-proteinase inhibitor
    h. androgen receptor assay
      (HUMARA)
    h. anti-CMV antibody
    h. anticytomegalovirus antibody
    h. cartilage glycoprotein 39
    CD4, immunoglobulin G,
      recombinant h.
    chickenpox immune globulin (h.)
    h. cloned DNA
    h. cutaneous leishmaniasis
    cytomegalovirus immune globulin
      intravenous, h.
    h. dermatosparaxis type Ehlers-
      Danlos syndrome
    h. diploid cell rabies vaccine
      (HDCV)
    h. diploid cell vaccine (HDCV)
    h. embryonic lung fibroblast
    h. gamma globulin
    h. granulocytic ehrlichiosis
    h. growth hormone (HGH)
    h. herpesvirus 1–7 (HHV)
    h. herpesvirus 6 (HHV-6)
    h. herpesvirus 8 (HHV-8)
    h. herpesvirus 6A (HHV-6A)

NOTES

H

human (continued)
  h. herpesvirus 6B (HHV-6B)
  h. host defense defect
  h. immune status survey (HISS)
  h. immunodeficiency virus (HIV)
  h. immunodeficiency virus-1 (HIV-1)
  h. immunodeficiency virus-2 (HIV-2)
  h. immunodeficiency virus antigen testing
  h. immunodeficiency virus deoxyribonucleic acid amplification assay
  h. immunodeficiency virus DNA amplification
  h. immunodeficiency virus immunoglobulin (HIVIG)
  h. leukemia-associated antigen
  h. leukocyte antibody (HLA)
  h. leukocyte antigen (HLA)
  h. leukocyte antigen allele
  h. lymphocyte antigen (HLA)
  measles immune globulin (h.)
  h. measles immune serum
  h. monocyte chemoattractant protein-1
  h. normal immunoglobulin
  h. nude defect
  h. papillomavirus (HPV)
  h. papillomavirus infection
  h. parvovirus (HPV)
  h. parvovirus B19
  h. pertussis immune serum
  poliomyelitis immune globulin (h.)
  rabies immune globulin, h.
  h. RD
  h. recombinant deoxyribonuclease
  h. rhabdomyosarcoma
  h. scarlet fever immune serum
  h. skin equivalent (HSE)
  h. skin nurse cell (HSNC)
  specific immune globulin (h.)
  h. stromelysin aggregated proteoglycan (H-SLAP)
  h. stromelysin aggregated proteoglycan test
  h. T-cell leukemia/lymphoma virus (HTLV)
  h. T-cell leukemia virus (HTLV)
  h. T-cell leukemia virus I (HTLV I)
  h. T-cell leukemia virus III (HTLV III)
  h. T-cell lymphotrophic virus (HTLV)
  h. T-cell lymphotrophic virus type I (HTLV-I)
  h. T-cell lymphotrophic virus type II (HTLV-II)
  h. T-cell lymphotrophic virus type III (HTLV-III)
  tetanus immune globulin, h.
  h. thymus lymphocyte antigen
  h. umbilical vein endothelial cell (HUVEC)
humanized BTI-322
humanus
  Pediculus h.
HUMARA
  human androgen receptor assay
Humatin
Humatrix
  H. Microclysmic Gel
  H. Microclysmic Gel filler
Humatrope
HuMax-CD4
humectant
Humibid LA
humidified oxygen
humidifier
  h. fever
  h. lung
humidity
humid tetter
humoral
  h. antibody
  h. defect
  h. host
  h. immune response
  h. immunity
  h. immunity status panel
hump
  buffalo h.
  dowager h.
Hunermann disease
Hunstad
  H. hand
  H. tumescent liposuction system
Hunter
  H. glossitis
  H. mucopolysaccharidosis
  H. robe
  H. syndrome
hunterian chancre
Hunter-Thompson syndrome
hunting
  h. phenomenon
  h. reaction
Hunt syndrome
Huriez syndrome
Hurler
  H. disease
  H. syndrome

Hurler-Scheie
    H.-S. mucopolysaccharidosis
    H.-S. syndrome
Hurst disease
HUS
    hemolytic uremic syndrome
Hutchinson
    chilblain lupus erythematosus of H.
    freckle of H.
    H. freckle
    H. mask
    melanotic freckle of H.
    H. sign
    H. summer protoporphyria
    H. summer prurigo
    H. teeth
    H. triad
Hutchinson-Gilford
    H.-G. progeria
    H.-G. syndrome
HUVEC
    human umbilical vein endothelial cell
HUVS
    hypocomplementemic urticarial vasculitis
    syndrome
Huxley layer
HVD
    hypoxic ventilatory drive
HVPT
    hyperventilation provocation test
HVS
    herpesvirus saimiri
    hyperventilation syndrome
Hyalase
Hyalgan
hyaline
    h. articular cartilage
    h. basement membrane
    h. degeneration
hyalinosis
    h. cutis et mucosa
    systemic h.
hyalinum
    Scytalidium h.
hyalohyphomycosis
Hyalomma variegatum
hyaluran
hyaluronan
    h. hexasaccharides
    h. injection
    h. oligosaccharide

hyaluronate
    h. injection
    sodium h.
hyaluronate-polylysine complex
hyaluronic
    h. acid
    h. acid injection
hyaluronidase
    h. activity
    h. deficiency
hybrid
    h. antibody
    h. capture assay (HCA)
    H. Capture II DNA-based test for
      human papillomavirus
    h. cell
    SV40-adenovirus h.
    h. total arthroplasty
hybridization
    h. buffer
    clonospecific oligoprobe h.
    deoxyribonucleic acid h.
    DNA h.
    fluorescence in situ h. (FISH)
    sequence-specific oligonucleotide
      probe h. (SSOP)
    in situ h. (ISH)
    h. test
hybridoma antibody
hyCare G hydrogel dressing
Hycodan
Hycomine
Hycor rheumatoid factor IgA ELISA
    autoimmune test
Hycort
    H. Topical
Hycotuss
Hy-C trial
hyCure collagen hemostatic wound
    dressing
hydantoin
    h. anticonvulsant
    DMDM h.
hydantoin/EDTA
hydatid rash
Hyde disease
Hydeltrasol injection
Hydeltra-TBA injection
Hyderm
hydradenitis
hydradenoma

NOTES

H

hydralazine-associated lupus-like syndrome
hydralazine syndrome
Hydramyn Syrup
hydrarthrosis
    intermittent h.
Hydrasorb foam wound dressing
hydrate
    chloral h.
    tacrolimus h.
hydrated petrolatum
Hydrate Injection
hydration
    adequate h.
    vigorous h.
hydrazine
    isonicotine h. (INH)
Hydrea
Hydrisinol
hydro
    Cutinova H.
hydroa
    h. estivale
    h. febrile
    h. gestationis
    h. gravidarum
    h. herpetiforme
    h. puerorum
    h. vacciniforme
    h. vesiculosum
hydrobromide
    homatropine h.
hydrocarbon
    aliphatic h.
    aromatic h.
hydrocephalus
hydrochloric acid
hydrochloride (HCl)
    amantadine h.
    amitriptyline h.
    amprolium h.
    aneurin h.
    bacampicillin h.
    benzphetamine h.
    bupivacaine h.
    butenafine h.
    chloroguanide h.
    chloroprocaine h.
    chlorpromazine h.
    chlortetracycline h.
    ciprofloxacin h.
    Cleocin h.
    clonidine h.
    cyclizine h.
    cyproheptadine h.
    cytarabine h.
    daunorubicin h.
    demeclocycline h.

    diphenhydramine h.
    diphenidol h.
    dyclonine h.
    eflornithine h.
    epinephrine h.
    ethambutol h.
    ethylnorepinephrine h.
    etidocaine h.
    fluoxetine h.
    fluphenazine h.
    halofantrine h.
    hydroxyzine h.
    isoxsuprine h.
    levocabastine h.
    lidocaine h.
    lomefloxacin h.
    mechlorethamine h.
    meclizine h.
    mefloquine h.
    mepivacaine h.
    methapyrilene h.
    minocycline h.
    Mustargen H.
    naftifine h.
    naloxone h.
    olopatadine h.
    oxymetazoline h.
    oxytetracycline h.
    pararosaniline h.
    paroxetine h.
    phenoxybenzamine h.
    phenylephrine h.
    phenylpropanolamine h.
    piperazine h.
    pramoxine h.
    prazosin h.
    procaine h.
    promethazine h.
    propranolol h.
    ranitidine h.
    rimantadine h.
    sertraline h.
    spectinomycin h.
    terbinafine h.
    tetracaine h.
    tetrahydrozoline h.
    vancomycin h.
hydrochlorothiazide (HCTZ)
hydrocodone bitartrate
Hydrocol hydrocolloid dressing
hydrocolloid
    BGC Matrix h.
    CombiDERM ACD h.
    Comfeel h.
    Curaderm h.
    Cutinova Thin h.
    DermAssist h.
    Dermatell h.

h. dressing
DuoDerm CGF h.
ExuDerm h.
Nu-Derm h.
RepliCare h.
Restore h.
SignaDress Sterile h.
Tegasorb Thin h.
Triad h.
Ultec h.
hydrocortisone
h. acetate
h. acetate cream
acetic acid, propanediol diacetate, and h.
bacitracin, neomycin, polymyxin b, and h.
Bactine H.
benzoyl peroxide and h.
h. butyrate
chloramphenicol, polymyxin b, and h.
clioquinol and h.
colistin, neomycin, and h.
iodoquinol and h.
lidocaine and h.
neomycin and h.
neomycin, polymyxin b, and h.
oxytetracycline and h.
polymyxin b and h.
h. sodium succinate
urea and h.
h. valerate
Hydrocortone
H. acetate
H. Phosphate
Hydrocort Topical
hydrocystoma
hydrofluoroalkane
hydrofluoroalkane-134a
hydrogel
h. dressing
Tegagel h.
hydrogen
h. breath test
h. peroxide
hydroid
feather h.
hydrolase
LTA$_4$ h.
hydrolysis of surfactant
hydrolyze

Hydropel
hydroperoxyeicosatetraenoic acid
Hydrophen
Hydrophiinae
hydrophila
Aeromonas h.
hydrophilic
h. petrolatum
h. polymer dressing
hydrophobia
hydrophobic
hydropic change in pneumocyte
hydroquinone
h. cream
h. USP and glycolic acid
HydroSKIN
Hydrosone
Hydro-Tex Topical
hydrotherapy
hydrous wool fat
hydroxide
dysprosium ferric h.
lactic acid with ammonium h.
potassium h. (KOH)
sodium h.
3-hydroxy-3-methylglutaryl coenzyme A (HMG-CoA)
3-hydroxy-3-methyl glutaryl coenzyme A reductase inhibitor
hydroxyapatite (HA)
h. chondrocalcinosis
h. crystal deposition
hydroxychloroquine (HCQ)
h. sulfate
h. therapy
hydroxycitronellal
hydroxyeicosatetraenoic acid (HETE)
5-hydroxyindoleacetic acid
hydroxyl
16-hydroxylated metabolite
hydroxylation
5-hydroxy-L-tryptophan
hydroxylysine content of collagen
hydroxylysylpyridinoline
crosslink h.
hydroxyprogesterone caproate
hydroxyproline
hydroxypropyl cellulose
hydroxyquinoline sulfate
hydroxyurea
hydroxyzine
h. HCl

NOTES

H

hydroxyzine *(continued)*
 h. hydrochloride
 theophylline, ephedrine, and h. (TEH)
HyFil hydrogel dressing
hyfrecator
 Birtcher h.
Hy-Gestrone injection
hygiene
 bronchial h.
hygroma
 cystic h.
hygroscopicity
hylan G-F 20
HYLL
 healthy years of life lost
Hylutin injection
Hymenolepis
 H. fraterna
 H. nana
Hymenoptera
 Hymenoptera sting
 Hymenoptera venom
 Hymenoptera venom anaphylaxis
Hymenopterous vespid
hyomagnesemia
Hypafix
Hy-Pam Oral
hyper
 h.-IgE syndrome
Hyperab
hyperabduction
hyperacanthosis
hyperacute organ rejection
hyperaldosteronism
 primary h.
hyperalgesia
 zone of h.
hyperalgia
 thermal h.
hyperalimentation
hyperandrogenism, insulin resistance, and acanthosis nigricans (HAIR-AN)
hyperbaric
 h. oxygen (HBO)
 h. oxygen therapy
hyperbilirubinemia
hypercalcemia
 familial hypocalciuric h.
hypercalciuria
hypercapnia
 permissive h.
hypercarbia
hypercarotenemia
hypercholesteremic xanthoma
hypercholesterolemia
 familial h.
hypercoagulable state

hypercortisolism
hyperekplexia
hyperelastica
 cutis h.
hyperemia
 zone of h.
hypereosinophilia
hypereosinophilic syndrome (HES)
hyperephidrosis
hyperergia
hyperergic encephalitis
hyperesthesia
hyperesthetic zone
hyperextensibility
hyperextensible skin type I–VIII
hyperextension
hyperfiltration
 glomerular h.
hypergammaglobulinemia
 M-component h.
 polyclonal h.
 h. of Waldenström
hypergammaglobulinemic purpura
Hypergel hydrogel dressing
hypergia
hypergic
hyperglobulinemia
hyperglobulinemic purpura
hypergranulosis
hypergranulotic dyscornification
HyperHep
hyperhidrosis
 emotional h.
 generalized h.
 gustatory h.
 h. lateralis
 h. oleosa
 primary h.
 unilateral h.
hyperhistidinemia
hyperhistidinuria
hyperhomocystinemia
hyperhydration
hyperhydrosis
hypericin
hyperidrosis
hyper-IgE (HIE)
 hyperimmunoglobulin E
hyper-IgM
 immunodeficiency with h.-I.
 h.-I. syndrome (HIM)
hyperimmune
 h. bovine colostrum IgC concentrate
 h. gamma globulin preparation
 h. serum
 h. state

hyperimmunization
hyperimmunoglobulin E (hyper-IgE)
hyperimmunoglobulinemia
    h. D, E syndrome
    h. syndrome (HID)
hyperinfection
hyperinflation
Hyperion
    H. Advanced alginate dressing
    H. bordered hydrocolloid dressing
    H. hydrophilic wound gel hydrogel
      dressing
    H. thin hydrocolloid dressing
    H. wound cleanser
hyperirritability
hyperirritable skin
hyperkalemia
hyperkeratinization
hyperkeratomycosis
hyperkeratosis, pl. **hyperkeratoses**
    dystrophic palmoplantar h.
    h. eccentrica
    epidermolytic h.
    h. excentrica
    h. figurata centrifuga atrophica
    focal acral h.
    h. follicularis et parafollicularis
    h. follicularis et parafollicularis in
      cutem penetrans
    h. follicularis vegetans
    generalized epidermolytic h.
    honeycomb h.
    h. lenticularis perstans
    h. lingua
    multiple minute digitate h.
    subungual h.
    h. subungualis
    h. universalis congenita
hyperkeratotic
    h. epidermis
    h. scabies
    h. spicule
hyperleukocytosis
hyperlinearity
    palmar h.
    plantar h.
hyperlinear palm
hyperlipemic xanthoma
hyperlipidemia
    familial combined h.
    Frederickson type IIa, IIb h.

hyperlipoproteinemia
    medication-induced h.
    multiple-type h.
    primary h.
    secondary h.
hyperliposis
hypermelanization
hypermelanosis
    linear and whorled nevoid h.
    nevoid h.
hypermelanotic
hypermobile-type Ehlers-Danlos
  syndrome
hypermobility syndrome
hypermutation
    somatic h.
hyperneocytosis
hyperonychia
hyperorthocytosis
hyperostosis
    ankylosing h.
    h. cranialis
    diffuse idiopathic skeletal h.
      (DISH)
    idiopathic skeletal h.
    sternoclavicular h.
    sternocostoclavicular h.
hyperostotica
    spondylosis h.
hyperostotic syndrome
hyperoxaluria
hyperparathyroidism
    secondary h.
hyperperistalsis
hyperpermeability
    dermal venular h.
hyperphenylalaninemia
hyperpigmentation
    bronze h.
    cutaneous h.
    familial progressive h. (FPH)
    hemosiderin h.
    industrial h.
    longitudinal nail h.
    marble cake h.
    mercury h.
    metal h.
    minocycline h.
    oral postinflammatory h.
    periorbital h.
    postinflammatory h.

NOTES

H

hyperpigmentation *(continued)*
    reticulate h.
    zebra-like h.
hyperplasia
    angiolymphoid h.
    basaloid folliculolymphoid h.
    benign h.
    congenital sebaceous gland h.
    crypt h.
    cutaneous lymphoid h. (CLH)
    fibrous h.
    focal epithelial h. (FEH)
    gingival h.
    goblet cell h.
    inflammatory fibrous h.
    intravascular papillary endothelial h.
    pseudoepitheliomatous h.
    psoriasiform epidermal h.
    rete ridge h.
    reticuloendothelial h.
    h. of sebaceous gland
    sebaceous senile h.
    senile sebaceous h.
    synovial h.
hyperplastic
    h. epidermis
    h. mucus-secreting goblet cell
    h. synovium (HS)
hyperprebetalipoproteinemia
hyperresponsiveness
    airway h. (AHR)
    bronchial h. (BHR)
hypersecretion
    mucus h.
hypersensitiveness
hypersensitivity
    h. angiitis
    atopic h.
    cell-mediated h.
    contact h.
    cutaneous basophil h. (CBH)
    delayed h. (DH)
    delayed-type h. (DTH)
    drug h.
    food h.
    immediate h.
    latex h.
    h. pneumonitis (HP)
    h. pneumonitis panel
    h. reaction
    reaginic h.
    h. skin testing
    tuberculin-type h.
    h. vasculitis
hypersensitization
hypersomnia
hypersplenism
hypersteatosis

hypersusceptibility
hypertelorism
    ocular h.
hypertension
    benign intracranial h.
    chronic thromboembolic
      pulmonary h. (CTEPH)
    mild h.
    portopulmonary h. (PPHTN)
    primary pulmonary h. (PPH)
    pulmonary h.
Hyper-Tet
hyperthyroidism
    clinical h.
    exogenous h.
    overt h.
hypertonia
hypertrichiasis
hypertrichophrydia
hypertrichosis
    h. lanuginosa
    nevoid h.
    h. partialis
    h. universalis
hypertriglyceridemia
    familial h.
hypertrophic
    h. cervical pachymeningitis
    h. cicatrix
    h. lichen planus
    h. lymphoid follicle
    h. osteoarthropathy
    h. ringworm
    h. rosacea
    h. scar
    h. smooth muscle layer
    h. tonsil
hypertrophica
    acne h.
hypertrophicum
    h. cutis
    eczema h.
    h. simplex
    strawberry h.
    verrucous h.
hypertrophicus
    corneus h.
    lichen corneus h.
    lichen planus h.
    lupus erythematosus h.
hypertrophy
    left ventricular h.
    progressive synovial h.
    submucosal gland h.
    h. of tongue papilla
hypertylosis
hyperuricemia
hyperuricuria

hypervaccination
hypervariable region
hyperventilation
    isocapnic h. (ISH)
    h. provocation test (HVPT)
    h. syndrome (HVS)
hyperviscosity syndrome
hypervitaminosis
    h. A, C, D, E
hyperzincuria
hypha, pl. **hyphae**
    spaghetti and meatballs appearance
    of spores and hyphae
hyphal form
hyphomycotic sycosis
hypoadrenalism
hypoallergenic
    h. diet
    h. product
hypoallergenicity
hypobaric hypoxia
hypocapnia
hypochondriasis
    monosymptomatic h.
hypochondrogenesis
hypochromic normocytic anemia
hypocomplementemia
hypocomplementemic
    h. glomerulonephritis
    h. urticarial vasculitis
    h. urticarial vasculitis syndrome
    (HUVS)
    h. vasculitis urticarial syndrome
hypoderm
hypodermatic
hypodermiasis
hypodermic
hypodermitis sclerodermiformis
hypodermolithiasis
hypodontia
hypoergia
hypoergic
hypofibrinogenemia
hypofibrinolytic
hypogammaglobinemia
hypogammaglobulinemia
    acquired h.
    primary h.
    secondary h.
    X-linked h.
hypogammaglobulinemic
hypoglycemia

hypogonadism
hypohidrosis
    postmiliarial h.
hypohidrotic ectodermal dysplasia
(HED)
hypolymphemia
hypomelanism
hypomelanosis
    congenital circumscribed h.
    guttate h.
    hereditary h.
    idiopathic guttate h.
    h. of Ito
hypometabolism brain lesion
hypomotility
    esophageal h.
hyponychial
hyponychium
hyponychon
hypoparathyroidism
    immunodeficiency with h.
hypophosphatasia
hypophosphatemia
hypophysitis
    lymphocytic h.
    lymphoid h.
hypopigmentation
    postinflammatory h.
    reticulate h.
hypopigmented
    h. macular eruption
    h. macule
hypopigmenter
hypopituitarism
hypoplasia
    cartilage-hair h.
    dermal h.
    focal dermal h.
    thymic h.
hypoprothrombinemia
hypopyon iritis
hyposensitivity
hyposensitization
    oral h.
hypostatica
    dermatitis h.
hypostaticum
    ulcus h.
hypostome
    barbed h.
hyposulfite
    sodium h.

NOTES

H

HypoTears
    H. PF solution
hypotension
    orthostatic h.
hypothalamic-pituitary-adrenal (HPA)
    h.-p.-a. system
hypothalamic-pituitary axis (HPA)
hypothalamo-pituitary adrenal (HPA)
hypothermic
    h. injury
    h. perfusion
hypothesis, pl. **hypotheses**
    cotriggering h.
    missing self h.
    Saunders-Zwilling h.
    unitarian h.
hypothetical
    h. mean organism
    h. mean strain (HMS)
hypothyroidism
    idiopathic h.
hypotonia
hypotonicity
hypotonic solution
hypotrichiasis
hypotrichosis
hypoventilation
hypovitaminosis
    h. A, B
hypovolemic shock
hypoxanthine, aminopterin and thymidine (HAT)
hypoxanthine-guanine
    h.-g. phosphoribosyltransferase (HGPRT)

h.-g. phosphoribosyltransferase deficiency
hypoxemia
    arterial h.
    rapid eye movement sleep-related h.
    REM sleep-related h.
    rest h.
hypoxia
    hypobaric h.
    neonatal h.
    synovial h.
hypoxic
    h. vasoconstriction
    h. ventilatory drive (HVD)
Hyprogest
    H. 250
    H. injection
Hyrexin-50 Injection
Hysone topical
hysterical
    h. edema
    h. reaction
hystriciasis
hystrix
    ichthyismus h.
    ichthyosis h.
Hy-Tape
HY-TEC automated allergy diagnostic system
Hytone Topical
Hyzine-50 Injection
HZ
    herpes zoster

I

  I antigen
  I cell
  I deficiency factor
  I invariant
  I pilus
  I region

I3

  prostacyclin I3

IA

  intraarticular

Ia

  Ia antigen
  Ia cell marker

Ia+

  immune-associated antigen-positive
  macrophage

IA-A-F

  idiopathic anaphylaxis-angioedema-
  frequent

IA-A-I

  idiopathic anaphylaxis-angioedema-
  infrequent

IACH

  immediate active cutaneous anaphylaxis

IA-G-F

  idiopathic anaphylaxis-generalized-
  frequent

IA-G-I

  idiopathic anyaphylaxis-generalized-
  infrequent

IAHIA

  immune adherence immunosorbent assay

Iamin

  I. gel wound dressing
  I. hydrogel dressing
  I. Wound Cleanser

IAPP

  islet amyloid polypeptide
  IAPP amylin

IA-Q

  idiopathic anaphylaxis-questionable

IAS

  illness attitude scale

iatrogenic

  i. calcinosis
  i. Cushing syndrome
  i. immunosuppression
  i. pneumothorax
  i. polymorphism

IA-V

  idiopathic anaphylaxis-variant

IB

  Excedrin IB
  Midol IB
  Motrin IB
  Pamprin IB
  Sine-Aid IB

I-B1 radiolabeled antibody
ibandronate
Ibaraki virus
IBD

  inflammatory bowel disease

IBIDS

  ichthyosis plus BIDS
  ichthyosis plus brittle hair, intellectual
  impairment, decreased fertility, short
  stature
  IBIDS syndrome

IBR

  infectious bovine rhinotracheitis
  IBR virus

IBS

  ichthyosis bullosa of Siemens
  inflammatory bowel syndrome
  irritable bowel syndrome

Ibuprin
ibuprofen

  Arthritis Foundation i.
  pseudoephedrine and i.

Ibuprohm
Ibu-Tab
IBV

  infectious bronchitis virus

IC

  immune complex
  inspiratory capacity

ICA

  islet cell antibody

ICAM

  intercellular adhesion module

ICAM-1

  intercellular adhesion molecule-1

ICC

  immunocytochemistry
  intraclass correlation coefficient

iccosomes
ICD

ICD-9 code

  irritant contact dermatitis

ICDRG

  International Contact Dermatitis Research
  Group

ICE

  immunoglobulin-complexed enzyme
  ICE disorder

ice

  i. compress
  i. cube test
  dry i.

ice-pick type scar

277

ICG
  indocyanine green
ichthammol
ichthyismus
  i. exanthematicus
  i. hystrix
Ichthyol
ichthyosiform
  i. dermatosis
  i. erythroderma
  i. sarcoidosis
ichthyosis
  acquired i.
  autosomal dominant lamellar i.
  autosomal recessive i.
  i. bullosa of Siemens (IBS)
  congenital erythrodermic i.
  i. congenita neonatorum
  i. fetalis
  follicular i.
  i. follicularis
  i. harlequin
  harlequin i.
  i. hystrix
  i. intrauterina
  lamellar i.
  i. lethalis
  i. linearis circumflexa (ILC)
  i. lingua
  nacreous i.
  nonbullous congenital
    erythrodermic i.
  i. palmaris et plantaris
  i. plus BIDS (IBIDS)
  i. plus brittle hair, intellectual
    impairment, decreased fertility,
    short stature (IBIDS)
  i. plus brittle hair, intellectual
    impairment, decreased fertility,
    short stature syndrome
  recessive X-linked i.
  i. sauroderma
  i. scutulata
  i. sebacea
  i. sebacea corneae
  senile i.
  i. serpentina
  i. simplex
  i. spinosa
  i. thysanotrichica
  i. uteri
  i. vulgaris
  i. vulgaris ichthyotic
  X-linked i.
ichthyotic
  ichthyosis vulgaris i.
ICM-3
icosahedral

ICOS molecule
ICP
  intracranial pressure
ICS
  inhaled corticosteroid
icteric
icteroid
icterus
  acquired hemolytic i.
  i. gravis
  i. melas
  i. neonatorum
  i. praecox
ICU
  immunological contact urticaria
ID
  immune deficiency
  immunodiffusion
  infecting dose
  infectious disease
IDA
  idiopathic destructive arthritis
idarubicin
IDD
  excess incidence
IDDM
  insulin-dependent diabetes mellitus
IDEC-114, -131
identical twin donor
identification
  i. bracelet
  i. tag
identity
  reaction of partial i.
idioagglutinin
idioheteroagglutinin
idioheterolysin
idioisoagglutinin
idioisolysin
idiolysin
idiopathic
  i. acute eosinophilic pneumonia
  i. anaphylaxis-angioedema-frequent
    (IA-A-F)
  i. anaphylaxis-angioedema-infrequent
    (IA-A-I)
  i. anaphylaxis-generalized-frequent
    (IA-G-F)
  i. anaphylaxis-questionable (IA-Q)
  i. anaphylaxis-variant (IA-V)
  i. anyaphylaxis-generalized-infrequent
    (IA-G-I)
  i. aortitis
  i. atrophoderma
  i. atrophoderma of Pasini and
    Pierini
  i. calcinosis cutis
  i. clubbing

i. cold agglutinin disease
i. cold urticaria
i. destructive arthritis (IDA)
i. eczematous disease
i. environmental intolerance (IEI)
i. flush
i. giant esophageal ulcer
i. guttate hypomelanosis
i. hirsutism
i. hypereosinophilic syndrome (IHES)
i. hypertrophic osteoarthritis
i. hypothyroidism
i. inflammatory myopathy (IIM)
i. late-onset eczema
i. livedo reticularis
i. lobular panniculitis
i. nephrotic syndrome
i. panhypopituitarism
i. panuveitis
i. periostosis
i. polyserositis
i. posterior uveitis
i. pulmonary fibrosis (IPF)
i. pulmonary hemosiderosis
i. recurrent palmoplantar hidradenitis
i. roseola
i. skeletal hyperostosis
i. thrombocytopenic purpura (ITP)
idiopathica
    livedo reticularis i.
idiopeptide
idiosyncrasy
idiosyncratic
    i. drug reaction
    i. sensitivity
idiotope
    set of i.'s
idiotype
    i. antibody
    i. autoantibody
    cross-reactive i.
idiotypic
    i. antigen
    i. antigenic determinant
IDM
    infant of diabetic mother
idoxuridine (IDUR)
id reaction
idrosis

IDSA
    Infectious Disease Society of America
IDUR
    idoxuridine
iduronic acid
I:E
    inspiratory to expiratory ratio
IEC
    intestinal epithelial cell
IEF
    isoelectric focusing
IEI
    idiopathic environmental intolerance
IEM
    immune electron microscopy
IF
    immunofluorescence
IFA
    silver stain
IF-A
    inflammatory factor of anaphylaxis
IFE
    immunofixation electrophoresis
Ifex
IFN
    interferon
IFN-alpha
    interferon alpha
IFN-beta
    interferon beta
IFN-gamma
ifosfamide
Ig
    immunoglobulin
        Ig class
IgA
    immunoglobulin A
        IgA antibody
        IgA antiendomysial antibody
        IgA antigliadin antibody
        IgA deficiency
        IgA dermatosis
        IgA nephropathy
        serum IgA
IgD
    immunoglobulin D
IgE
    immunoglobulin E
        IgE antibody
        latex-specific IgE
        IgE radioallergosorbent test
        total serum IgE

NOTES

IgE-dependent immunologic drug reaction
IgE-mediated
>I.-m. food allergy
>I.-m. response
IgE-sensitized cell
IGF-1
>insulin-like growth factor-1
IgG
>immunoglobulin G
>aggregated human IgG
>IgG antibody
>IgG avidity test
>biotinylated antihuman IgG
>*Candida albicans* IgG
>circulating antiepidermal BMZ IgG
>IgG complex
>IgG heavy chain
>IgG RF
>IgG subclass determination
>IgG subclass level
>IgG titer
IgG1
>immunoglobulin G1
IgG4
>immunoglobulin G4
IgG-coated erythrocyte
IgG-RF complement aggregate
IGIV
>immunoglobulin, intravenous
>Nordimmun IGIV
IgM
>immunoglobulin M
>IgM anticardiolipin antibody
>indirect enzyme immunoassay for anti-*Mycoplasma pneumoniae* IgM
>IgM nephropathy
>IgM RF
>IgM rheumatoid factor
>serum IgM
>X-linked immunodeficiency with hyper IgM
IgM-coated cell
igne
>erythema ab i. (EAI)
ignea
>zona i.
ignis
>sacer i.
ignorance
>clonal i.
IGT
>impaired glucose tolerance
IH
>infectious hepatitis
IHC
>immunohistochemistry

IHES
>idiopathic hypereosinophilic syndrome
IIa
>glycoprotein IIa (GPIIa)
IIb
>glycoprotein IIb (GPIIb)
IIb-IIIa
>glycoprotein IIb-IIIa (GPIIbIIIa)
IIEF
>International Index of Erectile Function
IIF
>indirect immunofluorescence
IIM
>idiopathic inflammatory myopathy
IL
>interleukin
IL-1
>interleukin-1
>IL-1, -2, -3, -4, -10, -13 cytokine
>IL-1 interleukin
>IL-1 receptor
IL-1–15
>interleukin-1–15
IL-2
>interleukin-2
>IL-2 receptor alpha chain (CD25) deficiency
>IL-2 receptor alpha chain gene
>IL-2 receptor-b and cytotoxic activity
IL-10
>interleukin-10
>IL-10 gene promoter
IL-11
>interleukin-11
IL-12
>interleukin-12
>IL-12 receptor beta-1 mutation
IL-12p40 deficiency
IL-1-beta cytokine
IL-1-alpha
>interleukin-1-alpha
ILC
>ichthyosis linearis circumflexa
ILD
>interstitial lung disease
Ilhéus
>I. encephalitis
>I. fever
>I. virus
iliacus
ilii
>osteitis condensans i.
iliopectineal
>i. bursitis
>i. ligament

iliopsoas
    i. bursitis
    i. hemorrhage
iliotibial band syndrome
Ilizarov external fixation
ill
    louping i.
illinition
illness
    i. attitude scale (IAS)
    environmental i.
    opportunistic i. (OI)
    roseola-like i.
Illouz cannula
illuminator
    BLU-U blue light photodynamic
    therapy i.
ILO
    International Labor Organization
    ILO pneumoconiosis classification
iloprost
Ilosone
    I. Oral
    I. Pulvules
Ilotycin Ophthalmic
IL-1ra
ILSI
    International Life Science Institute
ILVEN
    inflamed linear verrucous epidermal
    nevus
IM
    infectious mononucleosis
    IM Jaws alligator forceps
images
    store and forward i.
imaging
    ImmuRAID antibody i.
    laser Doppler perfusion i.
    magnetic resonance i. (MRI)
    magnetization transfer i. (MTI)
    videomicroscopic i.
    volumetric magnetization transfer i.
imbalance
    endocrine hormone i.
    protease-antiprotease i.
imbedded stinger
imbricata
    tinea i.
IMC
    index of marrow conversion
I-Methasone

imglucerase
imidazole
    i. carboxamide
    pyrindinyl i.
imidazolidinyl urea
imipenem and cilastatin
imipenem/cilastatin
imipramine
imiquimod
Imitrex
    I. injection
    I. Oral
immediate
    i. active cutaneous anaphylaxis
    (IACH)
    i. allergy
    i. antigen release
    i. contact urticaria
    i. contagion
    i. hypersensitivity
    i. hypersensitivity reaction
    i. phase reaction (IPR)
    i. skin reactivity
    i. tanning
    i. telogen release
    i. transfusion reaction
    i. wheal reaction
immersion
    excessive water i.
    i. foot
    oil i.
immitis
    Coccidioides i.
    Dirofilaria i.
immobilizing antibody
immortalization
immortalized human hepatocyte
ImmTher
immune
    i. adherence
    i. adherence immunosorbent assay
    (IAHIA)
    i. adherence phenomenon
    i. adhesion test
    i. adsorption
    i. agglutination
    i. agglutinin
    i. bacteriolysis
    i. complex (IC)
    i. complex assay
    i. complex clearance
    i. complex disease

NOTES

immune *(continued)*
    i. complex disorder
    i. complex glomerulonephritis
    i. complex immunologic drug reaction
    i. complex-mediated drug reaction
    i. complex nephritis
    i. complex vasculitis
    i. deficiency (ID)
    i. deposit
    i. deviation
    i. dysregulation
    i. electron microscopy (IEM)
    i. elimination
    i. engagement
    i. globulin, intramuscular
    i. globulin, intravenous
    i. hemolysin
    i. hemolysis
    i. inflammation
    i. interferon
    i. memory
    i. neutropenia
    i. opsonin
    i. paralysis
    i. precipitation
    i. privileged site
    i. protein
    i. response (Ir)
    i. response gene
    i. serum (IS)
    i. serum globulin
    i. suppressor (Is)
    i. suppressor gene
    i. surveillance
    i. system
    i. system modulator
    i. theory
    i. thrombocytopenia
    i. tolerance
immune-associated antigen-positive macrophage (Ia+)
immune-derived amyloidosis
immune-mediated
    i.-m. coagulation disorder
    i.-m. disease
    i.-m. membranous nephritis
    i.-m. thyroiditis
Immunex
immunifacient
immunity
    acquired i.
    active i.
    adoptive i.
    antiviral i.
    artificial active i.
    artificial passive i.
    bacteriophage i.

    cell-mediated i. (CMI)
    concomitant i.
    i. deficiency
    endogenous antitumor i.
    general i.
    group i.
    herd i.
    host i.
    humoral i.
    infection i.
    innate i.
    local i.
    maternal i.
    natural i.
    passive i.
    relative i.
    specific active i.
    specific passive i.
immunization
    active i.
    Heptavax i.
    passive i.
    i. requirement
    Standards for Pediatric I. (SPI)
    viral i.
immunize
Immuno
    Gammabulin I.
immunoadjuvant
immunoagglutination
immunoassay
    antinuclear antibody screening by enzyme i.
    double antibody i.
    enzyme i. (EIA)
    enzyme-linked i. (EIA)
    fluorescence polarization i. (FPIA)
    fluorescent enzyme i. (FEIA)
    ImmunoCard i.
    solid phase i. (SPIA)
    thin-layer i.
    urine myoglobin i.
immunobead assay
immunoblast
immunoblastic sarcoma of B, T cell
immunoblot
immunoblotting
immunobullous disease
Immuno-C
ImmunoCAP
ImmunoCard
    I. immunoassay
    I. STAT! Rotavirus test
    I. used for diagnosis of *Helicobacter pylori*
immunochemical
    i. abnormality

i. assay
i. relative
immunochemistry
immunocompetence
immunocompetent
i. cell
i. tissue therapy
immunocomplex
immunocompromised host
immunoconglutinin
immunocyte
immunocyte-derived amyloidosis
immunocytochemical
immunocytochemistry (ICC)
immunodeficiency
acquired i.
common variable unclassifiable i.
i. disease
i. disorder
i. electrophoresis
partial albinism with i.
phagocytic dysfunction i.
phagocytic dysfunction disorders i.
secondary i.
severe combined i. (SCID)
i. syndrome
i. with hyper-IgM
i. with hypoparathyroidism
X-linked severe combined i.
(XSCID)
immunodeficient
immunodepressant
immunodepressor
immunodeterminants
immunodiagnosis
immunodiffusion (ID)
antinuclear antibody i.
double i.
radial i. (RID)
single radial i. (SRID)
i. technique
immunodominant
immunoelectrophoresis
crossed i. (CIE)
quantitative i. (QIE)
rocket i. (RIE)
two-dimensional i.
immunoenhancement
immunoenhancer
immunoferritin
immunofixation electrophoresis (IFE)
immunofluorescence (IF)

i. analysis
antinuclear antibody i.
cytometric indirect i.
direct i.
i. finding
indirect i. (IIF)
i. method
i. microscopy
i. technique
immunofluorescent
i. examination
i. stain
immunogen
immunogenetics
immunogenetic wild-type adenovirus
immunogenic
i. peptide
i. protein
immunogenicity
immunoglobulin (Ig)
i. A (IgA)
anti-D i.
antihuman parvovirus i. G
chickenpox i.
i. class
i. class switching
i. D (IgD)
i. delta chain
DiffGAM bovine anti-*Clostridium
difficile* i.
i. domain
i. E (IgE)
i. E-mediated food allergy
i. epsilon chain
i. E-sensitized cell
i. fold
i. G (IgG)
i. G1 (IgG1)
i. G4 (IgG4)
i. gene
i. gene rearrangement
i. G heavy chain
i. G rheumatoid factor (IgG RF)
i. G rheumatoid factor complement
aggregate
i. heavy chain
hepatitis B i. (H-BIG)
human immunodeficiency virus i.
(HIVIG)
human normal i.
intravenous i.
i. IV

NOTES

immunoglobulin *(continued)*
　i. light chain-origin amyloid
　　deposit (AL protein)
　lyophilized i. G
　i. M-coated cell
　measles i.
　i. membrane
　monoclonal i.
　i. M rheumatoid factor (IgM RF,
　　IgM rheumatoid factor)
　i. mu chain
　nephropathic i.
　pertussis i.
　poliomyelitis i.
　rabies i.
　i. replacement therapy
　$RH_o(D)$ i.
　secretory i.
　secretory i. A
　i. subclass
　subcutaneous i. (SCIG)
　i. superfamily
　i. supergene family
　tetanus i.
　thyroid-binding inhibitory i. (TBII)
　thyrotropin-binding inhibitory i.
　　(TBII)
　varicella-zoster i. (VZIG)
immunoglobulin-complexed
　i.-c. enzyme (ICE)
　i.-c. enzyme disorder
immunoglobulin, intravenous (IGIV)
immunoglobulin M (IgM)
immunoglobulin-secreting cell
immunogold electron microscopy
immunohematology
immunohistochemical
immunohistochemistry (IHC)
　Ki-67 i.
immunoisolating microreactor
immunolocalization
immunologic
　i. adjuvant
　i. complication
　i. contact urticaria
　i. disorder
　i. drug reaction
　i. feature
　i. high dose tolerance
　i. inflammatory disease
　i. memory
　i. organ damage
　i. pregnancy test
　i. response
immunological
　i. competence
　i. contact urticaria (ICU)
　i. defense

　i. deficiency
　i. enhancement
　i. mechanism
　i. paralysis
　i. surveillance
　i. tolerance
immunologically
　i. activated cell
　i. competent cell
　i. privileged site
immunologist
　American Association of I.'s (AAI)
immunology
　allergy and i. (AI)
　cancer i.
　therapeutic i.
immunometric technique
immunomodulating drug regimen
immunomodulation
immunomodulator
immunomodulatory
immunopathology
immunoperoxidase
immunophenotype
immunophilin-binding drug
immunophilin isomerase activity
immunopotentiation
immunopotentiator
immunoprecipitation assay
immunoproliferative
　i. disorder
　i. small intestinal disease (IPSID)
immunoprophylaxis
　passive i.
immunoproteasome
immunopurging
　complement-mediated tumor cell i.
immunoradiometric assay (IRMA)
immunoreactant
　proinflammatory i.
immunoreaction
immunoreactive
　i. hormone
　i. insulin (IRI)
**immunoreceptor tyrosine-based activation
　motif (ITAM)**
immunoregulation
immunoregulatory
　i. circuit
　i. defect
immunoselection
immunosenescence
immunosorbent
immunostimulatory
　i. DNA sequence (ISS)
　i. oligodeoxynucleotide (ISS-ODN)
immunosuppressant cocktail

immunosuppression
    iatrogenic i.
    postgrafting i.
    TGF-induced i.
    transforming growth factor-
      induced i.
immunosuppression-associated
  leukoencephalopathy
immunosuppressive
    i. agent
    i. drug
    i. therapy (IST)
immunosurveillance
immunosympathectomy
immunotherapy
    active specific i. (ASI)
    adoptive i.
    biological i.
    cancer i.
    cellular adoptive i.
    passive i.
    rush i.
    short-term i. (STI)
    specific injection i. (SIT)
    sublingual-swallow i.
    venom i. (VIT)
immunotolerance
immunotoxin
immunotransfusion
Immupath
ImmuRAID antibody imaging
ImmuRAIT-LL2 monoclonal antibody
Immuthiol
Imogam
Imovax
    I. Rabies intradermal vaccine
    I. Rabies intramuscular vaccine
impaction sampler
impactor
    Cascade i.
    rotating air i.
    rotating arm i.
impaired
    i. glucose tolerance (IGT)
    i. neutrophil chemotaxis
impairment
    chronic phase shoulder i.
    i., decreased fertility, short stature
    functional i.
    photosensitivity, ichthyosis, brittle
      hair, intellectual i.

    restrictive functional i.
    subacute phase shoulder i.
impending respiratory failure
imperfecta
    dentinogenesis i.
    lethal osteogenesis i.
    osteogenesis i.
    severe deforming osteogenesis i.
    Sillence type II–IV osteogenesis i.
Imperfecti
    Fungi I.
impermeable
impermeant solution additive
impetigines (*pl. of* impetigo)
impetiginization
impetiginize
impetiginous
    i. cheilitis
    cheilitis granulomatosa i.
    i. syphilid
impetigo, pl. impetigines
    Bockhart i.
    bullous i.
    i. circinata
    i. contagiosa
    i. contagiosa bullosa
    i. eczematodes
    follicular i.
    Fox i.
    i. furfuracea
    furfuraceous i.
    i. gestationis
    i. herpetiformis
    i. neonatorum
    nonbullous i.
    i. simplex
    i. staphylogenes
    i. syphilitica
    i. variolosa
    i. vulgaris
impingement
    i. sign
    i. syndrome
implant
    Avanta i.
    bovine collagen dermal i.
    cartilage i.
    collagen i.
    ePTFE i.
    expanded polytetrafluoroethylene i.
    flexible silicone i.
    Medpor surgical i.

NOTES

implant *(continued)*
  Neer II i.
  osteochondral i.
  perichondrial i.
  periosteal i.
  SoftForm facial i.
  Spectrum Designs facial i.
  Zyderm collagen i.
  Zyplast collagen i.
implantation
  collagen i.
  i. cyst
importance
  allergic i.
impregnated pad
impregnation
  silver i.
improper repair of DNA
ImuLyme vaccine
Imuran
IMX
  whole-body antibody technique
in
  in noma ulcer
  in situ
  in situ hybridization (ISH)
  in situ squamous cell carcinoma
  in toto
  in vitro
  in vitro anergy
  in vitro cytotoxic assay
  in vitro fibrillogenesis
  in vitro proliferative lymphocyte
    response
  in vitro purging
  in vitro test
  in vivo
  in vivo reaction
inactivate
inactivated
  Japanese encephalitis virus
    vaccine, i.
  i. poliovirus vaccine (IPV)
  poliovirus vaccine, i.
  i. serum
inactivation
  nonrandom X chromosome i.
inactivator
  anaphylatoxin i.
inadvertent trauma
inaperturate
Inc.
  Laser Photonics, I. (LPI)
incarnati
incarnatus
  pilus i.
  unguis i.
incentive spirometry

incidence
  excess i. (IDD)
incision
  elliptical i.
  Mercedes Benz i.
  Risdon i.
incisional biopsy
incisor
  overriding maxillary i.
inclusion
  i. body
  i. body disease
  i. body encephalitis
  i. body myositis
  i. cell
  i. conjunctivitis virus
  i. cyst
  cytoplasmic i.
  i. dermoid
  hematoxyphilic i.
  Rocha-Lima i.
incognito
  scabies i.
  tinea i.
incognitus
  Mycoplasma i.
incompatibility
  ABO i.
incompatible blood transfusion reaction
incomplete
  i. agglutinin
  i. antibody
  i. antigen
  i. neurofibromatosis
inconspicua
  Candida i.
incontinence of pigment
incontinentia
  i. pigmenti
  i. pigmenti achromians
increased sympathoadrenal activity
incrementi
  stadium i.
incrustation
incubation period (IP)
incubative stage
incubatory carrier
Indanyl carbenicillin
Inderal LA
Indermil
  I. tissue adhesive
  I. topical adhesive
indeterminate
  i. cell histiocytosis
  i. leprosy
index, pl. **indices, indexes**
  algofunctional Lequesne i.

American Rheumatism
  Association i.
apoptotic i.
Atopic Dermatitis Area and
  Severity I. (ADASI)
Atopic Dermatitis Severity I.
  (ADSI)
Bath AS Functional I.
body mass i. (BMI)
British Isles Lupus Assessment
  Group i. (BILAG)
chemotherapeutic i.
Disease Extent I. (DEI)
Eczema Area and Severity I.
  (EASI)
endemic i.
Health Assessment Questionnaire
  Disability I. (HAQ DI)
International Prognostic I.
Lansbury articular i.
Lequesne algofunctional i.
Lequesne functional i.
leukopenic i.
i. of marrow conversion (IMC)
metacarpal i.
organ system failure i. (OSFI)
phagocytic i.
plaque i.
psoriasis area and severity i.
  (PASI)
Reliable Change I.
Ritchie articular i.
SASSAD severity i.
SCORAD i.
semiquantitative disease extent i.
Singh i.
SLE Disease Activity I. (SLEDAI)
splenic i.
tension-time i.
tumor burden i. (TBI)
ultraviolet light i.
volume thickness i. (VTI)
Western Ontario and McMaster
  Universities Osteoarthritis I.
  (WOMAC)
Indian tick typhus
India rubber skin
indicanidrosis
indicator system
indices (*pl. of* index)
indicis
indifferent electrode

indigenous
indinavir sulfate
indirect
  i. agglutination
  i. agglutination test
  i. assay
  i. coelenterate dermatitis
  i. Coombs test
  i. Coombs titer
  i. enzyme immunoassay for anti-
    Mycoplasma pneumoniae IgM
  i. fluorescent antibody
  i. fluorescent antibody test
  i. hemagglutination test
  i. immunofluorescence (IIF)
indium chloride scan
indium-labeled scanning
Indocid PDA
Indocin
  I. IV injection
  I. SR Oral
Indocollyre
indocyanine green (ICG)
indolent
  i. bubo
  i. nonpitting edema
  i. papule
  i. ulcer
indomethacin
Indotec
induced
  i. phagocytosis
  i. sensitivity
inducer
  i. cell
  extracellular matrix
    metalloproteinase i. (EMMPRIN)
inducible
  i. nitric oxide synthase
  i. skin color
induction
  antilymphocyte i.
  lysogenic i.
  ovulation i.
  i. period
indurata
  acne i.
  tuberculosis cutis i.
indurated
  i. border
  i. chancre
  i. lymphangitis

NOTES

indurated *(continued)*
    i. papule
    i. plantar keratoma (IPK)
    i. welt
induratio
    i. penis plastica
induration
    brawny i.
indurativa
    tuberculosis cutis i.
induratum
    erythema i.
industrial
    i. dermatitis
    i. dermatosis
    i. folliculitis
    i. hyperpigmentation
    i. smog
Inerpan dressing
inertial suction sampler
infancy
    acropustulosis of i.
    capillary hemangioma of i.
    fibrous hamartoma of i.
    transient erythroporphyria of i.
    transient hypogammaglobulinemia
      of i.
Infanrix vaccine
infant
    i. of diabetic mother (IDM)
    sudden unexpected death in i.'s
      (SUDI)
    sudden unexplained death in i.'s
      (SUDI)
infantile
    i. acne
    i. acropustulosis
    i. acute hemorrhagic edema of the
      skin
    i. colic
    i. digital fibroma
    i. digital myofibroblastoma
    i. eczema
    i. gastroenteritis
    i. gastroenteritis virus
    i. myofibromatosis
    i. neuroblastoma
    i. perianal pyramidal protrusion
    i. purulent conjunctivitis
infantilis
    lipodystrophia centrifugalis
      abdominalis i.
    prurigo i.
    roseola i.
infantum
    acrodermatitis papulosa i.
    cholera i.
    dermatitis excoriativa i.

    dermatitis exfoliativa i.
    dermatitis gangrenosa i.
    granuloma gluteale i.
    lichen i.
    roseola i.
infarction
    diabetic muscle i. (DMI)
    myocardial i. (MI)
infarctive
    i. inflammatory disease
    i. lesion
Infazinc
infect
infected vascular gangrene
infecting dose (ID)
infection
    alopecia, nail dystrophy, ophthalmic
      complication, thyroid dysfunction,
      hypohidrosis, ephelides and
      enteropathy, and respiratory
      tract i. (ANOTHER)
    atrium of i.
    atypical mycobacterial i.
    bacterial i.
    banal bacterial i.
    beta-hemolytic streptococcus i.
    bloodstream i. (BSI)
    Candida i.
    candidal i.
    catheter-related bloodstream i. (CR-
      BSI)
    chlamydial i.
    chronic Epstein-Barr virus i.
    closed-space i.
    congenital HIV i.
    congenital human immunodeficiency
      virus i.
    cross i.
    cryptogenic i.
    dermatophyte fungal i.
    disseminated gonococcal i.
    documented bacterial i. (DBI)
    documented viral i. (DVI)
    droplet i.
    EBV i.
    ectothrix i.
    endemic fungal i.
    endogenous i.
    endothrix i.
    enteroviral i.
    environmental mycobacterial i.
    Epstein-Barr virus i.
    focal i.
    fungal i. (FI)
    fungous i.
    granulomatous bacterial i.
    group A beta-hemolytic
      streptococcal i.

group A streptococcus i.
guinea worm i.
Hantavirus i.
herpes simplex i.
herpes zoster i.
herpetic i.
hibernal epidemic viral i. (HEVI)
hospital-acquired i.
human papillomavirus i.
i. immunity
laryngeal i.
latent i.
loa loa i.
lower respiratory tract i. (LRTI)
mass i.
metazoan i.
mixed nail i.
mycobacterial i.
natural focus of i.
necrotizing i.
nondermatophyte fungal i.
nontuberculous mycobacterial i.
nosocomial i.
opportunistic systemic fungal i.
overwhelming postsplenectomy i.
  (OPSI)
paravaccinia virus i.
phycomycotic i.
pneumococcal i.
primary herpes simplex i.
protozoan i.
pyodermatous i.
pyogenic i.
recurrent i.
repeated respiratory i.
reservoir of i.
rhinocerebral i.
rickettsial i.
scalp i.
seatworm i.
secondary i.
Shigella i.
spirochete i.
Streptococcus i.
subcutaneous fungal i.
subcutaneous necrotizing i.
superficial i.
sycosiform fungous i.
systemic fungal i.
transcervical i.
transforming i.
transplacental i.

unusual opportunistic i.
upper respiratory tract i. (URTI)
urinary tract i. (UTI)
vaccinia i.
varicella-zoster i.
vesicular viral i.
Vincent i.
viral respiratory i.
Western blot i.
yeast i.
zoonotic i.
infection-immunity
infectiosity
infectiosum
  ecthyma i.
  erythema i. (EI)
infectious
  i. angioma
  i. arteritis virus of horses
  i. arthritis
  i. avian bronchitis
  i. bovine rhinotracheitis (IBR)
  i. bovine rhinotracheitis virus
  i. bronchitis virus (IBV)
  i. bulbar paralysis
  i. canine hepatitis
  i. disease (ID)
  I. Disease Society of America
    (IDSA)
  i. ectromelia virus
  i. eczematoid dermatitis
  i. eczematous dermatitis
  i. endocarditis
  exuberant i.
  i. granuloma
  i. hepatitis (IH)
  i. hepatitis virus
  i. labial dermatitis
  i. mononucleosis (IM)
  i. nucleic acid
  i. papilloma of cattle
  i. papilloma virus
  i. perichondritis
  i. plasmid
  i. polyneuritis
  i. porcine encephalomyelitis
  i. porcine encephalomyelitis virus
  i. rhinitis
  i. wart
infectiousness
infectiva
  polioencephalitis i.

NOTES

infective
infectivity
inferior fornix
infest
infestans
    Phytophathoria i.
infestation
    Cheyletiella i.
    environmental mite i.
    louse i.
    mite i.
    Pediculus humanus capitis i.
    ping-pong i.
    Pthirus pubis i.
infiltrate
    Assmann tuberculous i.
    diffuse pulmonary i.
    fixed pulmonary i.
    fluffy alveolar i.
    granulomatous dermal i.
    lymphoid i.
    patchy i.
    perivascular i.
    transient migratory i.
    transient pulmonary i.
infiltration
    adipose i.
    inflammatory i.
    lymphocytic i.
    peribronchiolar lymphocyte i.
infiltrative basal cell carcinoma
infiltrator
    showerhead i.
Infinity sensor
Inflamase
    I. Forte Ophthalmic
    I. Mild Ophthalmic
inflame
inflamed
    i. linear verrucous epidermal nevus
    (ILVEN)
    i. ulcer
inflammation
    acute i. (AI)
    allergic i.
    chronic jejunal i.
    diffuse i.
    focal i.
    immune i.
    interstitial i.
    intraocular i.
    mucosal i.
    necrotizing scleritis with adjacent i.
    necrotizing scleritis without
      adjacent i.
    neutrophilic i.
    neutrophil-mediated joint i.

    i. reaction
    urate-associated i.
inflammatory
    i. arthritis
    i. bowel disease (IBD)
    i. bowel syndrome (IBS)
    i. cascade
    i. cell
    i. dermatosis
    i. edema
    i. factor of anaphylaxis (IF-A)
    i. fibrous hyperplasia
    i. infiltration
    i. linear verrucous epidermal nevus
    i. lung disease
    i. macrophage
    i. plaque
    i. tinea capitis
    i. ulcer
inflation
inflatum
    Scopulariopsis i.
infliximab monoclonal antibody
inflorescence
influenza, pl. **influenzae**
    i. A
    A/Texas/36/91-like i.
    avian i.
    A-Wuhan/359/95-like i.
    i. B
    B/Beijing/184/93-like i.
    i. C
    equine i.
    Hong Kong i.
    sequela of i.
    Spanish i.
    swine i.
    i. virus
    i. virus hemagglutinin
    i. virus vaccine
influenzae
    Haemophilus i. type b (HIB)
influenzal meningitis
Influenzavirus
infolded
infranate
infrapatellar bursitis
infriction
infundibulofolliculitis
    disseminated recurrent i.
    recurrent i.
infundibulum
    tumor of the follicular i. (TFI)
infusion
    allogenic bone marrow cell i.
    continuous subcutaneous insulin i.
    (CSII)
    donor leukocyte i. (DLI)

donor lymphocyte i. (DLI)
ETOPOPHOS i.
etoposide phosphate i.
ingestion
L-tryptophan i.
ingestive
Ingram
I. regimen for psoriasis
I. technique
ingress
neutrophil i.
ingrowing hair
ingrown
i. hair
i. nail
inguinale
acanthoma i.
Epidermophyton i.
granuloma i.
lymphogranuloma i.
inguinalis
tinea i.
inguinal ligament
INH
isoniazid
isonicotine hydrazine
Inhal-Aid bronchodilator
inhalant
i. allergen
i. allergen extract
inhalation
Atrovent Aerosol I.
i. breath unit
NebuPent I.
smoke i.
inhaled
i. corticosteroid (ICS)
i. dander
inhaler
AeroBid-M Oral Aerosol I.
AeroBid Oral Aerosol I.
Beclovent Oral I.
Beconase AQ Nasal I.
Chiesi powder i.
Diskhaler i.
Diskus i.
dry powder i. (DPI)
FOII powder i.
Inhalet i.
InspirEase i.
Intal Oral I.
metered-dose i. (MDI)

Nebuhaler i.
Orion i.
pressurized metered-dose i. (pMDI)
Rondo i.
Rotahaler i.
Spinhaler i.
Turbuhaler i.
Vancenase AQ I.
Vancenase Nasal I.
Vanceril Oral I.
Inhalet inhaler
inheritance
pattern of i.
X-linked recessive i.
inherited
i. complement deficiency syndrome
i. epidermolysis bullosa
i. patterned lentiginosis
inhibin
inhibiting antibody
inhibition
allogenic i.
eicosanoid i.
i. factor
i. fluorescent antibody
hemagglutination i.
leukotriene i.
prostaglandin synthesis i.
xanthine i.
inhibitor
5-alpha reductase i.
$alpha_1$-trypsin i.
angiogenesis i.
caspase i.
C1 esterase i.
collagenase i.
COX-1 i.
COX-2 i.
cysteine proteinase i.
decarboxylase i.
factor VIII:C i.
functional C1 esterase i.
fusion i. (FI)
5G1.1 recombinant C5
complement i.
HIV protease i.
HMG-CoA reductase i.
human alpha-1-proteinase i.
3-hydroxy-3-methyl glutaryl
coenzyme A reductase i.
MAO i.
monoamine oxidase inhibitor

NOTES

inhibitor *(continued)*
    mast cell i.
    monoamine oxidase i. (MAO inhibitor)
    myosin ATPase i.
    nonnucleoside reverse transcriptase i. (NNRTI)
    nucleoside analog RT i. (NRTI)
    nucleoside reverse transcriptase i. (NTRI)
    phosphodiesterase isoenzyme i.
    polypeptide i.
    protein C1 esterase i.
    recombinant human tissue factor pathway i. (r-hT-FPI)
    secretory leukoprotease i.
    surface-targeted plasmin i.
    synthesis i.
    target of rapamycin i. (TOR inhibitor)
    tissue factor pathway i. (TFPI)
    TNF i.
    TOR i.
        target of rapamycin inhibitor
    transcriptase i.
    tyrosinase i.
    tyrosine kinase i.

Initiative
    Children's Vaccine I. (CVI)

injectable
    i. collagen
    i. dye
    tinzaparin sodium i.

injection
    Adlone I.
    Adrucil i.
    Aloprim I.
    Amcort I.
    A-methaPred i.
    Amikin i.
    amphotericin B lipid complex i.
    AquaMEPHYTON i.
    Aristocort Forte I.
    Aristocort Intralesional I.
    Aristospan Intraarticular I.
    Aristospan Intralesional I.
    Articulose-50 i.
    Bactocill i.
    Bena-D i.
    Benadryl I.
    Benahist i.
    Ben-Allergin-50 I.
    Benoject i.
    Bicillin C-R 900/300 i.
    Bicillin L-A i.
    Brethine i.
    Bricanyl i.
    Bronkephrine i.

Calciferol i.
Carbocaine i.
Celestone Phosphate I.
Cel-U-Jec I.
Ceredase i.
Chlor-Trimeton I.
Cipro i.
Cleocin Phosphate I.
collagen i.
conjunctival i.
Cophene-B i.
Cortone Acetate i.
Crysticillin A.S. i.
Cytoxan i.
Decadron I.
Dehist i.
depMedalone I.
Depoject I.
Depo-Medrol I.
Depopred I.
D.H.E. 45 i.
Diflucan i.
Dihyrex I.
Dinate I.
Diphenacen-50 I.
Dizac i.
D-Med I.
Doxychel i.
Dramilin I.
Duralone I.
Duralutin i.
Duranest i.
Dymenate I.
Floxin i.
Foscavir i.
Garamycin i.
Histaject i.
hyaluronan i.
hyaluronate i.
hyaluronic acid i.
Hydeltrasol i.
Hydeltra-TBA i.
Hydrate I.
Hy-Gestrone i.
Hylutin i.
Hyprogest i.
Hyrexin-50 I.
Hyzine-50 I.
Imitrex i.
Indocin IV i.
intraarticular i.
intralesional i.
intratendinous i.
Isocaine HCl i.
Jenamicin i.
Kantrex i.
Keflin i.
Kefurox i.

Kenaject I.
Kenalog I.
Key-Pred I.
Key-Pred-SP I.
Konakion i.
Levophed i.
Lyphocin i.
Marmine I.
Medralone I.
Metro IV I.
Minocin IV i.
Monistat IV I.
M-Prednisol I.
Nafcil i.
Nallpen i.
Nasahist B i.
ND-Stat i.
Nebcin i.
Neosar i.
Netromycin i.
Neucalm-50 I.
Neupogen i.
Neut i.
Nordryl i.
Novocain i.
Nydrazid i.
Octocaine i.
Oraminic II i.
Ornidyl i.
Osmitrol i.
Pentacarinat i.
Pentam-300 I.
Permapen i.
Pfizerpen i.
Pfizerpen-AS i.
Phenazine I.
Phenergan I.
Polocaine i.
Pontocaine i.
Predaject i.
Predalone i.
Predcor i.
Predicort-50 i.
Prednisol TBA i.
Pro-Depo i.
Prodrox i.
Prometh i.
Prorex I.
Prostaphlin i.
Prothazine i.
Retrovir i.

Rifadin I.
Sandimmune i.
sensitizing i.
Solu-Medrol I.
Spectam i.
subcutaneous i.
Supartz i.
Tac-3, -40 I.
Terramycin IM i.
Toposar i.
Toradol i.
Triam-A I.
Triam Forte I.
Triamonide I.
Tri-Kort I.
Trilog I.
Trilone I.
Trisoject I.
Trobicin i.
Unipen i.
Ureaphil I.
Valium i.
Vancocin i.
Vancoled i.
VePesid i.
V-Gan i.
Vibramycin i.
Vistaril I.
Vistazine I.
Vumon i.
Wellcovorin i.
Wycillin i.
Zantac i.
Zetran i.
Zinacef i.
Zovirax i.

injury
    cold-induced cell i.
    graft i.
    hepatic ischemia and reperfusion i.
    HIR i.
    hypothermic i.
    I/R i.
        ischemia-reperfusion injury
    ischemia-reperfusion i. (I/R injury)
    oligodendrocyte i.
    photoacoustic i.
    preservation perfusion i.
    preservation reperfusion i.
    reperfusion i.
    sinusoidal lining cell i.

NOTES

injury *(continued)*
> transfusion-related acute lung i. (TRALI)
> whiplash i.

ink-spot lentigo
innate immunity
inner
> i. canthus
> i. root sheath

innocent bystander cell
inoculability
inoculable
inoculate
inoculating
inoculation herpes
inoculum
> plantar i.

inosinic
> i. acid
> i. acid dehydrogenase

Inosiplex
inositol
> i. phospholipid turnover
> i. triphosphate
> i. triphosphate pathway

Inoviridae
INR
> International Normalization Ratio
> INR clotting test

INRO surgical prosthetic nail
insect
> i. bite
> biting i.
> i. dermatitis
> i. sting
> i. sting kit
> i. virus

insecticide
insensible perspiration
insensitive sweat
inserta
> variola i.

insidious onset
insipidus
> nephrogenic diabetes i.

insolation
Insomnal
inspiratory
> i. capacity (IC)
> i. to expiratory ratio (I:E)
> i. positive airway pressure (IPAP)
> i. "Velcro" crackle

InspirEase inhaler
Inspiron
instability
> microsatellite i. (MSI)

Instat collagen matrix sponge

Institute
> International Life Science I. (ILSI)

institutional review board (IRB)
instructive theory
instrument
> diamond fraise dermabrasion i.
> IOS immunodiagnostic testing i.
> ProLine endoscopic i.

insufficiency
> adrenal i.
> adrenocortical i.

insula
insulin
> i. allergy
> i. antagonist
> immunoreactive i. (IRI)
> i. lipoatrophy
> lispro i.
> i. reaction
> i. resistance
> single-peak pork i.
> i. skin test
> i. tumor

insulin-dependent diabetes mellitus (IDDM)
insulin-like
> i.-l. growth factor-1 (IGF-1)
> i.-l. growth factor BP3 complex

insusceptibility
intake
> caloric i.

Intal
> I. Nebulizer solution
> I. Oral Inhaler

Integra artificial skin
integrin
> 1, 2, 3 i.

integrin-mediated adhesion
integrity
> Braden score for skin i.

integument
integumentary system
integumentum
> i. commune

Intelligent dressing
intemum
> erysipelas grave i.

intense
> i. pulsed light (IPL)
> i. pulsed light source (IPLS)

intensity
> gray-scale i.

interaction
> adhesin-receptor i.
> B7:counterreceptor i.
> cell i. (CI)
> cell-cell i.
> cognate i.

drug i.
HLA intercellular i.
receptor-ligand i.
T-cell counter-receptor i.
intercellular
    i. adhesion module (ICAM)
    i. adhesion molecule-1 (ICAM-1)
    i. bridge
    i. edema
    i. machinery
    i. space
intercensal
intercritical gout
interdigital
    i. dermatitis
    i. maceration
interdigitale
    epidermophytosis i.
interdigitalis
    mycosis i.
interface
    dermoepidermal i.
    Monarch Mini Mask nasal i.
interference
    bacterial i.
interfering
    defective i. (DI)
interferon (IFN)
    i. alfa-2a
    i. alfa-2b
    i. alfa-2b and ribavirin combination
    pack
    i. alfa-n3
    i. alpha (IFN-alpha)
    antigen i.
    i. B-1b
    i. beta (IFN-beta)
    fibroblast i.
    i. gamma
    i. gamma-1b
    i. gamma receptor deficiency
    immune i.
    leukocyte i.
    natural i. alfa
    pegylated i.
    recombinant gamma i.
    therapeutic i.
    i. therapy

interferon-independent mechanism
interleukin (IL)
    IL-1 i.
interleukin-1 (IL-1)
interleukin-1–15 (IL-1–15)
interleukin-2 (IL-2)
    i.-2 adjunctive chemotherapy
interleukin-10 (IL-10)
interleukin-11 (IL-11)
interleukin-12 (IL-12)
    exogenous i.-12
interleukin-1-alpha (IL-1-alpha)
interlobularly artery
interlobular septa
intermedia
    beta-thalassemia i.
intermediate
    i. carcinoma
    i. cyclosporine
    i. filament
    i. leprosy
    reactive oxygen i. (ROI)
intermedius
    Streptococcus i.
intermetacarpal
intermittent
    i. carrier
    i. hair-follicle dystrophy
    i. hydrarthrosis
    i. mandatory ventilation
    i. positive pressure breathing
    (IPPB)
    i. sterilization
internal
    i. hair apparatus
    i. meningitis
International
    I. Contact Dermatitis Research
    Group (ICDRG)
    I. Index of Erectile Function
    (IIEF)
    I. Labor Organization (ILO)
    I. Life Science Institute (ILSI)
    I. Normalization Ratio (INR)
    I. Pancreas Transplant Registry
    (IPTR)
    I. Prognostic Index
    I. Society of Heart and Lung
    Transplantation (ISHLT)

NOTES

International *(continued)*
    I. Society for Heart and Lung
       Transplant biopsy
    I. Society for Heart and Lung
       Transplant grade
international
    i. normalized ratio clotting test
      (INR clotting test)
internum
    erysipelas i.
interpalpebral fissure
interpapillary ridge
**Interpersonal Support Evaluation List
(ISEL)**
interphalangeal
    distal i. (DIP)
    i. joint
    proximal i. (PIP)
interplant
interplanting
interpolation flap
interpretation
    patch test i.
interquartile range (IQR)
interrogans
    Leptospira i.
interspecific graft
interstitial
    i. fibrosis
    i. infiltration by histiocyte
    i. inflammation
    i. lung disease (ILD)
    i. nephritis
    i. pressure
interstitium
    lung i.
intertinctus
    strophulus i.
intertriginous
    i. area
    i. psoriasis
    i. region
intertrigo
    bacterial i.
    Candida i.
    diaper rash i.
    eczema i.
    i. eczema
    erythema i.
    monilial i.
    i. with ulceration
intertrochanteric
    varus i.
interval
    anterior atlantodental i. (AADI)
    i. mapping technique
    posterior atlantodental i. (PADI)

intervention
    avocational i.
    psychosocial i.
    vocational i.
interzone
intestinal
    i. biopsy
    i. bypass arthritis
    i. epithelial cell (IEC)
    i. fluke
    i. lipodystrophy
    i. mucosal dysfunction
    i. nematode
    i. polyp
    i. transplantation
    i. ulceration
intestinalis
    Pneumatosis i.
intestinotoxin
intimal
    i. arteritis
    i. collagen
intimitis
    proliferative i.
intine
intolerance
    carbohydrate i.
    cow-milk protein i.
    disaccharide i.
    drug i.
    gluten i.
    idiopathic environmental i. (IEI)
    lactose i.
intoxication
    anaphylactic i.
    bromide i.
    metal i.
intraalveolar hemorrhage
intraarticular (IA)
    Aristospan I.
    i. glucocorticoid
    i. injection
    i. ossicles
    i. osteoid osteoma
    i. tophus
intrabursal
intracellular
    i. calcium chelator
    i. crystalloid solution
    i. digestion
    i. edema
    i. toxin
intraclass correlation coefficient (ICC)
intracranial pressure (ICP)
intractable
    i. plantar keratosis
    i. pyoderma
    i. wheezing

intracutaneous
- i. nevus
- i. reaction
- i. test

intracytoplasmic inclusion cell
intradermal
- i. anesthetic
- i. melanocyte
- i. nevus
- i. reaction
- i. skin test
- i. test concentration

IntraDop probe
intraepidermal
- i. abscess
- i. acanthoma
- i. blistering disease
- i. bulla
- i. carcinoma
- i. microabscess
- i. microabscess of psoriasis
- i. neutrophilic IgA dermatosis
- i. nevus
- i. vesiculation

intraepithelial mast cell
intragastral provocation under endoscopy (IPEC)
intragraft pressure
intrahepatic
- i. cholestasis of pregnancy
- i. islet graft

intralesional
- Aristospan I.
- i. corticosteroid therapy
- i. injection

intralysosomal
intramural thrombus
intramuscular
- immune globulin, i.

in-transit metastasis
intraocular inflammation
intraosseous hemorrhage
intraperitoneal glucose tolerance test (IPGTT)
intrapsychic stress
IntraSite
- I. gel
- I. hydrogel dressing

intrasplenic transplantation (isp-Tx)
intrasynovial complement level
intratendinous injection
intrathoracic blood volume (ITBV)

intrauterina
- ichthyosis i.

intravascular
- i. endothelial proliferation
- i. endothelial proliferative lesion
- i. papillary endothelial hyperplasia
- i. ultrasound (IVUS)

intravenous
- cytomegalovirus immune globulin i. (CMV-IGIV)
- i. fluid
- Fungizone i.
- i. gamma globulin (IVGG)
- i. glucose tolerance test (IVGTT)
- immune globulin, i.
- i. immune serum globulin (IVIG)
- i. immunoglobulin
- immunoglobulin, i. (IGIV)
- respiratory syncytial virus immune globulin i. (RSV-IGIV)
- Rh immune globulin i. (RhIGIV)

intraventricular hemorrhage
intravesical
- i. oxychlorosene sodium
- i. silver nitrate

intrinsic
- i. affinity
- i. allergy
- i. association constant
- i. asthma
- i. muscle atrophy

Intron A
intron-exon boundary
Intropin
intrusion
- alpha wave i.

intubation
intussusception
inunct
inunction
inundation fever
InV
- I. allotype
- I. group antigen

invaccination
invadens
- aegleria i.

invaginata
- trichorrhexis i.

invagination
invariant
- i. chain

NOTES

invariant *(continued)*
    i. chain CS
    I i.
invasion
    angiolymphatic i.
    pagetic petrous bony i.
    stage of i.
invasionis
    stadium i.
invasive
    i. aspergillosis
    i. candidiasis
    i. squamous cell carcinoma
invecta
    Solenopsis i.
Inventory
    Beck Depression I. (BDI)
    Children's Depression I. (CDI)
    Minnesota Multiphasic
      Personality I. (MMPI)
    Psoriasis Life Stress I. (PLSI)
inversa
    acne i.
    junctional epidermolysis bullosa
      atrophicans i.
inverse
    i. anaphylaxis
    epidermolysis bullosa, i.
    i. pityriasis rosea
    i. psoriasis
    i. ratio ventilation (IRV)
inversus
    situs i.
inverted follicular keratosis
inveterata
    psoriasis i.
Invirase
invisible glove
involuting flat hemangioma
involution form
involvement
    cardiovascular i.
    juvenile rheumatoid arthritis with
      spinal i.
    kidney i.
    lung i.
    20-nail i.
    nervous system i.
    palm-sole i.
    peripheral nerve i.
    predominant DIP joint i.
    predominant distal interphalangeal
      joint i.
    psoriatic arthritis with spinal i.
    renal i.
    skin i.
    T-cell i.
    twenty-nail i.

INVOS Cerebral Oximeter
io
    I. moth larva
    I. moth larva sting
Iobid DM
ioderma
Iodex Regular
iodica
    purpura i.
iodide
    i. acne
    potassium i.
    propidium i.
    saturated solution of potassium i.
      (SSKI)
iodine
    i. bush
    i. eruption
    radiolabeled i.
iodized collodion
iodochlorhydroxyquin
iododerma
Iodoflex absorptive dressing
Iodoform gauze
iodophor
iodoquinol and hydrocortisone
Iodosorb absorptive dressing
Iofed PD
Iohist DM
Ionil
Ionil-T plus
ionizing radiation
iontophoresis
iontophoretic unit
IOS immunodiagnostic testing
   instrument
IP
    incubation period
IPAP
    inspiratory positive airway pressure
IPEC
    intragastral provocation under endoscopy
IPF
    idiopathic pulmonary fibrosis
IPGTT
    intraperitoneal glucose tolerance test
I-Phrine Ophthalmic solution
IPITx
    isolated pancreatic islet transplantation
IPK
    indurated plantar keratoma
IPL
    intense pulsed light
IPLS
    intense pulsed light source
IPPB
    intermittent positive pressure breathing

IPR
 immediate phase reaction
ipratropium
 i. bromide
 i. bromide aerosol
IPSID
 immunoproliferative small intestinal
  disease
IPTR
 International Pancreas Transplant
  Registry
IPV
 inactivated poliovirus vaccine
IQR
 interquartile range
Ir
 immune response
  Ir gene
IR502 psoriasis vaccine
IRB
 institutional review board
Irgasan
IRI
 immunoreactive insulin
irides (*pl. of* iris)
iridescent virus
iridis
 herpes i.
iridocyclitis
Iridoviridae
Iridovirus
I/R injury
iris, pl. **irides**
 erythema i.
 I. forceps
 herpes i.
 heterochromia irides
 i. lesion
 lichen i.
 syphilis of i.
iritis
 hypopyon i.
 plastic i.
IRMA
 immunoradiometric assay
iron
 i. deficiency
 i. deficiency anemia
 i. oxide pigment
 i. storage disease
irradiance
irradiate

irradiation
 allograft i.
 Cytoxan and total body i.
  (CY/TBI)
 therapeutic i.
 thoracoabdominal i. (TAI)
 thymic i. (TI)
 total body i. (TBI)
 total lymphoid i. (TLI)
 whole body i. (WBI)
irregular border
irrigation
 tidal i.
irrigator
 Grossan nasal i.
irritable bowel syndrome (IBS)
irritans
 Pulex i.
 Trombicula i.
irritant
 i. contact dermatitis (ICD)
 i. contact urticaria
 i. hand dermatitis
 mild i.
 i. patch-test reaction
 i. patch-test response
 primary i.
irritate
irritation
 crab larvae i.
 i. fibroma
IRV
 inverse ratio ventilation
IS
 immune serum
Is
 immune suppressor
  Is gene
Isaacs syndrome
Isambert disease
ISAtx247 immunosuppressive drug
ischemia
 cold i.
 digital i.
 donor-related warm i.
 transient cerebral i.
ischemia-reperfusion injury (I/R injury)
ischemic ulcer
ischial bursitis
ischidrosis
ischiogluteal bursitis

NOTES

Iscove
> I. complete medium
> I. modified Dulbecco medium

ISEL
> Interpersonal Support Evaluation List

isethionate
> pentamidine i.
> piritrexim i.

ISH
> isocapnic hyperventilation
> in situ hybridization

ISHLT
> International Society of Heart and Lung
> Transplantation
> ISHLT biopsy
> ISHLT grade

island
> i. disease
> i. fever
> i. pedicle flap
> i. of sparing

islet
> i. allograft rejection
> i. alpha cell
> i. amyloid polypeptide (IAPP)
> i. cell antibody (ICA)
> i. cell transplant
> i. composite graft
> i. transplantation

isoagglutination
isoagglutinin
isoagglutinogen
isoallotypic determinant
isoantibody
isoantigen
> Rh i.

Isocaine HCl injection
isocapnic
> i. condition
> i. hyperventilation (ISH)

Isoclor
isocoproporphyrin
isocyanate
> i. disease
> i. HDI
> i. MDI
> i. TDI

isocytolysin
Isodine
Isoelast adhesive short stretch bandage
isoelectric focusing (IEF)
isoenzyme
> PLA2 i. (types IIA, IV, V)

isoerythrolysis
isoetharine
> Arm-a-Med i.
> Dey-Lute i.

isoeugenol
isoflurane
isoform
> catabolin i.
> i. PDGF-A, -B

isogeneic graft
isograft
isohemagglutination
isohemagglutinin
> saline i.

isohemolysin
isohemolysis
isoimmune
> i. neonatal neutropenia
> i. neonatal thrombocytopenia

isoimmunization
isokinetic collection
isolate
isolated
> i. dyskeratosis follicularis
> i. limb perfusion
> i. pancreatic islet transplantation
> (IPITx)

isoleucyl-tRNA synthetase
isoleukoagglutinin
isologous graft
isolysin
isolysis
isolytic
isomeric response
isometric exercise
isomorphic
> i. effect
> i. phenomenon
> i. response

isoniazid (INH)
> rifampin and i.

isoniazid-induced hepatitis
isonicotine hydrazine (INH)
isopathy
isophagy
isophil antibody
isophile antigen
Isoplast adhesive short stretch bandage
isoplastic graft
isoprecipitin
isoprenaline
Isoprinosine
isopropyl
> i. alcohol
> i. ester
> i. myristate

isoproterenol
> Arm-a-Med I.
> Dey-Dose I.

Dispos-a-Med I.
nebulized i.
i. and phenylephrine
Isopto
I. Atropine Ophthalmic
I. Cetapred Ophthalmic
I. Frin Ophthalmic solution
I. Homatropine Ophthalmic
I. Hyoscine Ophthalmic
I. Plain solution
I. Tears solution
isopyknic
isosensitize
isoserum treatment
Isospora belli
isosporiasis
isothiocyanate
allyl i.
fluorescein i. (FITC)
rhodamine i.
isotransplantation
isotretinoin
Isotrex
isotype
isotypic
isoxsuprine hydrochloride
isozyme
glutathione-dependent, cytosolic i.
PLA$_2$ i.
Ispaghula
isp-Tx
intrasplenic transplantation
isradipine
israelii
Actinomyces i.
ISS
immunostimulatory DNA sequence
ISS-ODN
immunostimulatory oligodeoxynucleotide
IST
immunosuppressive therapy
isthmic spondylolisthesis
isthmus
I-Sulfacet Ophthalmic
Isuprel
Italian
I. cypress
I. cypress tree
ITAM
immunoreceptor tyrosine-based activation motif

ITBV
intrathoracic blood volume
itch
Absorbine Jock I.
baker's i.
barber's i.
barn i.
bath i.
Boeck i.
clamdigger's i.
coolie i.
copper i.
copra i.
Cortef Feminine I.
Cuban i.
dew i.
dhobie i.
Dogger Bank i.
frost i.
grain i.
grocer's i.
ground i.
jock strap i.
kabure i.
ked i.
lumberman's i.
mad i.
Malabar i.
i. mite
Moeller i.
Norway i.
poultryman's i.
prairie i.
rice i.
Saint Ignatius i.
seven-year i.
straw i.
summer i.
swamp i.
swimmer's i.
toe i.
vulvar i.
warehouseman's i.
washerwoman's i.
water i.
winter i.
itching
nasal i.
i. purpura
itch-scratch-lichenification cycle
itchy
i. red bump disease

NOTES

itchy *(continued)*
> i. soft palate
> i. throat

Ito
> hypomelanosis of I.
> nevus of I.
> I. nevus

Ito-Reenstierna test
ITP
> idiopathic thrombocytopenic purpura
> chronic ITP

itraconazole
I-Tropine Ophthalmic
I.V.
> Gammar-P I.V.
> Merrem I.V.

ivermectin
Iverson dermabrader
IVGG
> intravenous gamma globulin

IVGTT
> intravenous glucose tolerance test

IVIG
> intravenous immune serum globulin

IVUS
> intravascular ultrasound

ivy
> poison i.

IvyBlock Lotion
IX
> protoporphyrin IX (PPIX)

Ixodes
> *I. cookei*
> *I. dammini*
> *I. dammini* tick
> *I. hexagonus*
> *I. pacificus*
> *I. pacificus* tick
> *I. persulcatus*
> *I. ricinus*
> *I. ricinus* wood tick
> *I. scapularis*
> *I. spinipalpis*

ixodiasis
ixodic
Ixodidae

J
- J chain
- J chain gene
- J serovar-specific epitope

J5 lipopolysaccharide

Jaa
- J. Amp
- J. Pyral

jaagsiekte

Jaa-Prednisone

Jaccoud arthropathy

jacket
- yellow j.

Jackson-Lawler syndrome

Jackson-Sertoli syndrome

Jackson-Weiss syndrome

Jacobi poikiloderma

Jacobsen syndrome

Jacobson forceps

Jacob ulcer

Jacquet
- J. erosive diaper dermatitis
- J. erythema

Jadassohn
- anetoderma of J.
- J. anetoderma
- J. disease
- J. epithelioma
- nevus sebaceus of J. (NSJ)
- sebaceous nevus of J.
- J. sebaceous nevus
- J. testerma

Jadassohn-Bloch test

Jadassohn-Lewandowsky
- J.-L. law
- J.-L. syndrome

Jadassohn-Pellizzari anetoderma

Jadassohn-Tièche nevus

Jadelot
- J. furrow
- J. line

Jaeger plate

Jaffe-Campanacci syndrome

jail fever

JAK2
- Janus kinase 2

Jak
- Janus family tyrosine kinase
- Jak kinase

Jak3 deficiency

Jakob-Creutzfeldt disease

JAM
- joint alignment and motion

James C. White tar ointment

Jamestown Canyon virus (JCV)

Janeway lesion

Janus
- J. family tyrosine kinase (Jak)
- J. kinase 2 (JAK2)
- J. reaction

Japanese
- J. B encephalitis
- J. B encephalitis virus
- J. cedar
- J. cedar tree
- J. encephalitis virus vaccine (JE-VAX)
- J. encephalitis virus vaccine, inactivated
- J. hot foot dermatitis
- J. lacquer tree
- J. river fever
- J. sargassum
- J. sargassum allergy

japonica
- *Cryptomeria j.*
- encephalitis j.

japonicum
- *Schistosoma j.*

Jarisch-Herxheimer reaction

Jarisch ointment

JAS
- juvenile ankylosing spondylitis

jasmine

jaundice
- catarrhal j.
- homologous serum j.

jaw
- j. claudication
- j. cyst
- lumpy j.
- phossy j.
- pincer j.

JCV
- Jamestown Canyon virus

JC virus

JDMS
- juvenile dermatomyositis

JDMS/PM
- juvenile dermatomyositis/polymyositis

jeanselmei
- *Exophiala j.*
- *Exserohilum j.*

Jeanselme nodule

JEB
- junctional epidermolysis bullosa

jejuni
- *Campylobacter j.*

jelly
- Vaseline petroleum j.

J

jellyfish
box j.
Portuguese j.
j. sting
Jenamicin injection
Jerne
J. plaque assay
J. technique
Jessner
lymphocytic infiltrate of J.
J. Peel
J. syndrome
Jessner-Kanof
benign lymphocytic infiltrate of J.-K.
J.-K. disease
jet-bubble mechanism
jet nebulizer
JE-VAX
Japanese encephalitis virus vaccine
jeweler's forceps
JH
JH gene
JH virus
JIA
juvenile idiopathic arthritis
jigger
JKA cell
Jk antigen
Jo-1
Jo-1 antibody
Jobbins antigen
Job syndrome
jock strap itch
jodbasedow
j. disease
j. phenomenon
Joest body
jogger
j. nipples
j. toe
John
J. Bunn Mini-Mist nebulizer
J. Dory fish prick testing
johnin
Johnson
J. grass
J. smut
joint
acromioclavicular j.
active j.
j. alignment and motion (JAM)
apophyseal j.
atlantoaxial j.
carpometacarpal j.
Charcot j.
Clutton j.
coding j.

j. congruence
costovertebral-girdle j.
cricoarytenoid j.
distal radicular j. (DRUJ)
j. effusion
facetal j.
glenohumeral j.
j. histology
interphalangeal j.
Luschka j.
manubriosternal j.
metatarsophalangeal j.
occipitoaxial j.
patellofemoral j.
peripheral j.
prosthetic j.
j. protection technique
j. protection training
pseudoneuropathic j.
radiocarpal j.
j. space narrowing
sternoclavicular j.
sternocostal j.
subtalar j.
j. swelling
temporomandibular j.
trochleo-ginglymoid j.
jojoba oil
Jones criteria
Jones-Mote
J.-M. radiation
J.-M. reaction
Jonston
J. alopecia
J. area
Jopling classification
Jordan anomaly
jordanis
Legionella j.
josamycin
Joseph skin hook
Jouvence
JPD
juvenile plantar dermatitis
Jr
Aerolate Jr
Congess Jr
EpiPen Jr
JRA
juvenile rheumatoid arthritis
Js antigen
juccuya
judacia
Parietaria j.
judgment
clinical j.
jugulation

jun
    j. gene
    J. protooncogene
junction
    dermal-epidermal j. (DEJ)
    dermoepidermal j.
    j. nevus
    pannus-cartilage j.
junctional
    j. epidermolysis bullosa (JEB)
    j. epidermolysis bullosa atrophicans
      generalisata gravis
    j. epidermolysis bullosa atrophicans
      generalisata mitis
    j. epidermolysis bullosa atrophicans
      inversa
    j. epidermolysis bullosa atrophicans
      localisata
    j. epidermolysis bullosa progressiva
    j. epidermolysis bullosa with
      pyloric atresia
    j. nevus
    j. variant
June
    J. grass
    J. grass pollen
jungle
    j. rot
    j. yellow fever
Jüngling disease
Junin virus
Junior Strength Motrin
juniper
    j. mix
    j. mix tree
    j. tar
    Western j.
Juri flap
Jurkat
    J. cell
    J. cell migration
    J. T-cell line

Just Tears solution
jute
juvenile
    j. ankylosing spondylitis (JAS)
    j. aponeurotic fibroma
    j. biotin deficiency
    j. chronic arthritis
    j. chronic polyarthritis
    j. colloid milium
    j. dermatomyositis (JDMS)
    j. dermatomyositis/polymyositis
      (JDMS/PM)
    j. elastoma
    j. gout
    j. hyaline fibromatosis
    j. idiopathic arthritis (JIA)
    j. melanoma
    j. palmoplantar fibromatosis
    j. papillomatosis
    j. pityriasis rubra pilaris
    j. plantar dermatitis (JPD)
    j. plantar dermatosis
    j. rheumatoid arthritis (JRA)
    j. rheumatoid arthritis rash
    j. rheumatoid arthritis with spinal
      involvement
    j. spring eruption
    j. xanthogranuloma (JXG)
    j. xanthogranuloma histiocytosis
    j. xanthoma
juvenilis
    verruca plana j.
juxtaarticular
    j. node
    j. nodule
    j. osteopenia
    j. osteoporosis
juxtacrine stimulation
JXG
    juvenile xanthogranuloma

NOTES

Junel oral Contraceptive

K

K antigen
K cell
Euxyl K 400
K virus

k82 ImmunoCap test

KA

keratoacanthoma

Kabuki syndrome
kabure itch
Kaffir pox
kala azar
Kalcinate
kale
Kaletra

K. capsule
K. oral solution

Kalginate

K. alginate dressing
K. alginate wound cover

Kalischer disease
kallak
kallikrein

k. activity
basophil k.
plasma k.

Kaltostat alginate dressing
kanamycin

k. sulfate
k. and vancomycin (KV)

Kandahar sore
kangri cancer
Kank-A
kansasii

Mycobacterium k.

Kantrex

K. injection
K. Oral

Kanzaki disease
kaolin clotting time
Kaopectate
Kaplan

K. PenduLaser 115
K. PenduLaser 115 laser system

Kaplan-Meier method
kapok
Kaposi

K. disease
K. sarcoma (KS)
K. varicelliform eruption
K. xeroderma

kaposiform hemangioendothelioma
(KHE)
kappa-binding nuclear factor
kappa-deleting element

kappa light chain
Karapandzic flap
karaya

k. gum
k. gum dermatitis

Karnofsky score
Kartagener syndrome
Kasabach-Merritt

K.-M. phenomenon
K.-M. syndrome

Kashin-Beck disease
Kassowitz-Diday law
Katayama fever
Kathon
Kathon-CG
Kauffmann-White scheme
Kawasaki

K. disease (KD)
K. syndrome

Kaye scissors
Kayser-Fleischer ring
KD

Kawasaki disease

kD, kd, kdal

kilodalton

72-kD gelatinase
92-kD gelatinase
48-kd La autoantigen
38-kd P_0 protein
220-kD protein
52-kd Ro autoantigen
60-kd Ro autoantigen
kedani fever
ked itch
Keep Clear Anti-Dandruff Shampoo
Keflex
Keflin injection
Keftab
Kefurox injection
kefyr

Candida k.

Kefzol
Kelev strain rabies virus
Kell blood antibody type
Kell-Cellano blood group
Keller ultraviolet test
Kelley-Seegmiller syndrome
Kellgren

K. disease
K. score

Kellgren-Lawrence stage
kellicotti

Paragonimus k.

Kelly encephalomyelitis

K

keloid
    acne k.
    k. acne
    Addison k.
    Alibert k.
    k. formation
keloidal
    k. basal cell carcinoma
    k. blastomycosis
    k. folliculitis
    k. scarring
    k. type scar
keloidalis
    acne k. (AK)
    folliculitis k.
keloidosis
Kenacort
    K. Oral
    K. Syrup
    K. Tablet
Kenaject-40
Kenaject Injection
Kenalog
    K. H
    K. Injection
    K. in Orabase
    K. Topical
Kenalog-10, -40
Kendall correlation coefficient
Kenicef
Kenonel Topical
Kentucky bluegrass
Kenya tick typhus
Keragen
Keralyt Gel
Kerastick
    Levulan K.
keratiasis
keratic
keratin
    hard k.
    nail k.
    soft k.
keratinase
keratinization
    ectopic k.
keratinize
keratinized cell
keratinocyte
    apoptotic k.
    dyskeratotic k.
    k. growth factor-2 (KGF-2)
    subconfluent k.
keratinocytic adhesion
keratinous
    k. cyst
    k. material
    k. sheet

keratitides
    filamentary k.
keratitis
    k. deafness
    epithelial k.
    filamentary k.
    herpetic stromal k. (HSK)
    k. rosacea
keratitis-deafness cornification disorder
keratitis-ichthyosis-deafness (KID)
    k.-i.-d. syndrome
keratoacanthoma (KA)
    k. centrifugum marginatum
    eruptive k.
    Ferguson-Smith k.
    multiple k.
    solitary k.
keratoangioma
keratoatrophoderma
keratoconjunctivitis
    atopic k.
    epidemic k.
    herpetic k.
    k. sicca
    vernal k.
    virus k.
keratoconus
keratocyte
keratoderma
    k. blennorrhagica
    k. blennorrhagicum
    carnauba-wax-like k.
    k. climacterica
    k. climactericum
    k. eccentrica
    epidermolytic palmoplantar k.
    Howell-Evans k.
    lymphedematous k.
    mutilating k.
    k. palmaris et
    k. palmaris et plantaris
    palmoplantar k. (PPK)
    k. plantare sulcatum
    punctate k.
    punctate porokeratotic k.
    k. punctatum
    Richner-Hanhart k.
    senile k.
    symmetric k.
    k. symmetrica
    Unna-Thost k.
    Vorner variant of Unna-Thost k.
keratodermatitis
keratodermia
keratodermic sandal
keratodes
    erythema k.
keratoelastoidosis marginalis

keratogenesis
keratogenetic
keratogenous zone
keratohyaline granule
keratoid exanthema
keratolysis
    k. exfoliativa
    k. exfoliativa areata manuum
    k. neonatorum
    pitted k.
    k. plantare sulcatum
keratolytic
    k. agent
    k. paint
keratoma
    k. diffusum
    k. disseminatum
    k. hereditaria mutilans
    k. hereditarium mutilans
    indurated plantar k. (IPK)
    k. malignum
    k. malignum congenitale
    k. palmare et plantare
    k. plantare sulcatum
    senile k.
    k. senile
keratomalacia
keratomycosis lingua
keratonosis
keratopachyderma
keratopathy
    band k.
    epithelial k.
keratoplastic
keratosa
    acne k.
keratose
keratosic cone
keratosis, pl. **keratoses**
    actinic k.
    arsenical k.
    aural k.
    benign lichenoid k.
    k. blennorrhagica
    k. climactericum
    k. diffusa fetalis
    follicular k.
    k. follicularis
    k. follicularis contagiosa
    k. follicularis spinulosa decalvans
    gonorrheal k.
    intractable plantar k.

inverted follicular k.
k. labialis
lichenoid k.
k. lichenoides chronica
lichen planus-like k.
nevoid k.
nevus follicularis k.
k. nigricans
k. obliterans
oral k.
k. palmaris et plantaris
k. palmaris et plantaris of the
    Meleda type
k. palmaris et plantaris of Unna-
    Thost
k. palmoplantaris punctata
pedunculated seborrheic k.
k. pilaris
k. pilaris atrophicans
k. pilaris atrophicans faciei
k. pilaris rubra
k. rubra figurata
seborrheic k.
senile k.
k. senilis
smoker k.
solar k.
stucco k.
k. suprafollicularis
suramin k.
tar k.
k. universalis congenita
k. vegetans
keratotic
    k. angioma
    k. material
    k. papule
    k. plug
    k. scabies
keratouveitis
Keri moisturizer
kerion
    k. celsi
    Celsus k.
    tinea k.
kerionic
Kern determinant
kernicterus
keroid
kerosene
kerotherapy
ketanserin

K

NOTES

ketoconazole
ketone
    methyl ethyl k. (MEK)
ketoprofen
11-keto-reductase
ketorolac tromethamine
ketotifen
Ketotop
Ketron-Goodman disease
Kettle syndrome
Keutel syndrome
Kevadon
Keyes punch
keyhole limpet hemocyanin
Key-Pred Injection
Key-Pred-SP Injection
KF-1 antigen
KGF-2
    keratinocyte growth factor-2
KHE
    kaposiform hemangioendothelioma
khellin
    topical k.
Ki-67
    K. immunohistochemistry
    K. marker detection
KI antigen
KID
    keratitis-ichthyosis-deafness
    KID syndrome
Kidd
    K. blood antibody type
    K. blood group
Kidde apparatus
kidney
    k. allograft
    k. bean
    k. involvement
    Madin-Darby bovine k. (MDBK)
    k. transplantation (KTx)
Kienböck-Adamson point
Kienböck disease
Kiesselbach plexus
Kikuchi disease
Kilham rat virus
killed-virus vaccine
killer
    k. cell (K cell)
    k. cell inhibitory receptor (KIR)
    k. inhibitor receptors-human
      leukocyte antigen (KIR-HLA)
    k. inhibitor receptors-human
      leukocyte antigen complex
    lymphokine-activated k. (LAK)
killing test
kilodalton (kD, kd, kdal)
45-kilodalton protein
Kimura disease

kinase
    Bruton tyrosine k. (BTK, Btk)
    c-jun N-terminal k.
    conserved helix-loop-helix
      ubiquitous k. (CHUK)
    creatinine k.
    extracellular signal-regulated k.
    herpes simplex virus thymidine k.
      (HSVTK)
    Jak k.
    Janus k. 2 (JAK2)
    Janus family tyrosine k. (Jak)
    mitogen-activated protein k.
      (MAPK)
    phosphoinositide 3 k.
    protein k. A (PKA)
    serine-threonine k.
    sphigosine k.
    Tec family of cytoplasmic protein
      tyrosine k.
    tyrosine k.
Kindler syndrome
kindling
    limbic k.
Kinerase N6-furfuryladenine skin cream
Kineret
kinesiology
    applied k.
kinetics
    single-hit k.
Kinetin
kinetochore
kininase
kinin system
kinky-hair
    k.-h. disease
    k.-h. syndrome
kinky hair
Kinyoun stain
KIR
    killer cell inhibitory receptor
Kirby-Bauer agar
KIR-HLA
    killer inhibitor receptors-human leukocyte
    antigen
    KIR-HLA complex
Kirsten-MSV Ras oncogene
Kisenyi sheep disease virus
kissing
    k. bug
    k. bug bite
kit
    AlaBLOT k.
    Alatest Latex-specific IgE allergen
    test k.
    Arrow pneumothorax k.
    Carmol scalp treatment k.

Circulon System Step 1, 2 venous
  ulcer k.
Cleanmix DNA purification k.
Hermal k.
insect sting k.
Marblot test k.
Persona ovulation predicting k.
Pro-Vent arterial blood sampling k.
Quantikine ELISA k.
RNeasy mini k.
Screening Patch Test K.
Kitamura
  acropigmentatio reticular of K.
  K. reticulate acropigmentation
Klaron lotion
Klauder syndrome
Klebsiella
  K. oxytoca
  K. pneumoniae
  K. rhinoscleromatis
Klein
  K. cannula
  K. pump
Klein-Waardenburg syndrome
Klenow fragment
Klerist-D Tablet
Kligman ointment
Klinefelter syndrome
Klippel-Feil syndrome
Klippel-Trenaunay-Parkes-Weber
  syndrome
Klippel-Trenaunay syndrome
Klippel-Trenaunay-Weber syndrome
Klonopin
Klorominr Oral
Klout
Km
  K. allotype
  K. allotypic determinant
  K. antigen
knee
  housemaid k.
  knock k.
knemometry
Kniest dysplasia
knife
  chalazion k.
Knight-Taylor brace
knob
  adenovirus fiber k.
knobby skin
knock knee

knot
  surfer's k.
knotted hair
knottin scaffold
knuckle
  k. pad
Kobberling-Duncan disease
Kobberling-Dunnigan syndrome
Köbner
  K. disease
  K. effect
  K. epidermolysis bullosa
  K. phenomenon (KP)
  K. phenomenon by history (KP-h)
Koch
  K. bacillus
  K. law
  K. old tuberculin
  K. phenomenon
  K. postulate
kochia
Koebner
  K. effect
  K. phenomenon
  K. reaction
koebnerization
Koenen tumor
Koeppe nodule
Kogoj
  K. pustule
  spongiform pustule of K.
KOH
  potassium chloride stain
  potassium hydroxide
    KOH examination
    KOH preparation
    KOH scraping
Köhler
  K. disease
  K. line
Kohn pore
koilonychia
  occupational k.
kojic acid
Kolmer test
Kolmogorov-Smirnov test
Komed lotion
Konakion injection
Kondon's Nasal
Koongol virus
Koplik spot

K

NOTES

Korean
    K. hemorrhagic fever
    K. hemorrhagic fever virus
    K. yellow moth dermatitis
Kostmann syndrome
Kotonkan virus
KP
    Köbner phenomenon
KP-e
    experimentally induced Köbner
      phenomenon
KP-h
    Köbner phenomenon by history
Krabbe disease
kra-kra (*var. of* craw-craw)
Kramer-Collins Spore trap
kraurosis
    k. penis
    k. vulva
Krause gland
kringle 4 domain of plasminogen
Krisovski sign
Kromayer lamp
Kronofed
krusei
    Candida k.
Kruskal-Wallis test
krypton lasing medium
Krysolgan
KS
    Kaposi sarcoma
KT
    Orudis KT

KTP
    potassium titanyl phosphate
      KTP laser
KTx
    kidney transplantation
Kulchitsky cell
Kupffer cell
kurtosis
Kurunegala ulcer
Kuru syndrome
KV
    kanamycin and vancomycin
Kveim
    K. antigen
    K. test
Kveim-Stilzbach antigen
kwashiorkor
    marasmic k.
Kwell
    K. Cream
    K. Lotion
    K. Shampoo
Kwellada
Kyasanur
    K. Forest disease
    K. Forest disease virus
kyphoscoliosis type Ehlers-Danlos syndrome
kyphoscoliotic type
kyphosis
    cervicothoracic k.
Kyrle disease

L
- L dose
- L unit of streptomycin

LA
- long acting
- lupus anticoagulant
  - Comhist LA
  - Dalalone L.A.
  - Dexasone L.A.
  - Dexone LA
  - Entex LA
  - Guaifenex LA
  - Humibid LA
  - Inderal LA
  - Nolex LA
  - Partuss LA
  - Phenylfenesin L.A.
  - Solurex L.A.
  - Theoclear L.A.
  - Touro LA
  - Westrim LA
  - Zephrex LA

La
- La antigen
- La Crosse virus

LABD
- linear IgA bullous dermatosis

labeling
- affinity l.
- T-cell antibody l.

Labello Active

labia (*pl. of* labium)

labial
- l. herpes simplex virus
- l. melanotic macule

labialis
- herpes l.
- keratosis l.
- myxadenitis l.

labium, pl. **labia**

laboratory
- colony-stimulating factor developed by Venereal Disease Research L. (CSF-VDRL)
- Hollister-Stier L.
- Medical Research Council L.'s (MRCL)
- Venereal Disease Research L.'s (VDRL)

labrum
- glenoid l.

LAC
- lupus anticoagulant antibody

lacerate

laceration

Lachman test
Lac-Hydrin
lackluster skin
lacquer
- Penlac nail l.

Lacril Ophthalmic solution
lacrimal
Lacrisert
lactalbumin
- alpha l.

lactase
lactate
- aluminum l.
- ammonium l.
- l. dehydrogenase
- l. dehydrogenase virus

lactea
- crusta l.

lactenin
lactic
- l. acid
- l. acidosis
- l. acid and sodium-PCA
- l. acid with ammonium hydroxide
- l. dehydrogenase (LDH)
- l. dehydrogenase agent

LactiCare
- L.-HC
- L.-HC Topical

Lactinol
lactobacillary milk
Lactobacillus
- *L. acidophilus*
- *L. casei*

lactobin
lactoferrin
lactoglobulin
- beta l.

lactose
- l. intolerance
- l. malabsorption

lactovegetarian diet
lacuna
lacunae
- fibrocartilage-cell l.
- osteocyte l.

lacunata
- *Moraxella l.*

LAD
- leukocyte adhesion deficiency

LAD1
- leukocyte adhesion deficiency type 1

LAD2
- leukocyte adhesion deficiency type 2

LAD3
> leukocyte adhesion deficiency type 3

LAD4
> leukocyte adhesion deficiency type 4

LADA
> latent autoimmune diabetes of adults

ladder
>> nucleosome l.

Laelaps echidninus

Laemmli sample buffer

laeta
>> *Loxosceles l.*

LAF-3
> leukocyte antigen factor-3

Lafora disease

lag phase

LaGrange scissors

Lahey scissors

Lahore sore

laidlawii
>> *Acholeplasma l.*

LAK
> lymphokine-activated killer
>> LAK cell

lake
>> venous l.

Lalonde hook forceps

la main en lorgnette

LAMB
> lentigines, atrial myxoma, mucocutaneous
> myxomas, and blue nevi
>> LAMB syndrome

lambda
>> l. bacteriophage
>> l. light chain

Lambert-Eaton
>> L.-E. myasthenic syndrome (LEMS)
>> L.-E. syndrome

lamblia
>> *Giardia l.*

lamb's
>> l. quarter
>> l. quarters weed pollen

lame foliacée

lamella
>> cornoid l.

lamellar
>> l. body (LB)
>> l. congenital ichthyosiform
>> erythroderma
>> l. desquamation
>> l. dominant
>> l. dyshidrosis
>> l. dystrophy
>> l. exfoliation of the newborn
>> l. granule
>> l. ichthyosis

>> l. plate
>> l. scale

lamelliform

lamellipodia formation

lamina
>> basal l.
>> cell l.
>> l. densa
>> l. fusca
>> l. lucida
>> l. propria
>> l. propria immune cell
>> l. splendens

laminated epithelial plug

laminin

Lamisil
>> L. Oral
>> L. tablet
>> L. topical
>> L. topical cream

Lamis PressureFuse automatic pressure control

lamivudine
>> zidovudine and l.

lamotrigine

lamp
>> black light fluorescent l.
>> black ray l.
>> carbon arc l.
>> cold quartz l.
>> fluorescent sun l.
>> heat l.
>> hot quartz vapor l.
>> Kromayer l.
>> narrowband UVB l.
>> quartz l.
>> quartz-iodine l.
>> ultraviolet A, B l.
>> UVA l.
>> UVB l.
>> uviol l.
>> Wood l.
>> xenon arc l.

Lamprene

Lamprey cannula

Lanacort

Lan antigen

Lanaphilic Topical

Lancefield classification

lance-ovate macule

Lancereaux-Mathieu disease

lancet
>> Pharmacia l.
>> Phazet l.

Lander Dandruff Control

Landouzy
>> L. disease
>> L. purpura

Landry-Guillain-Barré syndrome
Landry syndrome
Landschutz tumor
Lane disease
Langenbeck retractor
Langer-Giedion syndrome
Langerhans
    L. cell
    L. cell granule
    L. cell histiocytosis (LCH)
Langer line
Langhans cell
langue au chat
Laniazid Oral
lanolin
    anhydrous l.
    l., cetyl alcohol, glycerin, and
      petrolatum
Lanophyllin-GG
lanosum
    Microsporum l.
Lansbury articular index
lansingensis
    Legionella l.
Lantiseptic skin care product
lanuginosa
    acquired hypertrichosis l.
    hypertrichosis l.
lanuginous
lanugo hair
Lanvisone topical
laparoscopic donor nephrectomy (LDN)
lapinization
lapinized
larbish
large
    l. artery disease
    l. cell lymphoma
    l. external transformation-sensitive
      fibronectin (LETS)
    l. granular lymphocyte (LGL)
    l. vessel vasculitis
large-joint inflammatory arthritis
large-molecular-weight drug
large-plaque
    parapsoriasis l.-p.
    l.-p. parapsoriasis
Lariam
Larrey-Weil disease

Larsen
    L. grading system
    L. syndrome
larva, pl. **larvae**
    brown-tail moth l.
    l. currens
    gypsy moth l.
    Io moth l.
    l. migrans
    l. migrans profundus
larvalis
    porrigo l.
laryngeal
    l. edema
    l. infection
    l. papillomatosis
laryngotracheitis
    avian infectious l.
laryngotracheobronchitis
    acute l.
Lasan
    L. cream
    L. Unguent
Laschal scissors
L-ascorbic acid
LaseAway
    Polytec PI L.
Lasègue sign
laser
    alexandrite l.
    ALEXlazr l.
    argon l.
    argon-pumped tunable-dye l.
    Athos l.
    Aura L.
    Candela l.
    carbon dioxide l.
    CO_2 l.
    Coherent UltraPulse CO_2 l.
    continuous-wave l.
    copper bromide l.
    copper vapor l.
    CW dye l.
    Derma K l.
    diode l.
    l. Doppler flowmetry (LDF)
    l. Doppler perfusion imaging
    l. Doppler velocimetry
    dye l.
    EpiTouch l.
    erbium l.
    FeatherTouch CO2 l.

L

NOTES

laser *(continued)*

flashlamp-pumped pulsed-dye l. (FLPD, FPDL)

flashscanner-enhanced CO_2 l.

frequency doubled neodymium:yttrium-aluminum-garnet l.

gallium-aluminum-arsenide 904-nm l.

GentleLASE l.

KTP l.

potassium titanyl phosphate laser

LightSheer l.

long-pulsed potassium-titanyl-phosphate l.

Luxar NovaPulse l.

LX 20 l.

medical free electron l. (MFEL)

Nd:YAG l.

neodymium:yttrium-aluminum-garnet l.

New Star model 130 l.

NLite l.

normal-mode ruby l. (NMRL)

PhotoDerm l.

photogenica l.

L. Photonics, Inc. (LPI)

l. plume

potassium titanyl phosphate l. (KTP laser)

pulsed-dye l. (PDL)

Q-switched alexandrite l.

Q-switched Nd:YAG l.

Q-switched neodymium:YAG l. (QSYAG)

Q-switched ruby l. (QSRL)

quasicontinuous-wave l.

ruby l.

ScleroPLUS flashlamp-pumped pulsed tunable dye l.

Sharplan SilkTouch flashscan surgical l.

Silk L.

SilkTouch l.

Skinlight erbium:YAG l.

l. skin resurfacing (LSR)

solid-state dye l.

Spectrum ruby l.

l. surgery

SurgiPulse XJ l.

titanium:sapphire l.

UltraPulse CO_2 l.

Vasculight l.

VersaLight l.

VersaPulse l.

Viridis pulsed l.

Xanar 20 Ambulase CO_2 l.

XeCl excimer l.

YAG l.

yttrium-aluminum-garnet l.

laser-assisted

l.-a. internal fabrication (LIFT)

l.-a. internal fabrication technique

"Laser bra" procedure

Laserflo laser Doppler

Lasertrolysis hair removal

Lasix

lasofoxifene

Lassa

L. hemorrhagic fever

L. virus

Lassar

L. betanaphthol paste

L. plain zinc paste

LAT

linker for activation of T cell

lata

condyloma l.

fascia l.

perianal condylomata l.

late

l. benign syphilis

l. cardiovascular syphilis

l. centrilobar necrosis

l. congenital syphilis

l. latent syphilis

l. onset neurofibromatosis

l. osseous syphilis

l. respiratory systemic syndrome (LRSS)

l. yaw

latency

latens

scarlatina l.

latent

l. allergy

l. allotype

l. autoimmune diabetes of adults (LADA)

l. class analysis

l. infection

l. microbism

l. period

l. rat virus

l. stage

l. syphilis

l. transforming growth factor

late-onset

l.-o. renal failure

l.-o. spondyloepiphyseal dysplasia

late-phase

l.-p. allergic reaction

l.-p. cutaneous reaction (LPCR)

l.-p. reaction (LPR)

l.-p. response

lateral
l. collateral ligament (LCL)
l. nail fold
lateralis
hyperhidrosis l.
nevus unius l.
onychia l.
lateris
nevus unius l.
laterosporus
Bacillus l.
latex
l. agglutination test
l. allergy
l. allergy test
l. ELISA for antigen protein (LEAP)
l. fixation reaction
l. fixation test
Hevea brasiliensis l.
l. hypersensitivity
l. particle agglutination
polystyrene l.
l. RIA panel
latex-fruit syndrome
latex-specific IgE
Laticaudinae
Latranal
latrodactism
Latrodectus
L. mactans
L. mactans antivenom
L. mactans bite
LATS
long-acting thyroid stimulator
lattice fiber
latticework
latum
condyloma l.
Diphyllobothrium l.
Laugier-Hunziger syndrome
laurel fever
Lauth violet
LAV
lymphadenopathy-associated virus
lava bean
lavage
bronchoalveolar l. (BAL)
law
Behring l.
Farr l.
Grotthus-Draper l.

Halsted l.
Jadassohn-Lewandowsky l.
Kassowitz-Diday l.
Koch l.
Marfan l.
Planck's l.
l. of priority
Profeta l.
von Behring l.
Lawrence-Seip syndrome
laxa
cutis l.
lax skin
layer
barrier l.
basal cell l.
Bowman l.
cornified l.
granular cell l.
Henle l.
horny cell l.
Huxley l.
hypertrophic smooth muscle l.
lucid l.
malpighian l.
mushroom-hook l.
palisade l.
prickle cell l.
Profore wound contact l.
spinous l.
squamous cell l.
4-layer bandage (FLB)
lazarine leprosy
Lazaro
mal de San L.
lazaroid
Lazarus (LZRS)
LazerSporin-C Otic
lazy
l. leukocyte syndrome (LLS)
l. NK cell
lazy-S closure
LB
lamellar body
LBL
lymphoblastic lymphoma
LBP
lipopolysaccharide binding protein
LBT
lupus band test
L-canavaline

L

NOTES

317

LCD
liquor carbonis detergens
LCH
Langerhans cell histiocytosis
LCL
lateral collateral ligament
LCM virus
LCP
leukocytapheresis
LCR-based HLA typing
LCV
leukocytoclastic vasculitis
LD
lethal dose
living donor
LDA
limiting dilution analysis
LDA-1 antigen
LDF
laser Doppler flowmetry
LDH
lactic dehydrogenase
LDH agent
LDL-C
low-density lipoprotein cholesterol
LDLT
living donor liver transplantation
LDN
laparoscopic donor nephrectomy
L-DOPA
levodopa
L+ dose
LDP-02 humanized monoclonal antibody
LE
lupus erythematosus
LE cell
LE cell phenomenon
discoid LE
LE factor
lead
12-l. electrocardiogram
l. poisoning
l. stomatitis
l. time
leaflet
mitral l.
tricuspid valvular l.
leaf litter
leak
proton l.
Le antigen
LEAP
latex ELISA for antigen protein
learned helplessness
lectin
mannan-binding l. (MBL)
mannose-binding l. (MBL)
l. pathway

lectularius
Cimex l.
LED
light-emitting diode
lupus erythematosus disseminatus
Ledderhose syndrome
Ledercillin VK Oral
leech
Leede-Rumpel phenomenon
leek
leflunomide
left
l. side down-head up position
l. ventricular hypertrophy
leg
Barbados l.
elephant l.
Legg-Calvé-Perthes disease
Legionella
L. anisa
L. birminghamensis
L. bozemanii
L. cincinnatiensis
L. dumoffii
L. feeleii
L. jordanis
L. lansingensis
L. longbeachae
L. maceachernii
L. micdadei
L. oakridgensis
L. pneumophila
legionellosis
Legionnaires disease
leg-raise maneuver
legume
Leicester
L. disease
L. score
Leichtenstern phenomenon
Leiden
factor V L.
Leiner
L. dermatitis
L. disease
leiodermia
leiomyoma
l. cutis
uterine l.
leiomyosarcoma
leiotrichous
Leishman anemia
Leishman-Donovan body
Leishmania
L. donovani
L. major
L. orientalis
L. tropica

leishmaniasis
> acute cutaneous l.
> American l.
> l. americana
> anergic l.
> anthroponotic cutaneous l.
> antimonial drug therapy for l.
> chronic cutaneous l.
> cutaneous l. (CL)
> diffuse cutaneous l.
> disseminated cutaneous l. (DCL)
> dry cutaneous l.
> human cutaneous l.
> lupoid l.
> mucocutaneous l. (MCL)
> nasopharyngeal l.
> New World l.
> Old World l.
> pseudolepromatous l.
> recidivans l. (RL)
> l. recidivans
> rural cutaneous l.
> l. tegumentaria diffusa
> l. tropica
> urban cutaneous l.
> visceral l. (VL)
> viscerotropic l. (VTL)
> wet cutaneous l.
> zoonotic cutaneous l.

leishmania test
leishmanid
leishmanin test
leishmaniosis
Leishman-Montenegro-Donovan intradermal test
leishmanoid
> dermal l.
> post-kala-azar dermal l.

Leloir disease
lemic
Lemierre disease
lemon
LEMS
> Lambert-Eaton myasthenic syndrome

lenercept
length
> restriction fragment l.

Lennert lymphoma
Lennhoff sign
lens
lenscale
lens-induced uveitis

lenticula
lenticularis
> dermatofibrosis l.

lenticular syphilid
lenticulopapular
lentigines (*pl. of* lentigo)
lentiginosis
> centrofacial l.
> generalized l.
> inherited patterned l.
> periorificial l.
> l. profusa

lentiginous
lentigo, pl. **lentigines**
> lentigines, atrial myxoma, mucocutaneous myxomas, and blue nevi (LAMB)
> lentigines, electrocardiographic defects, ocular hypertelorism, pulmonary stenosis, abnormalities of genitalia, retardation of growth, deafness (LEOPARD)
> genital l.
> ink-spot l.
> l. maligna
> l. maligna melanoma
> nevoid l.
> nevus spilus l.
> PUVA-induced l.
> reticulated black solar l.
> senile l.
> l. senilis
> simple l.
> l. simplex
> solar ink-spot l.
> Touraine centrofacial l.

lentil
Lentivirinae
lentivirus
lentogenic
Lenz-Majewski syndrome
leonine facies
leontiasis
LEOPARD
> lentigines, electrocardiographic defects, ocular hypertelorism, pulmonary stenosis, abnormalities of genitalia, retardation of growth, deafness
> LEOPARD syndrome

leopard skin
leper
Lepidoglyphus destructor

L

NOTES

319

Lepidoptera
lepidosis
Lépine-Froin syndrome
Leporipoxvirus
lepothrix
lepra
    l. alba
    l. alphoides
    l. alphos
    l. anaesthetica
    l. arabum
    l. bacillus
    l. cell
    l. conjunctivae
    l. graecorum
    l. maculosa
    l. mutilans
    l. nervorum
    l. nervosa
    l. tuberculoides
    Willan l.
leprae
    Mycobacterium l.
leprechaunism
leprid
leprologist
leprology
leproma
lepromatous
    l. leprosy
    l. nodule
    polar l.
    l. reaction
lepromin
    l. reaction
    l. test
leprosarium
leprose
leprosery
leprostatic
leprosum
    erythema nodosum l.
leprosus
    lichen l.
    pemphigus l.
leprosy
    anesthetic l.
    articular l.
    Asturian l.
    borderline lepromatous l.
    borderline tuberculoid l.
    diffuse lepromatous l.
    dimorphous l.
    dry l.
    histoid l.
    indeterminate l.
    intermediate l.
    lazarine l.

    lepromatous l.
    Lombardy l.
    Lucio l.
    macular l.
    maculoanesthetic l.
    Malabar l.
    mixed l.
    mutilating l.
    neural l.
    nodular l.
    paucibacillary l.
    polar lepromatous l.
    pure neural l.
    reactional l.
    smooth l.
    spotted l.
    subclinical l.
    subpolar lepromatous l.
    trophoneurotic l.
    tuberculoid l.
    uncharacteristic l.
    virchowian l.
    water-buffalo l.
leprotic
leprotica
    alopecia l.
leprous
leptochroa
leptodermic
Leptospira interrogans
leptospirosis
Leptothrix
Leptotrombidium akamushi
Lequesne
    L. algofunctional index
    L. functional index
Leredde syndrome
Leri-Weill syndrome
Leroy I cell
Lesch-Nyhan syndrome
Lescol fluvastatin sodium
Leser-Trélat sign
lesion
    acneform l.
    angel kisses l.
    angioinvasive l.
    angioproliferative l.
    annular distribution of l.
    arciform distribution of l.
    l. arrangement
    atrophic hyperkeratotic l.
    atrophie blanche l.
    blanchable red l.
    blistering l.
    blueberry muffin l.
    blue-gray l.
    brown-black l.
    bullous skin l.

bull's eye l.
Bywaters l.
coin-sized l.
l. color
l. configuration
l. consistency
cutaneous pustular l.
dermal l.
devil's bite l.
l. distribution
division (I–IV) l.
eczematous l.
elementary l.
en coup de sabre scalp l.
erysipelas-like skin l.
l. evolution
firm l.
genital papulosquamous l.
genitourinary l.
greasy scaly l.
gross l.
hemorrhagic l.
herpetiform distribution of l.
histologic l.
hypometabolism brain l.
infarctive l.
intravascular endothelial
  proliferative l.
iris l.
Janeway l.
lichenified l.
linear distribution of l.
l. margination
medium l.
metachronous tissue l.
l. morphology
mother l.
nickel and dime l.
nonblanchable, abnormally
  colored l.
nummular l.
ocular l.
oil drop l.
osseous l.
osteolytic bone l.
papulopustular l.
papulosquamous l.
papulovesicular l.
polycyclic distribution of l.
polypoid l.
precancerous l.
primary l.

proliferative l.
pruritic l.
pulmonary l.
purpuric l.
pustular l.
pyodermatous skin l.
raspberry l.
reticular l.
ripe l.
rolled shoulder l.
Romanus l.
salt and pepper l.
satellite l.
scaling skin-colored l.
secondary l.
silvery scaly l.
l. size
skin l.
skin-colored l.
slope-shouldered l.
smooth skin-colored l.
soft l.
space-occupying l.
special l.
squamous intraepithelial l. (SIL)
square-shouldered l.
stork-bite l.
l. surface characteristic
synchronous tissue l.
target l.
traumatic l.
ulcer l.
ulceronecrotic l.
varicelliform l.
vasculitic l.
Vaughn-Jackson l.
venular l.
vesicobullous l.
vesiculopustular l.
vulvar l.
weeping l.
white l.
wire-loop l.
yellow l.
zosteriform distribution of l.

LET
  leukocyte esterase test
lethal
  l. chondrodysplasia
  l. dose (LD)
  l. midline granuloma

L

NOTES

lethal *(continued)*
    l. midline granulomatosis
    l. osteogenesis imperfecta
lethalis
    epidermolysis bullosa l.
    ichthyosis l.
lethargica
    encephalitis l.
LETS
    large external transformation-sensitive
    fibronectin
Letterer-Siwe disease
Leu-3+ helper T cell
leu-CAM
    leukocyte cell adhesion molecule
leucin
leucine
    l. zipper motif
    l. zipper transcription factor
Leucomax
Leucotropin
leucovorin calcium
leukapheresis cycle
leukapheresis-induced amelioration
leukasmus
leukemia
    acute lymphoblastic l. (ALL)
    acute lymphocytic l. (ALL)
    acute myelogenous l. (AML)
    acute myeloid l. (AML)
    adult T-cell l. (ATL)
    aleukemic l.
    B-cell chronic lymphocytic l. (B-CLL)
    B-cell lymphocytic l.
    chronic lymphocytic l. (CLL)
    chronic myeloid l. (CML)
    chronic T-cell l.
    cutaneous B-cell lymphocytic l.
    l. cutis
    feline l.
    l. of fowl
    granulocytic l.
    hairy cell l. (HCL)
    lymphocytic l.
    lymphoid l.
    monocytic l.
    murine l.
    myeloid l.
    myelomonocytic l.
    null cell l.
    primary cutaneous B-cell
      lymphocytic l.
    prolymphocytic l. (PLL)
    secondary cutaneous B-cell
      lymphocytic l.
    T-cell large granuloma
      lymphocyte l.

    T-cell lymphocytic l.
    thymus-derived l.
leukemia/lymphoma
leukemic
    l. arthritis
    l. reticuloendotheliosis
leukemid
Leukeran
leukin
Leukine
leukoagglutinin
leukocidin
leukoclastic
leukocytactic
leukocytapheresis (LCP)
leukocytaxia
leukocyte
    l. adhesion deficiency (LAD)
    l. adhesion deficiency type 1
      (LAD1)
    l. adhesion deficiency type 2
      (LAD2)
    l. adhesion deficiency type 3
      (LAD3)
    l. adhesion deficiency type 4
      (LAD4)
    l. antigen factor-3 (LAF-3)
    l. attachment assay
    l. cell adhesion molecule (leu-CAM)
    l. chemotaxis
    l. chimerism
    l. common antigen
    l. concentrate
    l. esterase test (LET)
    l. factor antigen-1 (LFA-1)
    l. histamine release
    l. histamine release test
    l. interferon
    passenger l.
    polymorphonuclear l. (PML)
leukocyte-poor preparation
leukocytoclastic
    l. angiitis
    l. vasculitis (LCV)
leukocytolysin
leukocytolysis
leukocytolytic
leukocytosis
leukocytosis-promoting factor
leukocytotactic
leukocytotaxia
leukocytotoxin
leukoderma
    acquired l.
    l. acquisitum centrifugum
    chemical l.
    l. colli

contact l.
genital l.
occupational l.
patterned l.
syphilitic l.
leukodermatous
leukodermia
leukoencephalitis
acute epidemic l.
subacute sclerosing l.
leukoencephalopathy
cerebral autosomal dominant
arteriopathy with subcortical
infarcts and l. (CADASIL)
immunosuppression-associated l.
progressive multifocal l. (PML)
reversible posterior l. (RPLS)
leukokeratosis oris
leukolysin
leukolysis
leukolytic
leukonecrosis
leukonychia
apparent l.
partial l.
l. striata
leukopathia
acquired l.
l. punctata reticularis symmetrica
l. symmetrica progressiva
l. unguis
leukopathy
symmetric progressive l.
leukopenia
leukopenic
l. factor
l. index
leukoplakia
acquired dyskeratotic l.
Candida l.
candidal l.
hairy l.
oral hairy l. (OHL)
proliferative verrucous l.
l. vulva
leukoplakic vulvitis
leukoplasia
leuko-poor
l.-p. blood component
l.-p. red blood cell
leukorrhea
LeukoScan diagnostic agent

leukosialin
leukosis
avian l.
enzootic bovine l.
fowl l.
leukotactic
leukotaxia
leukotaxine
leukotaxis
leukotoxin
leukotrichia annularis
leukotrichous
leukotriene (LT)
l. antagonist
l. B4 (LTB$_4$)
l. C, E
l. inhibition
l. reduction
l. regulation
LeukoVAX
Leukovirus
leupeptin
LeuTech radiolabeled antibody
Leutrol
levalbuterol
levamisole
Levaquin
levarterenol bitartrate
Levay antigen
level
beta$_2$-microglobulin l.
Clark l. (I–V)
fibrinogen l.
free salicylate l.
gp91^{phox} l.
IgG subclass l.
intrasynovial complement l.
no observed adverse effect l.
(NOAEL)
peak serum l.
recommended exposure l. (REL)
serum complement l.
specific IgE antibody l.
total serum IgE l.
Lever
L. 2000
L. and Schamberg-Lever
classification
Leviviridae
levocabastine hydrochloride
levodopa (L-DOPA)
l. stain

NOTES

levofloxacin
levonorgestrel
Levophed injection
levothyroxine sodium
Levulan
    L. Kerastick
    L. photodynamic therapy
Levulin PDT system
Lewandowski
    nevus elasticus of L.
    rosacea-like tuberculid of L.
Lewandowski-Lutz
    L.-L. disease
    epidermodysplasia verruciformis
      of L.-L.
Lewandowsky nevus elasticus
Lewis
    L. blood antibody type
    L. blood group
    triple response of L.
    L. triple response
    L. X oligosaccharide
Lewis-Summer syndrome
Leyden disease
Leydig cell tumor
LF-15-0195
Lf
    limes fluctuating
    Lf dose
    Lf unit
LFA
    lymphocyte function-associated antigen
LFA-1
    leukocyte factor antigen-1
    lymphocyte function antigen-1
    lymphocyte function-associated antibody-1
    lymphocyte function-associated antigen-1
LFA-2
    lymphocyte function-associated antibody-2
LFA-3
    lymphocyte function-associated antibody-3
    lymphocyte function-associated antigen-3
LFT
    liver function test
LGL
    large granular lymphocyte
L-glutathione
LGV
    lymphogranuloma venereum
LGV-CFT
    lymphogranuloma venereum complement
    fixation test
LH 7:2 antigen
Lhermitte-Duclos disease
Lhermitte sign

L'Homme rouge
Liacopoulos phenomenon
liarozole
liasis
Liatest C4b-BP test
liberator
    histamine l.
Libman-Sacks
    L.-S. endocarditis
    L.-S. syndrome
Librium
lice (pl. of louse)
Lice-Enz Shampoo
lichen
    l. agrius
    l. albus
    l. amyloidosis
    l. chronicus simplex
    l. corneus hypertrophicus
    l. fibromucinoidosus
    l. framboesianus
    l. hemorrhagicus
    l. infantum
    l. iris
    l. leprosus
    l. myxedematosus
    myxedematous l.
    l. nitidus
    l. nuchae
    l. obtusus
    l. obtusus corneus
    l. pilaris
    l. pilaris seu spinulosus
    l. planopilaris (LPP)
    l. planus actinicus
    l. planus annularis
    l. planus et acuminatus atrophicans
    l. planus follicularis
    l. planus hypertrophicus
    l. planus-like keratosis
    l. planus overlap syndrome
    l. planus pemphigoid
    l. planus pigmentosus
    l. planus verrucosus
    l. ruber
    l. ruber acuminatus
    l. ruber moniliformis
    l. ruber planus
    l. ruber verrucosus
    l. sclerosus
    sclerosus l.
    l. sclerosus et atrophicans
    l. sclerosus et atrophicus (LS&A)
    l. sclerosus scleroatrophy
    l. scrofulosis
    l. scrofulosorum
    l. scrofulous
    l. simplex chronicus (LSC)

l. striatus
l. striatus epidermal nevus
l. strophulosus
l. syphiliticus
l. trichophyticus
tropical l.
l. tropicus
l. urticatus
Wilson l.
lichenificatio gigantea
lichenification
giant l.
lichenified
l. dermatitis
l. lesion
l. plaque
licheniformis
Bacillus l.
lichenization
lichenoid
l. acute pityriasis
l. amyloidosis
chronica parapsoriasis l.
l. chronic dermatosis
l. contact dermatitis
l. eczema
l. eruption
exudative discoid and l.
l. keratosis
parapsoriasis l.
l. phase
pityriasis l.
tuberculosis cutis l.
lichenoides
melanodermatitis toxica l.
parapsoriasis l.
pityriasis l.
tuberculosis cutis l.
lichen-type scale
Lich-Gregoire
L.-G. repair
L.-G. ureteroneocystostomy
Lich technique
licorice
Lidakol cream
Lida-Mantle HC topical
Liddle syndrome
Lidemol
Lidex-E topical
Lidex topical

lidocaine
bacitracin, neomycin, polymyxin b, and l.
l. and epinephrine
l. hydrochloride
l. and hydrocortisone
l. and prilocaine
Lidoderm
LidoPen
life
health-related quality of l.
quality of l. (QOL)
life-year
quality-adjusted l.-y. (QALY)
LIFT
laser-assisted internal fabrication
LIFT technique
ligament
alar l.
glenohumeral l.
iliopectineal l.
inguinal l.
lateral collateral l. (LCL)
l. of Struthers
transverse l.
ligamentosa
spondylitis ossificans l.
ligamentum nuchae
ligand
addressing l.
calcium-signal modulating cyclophilin B l. (CAML)
Fas l. (FasL)
Fas-Fas l.
nuclear factor kappa B l.
osteoprotegerin l.
peptide l.
P-selectin l.
receptor activator of nuclear factor kappa B l. (RANKL)
tumor necrosis factor-related apoptosis-inducing l. (TRAIL)
ligase chain reaction
LIGHT
homologous to lymphotoxin, shows inducible expression and competes with herpes simplex virus glycoprotein D for herpes virus entry mediator, a receptor expressed by T lymphocyte
light
actinic l.
bili l.

NOTES

L

325

light *(continued)*
    Boyd surgical l.
    Castle examination l.
    l. chain
    l. eruption
    l. exposure
    Hanalux Oslo l.
    intense pulsed l. (IPL)
    long-wavelength ultraviolet l. (UVA)
    l. microscopy
    midrange spectrum ultraviolet l.
    midrange-wavelength ultraviolet l. (UVB)
    oral administration of psoralen and subsequent exposure to long wavelength ultraviolet l. (PUVA)
    l. scatter technique
    l. treatment
    ultraviolet l.
    l. urticaria
    Wood l.
light-emitting diode (LED)
LightSheer
    L. diode laser system for permanent hair removal
    L. laser
    L. SC
    L. SC laser hair removal system
light-sparing effect
lignieresii
    Actinobacillus l.
lignocaine monoethylglycine xylidine excretion test
Likert scale
lilacinus
    Paecilomyces l.
lilac tree
lima bean
limb
    l. defect
    l. pain
limbal guttering
limb-girdle dystrophy
limbi (*pl. of* limbus)
limbic kindling
limb-mammary syndrome
limbus, pl. limbi
    limbi conjunctiva
    limbi palpebrales anteriores
    limbi palpebrales posteriores
lime
limes fluctuating (Lf)
liminal
liminaris
    alopecia l.
limitation of exposure

limited
    l. progressive systemic sclerosis
    l. Wegener granulomatosis
limiting
    l. dilution analysis (LDA)
    l. precursor cell (LPC)
limits
    permissible exposure l. (PELs)
limnophilus
    Paederus l.
Limulus lysate assay
lincomycin
lincosamide
lindane
Lindner body
line
    Beau l.
    l.'s of Blaschko
    Blaschko l.
    Borsieri l.
    Cantle l.
    cell l.
    cement l.
    l.'s of cleavage
    Dennie l.
    Dennie-Morgan l.
    erythroleukemia cell l.
    established cell l.
    Futcher l.
    Jadelot l.
    Jurkat T-cell l.
    Köhler l.
    Langer l.
    marionette l.
    Mees l.
    MOLT-18, human T cell l.
    Morgan l.
    Muehrcke l.
    Pastia l.
    pigmentary demarcation l.
    Ramos B-cell l.
    RA synoviocyte l.
    Relaxed Skin Tension L. (RSTL)
    Sergent white l.
    tram l.
    Voigt l.
    white l.
linea, pl. lineae
    l. alba
    l. albicans
    l. IgM dermatosis of pregnancy
    l. nigra
    lineae striae atrophicae
linear
    l. atrophoderma of Moulin
    l. atrophy
    l. distribution
    l. distribution of lesion

l. epidermal nevus
l. extensor erythema
l. focal elastosis
l. IgA bullous dermatosis (LABD)
l. IgA bullous disease
l. IgA bullous disease in children
l. lichen planus
l. petechia
l. porokeratosis
l. progressive systemic sclerosis
l. scleroderma
l. scleroderma variant
l. streaking
l. telangiectasis
l. and whorled nevoid
  hypermelanosis
linearis
morphea l.
linearity
Mantel-Haenszel test for l.
liner
Ac'cents permanent lash l.
linezolid
lingua, pl. **linguae**
exfoliatio areata l.
l. geographica
hyperkeratosis l.
ichthyosis l.
keratomycosis l.
l. nigra
nigrities l.
pityriasis l.
l. plicata
psoriasis l.
l. scrotalis
tylosis l.
lingula, pl. **lingulae**
liniment
Sloan l.
lining
synovial l.
linkage disequilibrium
linked suppression
linker
l. for activation of T cell (LAT)
tonofilament-cytoplasmic plaque l.
transmembrane l.
link-protein-stabilized aggregate
linnaean system of nomenclature
linoleic acid
Linomide

linter
cotton l.
Lioresal
LIP
lymphocytic interstitial pneumonitis
lip cosmetic
lipedematous alopecia
lipid
l. granulomatosis
5-lipoxygenase-generated l.
12-lipoxygenase-generated l.
l. liquid crystal
neutral l.
l. peroxidation
l. storage disease
lipide
lipid-free cleanser
lipidosis
glycolipid l.
Lipkote
Coppertone L.
lipoatrophia annularis
lipoatrophic diabetes
lipoatrophy
annular l.
centrifugal l.
Ferreira-Marques l.
insulin l.
partial l.
postinfection l.
semicircular l.
lipoblastomatosis
benign l.
lipochrome histiocytosis disease
lipocortin
lipodermatosclerosis
lipodystrophia centrifugalis abdominalis
  infantilis
lipodystrophy
acquired generalized l.
acquired partial face-sparing l.
congenital total l.
intestinal l.
localized l.
partial face-sparing l.
progressive l.
total l.
5-lipogenase
lipogranuloma
sclerosing l.
lipogranulomatosis subcutanea

L

NOTES

lipoid
>l. dermatoarthritis
>l. granuloma
>l. pneumonia
>l. proteinosis

lipoidica
>necrobiosis l.

lipoidosis cutis et mucosa
lipolytica
>*Candida l.*

lipoma
>l. arborescens
>atypical l.
>pleomorphic l.
>spindle cell l.
>synovial l.

lipomatodes
>fibroma l.
>molluscum l.
>nevus l.

lipomatosis
>benign symmetric l.
>encephalocraniocutaneous l. (ECCL)
>mediastinal l.
>multiple symmetric l.

lipomatosus
>nevus l.

lipomelanic reticulosis
lipomelanotic
Lipomel melanoma vaccine
Liponyssus bacoti
lipophagia granulomatosis
lipophagic granuloma
lipophilic yeast
lipophosphoglycan (LPG)
lipopolysaccharide (LPS)
>l. binding protein (LBP)
>J5 l.
>l. vaccine

lipopolysaccharide-induced arthritis (LPS-induced arthritis)
lipopolysaccharide-stimulated
lipoprotein
>l. lipase deficiency
>l. polymorphism
>very-low-density l. (VLDL)

liposarcoma
liposculpture
liposomal doxorubicin
liposome
>clodronate-containing l.

liposuction
>syringe-assisted l.

LipoTECA cream
lipoteichoic acid (LTA)
lipotrophy
>semicircular l.

lipovaccine

Lipovnik virus
lipoxin
>l. A4, B4

lipoxygenase
>l. interaction product
>l. pathway

5-lipoxygenase-activating protein (FLAP)
12-lipoxygenase-generated lipid
5-lipoxygenase-generated lipid
5-lipoxygenase (5-LO)
lips
>blubbery l.
>cracked l.
>dry l.
>glowing red l.
>pseudocolloid of l.

Lipschütz
>L. body
>L. cell
>L. ulcer

Lipsorex
lipstick
lip-switch
liquefaction
>l. degeneration
>l. necrosis

Liqui-Caps
>Vicks 44 Non-Drowsy Cold & Cough L.-C.

liquid
>l. air
>Anaplex L.
>Baker's P&S l.
>Barc L.
>bland aerosolized l.
>Children's Motion Sickness l.
>Chlorafed L.
>End Lice L.
>l. ethyl chloride
>Gordofilm L.
>Hayfebrol L.
>l. human serum
>Lotrimin AF Spray L.
>l. nitrogen (LN$_2$)
>Occlusal-HP L.
>L. paraffin
>L. petrolatum
>L. Pred
>L. Pred Oral
>Pyrinyl II L.
>Rhinosyn L.
>Rhinosyn-PD L.
>Ryna L.
>Sudafed Plus L.
>Tisit L.
>Triple X L.

liquidambar

Liquifilm
> L. Forte solution
> HMS L.
> L. Tears
> L. Tears solution

Liqui-Gels
> Robitussin Severe Congestion L.-G.

Liquimat lotion
Liquiprin
LiquiShield-A Skin Protectant
LiquiVent
liquor carbonis detergens (LCD)
Lisch nodule
lisofylline
lispro insulin
lissotrichic
list
> Interpersonal Support Evaluation L. (ISEL)

Lister
> L. scissors
> L. tubercle

listerial
Listeria monocytogenes
listeriosis
listerism
listhesis
> subaxial l.

listing
> UNOS transplant l.

lithium succinate
litmus paper
Littauer scissors
litter
> leaf l.

Little League elbow
LITx
> liver and intestinal transplantation

live
> bacillus Calmette-Guérin L.
> measles virus vaccine, l.
> l. oak
> l. oak tree
> l. oral polio vaccine
> l. oral poliovirus vaccine
> rubella virus vaccine, l.
> TICE Bacillus Calmette-Guérin l. (TICE BCG)
> varicella virus vaccine l.

livedo
> l. annularis
> lupus l.

> l. pattern
> l. racemosa
> l. reticularis
> l. reticularis idiopathica
> l. reticularis symptomatica
> l. telangiectatica
> l. vasculitis

livedoid
> l. dermatitis
> l. vasculitis

livedo-patterned disease
liver
> l. allograft
> l. allotransplantation
> bioartificial l. (BAL)
> l. disease
> ELAD artificial l.
> l. extract
> l. function test (LFT)
> l. and intestinal transplantation (LITx)
> l. and kidney transplantation (LKT)
> l. palm
> l. spot

liver-specific protein (LSP)
livid
lividity
living
> l. donor (LD)
> l. donor liver transplantation (LDLT)
> l. skin equivalent (LSE)

living-related
> l.-r. donor (LRD)
> l.-r. liver transplantation (LRT)

livor
Livostin Ophthalmic
lizard skin
LKT
> liver and kidney transplantation

LLNA
> local lymph-node assay

LLS
> lazy leukocyte syndrome

LMC
> lymphocyte-mediated cytotoxicity

LN
> lupus nephritis

LN$_2$
> liquid nitrogen

LNPF
> lymph node permeability factor

L

NOTES

(5-LO)
5-lipoxygenase (5-LO)
Loa
L. loa
loa
Filaria l.
Loa l.
l. loa infection
5-LO-activating protein
loading
mechanical l.
loaiasis
Lobana wound cleanser
lobar bronchus
lobenzarit disodium
loblolly
l. pine
l. pine tree
Lobo disease
lobomycosis
lobster
lobucavir
lobular panniculitis
local
l. anaphylaxis
l. immunity
l. lymph-node assay (LLNA)
l. reaction
localisata
junctional epidermolysis bullosa atrophicans l.
localized
l. acquired cutaneous pseudoxanthoma elasticum
l. albinism
l. angiokeratoma
l. cutaneous amyloidosis epidermolysis bullosa, l.
l. epidermolysis bullosa simplex
l. granuloma annulare
l. lipodystrophy
l. mucocutaneous candidiasis
l. neurodermatitis
l. pagetoid reticulosis
l. pemphigoid of Brunsting-Perry
l. progressive systemic sclerosis
l. pustular psoriasis
l. scleroderma
l. tuberculous meningitis
l. vitiligo
loci (*pl. of* locus)
Locilex
L. pexiganan acetate cream
L. topical cream
Locoid Topical
locomotor ataxia
Loctite 15494 ethyl cyanoacrylate glue

loculation
locus, pl. **loci**
histocompatibility l. (HL)
l. minoris resistentiae
T l.
locust
black l.
lod
logarithm of odds
lodgepole
l. pine
l. pine tree
Lodine
Lo dose
lodoxamide tromethamine
Loesche classification
Loewenthal reaction
Löffler syndrome
Lofgren syndrome
Löfqvist tourniquet
logarithmic phase
logarithm of odds (lod)
logic
hierarchical clustering discrimination l.
logit transformation
LogMAR visual acuity
loiasis
Loiasis filariasis
Lolium
L. perenne (Lol p)
L. perenne allergen
Lol p
Lolium perenne
Lol p allergen (I-III)
Lombardy
L. leprosy
L. poplar tree
lomefloxacin hydrochloride
Lomir
lomustine
London
L. Drugs Sport
L. Drugs Sunblock
L. Drugs Sunscreen
Lone Star tick
long
l. acting (LA)
l. incubation hepatitis
l. terminal repeat sequence (LTR)
l. thoracic nerve palsy
Long-Acting
Sinex L.-A.
long-acting thyroid stimulator (LATS)
longbeachae
Legionella l.
long-handled dressing reacher

longibrachiatum
    Trichoderma l.
longior
    Tyroglyphus l.
longitudinal
    l. hyperpigmented band
    l. melanonychia
    l. nail hyperpigmentation
long-pulsed potassium-titanyl-phosphate laser
long-wavelength ultraviolet light (UVA)
Loniten Oral
look
    Hippocratic l.
loop
    l. diuretic
    Roux-Y l.
Loo punch
loose
    l. anagen hair syndrome
    l. body
    l. skin
loose-jointedness
loperamide
lophate
lopinavir/ritonavir
    l. capsule
    l. oral solution
lopinavir and ritonavir
Loprox
Lopurin
Lorabid
loracarbef
loratadine and pseudoephedrine
lorgnette
    la main en l.
Loroxide
Lortat-Jacobs disease
loss
    chronic blood l.
    eyebrow l.
    eyelash l.
    hair l.
    hearing l.
    powered air l.
    weight l.
lost
    healthy years of life l. (HYLL)
Lotemax
loteprednol
lotio
    Balneol l.

lotion
    Active Dry L.
    alcoholic white shake l.
    Alpha Keri l.
    Aquanil l.
    A/T/S l.
    BlemErase L.
    calamine l.
    carbamide body l.
    Carmol 10 body l.
    Carmol scalp treatment l.
    Clear Confident antifungal topical l.
    clotrimazole/betamethasone dipropionate l.
    colored alcoholic shake l.
    Complex 15 l.
    desonide otic l.
    dihydroxyacetone self-tanning l.
    Fostril l.
    G-well L.
    IvyBlock L.
    Klaron l.
    Komed l.
    Kwell L.
    Liquimat l.
    Lotrimin AF L.
    Lotrisone l.
    Mosquitone l.
    Neutrogena On-The-Spot Acne L.
    nonalcoholic white shake l.
    Nova Perfecting L.
    Panscol L.
    Pen-Kera l.
    Pennsaid topical l.
    Scabene L.
    Sebasorb l.
    Shade UvaGuard sunscreen l.
    Skinvisible l.
    sulfacetamide sodium scalp treatment l.
    talc l.
    Tinver L.
    triamcinolone l. (TAL)
Lotriderm
Lotrimin
    L. AF Cream
    L. AF Lotion
    L. AF Solution
    L. AF Spray Liquid
    L. AF Spray Powder
Lotrisone lotion

L

NOTES

Lou Gehrig disease
Louis-Bar syndrome
louping
    l. ill
    l. ill virus
louse, pl. **lice**
    body l.
    clothes l.
    crab l.
    End Lice
    head l.
    l. infestation
    pubic l.
    scalp l.
    sucking l.
louse-borne
    l.-b. relapsing fever
    l.-b. typhus
lousiness
lousy
Lovibond
    L. angle
    L. profile sign
low
    l. absolute glomerular filtration rate
    l. air-loss bed
    l. avidity
    l. cyclosporine
    l. flow rate
    l. frequency transduction
    l. plasma albumin
    l. urine pH
    l. virulence vaccine
low-density lipoprotein cholesterol (LDL-C)
low-egg-passage vaccine
Löwenstein-Jensen agar
lower respiratory tract infection (LRTI)
low-grade fever
low-phenylalanine diet
low-tyrosine diet
Loxosceles
    L. laeta
    L. reclusa
    L. reclusa bite
loxoscelism
    necrotic cutaneous l.
    viscerocutaneous l.
lozenge
    zinc gluconate l.
LP
    AstraZeneca LP
Lp(a)
LPC
    limiting precursor cell
LPCR
    late-phase cutaneous reaction

LPG
    lipophosphoglycan
l-phenylalanine mustard
LPI
    Laser Photonics, Inc.
        LPI excimer laser system
LPP
    lichen planopilaris
LPR
    late-phase reaction
LPS
    lipopolysaccharide
LPS-induced arthritis
LR
    lymphatic reconstruction
LRD
    living-related donor
Lr dose
LRS
    lymphoreticular system
LRSS
    late respiratory systemic syndrome
LRT
    living-related liver transplantation
LRTI
    lower respiratory tract infection
LS&A
    lichen sclerosus et atrophicus
LSC
    lichen simplex chronicus
LSE
    living skin equivalent
L-selectin
LSP
    liver-specific protein
LSR
    laser skin resurfacing
LT
    leukotriene
LTA
    lipoteichoic acid
LTA$_4$
    L. hydrolase
    L. hydrolase gene disruption
LTB$_4$
    leukotriene B4
    dihydroxy leukotriene, LTB4
LTC$_4$
    cysteinyl leukotriene, L.
    L. synthase
LTD$_4$
LTE$_4$
LTR
    long terminal repeat sequence
L-tryptophan
    L.-t. ingestion
Lu antigen
Lubath oil

lubricant
lubricant/emollient
 Bag Balm l.
 Udder Butter l.
lubrication
 skin l.
lubricin
Lubriderm moisturizer
LubriTears solution
lucent cleft
lucida
 lamina l.
lucid layer
lucidum
 stratum l.
luciferase reporter gene
luciliae
 Crithidia l.
Lucio
 diffuse leprosy of L.
 L. leprosy
 L. leprosy phenomenon
Lucké
 L. adenocarcinoma
 L. carcinoma
 L. virus
lucotherapy
Ludiomil
Ludwig angina
Luer-Lok syringe
lues
 l. nervosa
 l. tarda
 l. venerea
luetic mask
Lufyllin
lugdunensis
 Staphylococcus l.
Luikart dissector
Lukes-Collins non-Hodgkin lymphoma classification
lumbar ganglionectomy
lumberman's itch
lumbricoides
 Ascaris l.
lumican
luminal antigen
Lumitene
lumpy
 l. jaw
 l. skin disease
Lunar bone density machine

lunata
 Curvularia l.
lunate
lunate-capitate
lunch-time peel
Lund-Browder
 L.-B. burn scale
 L.-B. classification
lung
 l. allograft
 bathtub refinisher's l.
 bird-breeder's l.
 bird fancier l.
 butterfly l.
 cheese washer's l.
 diffuse interstitial fibrosis of the l.
 l. disease
 enzyme worker's l.
 epoxy resin l.
 farmer's l.
 honeycomb l.
 humidifier l.
 l. interstitium
 l. involvement
 malt-worker's l.
 mushroom picker's l.
 mushroom worker's l.
 paprika splitter's l.
 pituitary snuff taker's l.
 plastic worker's l.
 smallpox handler's l.
 thresher's l.
lunula, pl. **lunulae**
 diffusion of the l.
 red l.
 spotted l.
 l. unguis
Lunyo virus
lupiform
lupinosa
 porrigo l.
lupoid
 l. acne
 l. hepatitis
 l. leishmaniasis
 l. sclerosis
 l. sycosis
 l. ulcer
luposa
 tuberculosis l.
 tuberculosis cutis l.

L

NOTES

lupus
- l. alopecia
- l. anticoagulant (LA)
- l. anticoagulant antibody (LAC)
- l. band test (LBT)
- Cazenave l.
- l. cerebritis
- chilblain l.
- cutaneous l.
- discoid l.
- drug-induced l.
- l. erythematodes
- l. erythematosus (LE)
- l. erythematosus cell
- l. erythematosus cell test
- l. erythematosus discoides
- l. erythematosus disseminatus (LED)
- l. erythematosus hypertrophicus
- l. erythematosus, neonatal
- l. erythematosus panniculitis
- l. erythematosus phenomenon
- l. erythematosus profundus
- l. erythematosus tumidus
- l. erythematous-like rash
- l. fibrosus
- l. glomerulonephritis
- l. livedo
- l. lymphaticus
- l. miliaris disseminatus faciei
- l. mutilans
- neonatal l.
- l. nephritis (LN)
- l. papillomatosus
- l. pernio
- l. profundus/panniculitis
- l. sebaceous
- l. sebaceus
- l. serpiginosus
- l. superficialis
- l. syndrome
- l. thrombophilia
- l. tuberculosus
- l. verrucosus
- l. vorax
- l. vulgaris

lupus-like syndrome
lupus-scleroderma overlap syndrome
Luschka joint
lusitaniae
- Candida l.

Lustra-AF
Lustra cream
Lutheran blood group
Lutz-Miescher disease
Lutzomyia
Lutz-Splendore-Almeida disease
Luxar NovaPulse laser

Luxiq ViaFoam betamethasone valerate foam
LVG
- lymphogranuloma venereum

lwoffi
- Acinetobacter l.

LXA$_4$ R
LX 20 laser
Ly antigen
Lyb antigen
lycopenemia
lycopodium
- granuloma l.

Lyderm
Lyell
- L. disease
- L. syndrome

Lymantria
- L. dispar
- L. dispar sting

Lyme
- L. arthritis
- L. borreliosis
- L. disease DNA detection
- L. disease (stage 1–3)

Lymephobia
LYMErix
lymph
- l. cell
- l. gland
- l. node
- l. node biopsy
- l. node permeability factor (LNPF)
- l. nodule
- vaccine l.
- l. varix

lymphadenitis
- dermatopathic l.
- necrotizing l.
- regional granulomatous l.
- tuberculosis l.

lymphadenoma
lymphadenomatosis
lymphadenopathy
- angioblastic l.
- angioimmunoblastic l. (AIL)
- dermatopathic l.
- drug-induced l.
- hilar l.
- persistent generalized l. (PGL)

lymphadenopathy-associated virus (LAV)
lymphadenosis
- benign l.
- l. benigna cutis
- l. cutis benigna

lymphangiectasia
lymphangiectasis

lymphangiectatica
    pachyderma l.
lymphangiectatic elephantiasis
lymphangiectodes
lymphangioendothelioma
    benign l.
lymphangioleiomyomatosis
lymphangioma
    acquired progressive l. (APL)
    l. capillare varicosum
    l. cavernosum
    cavernous l.
    l. circumscriptum
    l. cysticum
    solitary simple l.
    l. superficium simplex
    l. tuberosum multiplex
    l. xanthelasmoideum
lymphangiomyomatosis
lymphangiosarcoma
    postmastectomy l.
lymphangitis
    ascending l.
    l. carcinomatosa
    indurated l.
    penile sclerosing l.
    sclerosing l.
lymphapheresis
lymphatic
    l. cisternae
    l. malformation
    l. nevus
    l. reconstruction (LR)
lymphatics
    dermal l.
lymphaticus
    lupus l.
    nevus l.
    varix l.
lymphatolytic serum
lymphedema
    chronic hereditary l.
    hereditary l.
    l. praecox
    primary l.
    secondary l.
lymphedema-distichiasis syndrome
lymphedematous keratoderma
lymphoablative technique
lymphoblastic lymphoma (LBL)
lymphoblastoma
lymphocele

LymphoCide antibody
lymphocutaneous pattern
lymphocytapheresis
lymphocyte
    l. activation
    B l.
    l. chemoattractant activity
    cytotoxic T l. (CTL)
    l. function antigen-1 (LFA-1)
    l. function assay
    l. function-associated antibody-1
        (LFA-1)
    l. function-associated antibody-2
        (LFA-2)
    l. function-associated antibody-3
        (LFA-3)
    l. function-associated antigen (LFA)
    l. function-associated antigen-1
        (LFA-1)
    l. function-associated antigen-3
        (LFA-3)
    l. homing receptor
    homologous to lymphotoxin, shows
        inducible expression and competes
        with herpes simplex virus
        glycoprotein D for herpes virus
        entry mediator, a receptor
        expressed by T l. (LIGHT)
    l. immune globulin
    large granular l. (LGL)
    peripheral blood l. (PBL)
    l. recirculation
    sensitized l.
    l. serine esterase
    l. subset count
    T l.
    T-helper-2 l. (TH2)
    l. transformation
    transformed l.
    tumor-infiltrating l. (TIL)
lymphocyte-mediated cytotoxicity (LMC)
lymphocytic
    l. apoptosis
    l. choriomeningitis virus (LCM
        virus)
    l. disease
    l. hypophysitis
    l. infiltrate of Jessner
    l. infiltration
    l. infiltration of the skin
    l. interstitial pneumonitis (LIP)

L

NOTES

lymphocytic *(continued)*
    l. leukemia
    l. vasculitis
lymphocytoma
    Borrelia l.
    l. cutis
lymphocytopenia
lymphocytosis
    diffuse infiltrative l.
    l. syndrome
lymphocytotoxic antibody
lymphoderma
lymphoepithelioid lymphoma
lymphogenous metastasis
lymphogranuloma
    l. benignum
    l. inguinale
    l. venereum (LGV, LVG)
    l. venereum antigen
    l. venereum complement fixation
    test (LGV-CFT)
    l. venereum virus
lymphogranulomatosis
    l. benigna
    l. maligna
    Schaumann benign l.
Lymphogranuloma venereum
    conjunctivitis
lymphohistiocytic
lymphohistiocytosis
    familial erythrophagocytic l.
    familial hemophagocytic l. (FHL)
lymphoid
    l. cell
    l. hypophysitis
    l. infiltrate
    l. leukemia
lymphokine
    l.-activated killer cell
    production of l.
lymphokine-activated
    l.-a. killer (LAK)
    l.-a. killer cell
lympholeukocyte
lymphoma
    adult T-cell l.
    adult T-cell leukemia/l. (ATLL)
    African Burkitt l.
    angiocentric l.
    angiodestructive l.
    B-cell l.
    body cavity-based B-cell l.
    Burkitt l.
    cutaneous B-cell l.
    cutaneous T-cell l. (CTCL)
    donor-transmitted l.
    gingival l.
    granulomatous cutaneous T-cell l.

    high-grade small noncleaved cell
    malignant l.
    histiocytic l.
    Hodgkin l.
    large cell l.
    Lennert l.
    lymphoblastic l. (LBL)
    lymphoepithelioid l.
    malignant l.
    MALT l.
    mantle cell l.
    marginal zone B-cell l. (MZBL)
    Mediterranean l.
    mucosa-associated lymphoid
    tissue l.
    non-Hodgkin l. (NHL)
    null-type non-Hodgkin l.
    peripheral T-cell l.
    pleomorphic l.
    primary cutaneous B-cell l.
    primary cutaneous T-cell l.
    primary effusion l.
    pseudomalignant l.
    pulmonary l.
    retrovirus-associated l.
    Revised European-American L.
    (REAL)
    secondary cutaneous B-cell l.
    signet ring l.
    subcutaneous panniculitis-like T-
    cell l. (SPTL)
    subcutaneous T-cell l.
    T-cell l.
    U-cell l.
    undefined-cell l.
lymphomagenesis
lymphoma-leukemia
    adult T-cell l.-l.
lymphomatoid
    l. granulomatosis
    l. papulosis (LyP)
lymphomatosis
    avian l.
    fowl l.
    ocular l.
    visceral l.
lymphomatous erythroderma
lymphopathia venereum
lymphopenia
lymphopenic thymic dysplasia
lymphoplasmacytapheresis
lymphoplasmacytic
lymphoplasmacytoid lymphoma cell
Lymphoprep Tube
lymphoproliferative disease
lymphoreticular
    l. cell

l. disorder
l. system (LRS)
lymphoreticulosis
benign inoculation l.
lymphosarcoma
fascicular l.
sclerosing l.
lymphosarcomatosis
lymphostatic verrucosis
lymphotoxicity
lymphotoxin
lymphotrophism
lymphotropic retrovirus
Lynghya **dermatitis**
LYOfoam
L. A, C, T foam dressing
L. Extra foam dressing
Lyon effect
lyophilized
l. extract
l. immunoglobulin G
Lyovac antivenom
LyP
lymphomatoid papulosis
Lyphocin injection
Lyra laser system
lysate
lyse
lysin
lysinogen
lysinogenic
lysis
endothelial l.
host-cell l.
NK cell l.
reactive l.

lysogen
lysogenesis
lysogenic
l. bacterium
l. induction
l. strain
lysogenicity
lysogenization
lysogeny
lysosomal
l. enzyme
l. glycoprotein
l. proteinase
lysosome trafficking regulator (LYST)
lysosomotropic antimalarial drug
lysozyme
hen egg l. (HEL)
tear l.
lysozyme-associated amyloidosis
lyssa
Lyssavirus
LYST
lysosome trafficking regulator
lysyl oxidase
Lyt antigen
lytic
l. enzyme
l. Epstein-Barr virus
Lytta
L. vesicata
L. vesicata sting
lytta
lyze
LZRS
Lazarus

L

NOTES

M
  M antigen
  Back-Ese M
  CarraSorb M
  M cell
  M protein
M1
  streptococcal M1
2M
  A 2M
    2-microglobulin-origin amyloid
    deposit
M3
  streptococcal M3
MA
  monoarthritis
Maalox H2 Acid Controller
MAB
  monoclonal antibody
Mab
  MEDI-507 anti-CD2 M.
MAb-170 monoclonal antibody
MABP
  maltose-binding protein
MabThera monoclonal antibody
MAb therapy
MAC
  membrane attack complex
  membranolytic attack complex
  microcystic adnexal carcinoma
  Mycobacterium avium complex
  Mycobacterium avium-intracellulare
maceachernii
  Legionella m.
macerate
macerated
maceration
  interdigital m.
  plantar m.
machination
machine
  CPM m.
  G5 massage and percussion m.
  Lunar bone density m.
  Northland bone density m.
  PhotoDerm m.
  m. preservation (MP)
  Respitrace m.
  Sysmex SE-9500 m.
  m. worker dermatitis
machinery
  intercellular m.
Machupo virus
MacIsaac disease
MacMARCKS protein

Macritonin
Macrobid
macrocheilia, macrochilia
macrocheiria, macrochiria
macrocytase
macrodactylia
Macrodantin
macroglobulinemia
  Waldenström m. (WM)
macroglossia
macrolabia
macrolide antimicrobial agent
macromelia
macromolecule
  bacterial m.
  matrix m.
macronychia
macrophage
  activated m.
  alveolar m.
  armed m.
  associated m.
  m. colony-stimulating factor (M-
    CSF)
  dendritic m.
  m. fibroblast
  hemosiderin-laden m.
  immune-associated antigen-
    positive m. (Ia+)
  inflammatory m.
  m. inflammatory protein (MIP)
  marginal metallophilic m.
  marginal zone m.
  m. migration inhibition test
  scavenger m.
  system of m.
macrophage-activating factor (MAF)
macrophage-derived
  m.-d. chemokine (MDC)
  m.-d. tumor necrosis factor
macrophage-like synoviocyte
macrophagic myofasciitis
macrophagocyte
macroscopic agglutination test
macrovascular
macrovesicular steatosis
mactans
  Latrodectus m.
macula, pl. maculae
  m. atrophica
  cerebral m.
  m. cerulea
  m. gonorrhoica
  mongolian m.

M

macula *(continued)*
    Saenger m.
    m. solaris
macular
    m. amyloidosis
    m. atrophy
    m. erythema
    m. leprosy
    m. purpura
    m. rash
    m. syphilid
maculata
    parapsoriasis m.
    pityriasis m.
maculate
maculation
maculatum
    atrophoderma striatum et m.
macule
    ash-leaf m.
    atrophic m.
    café-au-lait m. (CALM)
    cayenne pepper-like m.
    confetti m.
    congenital hypomelanotic m.
    evanescent m.
    hypopigmented m.
    labial melanotic m.
    lance-ovate m.
    mongolian m.
maculoanesthetic leprosy
maculoerythematous
maculopapular rash
maculopapule
maculosa
    lepra m.
    purpura m.
    urticaria m.
maculosus
    herpes tonsurans m.
    nevus m.
Madajet XL local anesthesia
madarosis
Madelung disease
madescent
madidans
    eczema m.
Madin-Darby
    M.-D. bovine kidney (MDBK)
    M.-D. bovine kidney cell
mad itch
madre
    buba m.
Madura
    M. boil
    M. foot
madurae
    Actinomadura m.

Madurella
    M. grisea
    M. mycetomi
maduromycosis
mAECA
    monoclonal antiendothelial cell antibody
maedi virus
MAF
    macrophage-activating factor
mafenide acetate
Maffucci syndrome
mafosfamide
Magan
MAGE
    melanoma-associated gene
Magellan Monitor
maggot
    Congo floor m.
    m. therapy
magnesium
    m. salicylate
    m. sulfate
magnetic resonance imaging (MRI)
magnetic-resonance imaging-compatible hollow-fiber bioreactor
magnetization transfer imaging (MTI)
magnolia
magnus
    Peptostreptococcus m.
Magsal
MAI
    Mycobacterium avium-intracellulare
    MAI bacteremia
maintenance
    m. cyclosporine monotherapy (mCsA)
    m. dose
Majocchi
    M. disease
    M. granuloma
    M. purpura
    purpura annularis telangiectodes of M.
major
    m. agglutinin
    aphthae m.
    Babesia m.
    m. basic protein (MBP)
    erythema multiforme m.
    m. histocompatibility
    m. histocompatibility complex (MHC)
    m. histocompatibility complex class I (MHC class I)
    m. histocompatibility complex class II (MHC class II)

m. histocompatibility complex (MHC) class II allele DRB1, DRB3, DRB4, DRB5, and DQB1

m. histocompatibility complex restriction

Leishmania m.

m. outer membrane protein (MOMP)

thalassemia m.

variola m.

makeup

Covermark corrective m.

Dermablend m.

mal

m. de Cayenne

m. de los pintos

m. del pinto

m. de Meleda

m. de San Lazaro

m. morado

m. perforans

m. perforant

m. perforant du pied

Malabar

M. itch

M. leprosy

M. ulcer

malabarica

phlegmasia m.

malabsorption

fat m.

lactose m.

malachite green

malacoplakia

maladie du sommeil

malady

Mortimer m.

malaise

malakoplakia

malaleuca tree

malalignment

varus m.

malar

m. butterfly rash

m. erythema

malaria

apocrine m.

cerebral m.

m. prophylaxis

therapeutic m.

malariae

Plasmodium m.

malarial therapy

Malassezia

M. furfur

M. ovalis

M. pachydermatis

malathion

malayi

Brugia m.

MALDI-TOF

matrix-assisted laser desorption ionization-time of flight

male

m. pattern alopecia

m. pattern baldness

maleate

azatadine m.

brompheniramine m.

chlorpheniramine m.

dexchlorpheniramine m.

methysergide m.

malformation

arteriovenous m. (AVM)

capillary m.

cystic lymphatic m.

lymphatic m.

venous m.

Malherbe

calcifying epithelioma of M.

M. calcifying epithelioma

epithelioma of M.

M. tumor

malic acid

maligna

lentigo m.

lymphogranulomatosis m.

onychia m.

papulosis atrophicans m.

pustula m.

scarlatina m.

variola m.

malignancy

B-cell m.

myositis with m.

systemic m.

malignant

m. acanthosis nigricans

m. angioendotheliomatosis

m. atrophic papulosis

m. blue nevus

m. bubo

m. catarrhal fever

m. catarrhal fever virus

NOTES

M

malignant *(continued)*
    m. catarrh of cattle
    m. chondroid syringoma
    m. clear cell acrospiroma
    m. degeneration
    m. down
    m. dyskeratosis
    m. eccrine poroma
    m. eccrine spiradenoma
    m. fibrous histiocytoma (MFH)
    m. glomus tumor (MGT)
    m. hemangioendothelioma
    m. hemangiopericytoma
    m. histiocytosis
    m. lentigo melanoma
    m. lymphoma
    m. melanoma in situ
    m. mole syndrome
    m. neoplasia
    m. neoplastic disease
    m. neuroleptic syndrome
    m. nodular hidradenoma
    m. papillomatosis
    m. papillomatosis of Degos
    m. peripheral nerve sheath tumor
    m. potentially fatal asthma
    m. progression
    m. pustule
    m. pyoderma
    m. smallpox
    m. systemic mastocytosis
    m. transformation
maligne
    papulose atrophicante m.
malignum
    granuloma m.
    keratoma m.
malignus
    pemphigus m.
malingering
Malis scissors
Mallazine Eye drops
mallei (*pl. of* malleus)
mallei
    Malleomyces m.
mallein
malleinization
Malleomyces
    M. mallei
    M. pseudomallei
mallet toe
malleus, pl. **mallei**
Mallorca miliary actinic acne
malnutrition
    episodic m.
    protein-energy m.
malodorous sweat
Maloney leukemia virus

malpighian layer
malpighii
    stratum m.
MALT
    mucosa-associated lymphoid tissue
    MALT lymphoma
malt
Malta fever
maltase
    acid m.
Maltese cross
maltodextrin
    Calgitrol calcium alginate wound
      dressing with m.
maltophilia
    Stenotrophomonas m.
    Xanthomonas m.
maltose-binding protein (MABP, MBP)
malt-worker's lung
malum
    m. coxae senilis
    m. perforans
    m. perforans pedis
Malvern analyzer
MAM
    Mycoplasma arthritidis mitogen
mamanpian
mammary
    m. cancer virus of mice
    m. Paget disease
    m. tumor virus of mice
mammilla, pl. **mammillae**
mammilliform
mammillitis
    bovine herpes m.
    bovine ulcerative m.
    bovine vaccinia m.
Manchurian
    M. hemorrhagic fever
    M. typhus
Mancini technique
mandibulae
    torus m.
mandibular torus
mandibuloacral dysplasia
mandibulofacial dysostosis
Mandol
mandrillaris
    Balamuthia m.
maneuver
    all-fours m.
    Apley m.
    arm duration m.
    arm raises m.
    arm straighten m.
    chair-rise m.
    floor-sit m.
    Gower m.

leg-raise m.
neck-flexion m.
pick-up m.
Proetz m.
stool-step m.
straight-leg duration m.
straight-leg lift m.
supine-to-prone m.
supine-to-sit m.
touch object m.
Valsalva m.

manganese superoxide dismutase gene
mange
demodectic m.
follicular m.
sarcoptic m.
mango dermatitis
manifestation
allergic m.
clinical m.
cutaneous m.
extraglandular m. (EGM)
mucocutaneous m.
presenting clinical m.
manipulation
gene m.
Mankin histologic/histochemical scale
mannan-binding
m.-b. lectin (MBL)
m.-b. lectin deficiency
mannequin
mannitol
mannose-binding
m.-b. lectin (MBL)
m.-b. protein
mannose binding molecule
mannosidosis
Mann-Whitney U test
man-of-war
Portuguese m.-o.-w.
MANOVA
multivariate analysis of variance
Manson
M. hemoptysis
M. pyosis
M. schistosomiasis
Mansonella
M. ozzardi
M. streptocerca
mansoni
Schistosoma m.

mansonii
Cladosporium m.
Mantadil
Mantel-Haenszel
M.-H. test
M.-H. test for linearity
M.-H. weighted odds ratio
M_1 antigen
mantle
Acid M.
m. cell lymphoma
Mantoux
M. pit
M. test
manubriosternal joint
manum
manus
tinea pedis et m.
manuum
keratolysis exfoliativa areata m.
tinea m.
MAO inhibitor
MAP
mitogen-activated protein
mitogen-activating protein
multiantigenic peptide
map
proteomic m.
Mapharsen organic arsenic
MAPK
mitogen-activated protein kinase
maple
m. bark disease
box elder m.
red m.
sugar m.
m. tree
m. tree pollen
maple-bark stripper's disease
MAPMAKER/QTL
mapping
epitope m.
fluorescence overlay antigen m.
(FOAM)
Maprotiline
Maranox
marasmic kwashiorkor
marasmus
Marax
Marbaxin

M

NOTES

marble
    m. cake hyperpigmentation
    m. skin
marblization
Marblot test kit
Marburg
    M. virus
    M. virus disease
Marcaine
Marcelle Sunblock
marcescens
    Serratia m.
Marcillin
Marek
    M. disease
    M. disease virus
Marena compression garment
Marezine
marfamoid hypermobility syndrome
Marfan
    M. law
    M. syndrome
marfanoid
    m. habitus
    m. hypermobility syndrome
margarine disease
margin
    free m.
    hidden m.
marginal
    m. alopecia
    m. band
    m. donor
    m. metallophilic macrophage
    m. nevus
    m. zone B-cell lymphoma (MZBL)
    m. zone macrophage
marginalis
    alopecia m.
    keratoelastoidosis m.
marginata
    alopecia m.
margination
    lesion m.
marginatum
    eczema m.
    erythema m.
    keratoacanthoma centrifugum m.
Marie-Bamberger syndrome
Marie-Strümpell disease
marine
    m. animal sting
    m. dermatitis
Marinesco-Sjögren syndrome
Marinesco succulent hand
Marinol
marinum
    Mycobacterium m.

marionette line
Marjolin ulcer
mark
    beauty m.
    dhobie m.
    ecchymotic m.
    erythematous m.
    port-wine m.
    strawberry m.
    stretch m.
    Unna m.
    washerman's m.
marked localized reaction
marker
    allotypic m.
    bone formation m.
    bone resorption m.
    bone turnover m.
    cell surface m.
    D'Assumpeau rhytidoplasty m.
    DR/MLC cell m.
    erythrocyte sheet rosette cell m.
    FAB-1 cell m.
    m. gene
    genetic m.
    highly polymorphic
      microsatellite m.
    Ia cell m.
    pan T-cell m.
    peroxidase cell m.
    serum m.
    solid-tumor m.
    Sudan cell m.
    surrogate m.
    T-cell m.
    tumor m.
market men disease
marking
    bronchovascular m.
Markov state-transition model
Marmine
    M. Injection
    M. Oral
marmorata
    cutis m.
marmorated
marmorization
marmoset virus
marneffei
    Penicillium m.
Maroteaux-Lamy
    M.-L. mucopolysaccharidosis
    M.-L. syndrome
marrow
    m. failure syndrome
    m. space
Marseilles fever
Marshall syndrome

Marshall-White syndrome
marsh elder
marsupialization
Marthritic
Marzola flap
Mas antigen
mascara
    solvent-based m.
    water-based m.
maschalephidrosis
maschalyperidrosis
mask
    Acnomel Acne M.
    m. burn
    Hutchinson m.
    luetic m.
    Neutrogena Acne M.
    PEP m.
    m. of pregnancy
    Swiss Therapy eye m.
    tropical m.
masked virus
Mason-Pfizer virus
masoprocol cream
masque biliaire
MASS
    mitral valve prolapse, aortic anomalies,
    skeletal changes, and skin changes
    MASS syndrome
mass
    body m.
    m. infection
    m. median aerodynamic diameter
    (MMD)
massive cerebral edema
massive-dose desensitization
Masson
    M. intravascular endothelial
    proliferation
    M. nevus
    M. pseudoangiosarcoma
    M. trichrome
    M. trichrome stain
mast
    m. cell
    m. cell degranulation test
    m. cell inhibitor
    m. cell proteinase
Mastadenovirus
mastectomy
    radical m.
master regulator gene

Mastisol
mastitis
    bovine m.
mastocyte
mastocytoma
    solitary m.
mastocytosis
    benign systemic m.
    cutaneous m.
    diffuse cutaneous m.
    malignant systemic m.
    papular m.
    pseudoxanthomatous m.
    m. syndrome
    systemic m.
    telangiectatic systemic m.
mastoiditis
Masugi nephritis
mat
    m. burn
    Harris pressure m.
    telangiectatic m.
Matarasso facelift scissors
matchbox sign
matched
    m. related donor (MRD)
    m. unrelated donor (MURD)
    m. unrelated donor stem cell
    transplant (mini-MUD)
material
    absorbent gelling m. (AGM)
    cross-reacting m.
    DermAssist wound filling m.
    Epicel skin graft m.
    keratinous m.
    keratotic m.
    periodic acid-Schiff-positive m.
    m. safety data sheet (MSDS)
    test m.
maternal immunity
maternus
    nevus m.
matricectomy
matrices (*pl. of* matrix)
Matrigel
matrilin-1
matrilysin
    a disintegrin and m. (ADAM)
matrix, pl. **matrices**
    M. collagen
    m. component
    distal nail m.

M

NOTES

matrix *(continued)*
    extracellular m. (ECM)
    fibrin m.
    hair m.
    m. macromolecule
    m. metalloproteinase (MMP)
    m. metalloproteinase-2 (MMP-2)
    m. metalloproteinase-3 (MMP-3)
    m. metalloproteinase-7 (MMP-7)
    m. metalloproteinase-8 (MMP-8)
    m. metalloproteinase-9 (MMP-9)
    m. metalloproteinase-10 (MMP-10)
    nail m.
    proximal nail m.
    m. synthesis
    m. unguis
    variance-covariance m.
matrix-assisted laser desorption ionization-time of flight (MALDI-TOF)
matrix-degrading enzyme
matter
    particulate m.
matting
    telangiectatic m. (TM)
mattress
    AkroTech m.
    convoluted foam m.
    Roho m.
    vinyl-alternating air m.
Matuhasi-Ogata phenomenon
maturation
    affinity m.
    m. B cell
mature bacteriophage
maturity-onset diabetes of the young (MODY)
Maurer optimization test
Mauriac syndrome
Mauserung phenomenon
max
    VO$_2$ m.
        maximal oxygen consumption
Maxacalcitol
Maxafil
Maxair Autohaler
Maxaquin Oral
Max-Caro
Maxenal
Maxidex
Maxiflor topical
maximal
    m. oxygen consumption (VO$_2$ max)
    m. ventilation (MV)
    m. voluntary ventilation (MVV)
maximum
    m. breathing capacity (MBC)

    M. Strength Desenex Antifungal Cream
    M. Strength Nytol
    m. temperature
Maxi-Myst bronchodilator
Maxipime
Maxitrol Ophthalmic
Maxivate Topical
Maxivent
Maxon suture
Maxorb
    M. alginate wound cover
    M. alginate wound dressing
Mayaro virus
Mayer hemalum
mayfly, may fly
maynei
    Euroglyphus m.
Mayo
    M. classification of rheumatoid elbow
    M. modified total elbow arthroplasty
mazamorra
Mazon Medicated Soap
Mazzotti
    M. reaction
    M. test
MBC
    maximum breathing capacity
    minimal bactericidal concentration
MBL
    mannan-binding lectin
    mannose-binding lectin
MBP
    major basic protein
    maltose-binding protein
    myelin basic protein
McArdle disease
MCC
    measure mucociliary clearance
MCCN
    mesangiocapillary glomerulonephritis
McCune-Albright syndrome
MCF
    monocyte chemotactic factor
McKeever and MacIntosh hemiarthroplasty
McKenzie test
McKrae herpesvirus
McKusick
    oculocerebral syndrome of Cross and M.
    M. syndrome
McKusick-Kaufman syndrome
MCL
    mucocutaneous leishmaniasis
3M Clean Seals bandage

McLeod phenotype
McMurray sign
MCN
  minimal change nephropathy
McNemar
  M. test
  M. test of significance
M-component hypergammaglobulinemia
MCP
  monocyte chemotactic protein
MCP-1
  monocyte chemoattractant protein-1
  monocyte chemotactic peptide-1
m-cresyl acetate
mCsA
  maintenance cyclosporine monotherapy
M-CSF
  macrophage colony-stimulating factor
MCTD
  mixed connective tissue disease
MCV
  molluscum contagiosum virus
MDBK
  Madin-Darby bovine kidney
  MDBK cell
MDC
  macrophage-derived chemokine
MDI
  metered-dose inhaler
  isocyanate MDI
MDR-TB
  multidrug-resistant tuberculosis
MDS
  myelodysplastic syndrome
MDT
  multidrug therapy
meadow
  m. dermatitis
  m. fescue
  m. fescue grass
  m. foxtail
  m. foxtail grass
meadow-grass
  m.-g. dermatitis
  m.-g. dermatosis
meal
  rye m.
  soybean m.
mean
  m. forced expiratory flow during
    the middle of FVC (FEF$_{25-75\%}$)
  standardized response m. (SRM)

measles
  atypical m.
  bastard m.
  black m.
  confluent m.
  m. convalescent serum
  French m.
  German m.
  m. immune globulin (human)
  m. immunoglobulin
  modified m.
  m., mumps, and rubella vaccine
    (MMR)
  m., mumps and rubella vaccines,
    combined
  three-day m.
  tropical m.
  m. virus
  m. virus vaccine
  m. virus vaccine, live
measure
  CD4+ M.
  European Consensus Lupus
    Activity M. (ECLAM)
  m. mucociliary clearance (MCC)
  Systemic Lupus Activity M.
    (SLAM)
Measurin
meatus
mebendazole
Mecca balsam
mechanica
  acne m.
mechanical
  m. abrasion
  m. acne
  m. alopecia
  m. loading
  m. pleurodesis
  m. vector
  m. ventilation (MV)
  m. ventilator
  m. vessel blockage
mechanic hand
mechanism
  m. of action
  defense m.
  genomic glucocorticoid m.
  immunological m.
  interferon-independent m.
  jet-bubble m.
mechanoblister

M

NOTES

mechanobullous disease
mechlorethamine hydrochloride
Mecholyl skin test
Meclan topical
meclizine hydrochloride
meclocycline sulfosalicylate
meclofenamate sodium
Meclomen Oral
MED
    minimal erythema dose
    minimum effective dose
Mederma
MEDI-493
media
    acute otitis m. (AOM)
    chronic otitis m.
    otitis m.
    pneumococcal otitis m.
    radiographic contrast m. (RCM)
    secretory otitis m.
medial
    m. canaliform dystrophy
    m. hemijoint articular space
median
    m. canaliform dystrophy
    m. effective concentration (EC_{50})
    m. nail dystrophy
    m. nerve
    m. raphe cyst of the penis
    m. rhomboid glossitis (MRG)
    m. survival time (MST)
mediana
    glossitis rhombica m.
    glossitis rhomboidea m.
MEDI-507 anti-CD2 Mab
mediastinal
    m. amyloidosis
    m. lipomatosis
mediastinoscopy
mediate contagion
mediation
    fibroblast m.
mediator
    m. cell
    downstream m.
    vasoactive m.
medical
    M. Dynamics 5990 needle
      arthroscope
    m. free electron laser (MFEL)
    M. Research Council (MRC)
    M. Research Council Laboratories
      (MRCL)
    m. therapy
medicamentosa
    acne m.
    alopecia m.
    dermatitis m.

    dermatosis m.
    embolia cutis m.
    rhinitis m.
    stomatitis m.
    urticaria m.
medicamentosus
medication-induced hyperlipoproteinemia
medicinal eruption
medicine
    complementary and alternative M.
      (CAM)
    environmental M.
    European Confederation for
      Laboratory M. (ECLM)
    evidence-based m. (EBM)
    Reese's Pinworm M.
    sports M.
Medi-Facts system
Medifil collagen
Medihaler-Epi Ergotamine
Medihaler-Iso
Medihoney
Medi-Mist nebulizer
medina worm
medinensis
    Dracunculus m.
Medin poliomyelitis
Mediplast Plaster
Medipore Dress-it dressing
Medipren
Medi-Quick Topical Ointment
Medi-Strumpf support hose
Mediterranean
    M. erythematous fever
    M. exanthematous fever
    M. lymphoma
    M. spotted fever
medium
    dermatophyte test m. (DTM)
    Dulbecco m.
    excimer lasing m.
    fibroblast-conditioned m. (FCM)
    HAT m.
    He-Ne lasing m.
    Iscove complete m.
    Iscove modified Dulbecco m.
    krypton lasing m.
    m. lesion
    Sabouraud m.
    Thayer-Martin m.
    Tissue-Tek OCT m.
medi virus
Medix ultrasonic nebulizer
Medlar body
Medpor surgical implant
Medralone Injection
Medrol
    M. Dosepak

M. Oral
M. Veriderm
medrysone
medulla
medullary
m. carcinoma flush
m. reticulosis
MedWatch
Mees
M. line
M. stripe
MEF
middle ear fluid
mefenamic acid
mefloquine hydrochloride
Mefoxin
Megabombus **sting**
Megace
megacins
megacystic microcolon syndrome
megaloblastic anemia
megalonychia
megalonychosis
Megalopyge
M. opercularis
M. opercularis sting
megaterium
Bacillus m.
megestrol acetate
meglumine diatrizoate enema study
MEGX
monoethylglycinexylidide
MEGX test/score
meibomian
m. gland
m. gland dysfunction
Meinicke test
Meirowsky phenomenon
Meischer syndrome
Meissner corpuscle
MEK
methyl ethyl ketone
mekongi
Schistosoma m.
Melacine vaccine
Melanex
M. solution
melanidrosis
melanin
hair m.
m. synthesis

m. transfer
white m.
melaninogenica
Prevotella m.
melanism
melanoacanthoma
oral m.
melanoacanthosis
melanoblast
melanoblastoma
melanocarcinoma
melanocomous
melanocyte
cultured autologous m.
intradermal m.
melanocyte-stimulating hormone (MSH)
melanocytic nevus
melanocytosis
oculodermal m.
melanoderma
m. cachecticorum
m. chloasma
parasitic m.
racial m.
Riehl m.
senile m.
melanodermatitis toxica lichenoides
melanodermia
melanodermic
melanodermicum
erythema chronicum figuratum m.
melanogenesis
melanohidrosis
melanoid
melanoleukoderma colli
melanoma
acral lentiginous m. (ALM)
amelanotic m.
benign juvenile m.
m. cell adhesion molecule (Mel-CAM)
Cloudman m.
conventional cutaneous malignant m. (CCMM)
desmoplastic malignant m.
halo m.
juvenile m.
lentigo maligna m.
malignant lentigo m.
minimal deviation m.
multiple primary m. (MPM)
nevoid malignant m. (NMM)

M

NOTES

melanoma *(continued)*
    nodular malignant m.
    spindle cell m.
    spitzoid malignant m.
    subungual m.
    superficial malignant m.
    superficial spreading m. (SSM)
    m. warning sign
melanoma-associated gene (MAGE)
melanoma-specific antigen
melanomatosis
melanomatous
melanonychia
    longitudinal m.
    m. striata
melanopathy
melanophage
    perifollicular m.
melanophore
melanoplakia
melanoprotein
melanorrhoea
    Anacardium m.
melanosis
    addisonian m.
    m. cachecticorum
    m. circumscripta precancerosa
    m. corii degenerativa
    m. diffusa congenita
    Dubreuilh precancerous m.
    generalized m.
    neonatal pustular m.
    neurocutaneous m.
    oculodermal m.
    pustular m.
    Riehl m.
    tar m.
    transient neonatal pustular m.
    universal acquired m.
melanosity
melanosome
melanotic
    m. ameloblastoma
    m. carcinoma
    m. freckle
    m. freckle of Hutchinson
    m. pigment
    m. progonoma
    m. protoporphyria
    m. prurigo of Borda
    m. prurigo of Hebra
    m. prurigo of Pierini
    m. sarcoma
    m. whitlow
melanotrichia
melanotrichous
melas
    icterus m.

melasma
    m. gravidarum
    m. universale
melatonin
Mel-CAM
    melanoma cell adhesion molecule
Meleda
    M. disease
    mal de M.
Meleney
    chronic undermining ulcer of M.
    M. chronic undermining ulcer
    M. gangrene
melioidosis
    Whitmore m.
Melkersson-Rosenthal syndrome
Melkersson syndrome
Mellaril
mellifera
    Apis m.
mellitus
    diabetes m.
    insulin-dependent diabetes m.
      (IDDM)
    noninsulin-dependent diabetes m.
      (NIDDM)
    type 1 diabetes m. (T1DM)
    type 2 diabetes m. (T2DM)
Melnick-Fraser syndrome
Meloidae
melorheostosis
meloxicam tablet
melphalan
Melzer reagent
membrane
    antiglomerular basement m. (anti-
      GMB)
    m. attack complex (MAC)
    basal cell m.
    basement m.
    bronchial mucous m.
    Bruch m.
    collodion m.
    croupous m.
    diphtheritic m.
    false m.
    m. filter
    focal rupture of basement m.
    glomerular basement m. (GBM)
    hyaline basement m.
    immunoglobulin m.
    mucous m.
    PAN m.
    plasma m.
    m. ruffling
    semiimpermeable m.
    Seprafilm bioresorbable m.
    subbasement m. (SBM)

subepithelial basement m. (SBM)
synovial m.
tuberculosis of serous m.
tympanic m. (TM)
membrane-bound cytochrome b$_{558}$
membrane-coating granule
membrane-type matrix metalloproteinase
membranolytic attack complex (MAC)
membranoproliferative glomerulonephritis
membranous
m. aplasia cutis
m. desquamation
m. glomerulonephritis
m. lupus nephritis
m. nephropathy (MN)
memory
B-cell m.
immune m.
immunologic m.
MEN
multiple endocrine neoplasia
multiple endocrine neoplasms
MEN syndrome
MEN 1
multiple endocrine neoplasia type 1
men
Anti-Acne Formula for M.
men who have sex with m.
(MSM)
Menadol
MEND
minimum effective naproxen dose
Mendelson syndrome
Menest
Mengo
M. encephalitis
M. virus
Meni-D
méningéale
tache m.
meningeal stage
meningioma
cutaneous m.
meningitic streak
meningitidis
Neisseria m.
meningitis, pl. **meningitides**
African m.
bacterial m. (BM)
basal m.
m. of the base
basilar m.

benign recurrent
endothelioleukocytic m.
brucellar m.
m. carcinomatosa
cerebrospinal m.
chemical m.
chronic posterior basic m.
curable serous m.
epidemic cerebrospinal m.
external m.
gummatous m.
Haemophilus influenzae m.
influenzal m.
internal m.
localized tuberculous m.
meningococcal m.
Mollaret m.
m. necrotoxica reactiva
occlusive m.
otitic m.
otogenic m.
plasmodial m.
posttraumatic rheumatic m.
m. sympathica
torula m.
torular m.
Wallgren aseptic m.
yeast m.
meningocele
atretic m.
rudimentary m.
meningococcal
m. arthritis
m. meningitis
m. polysaccharide vaccine, groups
A, C, Y, W-135
m. vaccine
meningococcemia
acute m.
meningoencephalitis
acute primary hemorrhagic m.
biundulant m.
cryptococcal m.
herpetic m.
mumps m.
meningooculofacial angiomatosis
meningosepticum
Flavobacterium m.
meningovascular neurosyphilis
meningovasculitis
meniscal fibrocartilage
meniscus, pl. **menisci**

M

NOTES

Menkes kinky hair syndrome
menocelis
Menomune-A/C/Y/W-135
menopausal flushing
Menorest
menstrual
    m. acne
    m. dermatosis
menstrualis
    herpes m.
mentagra
    acne m.
    Alibert m.
mentagrophytes
    Trichophyton m.
mentalis
    herpes m.
mental retardation, overgrowth, remarkable face, and acanthosis nigrans (MORFAN)
Mentax cream
menthol
    camphorated m.
Mentholatum
men who have sex with men (MSM)
MEP
    mucoid exopolysaccharide
meperidine
mephenytoin
Mephyton Oral
Mepitel contact layer sheet
mepivacaine hydrochloride
Mepore absorptive dressing
meprobamate
Mepron
mequinol and tretinoin
meralgia paresthetica
merbromin
2-mercaptoethane sulphonate sodium (mesna)
Mercapto mix
6-mercaptopurine (6-MP)
Mercedes
    M. Benz incision
    M. pattern
mercurials
    organic m.
mercurial stomatitis
mercuric oxide
mercurochrome
mercury
    ammoniated m.
    m. arc
    m. granuloma
    m. hyperpigmentation
    m. poisoning
meridian

Merkel
    M. cell
    M. cell carcinoma
    M. cell tumor
Merkel-cell-neurite complex
Merkel-Ranvier
    tactile cell of M.-R.
Merlenate topical
merocrine gland
meropenem
merosin deficiency dystrophy
merozygote
Merrem I.V.
Mersol
Merthiolate
Meruvax II
mesalamine
Mesalt debridement dressing
mesangial complex formation
mesangiocapillary glomerulonephritis (MCCN)
mesangium
Mesantoin
mesenchymal
    m. precursor
    m. progenitor cell
    m. tissue
mesenchyme
    synovial m.
mesentericography
    selective m.
mesenteric vasculitis
mesh
    absorbable m.
meshwork
    coagulation m.
mesilate
    nafamostat m.
mesna
    2-mercaptoethane sulphonate sodium
Mesnex
mesoderm
mesodermal
    m. dysplasia
    m. nevus
mesodermogenic neurosyphilis
mesogenic
mesophilic
mesosyphilis
mesothelial cell
mesothelioma
mesquite tree
messenger RNA (mRNA)
Mestranol
mesylate
    bitolterol m.
    dihydroergotamine m.
    saquinavir m.

MET
   minimum elicitation threshold
Metabisulfite
metabolic
   m. acidosis
   m. alteration
   m. bone disease
   m. disorder
   m. enthesopathy
   m. remission
   m. study
metabolism
   aberrant glycosaminoglycan m.
   amino acid m.
   arachidonic acid m.
   chylomicron m.
   copper m.
   glycosphingolipid m.
   P450 m.
   phenylalanine m.
   purine m.
   transcellular m.
   tyrosine m.
metabolite
   arachidonic acid m.
   16-hydroxylated m.
   oxygen m.
metacarpal index
metacarpophalangeal (MP)
   m. joint subluxation
metachromasia
metachronous tissue lesion
metaguazone
metal
   m. dermatitis
   m. fume fever
   m. hyperpigmentation
   m. intoxication
metal-catalyzed oxidative cleavage
metalloenzyme
metalloproteinase
   matrix m. (MMP)
   membrane-type matrix m.
   punctated m.
   tissue inhibitor of m. (TIMP)
metalloproteinase-2
   matrix m. (MMP-2)
metalloproteinase-3
   matrix m. (MMP-3)
metalloproteinase-7
   matrix m. (MMP-7)

metalloproteinase-8
   matrix m. (MMP-8)
metalloproteinase-9
   matrix m. (MMP-9)
metalloproteinase-10
   matrix m. (MMP-10)
metalloscopy
Metamucil
metaphyseal dysplasia
metaphysis, pl. **metaphyses**
metaplasia
   agnogenic myeloid m. (AMM)
   goblet cell m.
metaplastic mucus-secreting cell
Metaprel
metaproterenol
   Arm-a-Med M.
   Dey-Dose M.
   m. sulfate
metaraminol bitartrate
metargidin
Metasep
metastasis, pl. **metastases**
   biochemical m.
   contact m.
   hematogenous m.
   in-transit m.
   lymphogenous m.
   miliary m.
   tumor, node, m. (TNM)
metastatic
   m. calcification
   m. calcinosis cutis
   m. granuloma
   m. mumps
   m. tuberculous abscess
metatarsal (MT)
metatarsalgia
metatarsophalangeal (MTP)
   m. joint
metatypical carcinoma
Metazoa
metazoal parasite
metazoan infection
metazoonosis
Metchnikoff theory
Meted
meter
   AccuTrax Peak Flow M.
   Assess peak flow m.
   Astech peak flow m.
   AsthmaMentor Peak Flow M.

M

NOTES

meter *(continued)*
    Mini-Wright peak flow m.
    peak flow m.
    Pocketpeak peak flow m.
    TruZone peak flow m.
metered-dose inhaler (MDI)
methacholine
    m. bronchoprovocation challenge
    m. chloride
    m. chloride skin test
Methacin
methacrylate
    butyl m.
    ethyl m.
    polymethyl m.
methandrostenolone
methapyrilene hydrochloride
methdilazine
methenamine
methicillin-resistant *Staphylococcus*
    aureus **(MRSA)**
methicillin sodium
methionine
methocarbamol
method
    ABC m.
    avidin-biotin-peroxidase complex m.
    Brehmer m.
    Buehler m.
    Cox-Spjotvoll m.
    Dick m.
    dipstick m.
    disk sensitivity m.
    double antibody m.
    Fisher m.
    Genant m.
    heteroduplexing m.
    histoblot m.
    immunofluorescence m.
    Kaplan-Meier m.
    multinomial (polytomous) logistic
        regression m.
    Ouchterlony m.
    pencil m.
    potato-peeler m.
    prick-test m.
    Ranawat triangle m.
    Sakaguchi-Kauppi m.
    Schick m.
    TUNEL m.
    van der Heijde modification of
        Sharp m.
    volumetric m.
methotrexate (MTX)
methoxsalen
methoxycinnamate
    octyl m.
    m. and oxybenzone

methoxypromazine
methoxypsoralen
5-methoxypsoralen (5-MOP)
8-methoxypsoralen (8-MOP)
methyl
    m. ethyl ketone (MEK)
    m. nicotinate
    m. salicylate
methylation
    stochastic m.
methylbenzethonium chloride
methylcellulose
methylchloroisothiazoli-
    none/methylisothiazolinone
methyldopa
methylene blue
methylmalonic
methylmethacrylate
methylprednisolone
    m. acetate (MPA)
    pulse m.
methylrosaniline chloride
methylxanthine
methysergide maleate
Meticorten Oral
Metimyd Ophthalmic
Metoprolol in Dilated Cardiomyopathy
    Trial
Metreton Ophthalmic
MetroCream
MetroGel Topical
MetroGel-Vaginal
Metro IV Injection
MetroLotion
metronidazole
Metzenbaum scissors
Mexican tea
mexiletine
Meyerson nevus
Meyhoeffer curette
Mezlin
mezlocillin sodium
MF
    mycosis fungoides
MFEL
    medical free electron laser
MFG-IRAP retrovirus
MFH
    malignant fibrous histiocytoma
MG
    myasthenia gravis
mg
    milligram
MGC
    multinucleated giant cell
MGT
    malignant glomus tumor

MGUS
monoclonal gammopathy of unknown
significance
MHAQ
Modified Health Assessment
Questionnaire
MHA-TP
microhemagglutination-*Treponema
pallidum*
MHA-TP test
MHC
major histocompatibility complex
MHC antigen deficiency
chromosome 6, class III MHC
MHC class I, II
MHC class I, II deficiency
MHC molecule
MHC restriction
MI
myocardial infarction
Mi-2 antibody
Miacalcin
Miami STAR tissue expander
Mibelli
angiokeratoma of M.
M. angiokeratoma
M. disease
porokeratosis of M.
M. porokeratosis
M. syndrome
MIC
minimal inhibitory concentration
minimum inhibitory concentration
micaceous scale
Micanol cream
Micatin Topical
micdadei
Legionella m.
mice
back m.
mammary cancer virus of m.
mammary tumor virus of m.
New Zealand m.
pneumonia virus of m.
SCID m.
severe combined
immunodeficient m.
transgenic m.
micelle
Michel solution
miconazole

Micro
Retin-A M.
microabscess
intraepidermal m.
Munro m.
m. of mycosis fungoides
Pautrier m.
m. of psoriasis
Micro-Adson forceps with teeth
microaerophilic
microangiopathic hemolytic anemia
microaspiration
microbe
microbial
m. associates
m. genetics
m. persistence
m. vitamin
microbic
microbicidal
microbicide
Pro 2000 topical m.
Microbid
microbiologic
microbiologist
microbiology
microbiotic
microbism
latent m.
microceras
Dermatophagoides m.
microcheilia
microchimeric
m. antigen
m. cell
microchimerism
microcircular
microcirculatory disturbance
Micrococcus
micrococcus, pl. **micrococci**
coagulase-positive m.
microcontaminant
microcystic adnexal carcinoma (MAC)
microdermabrasion
MicroDigitrapper-HR, -S, -V
microdomain
microemulsion
cyclosporine m.
microenvironment
microevolution
microfibril
fibrillin-containing m.

M

NOTES

microfilaria
    degenerated m.
microfine
    zinc oxide m.
microfocus, pl. microfoci
MicroGard
2-microglobulin-origin amyloid deposit (A 2M)
micrognathia
microhemagglutination
microhemagglutination-*Treponema*
    m. pallidum (MHA-TP)
    m. pallidum test
microheterogeneity
microimmunofluorescence test (MIF)
MicroKlenz wound cleanser
microlymphocytotoxicity test
Micro-Mist nebulizer
microNefrin
micronodular tuberculid
micronychia
microorganism
micropapular tuberculid
microperfusion
microphage
microphagocyte
MicroPlaner soft tissue shaver
MicroPlus spirometer
Micropolyspora faeni
Micropore tape
microreactor
    immunoisolating m.
microsatellite
    m. instability (MSI)
    m. polymorphism
microscope
    electron m. (EM)
    epiluminescent skin surface m.
microscopic
    m. agglutination test
    m. polyangiitis (MPA)
microscopically controlled surgery
microscopy
    confocal laser scanning m.
    darkfield m.
    electron m.
    epiluminescence m. (ELM)
    field emission scanning electron m. (FESEM)
    immune electron m. (IEM)
    immunofluorescence m.
    immunogold electron m.
    light m.
    proton magnetic resonance m.
    surface m.
    transmission electron m. (TEM)
microshaver
    Stryker m.

microspherule
microspore
***Microsporidia* diagnostic procedure**
microsporidiosis
microsporina
    dermatomycosis m.
***Microsporon* (*var. of Microsporum*)**
microsporon
    Audouin m.
microsporosis
Microsporum, Microsporon
    M. audouinii
    M. canis
    M. canis, var distortum
    M. felineum
    M. ferrugineum
    M. fulvum
    M. furfur
    M. gypseum
    M. lanosum
    M. minutissimum
    M. nanum
microstomia
Microsulfon
microti
    Babesia m.
Micro-Trak
microtrauma
    postexertional m.
Microtrombidium
microtubule organizing center
microvascular abnormality
microvasculopathy
microvenular hemangioma
microvesicle
microvesicular steatosis
Microviridae
MID
    minimal infecting dose
midazolam
    benzodiazepine m.
middermal elastolysis
middle
    m. ear
    m. ear fluid (MEF)
midfoot
midge
    m. bite
    nimitti m.
midline
    m. granulomatosis
    m. lethal granuloma
Midol
    M. IB
    M. PM
midpoint skin test

midrange spectrum ultraviolet light
midrange-wavelength ultraviolet light
  (UVB)
Midrin
Miescher
    M. actinic granuloma
    M. cheilitis granulomatosa
    M. elastoma
    M. granulomatous cheilitis
Miescher-Leder granulomatosis
MIF
    microimmunofluorescence test
    migration-inhibitory factor
migrans
    annulus m.
    cutaneous larva m.
    erysipelas m.
    erythema chronicum m. (ECM)
    erythema nodosum m.
    larva m.
    ocular larma m.
    spiruroid larva m.
    ulcus m.
    visceral larva m.
migrant erysipelas
migrating cheilitis
migration
    m. inhibition test
    m. inhibitory factor test
    Jurkat cell m.
    transendothelial neutrophil m.
migration-inhibitory factor (MIF)
migratory
    m. glossitis
    m. panniculitis
Mikulicz
    M. aphtha
    M. disease
mild
    m. hypertension
    m. irritant
    silver protein, m.
Miles Nervine Caplets
milia (*pl. of* milium)
Milian
    M. citrine skin
    M. disease
    M. erythema
    M. sign
    M. syndrome
miliaria
    m. alba

    apocrine m.
    m. crystallina
    occlusion m.
    m. papulosa
    m. profunda
    m. propria
    pustular m.
    m. pustulosa
    m. rubra
    sebaceous m.
    m. vesiculosa
miliaris
    acne necrotica m.
    tuberculosis cutis m.
    variola m.
miliary
    m. acne
    m. fever
    m. metastasis
    m. papular syphilid
    m. sarcoid
    m. tuberculosis
milium, pl. milia
    colloid m.
    milia cyst
    milia en plaque
    juvenile colloid m.
    multiple eruptive milia
    m. neonatorum
    periocular milia
    pinhead-sized milia
    pinpoint-sized milia
milk
    acidophilus m.
    cow's m.
    m. crust
    m. factor
    goat's m.
    lactobacillary m.
    m. scall
    soy m.
    m. tetter
milkers'
    m. node
    m. nodule
    m. nodule virus
milk-induced colitis
milkpox
Millar asthma
Miller-Fisher variant
miller's asthma

M

NOTES

millet
    M. phlebectomy hook
    m. seed
mill fever
milligram (mg)
millipede sting
millipore
Mills-Reincke phenomenon
milphosis
Milroy disease
Milton
    M. disease
    M. edema
    M. urticaria
Milwaukee
    M. knee syndrome
    M. shoulder
    M. shoulder syndrome
mimicry
    molecular m.
    poxviral m.
mineralocorticoid
mineral oil
mineral-related nutritional disorder
Minerva cast
mini-allo
    allographic stem cell transplant
miniature scarlet fever
miniblade
    Beaver ES m.
    SP90 m.
minigene
Min-I-Jet
minimal
    m. bactericidal concentration (MBC)
    m. change nephropathy (MCN)
    m. deviation melanoma
    m. dose possible
    m. erythema dose (MED)
    m. infecting dose (MID)
    m. inhibitory concentration (MIC)
    m. lethal dose (MLD)
    m. phototoxic dose (MPD)
    m. pigment (MP)
    m. reacting dose (MRD)
minimal-pigment oculocutaneous albinism
mini-MUD
    matched unrelated donor stem cell
    transplant
minimum
    m. effective dose (MED)
    m. effective naproxen dose
    (MEND)
    m. elicitation threshold (MET)
    m. inhibitory concentration (MIC)
    m. temperature

MiniOX
    M. 1000
    M. 1A oxygen analyzer
Minipress
Miniscope MS-3
Mini Thin Asthma Relief
Mini-Wright peak flow meter
mink
    enteritis of m.
    m. enteritis virus
Minnesota
    M. antilymphoblast globulin
    M. Multiphasic Personality
    Inventory (MMPI)
Minocin
    M. IV injection
    M. Oral
minocycline
    m. hydrochloride
    m. hyperpigmentation
minor
    m. agglutinin
    aphthae m.
    M. Blue Dragon
    erythema multiforme m.
    M. iodine-starch test
    recurrent erythema multiforme m.
    variola m.
minoxidil
Minoxigaine
Mintezol
minus
    Spirillum m.
minute
    alveolar ventilation per m.
    oxygen consumption per m. (VO_2)
    physiological dead space ventilation
    per m.
    m. ventilation
minutissimum
    Corynebacterium m.
    Microsporum m.
miostagmin reaction
MIP
    macrophage inflammatory protein
mirabilis
    Proteus m.
Mirchamp sign
miscellaneous reaction
mismatch
    ABO m.
    CREG m.
    cross-reactive antigen group m.
missense mutation
missing self hypothesis
Mist
    AsthmaHaler M.
    Bronitin M.

Bronkaid M.
ENTsol M.
Primatene M.
Mitchell disease
mite
m. bite
m. control
dust m.
elevator grain dust m.
hair follicle m.
harvest m.
house dust m. (HDM)
house dust m. F, P
m. infestation
itch m.
nevus flammeus human granulocytic
ehrlichiosis m.
pyroglyphid m.
scabietic m.
soybean grain dust m.
m. typhus
wheat grain dust m.
mite-borne typhus
mithramycin
mitigata
variola m.
mitior
typhus m.
mitis
junctional epidermolysis bullosa
atrophicans generalisata m.
protoporphyria m.
prurigo m.
Mitis-type Ehlers-Danlos syndrome
mitochondria
mitochondrial
m. DNA syndrome
m. membrane potential
m. targeting sequence (MTS)
mitogen
Mycoplasma arthritidis m. (MAM)
pokeweed m. (PWM)
mitogen-activated
m.-a. protein (MAP)
m.-a. protein kinase (MAPK)
mitogen-activating protein (MAP)
mitogenesis
mitogenetic
mitogenic
mitoguazone
Mitraflex
M. Plus foam dressing

M. SC foam dressing
M. wound dressing
mitral
m. leaflet
m. valve prolapse, aortic
anomalies, skeletal changes, and
skin changes (MASS)
m. valve prolapse, aortic
anomalies, skeletal changes, and
skin changes syndrome
Mitrazol
Mitsuda
M. antigen
M. radiation
M. reaction
M. test
Mitutoyo digital caliper
mix
black rubber m.
caine m.
Carba m.
fragrance m. (FM)
juniper m.
Mercapto m.
paraben m.
thiuram m.
mixed
m. aerobic/anaerobic abscess
m. agglutination
m. agglutination reaction
m. agglutination test
m. asthma
m. chancre
m. connective tissue disease
(MCTD)
m. cryoglobulinemia
m. feather
m. hemangioma
m. hematopoietic chimerism
m. hepatic porphyria
m. inflammatory granuloma
m. leprosy
m. lymphocyte culture (MLC)
m. lymphocyte culture reaction
m. lymphocyte culture test
m. nail infection
m. porphyria
m. seborrheic-staphylococcal
blepharitis
m. sore
m. tumor

M

NOTES

mixed *(continued)*
    m. tumor of skin
    m. vespid antigen
mixed-linker PCR (ML-PCR)
mixing
    phenotypic m.
Mixter forceps
Miyagawa body
mizolastine
mizoribine
Mkar disease
ML3000
MLC
    mixed lymphocyte culture
       MLC test
MLD
    minimal lethal dose
MLNS
    mucocutaneous lymph node syndrome
ML-PCR
    mixed-linker PCR
MM
    multiple myeloma
    mycophenolate mofetil
       MM virus
3MM
    Whatman 3MM
MMD
    mass median aerodynamic diameter
MMF
    mycophenolate mofetil
MMP
    matrix metalloproteinase
MMP-2
    matrix metalloproteinase-2
MMP-3
    matrix metalloproteinase-3
MMP-7
    matrix metalloproteinase-7
MMP-8
    matrix metalloproteinase-8
MMP-9
    matrix metalloproteinase-9
MMP-10
    matrix metalloproteinase-10
MMPI
    Minnesota Multiphasic Personality
      Inventory
MMR
    measles, mumps, and rubella vaccine
      MMR vaccine
MMS
    Mohs micrographic surgery
MN
    membranous nephropathy
MNSs
    M. antigen
    M. blood group

MoAb
    monoclonal antibody
Mobic tablet
Mobidin
mobility
    syndrome of limited joint m.
      (SLJM)
Mobiluncus
moccasin
    m. foot
    m. snake bite
moccasin-type tinea pedis
model
    carrageenin-induced footpad
      inflammation m.
    Cholesky m.
    Markov state-transition m.
    Weibull regression m.
Modicon
modification
    posttranslational protein m.
modified
    m. Draize test
    M. Health Assessment
      Questionnaire (MHAQ)
    m. measles
    m. Rodman skin thickness score
    m. smallpox
    m. vaccinia virus Ankara strain
    m. varicella-like syndrome (MVLS)
modulation
    antigenic m.
modulator
    immune system m.
    selective estrogen receptor m.
      (SERM)
module
    CO-Oximeter m.
    intercellular adhesion m. (ICAM)
MODY
    maturity-onset diabetes of the young
MODY2-glucokinase
MODY3 HNF-1-alpha mutation
Moeller
    M. glossitis
    M. itch
moensin
mofetil
    mycophenolate m. (MM, MMF)
MOG
    myelin-oligodendrocyte glycoprotein
mohair
Mohs
    M. chemosurgery
    M. fresh-tissue technique
    M. micrographic surgery (MMS)
    M. procedure
moiety

moist
>m. gangrene
>Nasal M.
>m. papule
>m. tetter
>m. wart

Moi-Stir
moisture
>M. Ophthalmic drops
>m. vapor transmission rate (MVTR)

Moisturel moisturizer
moisturizer
>Aqua Care m.
>Betadine First Aid Antibiotics + M.
>body m.
>Eucerin Plus m.
>facial m.
>Keri m.
>Lubriderm m.
>Moisturel m.
>Nivea m.
>occlusive m.
>RoEzIt skin m.
>topical m.
>Vaseline Intensive Care m.

Mokola virus
molar
>mulberry m.

mold
>m. aeroallergen
>Alternaria m.
>m. control
>Smith-Pedersen m.
>m. spore

mole
>atypical m.
>hairy m.
>spider m.

molecular mimicry
molecule
>accessory m.
>adhesion m.
>antiapoptotic m.
>antiplatelet endothelial cell adhesion m. (anti-PCAM)
>apoptosis-associated m.
>B7 costimulatory m.
>cell adhesion m. (CAM)
>costimulatory m.
>effector m.

>endothelial-leukocyte adhesion m. (ELAM)
>Fas-Fas ligand m.
>Fas-L m.
>fusin m.
>heterotrimeric cell-membrane-bound m.
>ICOS m.
>leukocyte cell adhesion m. (leu-CAM)
>mannose binding m.
>melanoma cell adhesion m. (Mel-CAM)
>MHC m.
>multideterminant m.
>multimeric m.
>neural cell adhesion m. (NCAM)
>precursor m.
>soluble cell adhesion m.
>vascular cell adhesion m. (VCAM)

molecule-1
>endothelial leukocyte adhesion m. (ELAM-1)
>intercellular adhesion m. (ICAM-1)
>vascular cell adhesion m. (VCAM-1)

molgramostim
Mollaret
>M. HSV
>M. meningitis

molle
>fibroma m.
>heloma m.
>papilloma m.

Moll gland
mollusciformis
>nevus m.
>verruca m.

molluscoid neurofibroma
molluscous
molluscum
>m. body
>cholesterinic m.
>m. contagiosum
>m. contagiosum virus (MCV)
>m. corpuscle
>m. epitheliale
>m. fibrosum
>m. giganteum
>m. lipomatodes
>m. pendulum
>m. sebaceum

M

NOTES

molluscum *(continued)*
    m. varioliformis
    m. verrucosum
Moloney
    M. murine leukemia virus
    M. test
    M. virus
molt
MOLT-18, human T cell line
mometasone furoate
MOMP
    major outer membrane protein
Monarch Mini Mask nasal interface
monarthritis
monarticular
Monazole-7
Mondor disease
mongolian
    m. macula
    m. macule
    m. spot
mongolism
monilated
monilethrix
Monilia albicans
Moniliaceae
monilial
    m. granuloma
    m. intertrigo
    m. onychia
    m. paronychia
moniliasis
moniliforme
    Fusarium m.
moniliform hair
moniliformis
    lichen ruber m.
    Streptobacillus m.
Moniliformis soni
moniliid
Monistat
    M. IV Injection
    M. Vaginal
Monistat-Derm Topical
monitor
    AirWatch Asthma m.
    Digitrapper MkIII sleep m.
    EcoCheck oxygen m.
    Magellan M.
    NoxBOX m.
    Pick and Go m.
    TINA m.
    VenTrak respiratory mechanics m.
monitoring
    cytoimmunologic m.
    pulse oximetry m. (POM)
monkey
    m. B virus

    m. epithelium
    m. facies
monkeypox virus
monk's cowl
monoamine oxidase inhibitor (MAO inhibitor)
monoarthritis (MA)
    chronic m.
monoarticular
    m. antigen-induced arthritis
    m. arthritis of unknown etiology
monoassociated
monobactam
monobenzone
monochloroacetic acid
monochromatic light source
Monocid
monoclonal
    m. antibody (MAB, MoAb)
    m. antibody to CD4, 5a8
    m. antibody therapy (MAb therapy)
    m. antiendothelial cell antibody (mAECA)
    m. autoantibody
    m. B-cell neoplasm
    m. gammopathy
    m. gammopathy of unknown significance (MGUS)
    m. immunoglobulin
    m. peak
    m. protein
    m. protein, skin
7E3 monoclonal antiplatelet antibody
monocyte
    m. chemoattractant protein
    m. chemoattractant protein-1 (MCP-1)
    m. chemotactic factor (MCF)
    m. chemotactic peptide-1 (MCP-1)
    m. chemotactic protein (MCP)
monocyte-derived
    m.-d. cytokine
    m.-d. neutrophil chemotactic factor
monocyte-macrophage system
monocytic leukemia
monocytogenes
    Listeria m.
monocytopoiesis
    factor-inducing m.
monocytosis
    avian m.
monodisperse aerosol
Monodox Oral
monoecious
monoethylglycinexylidide (MEGX)
monogamous bivalency
Mono-Gesic

monohydrate
    cefadroxil m.
    cephalexin m.
monoinfection
monokine
monoleptic fever
monoLISA test
monomer
    Actin m.
monomeric
monomicrobic
monomorphous
mononeuritis multiplex
mononuclear
    m. cell
    m. phagocyte system (MPS)
mononucleosis
    infectious m. (IM)
    posttransfusion m. (PTM)
monooxygenase pathway
monophonic wheeze
monophosphate
    adenosine m. (AMP)
    cyclic adenosine m. (cAMP)
    cyclic guanosine m.
    cyclic nucleotide adenosine m.
    guanosine m. (GMP)
monoplast
monoplastic
monorecidive chancre
monosodium
    m. glutamate (MSG)
    m. urate (MSU)
    m. urate monohydrate crystal
monospecific antiserum
Monosporium apiospermum
monostearate
    glyceryl m.
monosymptomatic hypochondriasis
monosyphilide
monotherapy
    etanercept m.
    maintenance cyclosporine m.
    (mCsA)
monotypia
Mono-Vac test
monovalent antiserum
monoxide
    carbon m.
    diffusing capacity for carbon m.
    (DLCO)

monoxime
    butanedione m.
Monro
    foramen of M.
Monsel solution
monster
    Gila m.
montelukast
Montenegro
    M. reaction
    M. test
Monterey
    M. cypress
    M. cypress tree
montevideo
    Salmonella m.
Monurol
moon facies
5-MOP
    5-methoxypsoralen
8-MOP
    8-methoxypsoralen
morado
    mal m.
Moraxella
    M. catarrhalis
    M. lacunata
***Moraxella* conjunctivitis**
morbilli
morbilliform
    m. basal cell carcinoma
    m. eruption
    m. erythema
Morbillivirus
    equine M.
morbus
    cholera m.
    m. Darier
mordax
    calor m.
mordicans
    calor m.
MORFAN
    mental retardation, overgrowth,
    remarkable face, and acanthosis nigrans
    MORFAN syndrome
Morgan
    M. fold
    M. line
Morganella morganii
morganii
    Morganella m.

M

NOTES

morning
    m. glory anomaly
    m. stiffness
morphea
    acroteric m.
    m. acroterica
    Addison m.
    m. alba
    m. atrophica
    generalized m.
    m. guttata
    m. herpetiformis
    m. linearis
    m. pigmentosa
    m. pigmentosum
    m. profunda
    subcutaneous m.
    m. variant
morpheaform
    m. basal cell carcinoma
    m. sarcoid
morphealike
morphine sulfate
morphogenesis
morphogenic protein 6
morphologic classification
morphology
    dendritic m.
    lesion m.
    stellate m.
morphometric
morphonuclear
morpio, morpion, pl. morpiones
Morquio
    M. mucopolysaccharidosis
    M. syndrome
Morrey-Coonrad design
morrhuate
    sodium m.
Morrow-Brown needle
morsicatio buccarum
mortality
mortification
mortified
Mortimer malady
Morton neuroma
morula cell
morus
    nevus m.
MoRu-Viraten
Morvan disease
mosaic
    m. fungus
    m. skin
    m. wart
mosaicism
Moschcowitz disease
Mosco callus and corn remover

Moscow typhus
MOSD
    multiple organ system dysfunction
MOSF
    multiple organ system failure
mosquito
    m. bite
    m. forceps
mosquito-borne disease
Mosquitone lotion
mossy foot
moth
    m. dermatitis
    m. patch
moth-eaten
    m.-e. alopecia
    m.-e. baldness
mother
    m. dermatitis
    infant of diabetic m. (IDM)
    m. lesion
    m. yaw
Mother2Be
    M. skin treatment
motif
    immunoreceptor tyrosine-based activation m. (ITAM)
    leucine zipper m.
    nonmethylated CpG m.
motif-bearing cytokine
motion
    active range of m.
    continuous passive m. (CPM)
    joint alignment and m. (JAM)
    pain on m.
    passive m.
    m. sickness
motor
    m. deconditioning
    m. neuron weakness
    m. neuropathy
motorized cutter
Motrin
    M. IB
    M. IB Sinus
    Junior Strength M.
MOTT
    Mycobacteria other than tuberculosis
Mott cell
mottled
    m. opacity
    m. rarefaction
mottling
    netlike m.
moulage
mould
Moulin
    linear atrophoderma of M.

moult
mountain
    m. cedar
    m. cedar tree
mouse
    m. encephalomyelitis
    m. encephalomyelitis virus
    m. epithelium
    m. hepatitis
    m. hepatitis virus
    m. leukemia virus
    m. mammary tumor virus
    nude m.
    m. parotid tumor virus
    m. poliomyelitis
    m. poliomyelitis virus
    m. serum
    m. serum protein (MSP)
    m. thymic virus
    m. urine
    m. urine protein (MUP)
mousepox virus
mousse
    betamethasone m.
    RID M.
mousy odor
mouth
    burning m.
    dry m.
    m. erythema multiforme
    painful m.
    purse-string m.
    scabby m.
    sore m.
    trench m.
mouthwash
    Zephiran m.
movement
    alpha-nonrapid eye m. (alpha-NREM)
    genistein-inhibited m.
    herbimycin-inhibited m.
    nonrapid eye m. (nonREM, NREM)
    periodic leg m.
    rapid eye m. (REM)
moxa
moxalactam
Moxam
moxibustion
moxifloxacin HCl
Moynahan syndrome

MP
    machine preservation
    metacarpophalangeal
    minimal pigment
6-MP
    6-mercaptopurine
MPA
    methylprednisolone acetate
    microscopic polyangiitis
MPD
    minimal phototoxic dose
M-plasty
MPM
    multiple primary melanoma
        MPM Antimicrobial wound cleanser
        MPM composite dressing
        MPM conductive gel pad
        MPM GelPad impregnated gauze
        MPM hydrogel dressing
MPO
    myeloperoxidase
        MPO bone marrow stain
        MPO deficiency
M-Prednisol Injection
MPS
    mononuclear phagocyte system
    myofascial pain syndrome
MPT
    multiple parameter telemetry
    multiple puncture test
MR
    multicentric reticulohistiocytosis
    muscle-relaxant
        MR drug
MRC
    Medical Research Council
MRCL
    Medical Research Council Laboratories
MRD
    matched related donor
    minimal reacting dose
MRG
    median rhomboid glossitis
MRI
    magnetic resonance imaging
MRI-compatible hollow-fiber bioreactor
mRNA
    messenger RNA
        cathepsin K mRNA
MRSA
    methicillin-resistant *Staphylococcus aureus*

M

NOTES

MR-VAX II
MS-3
    Miniscope M.
MSA
    myositis-specific autoantibody
MS-1, -2 agent
MSD Enteric-Coated ASA
MSDS
    material safety data sheet
Mseleni disease
MSG
    monosodium glutamate
MSH
    melanocyte-stimulating hormone
      alpha-MSH
        alpha-melanocyte-stimulating
        hormone
      beta-MSH
MSI
    microsatellite instability
MSM
    men who have sex with men
MSP
    mouse serum protein
MST
    median survival time
MSTA Mumps
MSU
    monosodium urate
MT
    metatarsal
MTB
    Mycobacterium tuberculosis
MTC
    multilocular thymic cyst
MTD
    Mycobacterium Tuberculosis Direct
      MTD Test
MTI
    magnetization transfer imaging
MTP
    metatarsophalangeal
MTP-PE
MTS
    mitochondrial targeting sequence
MTX
    methotrexate
Mu antigen
mucate
    acetaminophen and
      isometheptene m.
Mucha disease
Mucha-Habermann
    M.-H. disease
    M.-H. syndrome
Much granule
mucicarmine stain

mucin clot test
mucinoid
mucinosa
    alopecia m.
mucinosis, pl. **mucinoses**
    acral persistent papular m.
    cutaneous focal m.
    follicular m.
    papular m.
    plaque-like cutaneous m.
    reticular erythematous m. (REM)
mucinous
    m. cyst
    m. degeneration
    m. eccrine carcinoma
Muckle-Wells syndrome
mucocele
mucociliary clearance
mucocutaneous
    m. candidiasis
    m. disease
    m. leishmaniasis (MCL)
    m. lymph node syndrome (MLNS)
    m. manifestation
    m. sporotrichosis
Muco-Fen-LA
mucogenicum
    Mycobacterium m.
mucoid
    m. degeneration
    m. exopolysaccharide (MEP)
mucolipidosis
mucolytic
Mucomyst
mucopolysaccharide
mucopolysaccharidosis,
   pl. **mucopolysaccharidoses**
    Hunter m.
    Hurler-Scheie m.
    Maroteaux-Lamy m.
    Morquio m.
    Sanfilippo m.
    Scheie m.
    Sly m.
    type I–VII m.
    X-linked m.
mucopurulent
mucormycosis
Mucor racemosus
mucosa, pl. **mucosae**
    hyalinosis cutis et m.
    lipoidosis cutis et m.
    nevus spongiosus albus m.
    oral m.
    reddening of oropharyngeal m.
    ulceration of oral m.
    upper respiratory tract m.

mucosa-associated
> m.-a. lymphoid tissue (MALT)
> m.-a. lymphoid tissue lymphoma

mucosal
> m. disease
> m. disease virus
> m. inflammation
> m. mast cell
> m. neuroma
> m. sloughing

mucositis
> genital plasma cell m.
> plasma cell m.

Mucosol

mucosum
> stratum m.

mucous
> m. cyst
> m. desiccation
> m. membrane
> m. membrane pemphigoid
> m. membrane ulceration
> m. papule
> m. patch
> m. plaque
> m. plug
> m. plugging
> m. stool

mucus
> balls of m.
> m. hypersecretion
> oyster mass of m.
> thick and sticky m.

Mudd acne

mud fever

Muehrcke
> M. band
> M. line
> M. sign

Mueller-Hinton agar

Muerto Canyon virus

mugwort weed pollen

mu-heavy chain disease

Muir-Torre syndrome

mulberry
> black m.
> m. molar
> paper m.
> m. pattern
> m. rash
> red m.

> m. spot
> white m.

Mulibrey nanism

Muller phlebectomy hook

multiantigenic peptide (MAP)

multibacillary

MultiBoot

multicellular helminth

multicentric
> m. disease
> m. reticulohistiocytosis (MR)

multideterminant molecule

Multidex filler

multidigit dactylitis

multidrug-resistant tuberculosis (MDR-TB)

multidrug therapy (MDT)

multifactorial

multifidus

multifocal
> m. demyelinating motor neuropathy
> m. histiocytosis
> m. Langerhans cell

multiforme
> atypical erythema m.
> bullous erythema m.
> chronic erythema m.
> drug-associated erythema m.
> erythema m. (EM)
> granuloma m.
> Hebra erythema m.
> herpes-associated erythema m. (HAEM)
> herpes simplex-associated erythema m. (HAEM)
> mouth erythema m.
> oral erythema m.
> postherpetic erythema m.

multiformis
> dermatitis m.
> protoporphyria chronica m.

multifunctional extracellular glycoprotein

multigemini
> pili m.

multiinfection

MultiLight system

multilineage
> m. colony-stimulating factor
> m. reconstitution

multilocularis
> *Echinococcus m.*

multilocular thymic cyst (MTC)

NOTES

multimembrane spanner
multimer
multimeric molecule
multinomial (polytomous) logistic
  regression method
multinucleate cell angiohistiocytoma
multinucleated giant cell (MGC)
MultiPad absorptive dressing
multipartial
multiple
  m. benign cystic epithelioma
  m. chemical sensitivity
  m. drug allergy syndrome
  m. endocrine neoplasia (MEN)
  m. endocrine neoplasia type 1
    (MEN 1)
  m. endocrine neoplasms (MEN)
  m. epiphyseal dysplasia
  m. eruptive milia
  m. hamartoma syndrome
  m. hereditary hemorrhagic
    telangiectasis
  m. idiopathic hemorrhagic sarcoma
  m. keratoacanthoma
  m. lentigines syndrome
  m. minute digitate hyperkeratosis
  m. mucosal neuroma
  m. mucosal neuroma syndrome
  m. myeloma (MM)
  m. myositis
  m. organ system dysfunction
    (MOSD)
  m. organ system failure (MOSF)
  m. parameter telemetry (MPT)
  m. primary melanoma (MPM)
  m. puncture test (MPT)
  m. puncture tuberculin test
  m. sclerosis
  m. serositis
  skin test antigens, m.
  m. sulfatase deficiency
  m. sulfatase deficiency syndrome
  m. symmetrical lipomatosis
  m. symmetric lipomatosis
  m. trichoepithelioma
multiple-type hyperlipoproteinemia
multiplex
  lymphangioma tuberosum m.
  mononeuritis m.
  m. nevus
  steatocystoma m.
  m. steatocystoma
  trichoepithelioma papillosum m.
  xanthoma tuberosum m.
multipotent hematopoietic cell
MultiPulse laser system
multisegmented

Multitest
  M. CMI
  M. test
multivalent
  m. antigen
  m. antiserum
  m. vaccine
multivariant
multivariate
  m. analysis of variance
    (MANOVA)
  m. logistic regression
multocida
  Pasteurella m.
mummification necrosis
mumps
  m. meningoencephalitis
  metastatic m.
  MSTA M.
  m. sensitivity test
  m. skin test antigen
  m. virus
  m. virus vaccine
Mumpsvax
Munchausen syndrome
Munro
  M. abscess
  M. microabscess
mu-opioid
MUP
  mouse urine protein
mupirocin
  m. ointment
muramyl-tripeptide
MURD
  matched unrelated donor
murex hybrid capture assay
Murex Suds
muriform
murine
  m. hepatitis
  m. homolog
  m. leukemia
  m. sarcoma virus
  M. solution
  m. thymoma
  m. typhus
murmur
  Carey Coombs m.
Murocel Ophthalmic solution
muromonab-CD3
Murray
  M. test
  M. Valley encephalitis (MVE)
  M. Valley encephalitis virus
  M. Valley rash
Murutucu virus
muscarinic receptor autoantibody

muscle
 accessory m.
 airway smooth m. (ASM)
 arrectores pilorum m.
 arrector pili m.
 m. biopsy
 bronchial smooth m.
 cutaneous m.
 dermal m.
 sacrospinalis m.
 m. self-antigen
 sternocleidomastoid m.
 m. weakness
muscle-relaxant (MR)
 m.-r. drug
Muscle-Wells syndrome
musculamine
muscular dystrophy
musculotendinous
 m. damage
 m. unit
musculus
 Mus m.
mushroom
 m. dust
 m. picker's lung
 m. worker's lung
mushroom-hook layer
musician's overuse syndrome
musk ambrette
Mus musculus
mussel
 blue m.
mustard
 l-phenylalanine m.
 nitrogen m.
 topical nitrogen m. (NH2)
 yellow m.
Mustargen Hydrochloride
Mustargen-MSD
mustelae
 Helicobacter m.
mutagen
 frame-shift m.
mutagenicity
mutant
 conditional-lethal m.
 conditionally lethal m.
 suppressor-sensitive m.
 temperature-sensitive m.
mutation
 addition-deletion m.

 CKR5 m.
 factor V Leiden m.
 frame-shift m.
 IL-12 receptor beta-1 m.
 missense m.
 MODY3 HNF-1-alpha m.
 novel missense m.
 point m.
 reading-frame-shift m.
 somatic m.
 transition m.
 transversion m.
mutilans
 m. arthritis
 arthritis m.
 keratoma hereditaria m.
 keratoma hereditarium m.
 lepra m.
 lupus m.
 psoriatic arthritis m.
mutilating
 m. keratoderma
 m. keratoderma of Vohwinkel
 m. leprosy
mutism
 tacrolimus-associated m.
MV
 maximal ventilation
 mechanical ventilation
MVE
 Murray Valley encephalitis
 MVE virus
MVLS
 modified varicella-like syndrome
MVTR
 moisture vapor transmission rate
MVV
 maximal voluntary ventilation
myalgia
 eosinophilic m.
 epidemic m.
Myambutol
Myapap drops
myasthenia
 m. gravis (MG)
 m. gravis syndrome
Mycelex-7, -G
Mycelex troche
mycelium
mycetoma
 actinomycotic m.
 Bouffardi black m.

NOTES

M

mycetoma *(continued)*
 Bouffardi white m.
 Brumpt white m.
 Carter black m.
 eumycotic m.
 Nicolle white m.
 Vincent white m.
mycetomi
 Madurella m.
mycid
Mycifradin
 M. Sulfate Oral
 M. Sulfate Topical
Mycitracin Topical
Myclo-Derm
Myclo-Gyne
mycobacteria
 m. HSP
 nontuberculous m.
mycobacterial
 m. abscess
 m. infection
***Mycobacteria* other than tuberculosis (MOTT)**
mycobacteriosis
 environmental m.
Mycobacterium
 M. abscessus
 M. avium
 M. avium complex (MAC)
 M. avium-intracellulare (MAC, MAI)
 M. avium-intracellulare bacteremia
 M. balnei
 M. bovis
 M. chelonae
 M. fortuitum
 M. gordonae
 M. haemophilum
 M. kansasii
 M. leprae
 M. marinum
 M. mucogenicum
 M. peregrinum
 M. phlei
 M. smegmatis
 M. thermoresistable
 M. tuberculosis (MTB)
 M. tuberculosis detection
 M. Tuberculosis Direct (MTD)
 M. tuberculosis Direct Test
 M. ulcerans
 M. vaccae
 M. xenopi
Mycobutin
mycodermatitis
Mycogen II Topical
Mycolog-II Topical

mycology
Myconel Topical
mycophage
mycophenolate mofetil (MM, MMF)
Mycoplasma
 M. arthritidis
 M. arthritidis mitogen (MAM)
 M. faucium
 M. genitalium
 M. hominis
 M. incognitus
 M. pneumoniae
mycoplasma
 m. disease
 m. IgM titer
 m. pneumonia of pig
mycoplasmal pneumonia
mycosis, pl. **mycoses**
 m. cutis chronica
 deep m.
 m. favosa
 m. framboesioides
 m. fungoides (MF)
 m. fungoides d'emblée
 m. fungoides palmaris et plantaris
 Gilchrist m.
 m. interdigitalis
 opportunistic systemic m.
 Posada m.
 pulmonary m.
 rare m.
 subcutaneous m.
mycostatic
Mycostatin
 M. Oral
 M. pastilles
 M. topical
mycotic dermatitis
mycovirus
Mydfrin Ophthalmic solution
mydriatic
myelin-associated glycoprotein antibody detection
myelin basic protein (MBP)
myelin-oligodendrocyte glycoprotein (MOG)
myelitic enterovirus
myelitis
 amyotrophic syphilitic m.
 transverse m.
myeloablative conditioning
myeloblastic protein
myeloblastosis
 avian m.
myelodysplastic syndrome (MDS)
myelofibrosis
 cutaneous m.

myeloid
>m. colony
>m. leukemia
>m. stem cell

myeloma
>m. growth factor
>multiple m. (MM)
>plasma cell m.

myelomatosis
myelomonocytic leukemia
myelonecrosis
myelopathy
>vacuolar m.

myeloperoxidase (MPO)
>m. bone marrow stain (MPO bone marrow stain)
>m. deficiency

myeloperoxidase-hydrogen peroxide halide system
myeloproliferative disease
myeloradiculopathy
myeloradiculopolyneuronitis
myelosis
myelosuppression
>azathioprine-induced m.

myelosuppressive
myelosyphilis
myiasis
>botfly facultative m.
>botfly obligate m.
>creeping m.
>facultative m.
>obligate m.
>m. oestruosa
>subcutaneous m.
>tumbu fly m.
>wound m.

Myminic Expectorant
myoadenylate
>m. deaminase
>m. deaminase deficiency

myoblast
myoblastoma
>granular cell m.

myocardial
>m. dysfunction
>m. infarction (MI)

myocarditis
>clinical m.
>giant cell m.

Myochrysine

myoclonus
>nocturnal m.
>progressive encephalomyelitis with rigidity and m. (PERM)

Myocrisin
myocyte
>Anitschkow m.

myoD
myoepithelial sialadenitis
myoepithelioma
myoepithelium
myofascial pain syndrome (MPS)
myofasciitis
>macrophagic m.

myofibril
myofibroblast
myofibroblastoma
>infantile digital m.

myofibromatosis
>infantile m.

myogenic paralysis
myoglobin
>quantitative immunoassay for urine m.
>m. release

myoglobinuria
myoma
myonecrosis
>clostridial m.
>m. syndrome

myopathy
>drug-related m.
>idiopathic inflammatory m. (IIM)
>sarcoid-like granulomatous m.
>steroid m.
>vacuolar m.

myophosphorylase deficiency
myorelaxant drug
myosin
>m. ATPase inhibitor
>m. light chain

myositis
>acute disseminated m.
>childhood m.
>dermatomyositis sine m.
>eosinophilic m.
>epidemic m.
>giant cell m.
>inclusion body m.
>multiple m.
>nodular m.
>orbital m.

M

NOTES

myositis *(continued)*
    m. ossificans
    overlap m. (OVLP)
    m. with malignancy
myositis-associated autoantibody
myositis-specific
    m.-s. antibody
    m.-s. autoantibody (MSA)
myosynovitis
Myoviridae
Myphetapp
myringitis
    m. bulbosa
    bullous m.
myringodermatitis
myringotomy with aspiration
myristate
    isopropyl m.
myrmecia wart
myrmekiasm
myrtle
    wax m.
Mytrex F topical
myxadenitis labialis

myxedema
    circumscribed m.
    generalized m.
    pretibial m. (PTM)
myxedematosus
    lichen m.
myxedematous
    m. arthropathy
    m. facies
    m. lichen
myxoid
    m. cyst
    m. pseudocyst
myxolipoma
myxoma
    cardiocutaneous m.
    nerve sheath m.
myxomatosis virus
myxomatous degeneration
myxosarcoma
myxovirus
MZBL
    marginal zone B-cell lymphoma
M-Zole 7 Dual Pack

N

nitrogen
Alferon N
N segment
nabumetone
NAC
nasal allergen challenge
NACDG
North American Contact Dermatitis Group
N-acetyl-4-S-cysteaminyl phenol
N-acetylcysteine
N-acetylneuraminic acid
nacreous ichthyosis
Nadinola
nadolol
Nadopen-V
NADPH
nicotinamide adenine dinucleotide phosphate
NADPH oxidase
NADPH oxidase system
Naegeli
chromatophore nevus of N.
N. syndrome
Naegeli-Franceschetti-Jadassohn syndrome
Naegleria fowleri
NAEP
National Asthma Education Program
naeslundii
Actinomyces n.
naevoid (*var. of* nevoid)
naevus (*var. of* nevus)
NAF
neutrophil-activating factor
nafamostat mesilate
nafate
cefamandole n.
Nafcil injection
nafcillin sodium
Nafrine
naftifine hydrochloride
Naftin
N. cream
N. topical
Naga sore
nail
athletic n.
azure lunula of n.
n. biting
blue n.
brittle n.
n. change
Chevron n.

claw n.
n. clubbing
clubbing of n.
convex n.
double-edge n.
egg shell n.
n. fold
n. fold capillaroscopy
n. fold capillaroscopy abnormality
n. fold capillary loop abnormality
geographic stippling of n.
green n.
green-striped n.
n. groove
half-and-half n.
herringbone n.
Hippocratic n.
n. horn
ingrown n.
INRO surgical prosthetic n.
n. keratin
n. matrix
omega n.
Ony-Clear N.
parrot-beak n.
pincer n.
n. pit
pitted n.
pitting of n.
n. pitting
n. plate
Plummer n.
n. polish
racket n.
ram's horn n.
reedy n.
ringworm of n.
n. root
sculptured n.
n. shedding
shell n.
n. skin
splitting n.
spoon n.
stippled n.
sulcus of matrix of n.
Terry n.
trumpet n.
turtleback n.
n. wall
n. wart
yellow n.
nailbed cancer
20-nail involvement
nail-patella-elbow syndrome

nail-patella syndrome
Nairobi sheep disease virus
Nairovirus
naive B cell
Na⁺-K⁺
sodium-potassium
Na⁺-K⁺ ATPase pump
naked
n. DNA encoding
n. plasmid DNA
n. tubercle
n. virus
Nalcrom
Naldecon
Naldecon-EX Children's Syrup
Naldelate
Nalebuff classification
Nalfon
Nalgest
nalidixic acid
Nallpen injection
naloxone hydrochloride
Nalspan
NAME
nevi, atrial myxoma, myxoid
neurofibromas, and ephelides
nevi, atrial myxomas, myxomas of skin
and mammary glands, and ephelides
NAME syndrome
nana
Hymenolepis n.
NANB
non-A non-B
NANB hepatitis
nanism
Mulibrey n.
Nanophyetus salmincola
nanum
Microsporum n.
NAP
neutrophil-activating protein
nape nevus
Naphcon-A
naphthylalkalone
napkin
n. dermatitis
n. psoriasis
n. rash
Naprelan
Naprosyn
naproxen sodium
NAPRTCS
North American Pediatric Renal
Transplant Cooperative Study
NAR
nonanaphylactic reaction

NARES
nonallergic rhinitis with eosinophilia
syndrome
Narins cannula
naris, pl. **nares**
narium
narrowband
n. UVB (NBUVB)
n. UVB lamp
n. UVB therapeutic light exposure
narrowing
joint space n.
Nasabid
Nasacort AQ
Nasahist
N. B
N. B injection
nasal
n. allergen challenge (NAC)
n. allergy
n. antigen challenge test
n. cannula dermatitis
n. canthus
n. congestion
n. congestion score (NCS)
n. glioma
n. herpes
n. itching
Kondon's N.
N. Moist
n. mucosal ulceration
Otrivin N.
n. polyp
n. provocation test
n. scraping
N. & Sinus Relief
n. smear
n. solar dermatitis
n. symptom score (NSS)
n. turbinate
Tyzine N.
n. verge
Nasalcrom Nasal solution
Nasalide Nasal Aerosol
Nasarel Nasal Spray
NASBA
nucleic acid sequence based amplification
nasi
acne necroticans et exulcerans
serpiginosa n.
alae n.
granulosis rubra n.
vestibulum n.
Nasik vibrio
nasoantral window
nasobronchial reflex
nasociliary
nasolabial fold (NLF)

Nasonex
nasopharyngeal
  n. aspirate (NPA)
  n. biopsy
  n. carcinoma
  n. leishmaniasis
  n. ulcer
nasopharyngoscopy
NASTRA
  North American Study of Treatment for
  Refractory Ascites
  NASTRA study
Nasu-Hakola disease
Natacyn Ophthalmic
natamycin
natiform skull
National
  N. Asthma Education Program
  (NAEP)
  N. Center for Health Statistics
  (NCHS)
  N. Committee for Clinical
  Laboratory Standards (NCCLS)
  N. Immunization Program (NIP)
  N. Institute of Arthritis and
  Metabolic Diseases (NIAMD)
  N. Institute of Arthritis,
  Musculoskeletal and Skin
  Disorders (NIAMS)
  N. Institutes of Health (NIH)
  N. Marrow Donor Program
  (NMDP)
  N. Vaccine Advisory Committee
  (NVAC)
native
  n. anergy
  n. type anti-DNA antibody
natural
  n. anergy
  n. antibody
  n. cytotoxicity receptor
  n. focus of infection
  n. hemolysin
  n. immunity
  n. interferon alfa
  n. killer (NK)
  n. killer cell
  n. killer cell activation
  n. killer cell-stimulating factor
  (NKSF)
  n. killer-mediated cytotoxicity
  n. rubber latex allergy

Naturale
  Tears N.
Nature's Tears solution
nausea
  epidemic n.
Nauseatol
Nausex
navy bean
Naxen
NBCCS
  nevoid basal cell carcinoma syndrome
NBT
  nitroblue tetrazolium
  NBT mosaic pattern
NBUVB
  narrowband UVB
NCA
  nonspecific cross-reacting antigen
NCAM
  neural cell adhesion molecule
NCB
  needle-core biopsy
NCCLS
  National Committee for Clinical
  Laboratory Standards
NCHS
  National Center for Health Statistics
NCS
  nasal congestion score
  nerve conduction study
ND
  Newcastle disease
  Congestac ND
  ND virus
N.D.
  Chlor-Tripolon N.D.
Nd
  neodymium
ND-Stat
  N.-S. injection
Nd:YAG
  neodymium:yttrium-aluminum-garnet
  Nd:YAG laser
near-fatal asthma
Nebcin injection
Nebraska calf scours virus
Nebuhaler inhaler
nebules
  Ventolin n.
nebulin
nebulization
nebulize

NOTES

nebulized
    n. bronchodilator
    n. isoproterenol
nebulizer
    Aerochamber n.
    AeroSonic personal ultrasonic n.
    AeroTech II n.
    Ailos n.
    DeVilbiss Pulmon-Aid n.
    Fisoneb ultrasonic n.
    jet n.
    John Bunn Mini-Mist n.
    Medi-Mist n.
    Medix ultrasonic n.
    Micro-Mist n.
    Pulmo-Aide n.
    Respirgard II n.
    Schuco 2000 n.
    Shuco-Myst n.
    Twin Jet n.
    ultrasonic n.
    Wright n.
NebuPent Inhalation
NEC
    necrotizing enterocolitis
Necator americanus
necatoriasis
neck
    n. dermatitis
    farmer's n.
    fiddler n.
    sailor's n.
neck-flexion maneuver
necklace
    Casal n.
    n. of pearls
    n. of Venus
necrobiosis
    n. granulomatosis
    n. lipoidica
    n. lipoidica diabeticorum
necrobiotic
    n. granuloma
    n. xanthogranuloma
necrogenic
    n. tubercle
    n. wart
necrogenica
    verruca n.
necrolysis
    epidermal n.
    toxic epidermal n. (TEN)
necrolytic migratory erythema
necrosis
    acute retinal n. (ARN)
    acute tubular n.
    aseptic n.
    aspirin-induced papillary n.

    avascular n. (AVN)
    caseation n.
    central fibrinoid n.
    centrilobar n. (CLN)
    cold-induced n.
    coumarin n.
    fat n.
    fibrinoid n.
    late centrilobar n.
    liquefaction n.
    mummification n.
    neutrophilic n.
    papillary n.
    piecemeal n.
    n. progrediens
    progressive outer retinal n. (PORN)
    radium n.
    subcutaneous fat n.
    traumatic fat n.
necrosum
    vaccinia n.
necrotic
    n. arachnidism
    n. center
    n. cutaneous loxoscelism
    n. excoriation
    n. pocket
    n. tissue
    n. ulcer
necrotica
    acne n.
    dermatitis nodularis n.
necroticans
    erythema n.
necrotisans
    sycosis nuchae n.
necrotized chilblain
necrotizing
    n. angiitis
    n. enterocolitis (NEC)
    n. fasciitis
    n. granuloma
    n. infection
    n. lymphadenitis
    n. scleritis with adjacent inflammation
    n. scleritis without adjacent inflammation
    n. sialometaplasia
    n. vasculitis
nectary of floral unit
nedocromil sodium
needle
    Accuhair n.
    ADG n.
        adjustable-length gauge needle
    adjustable-length gauge n. (ADG, ADG needle)

Allerprick n.
n. arthroscopy
n. biopsy
Colorado microdissection n.
Davis and Geck systemic plastic reconstruction P3 or PS3 n.
Davis and Geck systemic PR and PRE P3 or PS3 n.
Ethicon P and PS n.
FS reverse cutting n.
Hagedorn n.
Morrow-Brown n.
No-Kor n.
Osterballe precision n.
Parker-Pearson n.
precision-point n.
Pricker n.
reverse cutting n.
for skin reverse cutting n.
Stallerpointe n.
Thomas n.
Wyeth bifurcated n.
needle-core biopsy (NCB)
Needleman-Wunsch algorithm
needlestick
Neer II implant
Neethling virus
Nef protein
NEG
nonenzymatic glycation
negative
n. anergy
n. control test
n. crossmatch
n. nevus
n. patch test
n. phase
n. predictive value (NPV)
n. reaction
n. schick test
n. selection
n. strand virus
NegGram
Negishi virus
Negri
N. body
N. corpuscle
NEH
neutrophilic eccrine hidradenitis
Neisseria
N. gonorrhoeae

N. meningitidis
N. meningitidis B
Neisseria gonorrhoeae
nelfinavir
Nellcor Symphony N-3000 pulse oximeter
Nelson syndrome
nematocyst
venom-bathed n.
nematode
n. dermatitis
filarial n.
intestinal n.
neoangiogenesis
neoangiomatous
neoantigen
neoarsphenamine organic arsenic
NEOB
New England Organ Bank
Neocate formula
Neo-Cortef
N.-C. Ophthalmic
N.-C. Topical
NeoDecadron Ophthalmic
NeoDerm
Neo-Dexameth Ophthalmic
neodymium (Nd)
neodymium:yttrium-aluminum-garnet (Nd:YAG)
n.-a.-g. laser
neoepidermis
neoepithelium
neoepitope
aggrecanase-induced aggrecan n.
NeoFed
neoformans
Cryptococcus n.
Saccharomyces n.
Neo-fradin Oral
neomembrane
Neo-Metric
Neomixin topical
neomycin
n. dermatitis
n. and hydrocortisone
n. and polymyxin b
n., polymyxin b, and dexamethasone
n., polymyxin b, and gramicidin
n., polymyxin b, and hydrocortisone

N

NOTES

neomycin *(continued)*
  n., polymyxin b, and prednisolone
  n. sulfate
neonatal
  n. acne
  n. anemia
  n. biotin deficiency
  n. calf diarrhea virus
  n. citrullinemia
  erythema multiforme n.
  n. herpes
  n. herpes simplex virus
  n. hypoxia
  n. lupus
  n. lupus erythematosus (NLE)
  lupus erythematosus, n.
  n. pustular melanosis
  n. skin allograft
  n. systemic candidiasis
  n. tyrosinemia
neonatalis
  herpes n.
neonatal-onset multisystem inflammatory disease (NOMID)
neonate
neonatorum
  acne n.
  adiponecrosis subcutanea n.
  anemia n.
  blennorrhea n.
  dermatitis exfoliativa n.
  edema n.
  erythema toxicum n.
  ichthyosis congenita n.
  icterus n.
  impetigo n.
  keratolysis n.
  milium n.
  ophthalmia n.
  pemphigus n.
  scleredema n.
  sclerema n.
  seborrhea squamosa n.
Neopap
neoplasia
  cutaneous n.
  malignant n.
  multiple endocrine n. (MEN)
  multiple endocrine n. type 1 (MEN 1)
  vulvar intraepithelial n.
neoplasm
  monoclonal B-cell n.
  multiple endocrine n.'s (MEN)
  plasma cell n.
  Revised European-American Classification of Lymphoid N. (REAL)

neoplastic
  n. angioendotheliomatosis
  n. cell
  n. disease
neoplastica
  acrokeratosis n.
  alopecia n.
NEOPO
  Northeast Organ Procurement Organization
Neo-Polycin ointment
neopterin
Neoral Oral
Neosar injection
Neospora canium
Neosporin
  N. Cream
  N. Ophthalmic Ointment
  N. Ophthalmic Solution
  N. Topical Ointment
Neosten
NeoStrata
  N. gel
  N. HQ
NeoSynalar
Neo-Synephrine
  N.-S. 12 Hour Nasal solution
  N.-S. Ophthalmic solution
Neo-Tabs Oral
Neothylline
Neotopic
Neotricin HC Ophthalmic Ointment
Neova Eye Therapy
neovascularization
Neo-Zol
nephelometry
nephrectomy
  laparoscopic donor n. (LDN)
nephritic factor
nephritis, pl. **nephrides**
  acute interstitial n.
  antibasement membrane n.
  antikidney serum n.
  immune complex n.
  immune-mediated membranous n.
  interstitial n.
  lupus n. (LN)
  Masugi n.
  membranous lupus n.
  nephrotoxic serum n. (NSN)
  polyoma virus-associated interstitial n.
  scarlatinal n.
  serum n.
  silent lupus n.
  streptococcal n.
  transfusion n.
  tuberculous n.

tubulointerstitial n. (TIN)
World Health Organization
  classification of lupus n. (I, IIA,
  IIB, III, IV, V)
nephritogenic
  n. effector
  n. process
Nephrocaps
nephrogenic diabetes insipidus
nephrogenicity
nephrolithiasis
nephrolysin
nephrolysis
nephrolytic
nephropathia epidemica
nephropathic
  n. immune response
  n. immunoglobulin
nephropathy
  amyloidotic n.
  Berger IgA n.
  chronic allograft n. (CAN)
  chronic cyclosporine n.
  chronic transplant n. (CTN)
  familial juvenile hyperuricemic n.
  IgA n.
  IgM n.
  membranous n. (MN)
  minimal change n. (MCN)
  urate n.
nephrosis
  hemoglobinuric n.
  toxic n.
nephrotic-range proteinuria
nephrotic syndrome
nephrotoxicity
  chronic n.
nephrotoxic serum nephritis (NSN)
nephrotoxin
NERDS
  nodules, eosinophilia, rheumatism,
    dermatitis, and swelling
  NERDS syndrome
nerve
  common peroneal n.
  n. compression-degeneration
    syndrome
  n. conduction study (NCS)
  n. conduction velocity
  n. deafness
  n. entrapment
  n. entrapment syndrome

femoral n.
n. growth factor (NGF)
n. growth factor antiserum
median n.
peripheral n.
phrenic n.
radial n.
sciatic n.
n. sheath
n. sheath myxoma
sinuvertebral n.
tibial n.
ulnar n.
vagus n.
Nervocaine
nervorum
  lepra n.
  vasa n.
nervosa
  lepra n.
  lues n.
  onychalgia n.
  purpura n.
  rhinitis n.
nervosus
  nevus n.
nervous
  n. exhaustion
  n. system
  n. system involvement
Nesacaine-MPF
nests of nevus cells
Netherton syndrome (NS)
N-ethyl-o-crotonotoluide
netilmicin sulfate
netlike mottling
Netromycin injection
netted pattern
nettle rash
Nettleship disease
Nettleship-Falls ocular albinism
Nettleship-Falls-type ocular albinism
nettling hair
Network
  People of Color Against AIDS N.
    (POCAAN)
Neucalm
Neucalm-50 Injection
Neufeld
  N. capsular swelling
  N. reaction
Neumann disease

N

NOTES

Neupogen injection
neural
  n. cell adhesion molecule (NCAM)
  n. foramina
  n. leprosy
  n. nevus
  n. theory
  n. tissue
neuralgia
  postherpetic n. (PHN)
  red n.
neural-mediated flushing
neuraminidase
neurapraxia
neurasthenia
neuridine
neurilemmoma, neurolemmoma
neuritic atrophoderma
neuriticum
  atrophoderma n.
  eczema n.
neuritis
  optic n.
  peripheral n.
neuroallergy
neuroarthropathy
Neurobehavioral Cognitive Status examination
neuroblastoma
  infantile n.
NeuroCell-HD, -PD
neurocirculatory asthenia
neurocristic hamartoma
neurocutaneous
  n. melanosis
  n. syndrome
neurocysticercosis
neurodegenerative disease
neurodermatitic
neurodermatitis
  circumscribed n.
  n. disseminata
  disseminated n.
  exudative n.
  genital n.
  localized n.
  nodular n.
  nummular n.
neurodermatosis
neurodermite dissemine
neuroectodermal
  n. defect
  n. melanolysomonal disease
neuroendocrine tumor
neuroepidermal
neurofibroma
  molluscoid n.

  pacinian n.
  plexiform n.
neurofibromatosis
  abortive n.
  central type n.
  classic n.
  elephantiasis n.
  incomplete n.
  late onset n.
  segmental n.
  n. (types 1-8)
  n., type 1 syndrome
  variant n.
neurofibrosarcoma
neurofilament promoter
neuroid nevus
neuroimmune dysfunction
neuroimmunomodulation
neurokinin
  n. A, B
neurolabyrinthitis
  viral n.
neurolemmoma (*var. of* neurilemmoma)
neuroleprosy
neurolipomatosis dolorosa
neurologic
  n. disorder
  n. genodermatosis
neurolues
neurolymphomatosis gallinarum
neurolysin
neuroma
  amputation n.
  n. cutis
  encapsulated n.
  Morton n.
  mucosal n.
  multiple mucosal n.
  palisaded encapsulated n.
  plexiform n.
  traumatic n.
  Verneuil n.
neuromatosa
  elephantiasis n.
neuromatosis elephantiasis
neuromatous
neuromelanin
neuromyelitis optica
neuromyoarterial glomus
neuromyopathy
  peripheral n.
neuromyotonia
neuron
  GABAergic n.
neuronevus
neuronophage
neuronophagia

neuron-specific
- n.-s. enolase (NSE)
- n.-s. enolase stain

Neurontin

neuropathic
- n. amyloidosis
- n. arthritis
- n. arthropathy
- n. foot
- n. joint disease

neuropathica
- plica n.

neuropathy
- asymmetric peripheral sensory n.
- entrapment n.
- hereditary sensory radicular n.
- motor n.
- multifocal demyelinating motor n.
- posterior interosseous n.

neuropeptide

neuropsychiatric
- n. disease
- n. symptom
- n. syndrome of systemic lupus erythematosus (NPSLE)
- n. systemic lupus erythematosus (NPSLE)

neurorelapse

neuroretinitis

Neuro-smooth needle holder

Neurospora sitophila

neurosurgery needle holder

neurosyphilis
- ectodermogenic n.
- meningovascular n.
- mesodermogenic n.
- parenchymatous n.
- paretic n.
- tabetic n.

neurotabes diabetica

neurothekeoma

neurotica
- alopecia n.

neurotic excoriation

neurotoxicity
- cyclosporine-induced n.

neurotoxin
- eosinophil-derived n.

neurotransmitter
- GABA inhibitory n.
- nociceptive n.

neurotrophic
- n. ulcer
- n. virus

neurotropic virus

neurovaccine

neurovirus

Neut injection

neutral
- n. lipid
- n. lipid storage
- n. lipid storage disease
- n. protease
- n. proteinase

neutralization
- serum n.
- n. test
- viral n.

neutralizing (Nt)
- n. murine monoclonal antitumor necrosis factor antibody

Neutrexin

Neutrogena
- N. Acne Mask
- N. Hand cream
- N. Healthy Scalp Anti-Dandruff
- N. On-The-Spot Acne Lotion
- N. T/Derm
- T/Gel N.
- N. T/Gel
- T/Sal N.

neutropenia
- autoimmune n.
- cyclic n.
- immune n.
- isoimmune neonatal n.

neutrophil
- n. antibody and transfusion reaction
- n. chemotactant factor
- n. chemotaxis
- n. dysplasia
- n. elastase
- n. ingress
- polymorphonuclear n. (PMN)
- n. polynucleosis
- rolling n.

neutrophil-activating
- n.-a. factor (NAF)
- n.-a. peptide-1
- n.-a. protein (NAP)

neutrophilic
- n. eccrine hidradenitis (NEH)
- n. inflammation

N

NOTES

neutrophilic *(continued)*
    n. intraepidermal IgA dermatosis
    n. necrosis
neutrophil-mediated joint inflammation
neutrophil-specific (secondary) granule deficiency
NeuVisc
nevi *(pl. of* nevus)
nevirapine
nevocellular nevus
nevocyte
nevocytic nevus
nevoid, naevoid
    n. anomaly
    n. basal cell carcinoma
    n. basal cell carcinoma syndrome (NBCCS)
    n. elephantiasis
    n. hyperkeratosis of nipple and areola
    n. hypermelanosis
    n. hypertrichosis
    n. keratosis
    n. lentigo
    n. malignant melanoma (NMM)
    n. telangiectasia
nevolipoma
nevomelanocytic (NM)
nevose
nevoxanthoendothelioma
nevus, naevus, pl. **nevi**
    n. acneiformis unilateralis
    acquired melanocytic n.
    active n.
    amelanotic n.
    n. anemicus
    n. angiectodes
    n. angiomatodes
    angiomatoid Spitz n.
    angiomatous n.
    n. arachnoideus
    n. araneosus
    n. araneus
    nevi, atrial myxoma, myxoid neurofibroma, and ephelides syndrome
    nevi, atrial myxoma, myxoid neurofibromas, and ephelides (NAME)
    nevi, atrial myxomas, myxomas of skin and mammary glands, and ephelides (NAME)
    n. avasculosus
    balloon cell n.
    basal cell n.
    bathing-trunk n.

Becker n.
blue rubber-bleb n.
Blue + Spitz n.
capillary n.
n. cavernosus
n. cell
n. cell, A-, B-, C-type
cellular blue n.
n. cerebelliformis
combined nevi
comedo n.
comedones epidermal n.
comedonicus n.
n. comedonicus
common blue n.
compound n.
congenital giant pigmented n.
connective tissue n.
deep penetrating n.
n. depigmentosus
dermoepidermal n.
dysplastic n.
ECN-BLITZ n.
n. elasticus of Lewandowski
epidermal n.
epidermic-dermic n.
epithelial n.
epithelioid blue n.
epithelioid cell n.
epithelioid combined nevi (ECN)
epithelioid combined nevi deep penetrating n. (ECN-DPN)
n. epitheliomatocylindromatosus
erectile n.
fatty n.
faun tail n.
n. fibrosus
flame n.
n. flammeus
flammeus n.
n. flammeus human granulocytic ehrlichiosis mite
n. flammeus nuchae
n. follicularis keratosis
n. fragarius
n. fuscoceruleus
n. fuscoceruleus acromiodeltoideus fuscoceruleus ophthalmomaxillaris
garment n.
giant congenital pigmented n.
hair follicle n.
hairy n.
halo n.
hard n.
hepatic n.
honeycomb n.

inflamed linear verrucous
epidermal n. (ILVEN)
inflammatory linear verrucous
epidermal n.
intracutaneous n.
intradermal n.
intraepidermal n.
Ito n.
n. of Ito
Jadassohn sebaceous n.
Jadassohn-Tièche n.
junction n.
junctional n.
lentigines, atrial myxoma,
mucocutaneous myxomas, and
blue nevi (LAMB)
lichen striatus epidermal n.
linear epidermal n.
n. lipomatodes
n. lipomatodes superficialis
n. lipomatosus
n. lipomatosus cutaneus superficialis
lymphatic n.
n. lymphaticus
n. maculosus
malignant blue n.
marginal n.
Masson n.
n. maternus
melanocytic n.
mesodermal n.
Meyerson n.
n. mollusciformis
n. morus
multiplex n.
nape n.
negative n.
n. nervosus
neural n.
neuroid n.
nevocellular n.
nevocytic n.
nevus-cell n.
nodular connective tissue disease n.
nonpigmented n.
nuchal n.
n. oligemicus
oral epithelial n.
organoid n.
Ota n.
n. of Ota
n. papillaris

n. papillomatosus
pigmented hair epidermal n.
n. pigmentosus
n. pigmentosus et pilosus
n. pilosus
plane n.
plexiform spindle cell n. (PSCN)
polyploid n.
port-wine n.
n. profundus
raspberry n. _n. of Reed_
resting n.
n. sanguineus
scarf n.
sebaceous n.
n. sebaceous
n. sebaceus
n. sebaceus of Jadassohn (NSJ)
segmental n.
soft n.
speckled lentiginous n.
spider n.
n. spilus
n. spilus lentigo
n. spilus tardus
spindle and epithelioid cell n.
Spitz n.
n. spongiosus albus mucosa
stellar n.
stocking n.
straight hair n.
strawberry n.
subcutaneous n.
n. sudoriferous
Sutton n.
n. syringocystadenomatosus
papilliferus
n. syringocystadenosus papilliferus
systematized n.
Tieche n.
n. unilateralis comedonicus
n. unius lateralis
n. unius lateris
Unna n.
vascular n.
n. vascularis
n. vascularis fungosus
n. vasculosus
n. venosus
venous n.
n. verrucosus
verrucous n.

NOTES

N

nevus *(continued)*
n. vinosus
vulvar n.
Werther n.
white sponge n.
woolly-hair n.
zoniform n.
zosteriform lentiginous n. (ZLN)
nevus-cell nevus
New
N. Beginnings topical gel sheeting
N. Decongestant
N. England Organ Bank (NEOB)
N. Star model 130 laser
N. World leishmaniasis
N. Zealand mice
newborn
bullous impetigo of n.
hemolytic anemia of n.
hemolytic disease of n.
lamellar exfoliation of the n.
spontaneous gangrene of n.
subcutaneous fat necrosis of n.
transient bullous dermolysis of
the n.
Newcastle
N. disease (ND)
N. disease virus
Newman-Keuls test
newsprint
nexin-1
protease n.
nexine
Nezelof
N. syndrome
N. type of thymic alymphoplasia
NF1
NFAT
nuclear factor of activated T cell
NF-ATc protein
NF-κB
nuclear factor-kappa B
NGF
nerve growth factor
NGF antiserum
N.G.T. Topical
NH2
topical nitrogen mustard
NHBD
nonheart-beating donor
NHBD transplantation
NHL
non-Hodgkin lymphoma
Niacels
niacinamide
niacin deficiency

NIAMD
National Institute of Arthritis and
Metabolic Diseases
NIAMS
National Institute of Arthritis,
Musculoskeletal and Skin Disorders
NiCad
nickel-cadmium
nickel
n. allergy
n. and dime lesion
n. hand dermatitis
n. sensitivity
n. sulfate
nickel-cadmium (NiCad)
Niclocide
niclosamide
Nicobid
Nicolar
Nicolau syndrome
**Nicolle-Novy-MacNeal medium culture
(NNN)**
Nicolle white mycetoma
**nicotinamide adenine dinucleotide
phosphate (NADPH)**
nicotinate
methyl n.
nicotine stomatitis
Nicotinex
nicotinic acetylcholine receptor
Nico-Vert
NICU
nonallergic contact urticaria
nonconimmunological contact urticaria
NidaGel
NIDDM
noninsulin-dependent diabetes mellitus
nidogen
Nidryl Oral
nidulans
Aspergillus n.
Nieden syndrome
Niemann-Pick disease
nifedipine
nifurtimox
niger
Aspergillus n.
Peptococcus n.
NightBird nasal CPAP
night blindness
Night Cast R
Nighttime
Arthritis Foundation N.
nigra
acanthosis papulosa n.
dermatosis papulosa n.
linea n.
lingua n.

pityriasis n.
seborrhea n.
tinea n.
trichomycosis n.

nigrans
familial acanthosis n.
mental retardation, overgrowth,
remarkable face, and
acanthosis n. (MORFAN)

nigricans
acanthosis n. (AN)
drug-induced acanthosis n.
hyperandrogenism, insulin resistance,
and acanthosis n. (HAIR-AN)
keratosis n.
malignant acanthosis n.
pseudoacanthosis n.
Rhizopus n.
type A, B, C acanthosis n.

nigrities lingua
Nigrospora
NIH
National Institutes of Health
Nikolsky sign
Nilstat topical
NIMA
noninherited maternal antigen
Nimble Fingers glove
nimitti midge
nimodipine
Nimotop
nines
rule of n.
n. rule
ninth-day erythema
NIP
National Immunization Program
Nipah
nipper
Amico nail n.
nipples
jogger's n.
nit
nitazoxanide (NTZ)
2-nite
Sleepwell 2-n.
nitidus
lichen n.
nitrate
econazole n.
intravesical silver n.
oxiconazole n.

silver n.
sulconazole n.

nitric oxide
nitritoid reaction
nitroblue
n. tetrazolium (NBT)
n. tetrazolium tcst
nitrofurantoin
nitrofurazone
nitrogen (N)
liquid n. (LN$_2$)
n. mustard
2-(2-nitro-4-trifluromethylbenzoyl)-3-cyclohexanedione (NTBC therapy)
nitrotyrosine
nitrous oxide
Nivea moisturizer
Nix Creme Rinse
Nizoral
N. A-D Shampoo
N. Oral
N. Topical
NK
natural killer
NK cell
NK cell activation
NK cell lysis
NK cell-mediated cytotoxicity
NKSF
natural killer cell-stimulating factor
NLE
neonatal lupus erythematosus
NLF
nasolabial fold
N-linked pattern
NLite laser
NLS
nuclear localization signal
NM
nevomelanocytic
NMDP
National Marrow Donor Program
NMM
nevoid malignant melanoma
NMR
NMRL
normal-mode ruby laser
NMSC
nonmelanoma skin cancer
NNN
Nicolle-Novy-MacNeal medium culture

NOTES

N

NNRTI
  nonnucleoside reverse transcriptase
  inhibitor
no
  no observed adverse effect level
    (NOAEL)
  No Pain-HOT PACKS
  No Pain-HP
  No Sting barrier film
NO-AD Sunscreen
NOAEL
  no observed adverse effect level
NOAR
  Norfolk Arthritis Register
Nocardia
  N. asteroides
  N. brasiliensis
  N. caviae
  N. farcinica
  N. tenuis
  N. transvalensis
nocardia
nocardiosis
nociception
nociceptive neurotransmitter
nocodazole
nocturnal
  n. asthma
  n. hemoglobinuria
  n. myoclonus
  n. wheezing
nodal fever
node
  Bizzozero n.
  Bouchard n.
  Heberden n.
  juxtaarticular n.
  lymph n.
  milkers' n.
  Osler n.
  Parrot n.
  Schmorl n.
  sentinel lymph n. (SLN)
nodi (*pl. of* nodus)
nodosa
  cutaneous polyarteritis n.
  dermatitis n.
  periarteritis n.
  polyarteritis n. (PAN)
  systemic polyarteritis n.
  tinea n.
  trichomycosis axillaris n.
  trichorrhexis n.
nodose
nodositas crinium
nodosity
nodosum
  erythema n. (EN)

nodous
nodular
  n. basal cell carcinoma
  n. chondrodermatitis
  n. connective tissue disease nevus
  n. elastosis
  n. episcleritis
  n. granulomatous vasculitis
  n. hidradenoma
  n. leprosy
  n. malignant melanoma
  n. migratory panniculitis
  n. myositis
  n. neurodermatitis
  n. nonsuppurative panniculitis
  n. non-X histiocytosis
  n. panencephalitis
  n. pattern
  n. pseudosarcomatous fasciitis
  n. pulmonary amyloidosis
  n. scabies
  n. scleritis
  n. sclerosing Hodgkin disease
    (NSHD)
  n. shadow
  n. subepidermal fibrosis
  n. synovitis
  n. syphilid
  n. tuberculid
  n. xanthoma
nodularis
  chondrodermatitis helicis n.
  dermatitis psoriasiformis n.
  prurigo n.
  trichomycosis axillaris n.
nodulated
nodulation
nodule
  apple jelly n.
  athlete's n.
  Bohn n.
  Busacca n.
  Caplan n.
  cutaneous n.
  cutaneous-subcutaneous n.
  dark-staining n.
  embolic n.
  n.'s, eosinophilia, rheumatism,
    dermatitis, and swelling (NERDS)
  n.'s, eosinophilia, rheumatism,
    dermatitis, and swelling syndrome
  glial n.
  Jeanselme n.
  juxtaarticular n.
  Koeppe n.
  lepromatous n.
  Lisch n.
  lymph n.

milkers' n.
paraumbilical n.
picker's n.
pulmonary necrobiotic n.
red papule and n.
rheumatoid n.
sharply circumscribed n.
Sister Mary Joseph n.
Stockman n.
subcutaneous granulomatous n.
subcutaneous rheumatoid n.
subepidermal calcified n.
noduli (*pl. of* nodulus)
nodulocystic acne
nodulosis
pulmonary n.
rheumatoid n.
noduloulcerative
n. basal cell carcinoma
n. syphilis
n. tertiary syphilis
nodulous
nodulus, pl. **noduli**
n. cutaneus
nodus, pl. **nodi**
noir
talon n.
noire
atrophie n.
tache n.
No-Kor needle
Nolahist
Nolamine
Nolex LA
noma
nomenclature
binary n.
linnaean system of n.
NOMID
neonatal-onset multisystem inflammatory
disease
nominal allotype
non-A
n.-A. non-B (NANB)
n.-A. non-B hepatitis
n.-A. non-B hepatitis virus
nonacetylated salicylate
nonacnegenic
nonadherent cell
non-A-E hepatitis
nonalcoholic white shake lotion

nonallergic
n. asthma
n. contact urticaria (NICU)
n. rhinitis with eosinophilia
syndrome (NARES)
No-Name Dandruff Treatment
nonamer
nonamide
nonanaphylactic reaction (NAR)
nonarticular syndrome
non-B
n.-B cell
non-A n.-B (NANB)
**nonblanchable, abnormally colored
lesion**
nonblanching purpura
nonbullous
n. congenital erythrodermic
ichthyosis
n. congenital ichthyosiform
erythroderma
n. impetigo
noncaseating granuloma
noncatecholamine
noncavitary
noncicatrizing alopecia
noncomedogenic
**nonconimmunological contact urticaria
(NICU)**
nonconjugative plasmid
noncorticosteroid antiinflammatory agent
noncross-reactive drug
noncytolytic
nondenaturing condition
nondermatophyte fungal infection
Non-Drowsy
Contac Cold N.-D.
Drixoral N.-D.
nondrug-related reaction
**noneczematous persistent papular gold
eruption**
nonenzymatic glycation (NEG)
nonesterified PABA
nonfunction
primary n. (PRNF)
nongenomic glucocorticoid effect
nongonococcal bacterial arthritis
nonheart-beating
n.-b. donor (NHBD)
n.-b. donor liver transplantation
nonhemophiliac patient

N

NOTES

nonhistone protein
non-Hodgkin lymphoma (NHL)
nonidentity
    reaction of n.
nonimmediate-type immunologic drug
  reaction
nonimmune
    n. agglutination
    n. serum
nonimmunity
nonimmunologic
    n. basis
    n. complication
    n. drug reaction
noninflammatory
    n. arthritis
    n. edema
noninherited maternal antigen (NIMA)
Nonin Onyx pulse oximeter
noninsulin-dependent diabetes mellitus
  (NIDDM)
nonirritating test substance
nonlinear IgA deposition
nonlymphocytic cell
nonmelanoma skin cancer (NMSC)
nonmeningeal
nonmethylated CpG motif
nonmyeloablative
    n. conditioning regimen
    n. HSCT
nonnecrotizing angiitis
Nonne-Milroy-Meige syndrome
nonneoplastic disease
nonneuropathic systemic amyloidosis
nonnucleoside reverse transcriptase
  inhibitor (NNRTI)
nonoccluded virus
nonocclusive dressing
nonoxynol-9 cream
nonpalpable purpura
nonparasitic sycosis
nonpathogenic fungus
nonpharmacologic measure of treatment
nonpigmented nevus
nonpoisonous
nonpolio enterovirus
nonprecipitable antibody
nonprecipitating antibody
nonprecipitation antibody
nonproductive cough
nonradicular
nonrandom X chromosome inactivation
nonrapid eye movement (nonREM,
  NREM)
nonREM
    nonrapid eye movement
    nonREM sleep
nonresponder tolerance

nonrestorative sleep
nonrheumatoid
    n. episcleritis
    n. scleritis
nonscarring alopecia
nonsecretor
nonsedating antihistamine
nonselective adenosine receptor
  antagonist
nonsense triplet
nonshedding dog
nonspecific
    n. absorption
    n. anergy
    n. climatic change
    n. cross-reacting antigen (NCA)
    n. dermatitis
    n. esterase (NSE)
    n. esterase stain
    n. protein
    n. therapy
nonsteroidal
    n. anti-inflammatory
    n. anti-inflammatory drug (NSAID)
nonstick gauze
nonsuction grasper
nonsyphilitic treponematosis
nonthrombocytopenic purpura
nontreponemal flocculation test
nontropical sprue
nontuberculous
    n. mycobacteria
    n. mycobacterial infection
nonunion
    ankylosis n.
    supracondylar n.
nonunited olecranon
nonvenereal
    n. bubo
    n. syphilis
    n. treponematosis
noon
    N. pollen unit
    n. unit
Noonan syndrome
norastemizole
Nordimmun IGIV
Norditropine
Nordryl
    N. Injection
    N. Oral
norepinephrine bitartrate
norethindrone
norfloxacin
Norfolk Arthritis Register (NOAR)
Norisodrine
Noritate cream
norlupinane

normal
>   n. animal
>   n. antibody
>   n. antitoxin
>   n. cornification
>   n. horse serum
>   n. opsonin
>   n. toxin

normal-mode ruby laser (NMRL)
Normlgel hydrogel dressing
normocapnia
normocholesteremic xanthoma
normochromic
normocomplementemic
normocytic
normolipemic xanthomatosis
normolipoproteinemic xanthomatosis
Noroxin Oral
Norpramin
Nor-tet Oral
North
>   N. American antisnakebite serum
>   N. American blastomycosis
>   N. American Contact Dermatitis Group (NACDG)
>   N. American Pediatric Renal Transplant Cooperative Study (NAPRTCS)
>   N. American Study of Treatment for Refractory Ascites study
>   N. Asian tick typhus
>   N. Queensland tick typhus

Northbent scissors
Northeast Organ Procurement Organization (NEOPO)
northern
>   N. blot analysis
>   n. rat flea
>   n. rat flea bite

Northland bone density machine
nortriptyline
Norvir
Norwalk
>   N. agent
>   N. virus

Norwalk-like agent
Norway itch
Norwegian scabies
Norwood classification system
nose
>   saddle n.

Nosema
>   N. connori
>   N. corneum
>   N. ocularum

nosematosis
nose-pad dermatitis
nosocomial
>   n. gangrene
>   n. infection
>   n. pneumonia (NP)

nosocomialis
>   phagedena n.

Nosopsyllus
>   N. fasciatus
>   N. fasciatus bite

nosotoxic
nosotoxin
nostras
>   cholera n.
>   n. elephantiasis
>   elephantiasis n.
>   piedra n.

Nostrilla
notalgia paresthetica
notatum
>   Penicillium n.

Notch signaling pathway
Nothnagel-type acroparesthesia
Notoedres
Novacet topical
Novafed
Novafil suture
Novahistine
Novamoxin
Nova Perfecting Lotion
Novasen
novel missense mutation
novo
>   de n.

Novo-AZT
Novobetamet
Novocaine
Novocain injection
Novo-Cimetine
Novo-Cromolyn
Novo-Difenac-K
Novo-Difenac-SR
Novo-Diflunisal
Novo-Dimenate
Novo-Doxylin
Novo E
Novo-Famotidine

N

NOTES

Novo-Flurprofen
Novo-Keto
Novo-Ketoconazole
Novo-Keto-EC
Novo-Methacin
Novo-Naprox
Novo-Nidazol
Novo-Pen-VK
Novo-Pheniram
Novo-Pirocam
Novo-Piroxicam
Novo-Prednisolone
Novo-Profen
Novo-Purol
Novo-Pyrazone
Novo-Ranidine
Novo-Rythro Encap
Novo-Sundac
Novo-Tetra
Novo-Tolmetin
noxa, pl. **noxae**
NoxBOX monitor
noxythiolin
NP
    nosocomial pneumonia
NP-27
NPA
    nasopharyngeal aspirate
NPSLE
    neuropsychiatric syndrome of systemic
      lupus erythematosus
    neuropsychiatric systemic lupus
      erythematosus
NPV
    negative predictive value
NR
    Tussi-Organidin NR
NREM
    nonrapid eye movement
NRTI
    nucleoside analog RT inhibitor
NS
    Netherton syndrome
NSAID
    nonsteroidal anti-inflammatory drug
      NSAID gastropathy
NSE
    neuron-specific enolase
    nonspecific esterase
      NSE stain
NSHD
    nodular sclerosing Hodgkin disease
NSJ
    nevus sebaceus of Jadassohn
NSN
    nephrotoxic serum nephritis
NSS
    nasal symptom score

Nt
    neutralizing
NTBC therapy
N-telopeptide urine test
N-Terface
    N.-T. contact layer sheet
    N.-T. contact layer wound dressing
    N.-T. gauze
NTPPH
    nucleoside triphosphate
      pyrophosphohydrolase
NTPPPH
    nucleoside triphosphate
      pyrophosphohydrolase
NTRI
    nucleoside reverse transcriptase inhibitor
NTZ
    nitazoxanide
    NTZ Long Acting Nasal Solution
Nu-Amoxi
Nu-Ampi
Nu-Beclomethasone
nuchae
    acne keloidalis n.
    cutis rhomboidalis n.
    erythema n.
    lichen n.
    ligamentum n.
    nevus flammeus n.
    sycosis n.
nuchal
    n. hemangioma
    n. nevus
Nu-Cimet
nuclear
    n. dot pattern
    n. factor
    n. factor of activated T cell
      (NFAT)
    n. factor-kappa B (NF-κB)
    n. factor kappa B ligand
    n. inclusion body
    n. lamin B1
    n. localization signal (NLS)
nucleated endothelial cell
nucleatum
    Fusobacterium n.
nuclei (*pl. of* nucleus)
nucleic
    n. acid probe
    n. acid sequence based
      amplification (NASBA)
nucleocapsid
nucleohistone
nucleoid
nucleolar staining
nucleoside
    n. analog RT inhibitor (NRTI)

n. phosphorylase
n. reverse transcriptase inhibitor (NTRI)
n. triphosphate pyrophosphohydrolase (NTPPH, NTPPPH)

nucleosome
    n. antibody
    n. ladder

nucleotidase

nucleotide
    antisense n.
    n. polymorphism
    sense n.

nucleotoxin

Nuclepore filter

nucleus, pl. **nuclei**
    droplet n.
    n. pulposus

Nucofed

nude
    n. bone graft transplantation
    n. mouse

Nu-Derm
    N.-D. hydrocolloid
    N.-D. hydrocolloid dressing
    Obagi N.-D.
    N.-D. System

Nu-Diclo

Nu-Diflunisal

Nu-Doxycycline

Nu-Famotidine

Nu-Flurprofen

Nu Gauze dressing

Nu-Gel
    N.-G. hydrogel sheet
    N.-G. hydrogel wound dressing
    N.-G. synthetic dressing

Nu-Hope skin barrier strip

Nu-Ibuprofen

Nu-Indo

Nu-Ketocon

Nu-Ketoprofen

Nu-Ketoprofen-E

null
    n. allele
    n. cell
    n. cell leukemia

null-type non-Hodgkin lymphoma

number
    chromosome n.

numbness

numerical taxonomy

nummular
    n. eczema
    n. eczematous dermatitis
    n. erythema
    n. lesion
    n. neurodermatitis
    n. syphilid

nummulare
    eczema n.

nummularis
    psoriasis n.

Nu-Naprox

Nu-Pen-VK

Nupercainal

Nu-Pirox

Nuprin

Nu-Ranit

nurse cell

Nursoy formula

nut
    Brazil n.

Nu-Tears II solution

Nu-Tetra

nutraceuticals

Nutracort Topical

Nu-Trake Weiss emergency airway system

Nutramigen formula

Nutraplus Topical

nutrient artery

nutritional
    n. deficiency dermatitis
    n. deficiency eczema
    n. disorder

Nutrol A D

Nutrotropin

NUVO barrier film

Nuvolase 660 laser system

NVAC
    National Vaccine Advisory Committee

Nydrazid injection

Nylexogrip cohesive long stretch bandage

nylon
    n. stocking dermatitis
    n. suture

nystagmus

nystatin and triamcinolone

Nystat-Rx

Nystex topical

Nyst-Olone II topical

Nytol
    Maximum Strength N.
    N. Oral

N

NOTES

O

O agglutinin
O antigen
O to T flap
O to Z flap

OA

occupationally induced asthma
ocular albinism
osteoarthritis

OAF

osteoclast-activating factor

oak

Gambel o.
live o.
o. moss absolute
poison o.
o. tree
o. tree pollen
western poison o.
white o.

oakridgensis

Legionella o.

OAS

oral allergy syndrome
OAS 1000

Oasis wound dressing
oat
oatmeal

colloidal o.
o. treatment

Obagi Nu-Derm
obconica

Primula o.

obesity

protein-energy-related o.
vitamin-related o.

objective synonym
obligate

o. aerobe
o. myiasis

obliterans

arteriosclerosis o.
balanitis xerotica o.
keratosis o.
thromboangiitis o. (TAO)

obliterative

o. airway disease
o. granulomatous fibrosis

O'Brien

O. actinic granuloma
O. scissors

obstruction

episodic bronchial o.
fixed airflow o.

severe o.
upper airway o.

obstructive

o. liver disease
o. purpura
o. sleep apnea (OSA)

obturator internus bursitis
obtusus

lichen o.

obvious physical exhaustion
OCA

oculocutaneous albinism

occidentale

Anacardium o.

occidentalis

Dermacentor o.

occipital

o. forelock
o. horn syndrome

occipitoaxial joint
occlude
occluded virus
occludens

zonula o.

Occlusal
Occlusal-HP Liquid
occlusion

o. miliaria
portal o.

occlusive

o. dressing
o. meningitis
o. moisturizer
o. patch test
o. phase
o. sheeting
o. therapy

occuloglandular syndrome
occult blood
occupational

o. acne
o. allergen
o. allergic alveolitis
o. dermatosis
o. exposure
o. immunologic lung disease
(OLD)
o. koilonychia
o. leukoderma
o. non-IgE-dependent asthma
o. rubber dermatitis
o. therapy (OT)
o. vitiligo

occupationally induced asthma (OA)

occupation-related syndrome
Ochrobacterium anthropi
ochrodermia
ochronosis
    endogenous o.
    exogenous o.
    ocular o.
ochronotic
    o. arthritis
    o. arthropathy
    o. spondylosis
Ockelbo disease
octamer
octapeptide
Octicair Otic
Octocaine injection
octreotide acetate
octulosonic acid
octyl methoxycinnamate
OcuClear Ophthalmic
OcuCoat PF Ophthalmic solution
Ocufen Ophthalmic
ocular
    o. adnexa
    o. albinism (OA)
    o. allergy
    o. atopic dermatitis
    o. cicatricial pemphigoid
    o. herpes simplex
    o. hypertelorism
    o. immune disease
    o. inflammatory disease
    o. inflammatory disorder
    o. larma migrans
    o. lesion
    o. lymphomatosis
    o. ochronosis
    o. pemphigus
    o. sarcoidosis
    o. toxicity
ocular-mucous membrane syndrome
ocular-scoliotic type Ehlers-Danlos
   syndrome
ocularum
    Nosema o.
oculi
    orbicularis o.
oculocerebral syndrome of Cross and
   McKusick
oculocutaneous
    o. albinism (OCA)
    o. telangiectasia
oculodermal
    o. melanocytosis
    o. melanosis
oculoglandular
oculoleptomeningeal amyloidosis
oculo-oral-genital syndrome

oculopharyngeal dystrophy
Ocu-Merox
Ocutricin
    O. HC Otic
    O. Topical Ointment
Ocu-Tropine Ophthalmic
odaxetic
ODD
    once-daily dosing
odds
    logarithm of o. (lod)
odeus
    herpes o.
Odland body
ODN
    oligodeoxynucleotide
odontoid process displacement
odonto-tricho-ungual-digital-palmar
   syndrome
odor
    o. control
    mousy o.
    volatile o.
odorans
    Alcaligenes o.
odoriferous
ODTS
    organic dust toxic syndrome
O'Duffy criteria
Odulimomab
oedema
    purpura en cocarde avec o.
Oesch
    O. perforation invagination stripper
    O. phlebectomy hook
Oesophagostomum
oestrosa
    dermamyiasis linearis migrans o.
oestruosa
    myiasis o.
OET
    open epicutaneous test
OFC
    open food challenge
Off-Ezy
officinalis
    poxvirus o.
ofloxacin
Ofuji
    O. disease
    papuloerythroderma of O.
Ohara disease
OHL
    oral hairy leukoplakia
Ohmeda hand-held oximeter
ohne Hauch
OHT
    orthotopic heart transplantation

OI
opportunistic illness
oidiomycin
oidiomycosis
"oid-oid" disease
oil
o. acne
Alpha-Keri o.
o. bath
o. of bergamot
Cade o.
Cajuput o.
citronella o.
clove o.
coal tar, lanolin, and mineral o.
Derma-Smoothe O.
o. drop change
o. drop lesion
o. drop sign
eucalyptus o.
evening primrose o.
fish o.
o. folliculitis
o. gland
o. immersion
jojoba o.
Lubath o.
mineral o.
patchouli o.
petitgrain o.
pine o.
RoBathol o.
silicone o.
trypsin, balsam Peru, and castor o.
Turpentine o.
o. vaccine
ylang-ylang o.
Oilated Aveeno
oil-based facial foundation
Oil-Free
O.-F. Acne Wash
Coppertone O.-F.
oiliness
oil-in-water
oil-spot discoloration
oily granuloma
ointment
20-10-5 o.
absorbent o.
A and D O.
AK-Spore H.C. Ophthalmic O.
Aloe Vesta antifungal o.

Amerigel topical o.
Baby's Own O.
Cavilon barrier o.
Cormax O.
Cortisporin Ophthalmic O.
Cortisporin Topical O.
Denavir o.
Efalith o.
emulsifiable o.
Hebra o.
James C. White tar o.
Jarisch o.
Kligman o.
Medi-Quick Topical O.
mupirocin o.
Neo-Polycin o.
Neosporin Ophthalmic O.
Neosporin Topical O.
Neotricin HC Ophthalmic O.
Ocutricin Topical O.
Panscol o.
rose water o.
Salacid O.
Septa Topical O.
tacrolimus o.
o. of tar
Terak Ophthalmic O.
Terramycin w/Polymyxin B
Ophthalmic O.
triamcinolone o. (TAO)
Tronothane o.
water-in-oil o.
water-repellent o.
water-soluble o.
Whitfield o.
ointment/dressing
Dermagran o.
Oka vaccine
OKT
Ortho-Kung T
OKT cell
OKT3
O. antibody
5 O. antilymphocyte therapy
Orthoclone O.
olamine
ciclopirox o.
Olay Sensitive Skin bar
OLD
occupational immunologic lung disease
old
o. ecchymosis

O

NOTES

395

old *(continued)*
    o. tuberculin (OT)
    O. World leishmaniasis
old-man's pemphigus
Olea europa
olecranon
    o. bursitis
    o. fossa
    nonunited o.
    o. procedure
    o. process
oleic acid
oleoresin
    capsaicin o.
    plant o.
oleosa
    hyperhidrosis o.
    seborrhea o.
oleosus
Oligella
oligemicus
    nevus o.
olighidria
oligoadenylate synthase
oligoarthritis
    asymmetric o.
    seronegative o.
oligoarthropathy
    asymmetric o.
oligoarticular seronegative rheumatoid arthritis
oligoclonal
oligocystic
oligodendrocyte
    o. destruction
    o. injury
oligodeoxynucleotide (ODN)
    antisense o.
    immunostimulatory o. (ISS-ODN)
    unmethylated o.
oligodynamic
oligoglysine
oligohidria
oligohidrosis
oligonucleotide
    antisense phosphorothioate o.
    o. probe
oligophrenia
    phenylpyruvic o.
oligoprobe
oligosaccharide
    asparagine-linked o.
    hyaluronan o.
    Lewis X o.
oligospermia
oligosymptomatic
oligotrichia
oligotrichosis

oligotyping
O-linked
    O.-l. pattern
    O.-l. saccharide
olivae
    vellus o.
olive
    Russian o.
    o. tree
    o. tree pollen
Ollendorf syndrome
Olmsted syndrome
olopatadine hydrochloride
olsalazine sodium
Olsen-Hegar needle holder
OLT
    orthotopic liver transplantation
Olux foam
omalizumab
Ombrelle sunscreen
omega-3, -6 fatty acid
omega nail
Omenn syndrome
omeprazole
OMERACT
    Outcome Measures in Rheumatology Clinical Trial
Ommaya reservoir
Omniderm
    O. synthetic dressing
    O. transparent film
Omnipen
Omnipen-N
omphalocele
Omsk
    O. hemorrhagic fever
    O. hemorrhagic fever virus
OMU
    ostiomeatal unit
once-daily dosing (ODD)
Onchocerca
    O. caecutiens
    O. volvulus
onchocerciasis
onchocercosis
oncofetal antigen
oncogene
    BNLF-1 o.
    Kirsten-MSV Ras o.
oncogenic virus
oncology
Oncolym radiolabeled monoclonal antibody
Onconase
oncornaviruses
oncostatin M (OSM)
Oncovin

Oncovirinae
oncovirus
oncus
Ondine curse, periodic breathing
one hand-two foot syndrome
ongles en raquette
onion mite dermatitis
Only
    Faces O.
onset
    insidious o.
    pauciarticular o.
Ontak protein
ontogeny
onychalgia nervosa
onychatrophia
onychatrophy
onychauxis
onychectomy
onychia
    Candida o.
    o. craquelé
    o. lateralis
    o. maligna
    monilial o.
    o. parasitica
    o. periungualis
    o. piannic
    o. punctata
    o. sicca
    syphilitic o.
onychitis
onychoclasis
onychocryptosis
onychodystrophy
onychogenic
onychogryphosis, onychogryposis
onychoheterotopia
onychoid
onychology
onycholysis
onychoma
onychomadesis
onychomalacia
onychomycosis
onychonosus
onychoosteodysplasia
onychopachydermoperiostitis
    psoriatic o. (POPP)
onychopathic
onychopathology
onychopathy

onychophagia
onychophagy
onychophosis
onychophyma
onychoptosis
onychorrhexis
onychoschizia
onychosis
onychotillomania
onychotomy
onychotrophy
Ony-Clear
    O.-C. Nail
    O.-C. Spray
o'nyong-nyong
    o.-n. fever
    o.-n. virus
Onyvul
onyx
onyxis
onyxitis
oocysts
    Cryptosporidium o.
oomycetes
oozing dermatitis
O&P
    ova and parasites
    test for O&P
opacification
    amorphous parenchymal o.
    corneal o.
    ground-glass o.
opacity
    mottled o.
opaline patch
Opcon-A
OPD
    optical penetration depth
open
    o. application test
    o. comedo
    o. epicutaneous test (OET)
    o. food challenge (OFC)
    o. lung biopsy
    o. patch test
    o. reduction and internal fixation
    (ORIF)
    o. tuberculosis
    o. wet dressing
opera-glass deformity
opercula

O

NOTES

opercularis
    Megalopyge o.
operculate
ophiasic alopecia areata
ophiasis
ophritis
ophryitis
ophryogenes
    ulerythema o.
Ophthacet Ophthalmic
Ophthalgan Ophthalmic
ophthalmia
    o. neonatorum
    spring o.
    sympathetic o.
Ophthalmic
    Achromycin O.
    Acular O.
    AK-Chlor O.
    AK-Cide O.
    AK-Dex O.
    AK-Homatropine O.
    AK-Neo-Dex O.
    AK-Poly-Bac O.
    AK-Pred O.
    AK-Sulf O.
    AKTob O.
    AK-Tracin O.
    AK-Trol O.
    Alomide O.
    Atropair O.
    Atropine-Care O.
    Atropisol O.
    Betimol O.
    Bleph-10 O.
    Blephamide O.
    Cetamide O.
    Cetapred O.
    Chloroptic O.
    Chloroptic-P O.
    Ciloxan O.
    Collyrium Fresh O.
    Dexacidin O.
    Dexasporin O.
    Econopred Plus O.
    Flarex O.
    Fluor-Op O.
    FML Forte O.
    Garamycin O.
    Genoptic S.O.P. O.
    Gentacidin O.
    Gentak O.
    Herplex O.
    HMS Liquifilm O.
    Ilotycin O.
    Inflamase Forte O.
    Inflamase Mild O.
    Isopto Atropine O.
    Isopto Cetapred O.
    Isopto Homatropine O.
    Isopto Hyoscine O.
    I-Sulfacet O.
    I-Tropine O.
    Livostin O.
    Maxitrol O.
    Metimyd O.
    Metreton O.
    Natacyn O.
    Neo-Cortef O.
    NeoDecadron O.
    Neo-Dexameth O.
    OcuClear O.
    Ocufen O.
    Ocu-Tropine O.
    Ophthacet O.
    Ophthalgan O.
    Ophthocort O.
    Osmoglyn O.
    Polysporin O.
    Polytrim O.
    Pred Forte O.
    Pred-G O.
    Pred Mild O.
    Sodium Sulamyd O.
    Sulf-10 O.
    Sulfair O.
    Tetrasine Extra O.
    Timoptic O.
    Timoptic-XE O.
    TobraDex O.
    Tobrex O.
    Vasocidin O.
    Vasosulf O.
    Vira-A O.
    Viroptic O.
    Visine L.R. O.
ophthalmica
    zona o.
ophthalmicus
    herpes zoster o.
ophthalmic zoster
ophthalmomaxillaris
    nevus fuscoceruleus
        acromiodeltoideus fuscoceruleus o.
ophthalmomyiasis
ophthalmopathy
    thyroid-associated o. (TAO)
Ophthocort Ophthalmic
opiates
opioid
O-plasty to Z-plasty
OPO
    optical parametric oscillator
    organ procurement organization
oppilation

opportunistic
- o. fungus
- o. illness (OI)
- o. organism
- o. pathogen
- o. systemic fungal infection
- o. systemic mycosis

opposition-versus-pressure relation

OPSI
- overwhelming postsplenectomy infection

opsinogen

OpSite
- O. Flexigrid adhesive dressing
- O. Flexigrid transparent film
- O. Plus composite dressing
- O. postop composite dressing
- O. semipermeable dressing

opsogen

opsonic
- o. deficiency
- o. receptor

opsonin
- common o.
- immune o.
- normal o.
- specific o.
- thermolabile o.
- thermostable o.

opsonization

opsonizing antibody

opsonocytophagic

opsonometry

opsonophagocytic defect

opsonophilia

opsonophilic

optic
- o. atrophy
- o. glioma
- o. neuritis

optica
- neuromyelitis o.

optical
- o. coherent tomography
- o. parametric oscillator (OPO)
- o. penetration depth (OPD)

OptiChamber

Opticrom

Opti-Flex

OptiHaler

Optimine

optimum temperature

Optimyd

Optipore Sponge wound cleanser

Opti 1 portable pH/blood gas analyzer

Optivar

OPV
- oral polio vaccine

Orabase
- O. HCA
- O. HCA Topical
- Kenalog in O.
- O. with benzocaine

Oracit

Orafen

Ora-Jel

oral
- Achromycin V O.
- o. administration of psoralen and subsequent exposure to long wavelength ultraviolet light (PUVA)
- Aller-Chlor O.
- o. allergy syndrome (OAS)
- AllerMax O.
- AL-Rr O.
- Amino-Opti-E O.
- Ansaid O.
- o. antihistamine
- Anxanil O.
- o. aphthous ulcer
- Aquasol E O.
- Aristocort O.
- Asacol O.
- Atarax O.
- Atolone O.
- Atozine O.
- Bactocill O.
- Banophen O.
- Beepen-VK O.
- Belix O.
- Benadryl O.
- Betapen-VK O.
- Bio-Tab O.
- Blocadren O.
- Brethine O.
- Bricanyl O.
- Calciferol O.
- o. calcitonin
- Calm-X O.
- o. candidiasis
- Cataflam O.
- o. cavity abnormality
- CeeNU O.
- Ceftin O.

NOTES

O

oral *(continued)*
Celestone O.
o. challenge
Chlo-Amine O.
Chlorate O.
Chlor-Trimeton O.
Cipro O.
Cleocin HCl O.
Cleocin Pediatric O.
Coly-Mycin S O.
o. condyloma planus
Cortone Acetate O.
Cytoxan O.
Decadron O.
Delta-Cortef O.
Deltasone O.
Diamine T.D. O.
Diflucan O.
Dimetabs O.
Dimetane O.
Dormarex 2 O.
Dormin O.
Doryx O.
Doxychel O.
Dramamine O.
Drisdol O.
Dynacin O.
E.E.S. O.
E-Mycin O.
o. epithelial nevus
o. (erosive) lichen planus
Eryc O.
EryPed O.
Ery-Tab O.
o. erythema multiforme
Erythrocin O.
o. erythromycin ethylsuccinate
Eryzole O.
Flagyl O.
o. florid papillomatosis
Floxin O.
Flumadine O.
Gantrisin O.
Gastrocrom O.
Genahist o.
o. hairy leukoplakia (OHL)
Hy-Pam o.
o. hyposensitization
Ilosone O.
Imitrex O.
Indocin SR o.
o. iron therapy
Kantrex O.
Kenacort o.
o. keratosis
Klorominr o.
Lamisil o.
Laniazid O.

Ledercillin VK O.
Liquid Pred O.
Loniten o.
Marmine o.
Maxaquin O.
Meclomen O.
Medrol o.
o. melanoacanthoma
Mephyton O.
Meticorten O.
Minocin O.
Monodox O.
o. mucosa
Mycifradin Sulfate O.
Mycostatin O.
Neo-fradin O.
Neoral O.
Neo-Tabs O.
Nidryl O.
Nizoral O.
Nordryl o.
Noroxin O.
Nor-tet o.
Nytol o.
Orasone O.
Panmycin O.
PCE O.
PediaCare o.
Pediapred o.
Pediazole O.
Penetrex O.
Pentasa O.
Pen-Vee K O.
Pepcid O.
Phenameth O.
Phendry O.
Phenergan O.
Phenetron O.
o. polio vaccine (OPV)
poliovirus vaccine, live, trivalent, o.
o. postinflammatory hyperpigmentation
Prednicen-M O.
Prelone o.
Prostaphlin O.
Prothazine O.
Protostat o.
Retrovir O.
Rifadin o.
Rimactane O.
Robicillin VK O.
Robitet o.
Salagen O.
Sandimmune O.
Siladryl o.
Sleep-eze 3 O.
Sominex O.

Sporanox O.
Sterapred O.
Sumycin O.
o. tattoo
Tega-Vert O.
Telachlor O.
Teldrin O.
Teline O.
Terramycin O.
Tetracap o.
Tetralan O.
Tetram O.
o. thrush
o. tolerance
Trisoralen O.
o. tuberculosis
Twilite o.
o. ulceration
Unipen O.
Uri-Tet O.
Valium O.
Valrelease o.
Vancocin o.
V-Cillin K o.
Veetids o.
VePesid o.
Vibramycin o.
Videx o.
Vistaril o.
Vivotif Berna o.
Voltaren o.
Voltaren-XR o.
Wellcovorin o.
Zantac o.
Zovirax o.
oral-ocular-genital syndrome
Oraminic II injection
orange
o. blossom
o. peel appearance
Orap
Orasone Oral
Orbasone system
orbiculare
Pityrosporum o.
orbicular eczema
orbicularis
alopecia o.
o. oculi
psoriasis o.
orbital
o. granuloma

o. inflammatory disease
o. myositis
o. pseudotumor
Orbivirus
orchard
o. grass
o. grass pollen
orchitis
allergic o.
ordinal designation of the exanthemata
Oregon ash
Orentreich punch
Orex
3′orf gene
orf virus
organ
o. culture
o. parking
o. procurement organization (OPO)
o. system failure index (OSFI)
o. transplantation system
o. xenograft
organ-cultured corneal tissue
Organex
organic
o. dust toxic syndrome (ODTS)
o. mercurials
Organidin
organism
calculated mean o. (CMO)
Cox o.
culprit o.
encapsulated o.
Gram-negative o.
Gram-positive o.
group JK o.
hypothetical mean o.
opportunistic o.
pleuro-pneumoniae-like o. (PPLO)
prokaryotic extracellular o.
transgenic o.
organization
Food Agricultural O. (FAO)
health maintenance o. (HMO)
International Labor O. (ILO)
Northeast Organ Procurement O.
  (NEOPO)
organ procurement o. (OPO)
organoid nevus
organotaxis
organotropic
organotropism

NOTES

O

organotropy
organ-specific
    o.-s. antigen
    o.-s. tolerance
Orgotein
Oriboca virus
Oriental
    O. boil
    O. button
    O. rat flea
    O. rat flea bite
    O. ringworm
    O. sore
    O. ulcer
orientalis
    Amycolatopsis o.
    furunculosis o.
    Leishmania o.
ORIF
    open reduction and internal fixation
orifice
    follicular o.
orificialis
    tuberculosis o.
    tuberculosis cutis o.
orificial tuberculosis
origin
    antirabies serum, equine o.
    fever of unknown o. (FUO)
Original
    Doan's, O.
Orimune
Orinidyl
Orion
    O. device
    O. inhaler
oris
    adenomatosis o.
    cancrum o.
    fetor o.
    leukokeratosis o.
Ormazine
Ornade
Ornex Cold
ornidazole
Ornidyl injection
ornithine-ketoacid transaminase 3 antibody
ornithine transcarbamylase deficiency
Ornithodoros
ornithosis virus
orofacial
    o. herpes simplex
    o. tuberculosis
orolabial herpes
oronasal

oropharyngeal
    o. candidiasis
    o. gonorrhea
oropharynx
orosomucoid
orotic aciduria
orotidinuria
Oroya fever
orphan
    chicken embryo lethal o. (CELO)
    o. disease
    o. drug
    enteric cytopathogenic bovine o. (ECBO)
    enteric cytopathogenic human o. (ECHO)
    enteric cytopathogenic monkey o. (ECMO)
    enteric cytopathogenic swine o. (ECSO)
    respiratory enteric o. (REO)
    o. virus
orris root
Orthoclone
    O. OKT3
    O. OKT3 anti-CD3 monoclonal antibody
Ortho-Ice Multipaks system
orthokeratinization
orthokeratosis
Ortho-Kung
    O.-K. T (OKT)
    O.-K. T cell
orthologue
orthomolecular therapy
Orthomune monoclonal antibody
Orthomyxoviridae virus
orthophosphate (P1)
orthopnea
Orthopoxvirus vaccinia
orthosis, pl. **orthoses**
    ankle-foot o. (AFO)
    patellar tendon-bearing o.
    spring-assisted knee extension o.
    thoraco-lumbar-sacral o.
orthostatic
    o. acrocyanosis
    o. hypotension
    o. purpura
orthotic
orthotopic
    o. heart transplantation (OHT)
    o. liver transplantation (OLT)
Orthovisc
Orudis KT
Oruvail

oryzae
>   *Aspergillus o.*
>   *Rhizopus o.*

orzihabitans
>   *Flavimonas o.*

OS
>   oxidative stress

OSA
>   obstructive sleep apnea

Oscar virus

oscillation
>   high frequency o.

oscillator
>   Hayek o.
>   optical parametric o. (OPO)

OSFI
>   organ system failure index

Osler
>   O. disease
>   O. hemangiomatosis
>   O. node
>   O. sign
>   O. syndrome II
>   O. triad

Osler-Weber-Rendu
>   O.-W.-R. disease
>   O.-W.-R. syndrome

OSM
>   oncostatin M

OSMED
>   otospondylometaphyseal dysplasia
>   OSMED syndrome

osmidrosis
osmiophilic crystal structure
Osmitrol injection
OsmoCyte pillow wound dressing
Osmoglyn Ophthalmic
osmolality
osmophil
osmotic shock
OspA primer-probe
OspB primer-probe
osseous
>   o. choristoma of the tongue
>   o. heteroplasia
>   o. lesion
>   o. syphilis
>   o. tumor
>   o. yaw

ossicles
>   intraarticular o.

ossificans
>   myositis o.

ossification
>   entheseal o.
>   paraarticular o.
>   periarticular o.

ossium
>   fibrogenesis imperfecta o.

osteitis
>   chronic recurrent multifocal o.
>   (CRMO)
>   o. condensans ilii
>   o. fibrosa
>   o. fibrosa cystica disseminata
>   o. pubis
>   synovitis, acne, pustulosis,
>   hyperostosis, o. (SAPHO, SAPHO
>   syndrome)

osteoarthritis (OA)
>   erosive o. (EOA)
>   facet joint o.
>   glenohumeral o.
>   idiopathic hypertrophic o.
>   patellofemoral o.
>   radiologic o. (ROA)

osteoarthropathy
>   hypertrophic o.
>   tabetic o.

osteoarticular candidiasis
Osteo Bi-Flex
osteoblast-lineage cell
osteocalcin
osteochondral implant
osteochondritis
>   o. dissecans
>   parrot syphilitic o.

osteochondrodysplasia
osteochondromatosis
osteoclast-activating factor (OAF)
osteoclast differentiation factor
osteoclastogenesis
osteocyte lacunae
osteodermatopoikilosis
osteodermatous
osteodermia
osteodystrophy
>   Albright hereditary o.

osteogenesis
>   o. imperfecta
>   o. imperfecta syndrome
>   o. imperfecta tarda

OsteoGram bone density test

O

NOTES

osteohypertrophic nevus flammeus
osteoid osteoma
osteolytic bone lesion
osteoma
    o. cutis
    intraarticular osteoid o.
    osteoid o.
osteomalacia
Osteomark urine-based test
osteomatoid
osteomatosis
osteomyelitis
    Aspergillus o.
    blastomycotic o.
    Candida o.
    candidal o.
    chronic multifocal o.
    coccidioidal o.
    pyogenic o.
    salmonella o.
    typhoid o.
    o. variolosa
osteon
osteonecrosis
osteonectin
osteoonychodysplasia
    hereditary o. (HOOD)
osteopenia
    juxtaarticular o.
    periarticular o.
osteopetrosis gallinarum
osteophyte
osteopoikilosis
osteopontin
osteoporosis
    age-related o.
    o. circumscripta
    glucocorticoid-induced o.
    juxtaarticular o.
    periarticular o.
    type I, II o.
osteoprotegerin ligand
osteosis cutis
osteotabes
osteotomy
    Bernese periacetabular o.
    periacetabular o.
    proximal femoral o.
Osterballe precision needle
ostia (*pl. of* ostium)
ostial
    porokeratotic eccrine o.
ostiomeatal unit (OMU)
ostium, pl. **ostia**
    pilosebaceous o.
ostracea
    parakeratosis o.

ostraceous
    o. psoriasis
    o. scale
ostreacea
    psoriasis o.
OT
    occupational therapy
    old tuberculin
Ota
    nevus of O.
    O. nevus
Ot antigen
Otic
    Acetasol HC O.
    AK-Spore H.C. O.
    AntibiOtic O.
    Bacticort O.
    Cortatrigen O.
    Cortisporin O.
    O. Domeboro
    Dri-Ear O.
    Drotic O.
    LazerSporin-C O.
    Octicair O.
    Ocutricin HC O.
    Otobiotic O.
    Otocort O.
    Otomycin-HPN O.
    Otosporin O.
    Pediotic O.
    Swim-Ear O.
    VoSol HC O.
oticus
    herpes zoster o.
otitic meningitis
otitis
    o. externa
    external o.
    o. media
Otobiotic Otic
Otocalm Ear
Otocort Otic
otogenic meningitis
Otomycin-HPN Otic
otomycosis
otoscopy
    pneumatic o.
otospondylometaphyseal dysplasia
  (OSMED)
Otosporin Otic
ototoxicity
Otrivin Nasal
Ouchterlony
    O. double diffusion technique
    O. method
    O. test
Oudin current
Out of Africa

Outcome Measures in Rheumatology Clinical Trial (OMERACT)
outer
    o. canthus
    o. root sheath
Outerbridge scale
output
    adequate urine o.
OVA
    chicken ovalbumin
    ovalbumin
    OVA antigen
ovalbumin (OVA)
    o. antigen
    chicken o. (OVA)
ovalbumin-derived epitope
ovalbumin-induced arthritis
ovale
    Pityrosporum o.
    Plasmodium o.
ovalis
    Malassezia o.
ova and parasites (O&P)
Ovarex MAb monoclonal antibody
Ovcon
overdosage
overdose
    drug o.
overexpression
    gene o.
overlap
    o. disease
    o. myositis (OVLP)
    o. syndrome
overlay
    PAL pump for air mattress o.
overmoisturization
overriding maxillary incisor
overt hyperthyroidism
overuse syndrome
overwhelming postsplenectomy infection (OPSI)
overwintering
Ovide Topical
ovine progressive pneumonia
ovinia
oviposit
OVLP
    overlap myositis
ovomucoid
ovulation induction
Owens Surgical dressing

oxacillin
    o. disk diffusion test
    o. sodium
oxalate crystal
oxalosis
oxamniquine
Oxandrin
oxandrolone
oxaprozin
oxazepam
oxeye, ox-eye
    e. daisy
Oxford unit
oxiconazole nitrate
oxidase
    lysyl o.
    NADPH o.
    urate o.
oxidative
    o. burst
    o. stress (OS)
oxide
    aluminum o.
    endothelial-derived nitric o.
    ethylene o. (ETO)
    mercuric o.
    nitric o.
    nitrous o.
    zinc o.
oxidized cellulose
OxiFlow
oximeter
    Cricket recording pulse o.
    INVOS Cerebral O.
    Nellcor Symphony N-3000 pulse o.
    Nonin Onyx pulse o.
    Ohmeda hand-held o.
    Oxypleth pulse o.
    OxyTemp hand-held pulse o.
    SpotCheck+ handheld pulse o.
oxipurinol
Oxistat topical
OX-K proteus antigen
Oxsoralen-Ultra
    O.-U. Oral
Oxsoralen-Ultra oral
OX-2, -19 test
oxtriphylline
Oxy
    O. Control
    O. Deep Pore
    O. Medicated Pads

O

NOTES

Oxy *(continued)*
  O. Night Watch
  O. Power Pads
  O. 10 Wash
Oxy-5
  O. Advanced Formula for Sensitive
  Skin
  O. Tinted
**Oxy-10 Advanced Formula for Sensitive
Skin**
oxybenzone
  methoxycinnamate and o.
Oxybutazone
Oxycel
oxychlorosene sodium
OxyContin
Oxyderm
Oxyfil oxygen refilling system
oxygen
  o. consumption per minute (VO_2)
  continuous low-flow o.
  fraction of inspired o. (FIO_2)
  o. free radical
  humidified o.
  hyperbaric o. (HBO)
  o. metabolite
  partial pressure of o. (PO_2)
  partial pressure alveolar o. (PAO_2)
  partial pressure arterial o. (PaO_2)
  supplemental o.
oxygenase
  enzyme heme o.

oxygenation
  extracorporeal membrane o.
  (ECMO)
oxygenator
oxyhemoglobin (HbO_2)
Oxyl
oxymetazoline hydrochloride
oxymetholone
oxyphenbutazone
Oxypleth pulse oximeter
oxysporum
  Fusarium o.
OxyTemp hand-held pulse oximeter
oxytetracycline
  o. hydrochloride
  o. and hydrocortisone
  o. and polymyxin b
OxyTip
oxytoca
  Klebsiella o.
oxyuriasis
Oxyuris vermicularis
oyster mass of mucus
oyster-shell crust
Oz
  O. antigen
  O. isotypic determinant
ozochrotia
ozone
ozzardi
  Mansonella o.

P

P antigen
P blood group antigen
P and PD
P & S plus

P1

orthophosphate

p24

p24 antigen
p24 antigen testing

P53

P53 tumor suppressor gene

P450

cytochrome P450
P450 metabolism

p56 Lck deficiency
PA

polyarthritis

PAB

para-aminobenzoate

PABA

paraaminobenzoic acid
PABA ester
esterified PABA
nonesterified PABA

PAC

papular acrodermatitis of childhood

Pacheco parrot disease virus
pachydactyly
pachyderma

p. lymphangiectatica
p. verrucosa
p. vesica

pachydermatis

Malassezia p.

pachydermatocele
pachydermatosis
pachydermatous
pachydermia
pachydermic
pachydermoperiostosis plicata
pachyglossia
pachyhymenia
pachyhymenic
pachylosis
pachymenia
pachymenic
pachymeningitis

hypertrophic cervical p.
rheumatoid p.

pachyonychia congenita
pachyotia
Pacific tick
pacificus

Ixodes p.

pacinian neurofibroma
Pacis BCG
pack

interferon alfa-2b and ribavirin
combination p.
M-Zole 7 Dual P.

packed red cell transfusion
Packets

ENTsol P.

PACKS

No Pain-HOT P.

paclitaxel
PACNS

primary angiitis of the central nervous
system

pad

Clearasil P.'s
grounding p.
herniated presacral fat p.
impregnated p.
knuckle p.
MPM conductive gel p.
Oxy Medicated P.'s
Oxy Power P.'s
STD-E P.'s
Tegaderm transparent dressing with
absorbent p.

PADI

posterior atlantodental interval

padimate O
PADPRP

poly (adenosine diphosphate-ribose)
polymerase

PAEC

pig aortic endothelial cell

Paecilomyces

P. lilacinus
P. variotii

Paederus

P. dermatitis
P. gemellus
P. gemellus sting
P. limnophilus
P. limnophilus sting

Paenibacillus popilliae
PAF

platelet activating/aggregating factor
platelet-activating factor
platelet-aggregating factor

PAF-AH

platelet-activating factor acetylhydrolase

PAFD

percutaneous abscess and fluid drainage

PAG

pregnancy alpha-2 glycoprotein

P

PAGE
    polyacrylamide gel electrophoresis
Paget
    P. abscess
    P. abscess syndrome
    P. cell
    P. disease
pagetic petrous bony invasion
pagetoid
    p. cell
    p. reticulosis
PAH
    p-aminohippurate
Pahvant
    P. Valley fever
    P. Valley plague
pain
    chronic widespread p.
    global rating of p.
    limb p.
    p. on motion
    paranasal sinus p.
    pleuritic chest p.
    p. spot
painful
    p. adiposity
    p. mouth
    p. piezogenic pedal papule
    p. tongue
painful-bruising syndrome
Pain-HP
    No P.-H.
painless thyroiditis
paint
    Castellani p.
    keratolytic p.
    SAL p.
    salicylic acid-lactic acid p.
paired venom gland
pairs
    recipient-donor p.
PAIS
    punctate area of increased signal
PAK
    pancreas-after-kidney
    pancreas after kidney transplant
    PAK transplant
Pak
    Benzamycin P.
    Shingles Relief P.
palatal
    p. clicking
    p. papillomatosis
palate
    ankyloblepharon, ectodermal defect, and cleft lip and/or p. (AEC)
    ectodermal dysplasia, ectrodactyly and cleft lip and/or p. (EEC)

    hard p.
    high-arched p.
    itchy soft p.
palatinus
    torus p.
pale
    p. cell acanthoma
    p. color
palestinensis
    Acanthamoeba p.
palindromic rheumatism
palisade
    p. cell
    p. layer
palisaded encapsulated neuroma
palisading
    p. granuloma
    p. histiocyte
palivizumab antibody
pallescense
pallesthesia
pallida
    Spirochaeta p.
pallidum
    microhemagglutination-*Treponema p.* (MHA-TP)
    Treponema p.
Pallister-Hall syndrome
Pallister mosaic aneuploid syndrome
pallor
palm
    black p.
    hyperlinear p.
    liver p.
    queen p.
    reddening of p.
    p. tree
    tripe p.
    triple p.
palmar
    p. aponeurosis
    p. crease
    p. erythema
    p. fascia
    p. fasciitis and polyarthritis syndrome
    p. hyperlinearity
    p. psoriasis
    p. subluxation
    p. syphilid
    p. wart
    p. xanthoma
palmare
    erythema p.
    xanthoma multiplex striatum p.
palmaris
    acanthosis p.
    pyosis p.

xanthochromia striata p.
xanthoma striata p.
palmellina
trichomycosis p.
palmitate
cetyl p.
clofazimine p.
palmoplantar
p. eccrine hidradenitis (PEH)
p. erythrodysesthesia syndrome
p. fibromatosis
p. keratoderma (PPK)
p. pustulosis
palmoplantaris
pustulosis p.
palm-sole involvement
Palomar E2000 ruby laser hair reduction
palpable purpura
palpebral
p. blotch
p. edema
palpebrarum
dermatolysis p.
pediculosis p.
xanthelasma p.
xanthoma p.
p. xanthoma
PAL pump for air mattress overlay
palsy
axillary nerve p.
Bell p.
facial nerve p.
long thoracic nerve p.
spinal accessory nerve p.
suprascapular nerve p.
transitory p.
Pamelor
pamidronate
p-aminohippurate (PAH)
pamoate
pyrantel p.
Pamprin IB
PAN
polyacrylonitrile
polyarteritis nodosa
PAN membrane
Panadol
Panafil
P. enzymatic debrider
P. enzymatic debriding agent

Panafil-White
P.-W. enzymatic debrider
P.-W. enzymatic debriding agent
panagglutinable
panagglutinins
panallergen
panama
Salmonella p.
panaritium
Panasol II home phototherapy system
panatrophy
p. of Gower
panbronchiolitis
P-ANCA
perinuclear antineutrophil cytoplasmic antibody
P-ANCA titer
pancreas
p. after kidney transplant (PAK)
p. transplant alone (PTA)
p. transplantation
pancreas-after-kidney (PAK)
pancreatic
p. disorder
p. lobular panniculitis
p. oncofetal antigen (POA)
pancreaticoduodenal transplantation
pancreaticoduodenectomy
pancreatitis
pancuronium bromide
pancytopenia
familial p.
Pandel
pandemic
pandemicity
panel
ABPA p.
acute bronchopulmonary aspergillosis p.
anergy p.
cellular immune p.
humoral immunity status p.
hypersensitivity pneumonitis p.
latex RIA p.
panel-reactive
p.-r. antibody (PRA)
p.-r. antibody testing
panencephalitis
nodular p.
subacute sclerosing p. (SSPE)
panhidrosis
panhypogammaglobulinemia

NOTES

P

panhypopituitarism
    autoimmune p.
    idiopathic p.
    secondary p.
panidrosis
panimmunity
panleukopenia virus of cats
panmictic
Panmycin Oral
panmyelophthisis
    familial p.
panniculalgia
panniculitides
panniculitis
    alpha$_1$ antitrypsin deficiency p.
    chemical p.
    cold p.
    connective tissue p.
    cytophagic histiocytic p.
    cytophagic lobular p.
    enzyme-related p.
    eosinophilic p.
    equestrian p.
    factitial p.
    gouty p.
    histiocytic cytophagic p. (CHP)
    idiopathic lobular p.
    lobular p.
    lupus erythematosus p.
    migratory p.
    nodular migratory p.
    nodular nonsuppurative p.
    pancreatic lobular p.
    physical lobular p.
    popsicle p.
    poststeroid p.
    relapsing febrile nodular
     nonsuppurative p.
    scleroderma septal p.
    sclerosing p.
    septal p.
    subacute nodular migratory p.
    traumatic p.
    vessel-based lobular p.
pannus
    p. cell
    cellular p.
    fibrous p.
    rheumatoid p.
pannus-cartilage junction
PanoGauze
    P. hydrogel-impregnated gauze
    P. impregnated gauze
panophthalmitis
Panoplex hydrogel dressing
PanOxyl-AQ
PanOxyl Bar
panreactive monoclonal antibody

Panretin topical gel
Panscol
    P. Lotion
    P. ointment
panspermia
pan T-cell marker
pantothenic acid deficiency
pantropic virus
pants paresthesia syndrome
panuveitis
    idiopathic p.
PAO$_2$
    partial pressure alveolar oxygen
PaO$_2$
    partial pressure arterial oxygen
pao ferro wood
Pap
    Papanicolaou
    Pap test
PAPA
    pyogenic sterile arthritis, pyoderma
    gangrenosum and acne
    PAPA syndrome
papain
Papanicolaou (Pap)
    P. test (Pap test)
papaverine
paper
    p. dermatitis
    Diazo p.
    litmus p.
    p. mulberry
    p. mulberry tree
    p. radioimmunosorbent test (PRIST)
    p. wasp
paper-thin scar
papilla, pl. **papillae**
    anogenital vestibular p.
    dermal p.
    hypertrophy of tongue p.
    vestibular p.
papillaris
    nevus p.
    pars p.
papillary
    p. atrophy
    p. dermis
    p. eccrine adenoma
    p. ectasia
    p. hidradenoma
    p. necrosis
    p. tumor
papillation
papilliferous
papilliferum
    hidradenoma p.
    syringoadenoma p.
    syringocystadenoma p.

papilliferus
  nevus syringocystadenomatosus p.
  nevus syringocystadenosus p.
papilliform
papillitis
papilloadenocystoma
papillocarcinoma
papilloma
  p. acuminatum
  basal cell p.
  canine oral p.
  p. diffusum
  p. durum
  hard p.
  p. inguinale tropicum
  p. molle
  Shope p.
  soft p.
  p. venereum
  p. virus
  zymotic p.
papillomatosis
  confluent and reticulate p.
  florid cutaneous p. (FCP)
  florid oral p.
  p. of Gougerot-Carteaud
  juvenile p.
  laryngeal p.
  malignant p.
  oral florid p.
  palatal p.
  recurrent respiratory laryngeal p.
  reticulated p.
papillomatosus
  lupus p.
  nevus p.
papillomatous
Papillomavirus
papillomavirus
  human p. (HPV)
  Hybrid Capture II DNA-based test
    for human p.
Papillon-Lèfevre syndrome
Papineau graft
Papovaviridae
papovavirus
pappataci
  p. fever
  p. fever virus
pappose
pappus
paprika splitter's lung

papula
papular
  p. acne
  p. acrodermatitis
  p. acrodermatitis of childhood
    (PAC)
  p. dermatitis
  p. dermatitis of pregnancy
  p. fever
  p. fibroplasia
  p. mastocytosis
  p. mucinosis
  p. sarcoid
  p. scrofuloderma
  p. stomatitis virus of cattle
  p. syphilid
  p. syphiloderma
  p. tuberculid
  p. urticaria
  p. xanthoma
papular-purpuric
  p.-p. gloves and socks syndrome
  p.-p. stocking and glove syndrome
papulation
  granular p.
  perifollicular p.
papulatum
  erythema p.
papule
  Celsus p.
  discrete umbilicated p.
  fibrous p.
  follicular p.
  Gottron p.
  indolent p.
  indurated p.
  keratotic p.
  moist p.
  mucous p.
  painful piezogenic pedal p.
  penile pearly p.
  persistent pearly penile p.
  piezogenic pedal p.
  polygonal p.
  prurigo p.
  pruritic p.
  purple-red p.
  red p.
  satellite erythematous p.
  split p.
  yellow p.
Papulex

NOTES

P

411

papuliferous
papuloerosive erythema
papuloerythematous
papuloerythroderma of Ofuji
papulonecrotica
    tuberculosis cutis p.
papulonecrotic tuberculid
papulopustular lesion
papulopustule
papulosa
    acne p.
    miliaria p.
    p. nigra dermatosis
    parakeratosis p.
    stomatitis p.
    urticaria p.
papulose atrophicante maligne
papulosis
    atrophic p.
    p. atrophicans maligna
    Bowenoid p.
    clear-cell p.
    lymphomatoid p. (LyP)
    malignant atrophic p.
papulosquamous
    p. dermatitis
    p. disorder
    p. eruption
    p. lesion
    p. syphilid
papulosum
    eczema p.
    erythema p.
papulovesicle
papulovesicular
    p. acrolocated syndrome
    p. lesion
    p. rash
Papworth heart donor survey
papyraceous scar
PAR
    protease-activated receptor
paraaminobenzoic acid (PABA)
paraaminosalicylate sodium
paraaminosalicylic acid
paraarticular ossification
paraben mix
parachlorometaxylenol (PCMX)
parachlorophenylalanine
parachroma
parachromatosis
paracoccidioidal granuloma
Paracoccidioides brasiliensis
paracoccidioidin skin test
paracoccidioidomycosis
paracrine
paradox
    thoracoabdominal p.

paradoxical
    p. pulse
    p. sleep
paradoxus
    pulsus p.
paraffin
    p. breast augmentation
    Liquid p.
paraffinoma
parafollicularis
    hyperkeratosis follicularis et p.
parafrenal abscess
paragonimiasis
Paragonimus
    P. kellicotti
    P. westermani
parahaemolyticus
    Haemophilus p.
parahidrosis
parainfluenza
    p. virus
parainfluenzae
    Haemophilus p.
parakeet feather
parakeratosis
    p. ostracea
    p. papulosa
    p. psoriasiformis
    p. pustulosa
    p. scutularis
    p. variegata
parallergic
paraluis-cuniculi
    Treponema p.-c.
paralysis, pl. paralyses
    acute atrophic p.
    acute flaccid p. (AFP)
    fowl p.
    immune p.
    immunological p.
    infectious bulbar p.
    myogenic p.
    parotitic p.
    phrenic nerve p.
    postdiphtheric p.
    Pott p.
    syphilitic spastic spinal p.
    tick p.
parameter
paramethasone acetate
paramyloidosis
Paramyxoviridae virus
Paramyxovirus
paranasal
    p. sinus drainage
    p. sinus pain
paraneoplastic
    p. acrokeratosis

p. pemphigus (PNP)
p. subacute cerebellar degeneration
p. syndrome
paraneoplastica
  acrokeratosis p.
parangi
Para-Pak Ultra Ecofix system
paraparesis
  areflexic p.
  HTLV-1-associated myelopathy or
    tropical spastic p. (HAM/TSP)
  tropical spastic p. (TSP)
parapertussis
  Bordetella p.
paraphenylenediamine (PPDA)
  p. dermatitis
paraphimosis
parapneumonic effusion
Parapoxvirus
paraproteinemia
parapsilosis
  Candida p.
parapsoriasis
  p. acuta et varioliformis
  p. en gouttes
  p. en plaque
  p. guttata
  guttate p.
  p. large-plaque
  large-plaque p.
  p. lichenoid
  p. lichenoides
  p. lichenoides et varioliformis acuta
  p. maculata
  poikilodermatous p.
  p. retiform
  retiform p.
  small plaque p.
  p. small-plaque
  p. variegata
pararama
pararosaniline hydrochloride
parascarlatina
parasitaria
parasite
  metazoal p.
  ova and p.'s (O&P)
parasitic
  p. cyst
  p. disease
  p. granuloma

p. melanoderma
p. sycosis
parasitica
  achromia p.
  glossitis p.
  onychia p.
parasiticum
  eczema p.
parasitophobia
parasitosis
  delusion of p.
parasympathetic nerve fiber
parasyphilis
parathyroidectomy
paratope
paratracheal region
paratrichosis
paratrimma
  erythema p.
paratripsis
paratriptic
paratyphi
  Salmonella p.
paratyphoid fever
paraumbilical nodule
paraungual
paravaccinia
  p. virus
  p. virus infection
Paravespula sting
parchment skin
Par Decon
parenchyma
parenchymal
  p. amyloidosis
  p. fibrosis
parenchymatous
  p. glossitis
  p. neurosyphilis
  p. syphilis
parenteral
  p. absorption
  Coly-Mycin M P.
  p. corticosteroid
  p. diphenhydramine
  p. gold
paresis
paresthesia
paresthetica
  meralgia p.
  notalgia p.
paretic neurosyphilis

NOTES

P

413

paridrosis
parietalis
    decidua p.
Parietaria-induced rhinoconjunctivitis
Parietaria judacia
Parinaud oculoglandular syndrome
Paris green
Parker-Pearson needle
Parker retractor
Parkes-Weber hemangiomatosis
parking
    organ p.
Parkinson disease
Parkland
    P. burn resuscitation formula
    P. formula for fluid resuscitation
      for burn trauma
Park-Williams bacillus
paromomycin
    p. sulfate
paronychia
    acute p.
    bacterial p.
    Candida p.
    candidal p.
    chronic p.
    herpetic p.
    monilial p.
paronychial
    p. wart
paronychomycosis
paronychosis
parotid
    p. gland
    p. sialography
parotiditis
    epidemic p.
parotitic paralysis
parotitis
paroxetine
    p. HCl
    p. hydrochloride
paroxysmal
    p. cold hemoglobinuria
    p. flushing
    p. hand hematoma
    p. nocturnal hemoglobinuria (PNH)
    p. pruritus
    p. sneezing
paroxysm of coughing
PARP autoantibody
parrot
    p. feather
    P. node
    P. pseudoparalysis
    P. sign
    P. syndrome
    p. syphilitic osteochondritis

    P. ulcer
    p. virus
parrot-beak nail
Parry-Romberg syndrome
pars
    p. papillaris
    p. reticularis
parsley
parsnip
Parsol
    P. 1789
    P. 1789 sunscreen
parthenium dermatitis
partial
    p. agglutinin
    p. albinism
    p. albinism with immunodeficiency
    p. antigen
    p. combined immunodeficiency
      disorder
    p. face-sparing lipodystrophy
    p. leukonychia
    p. lipoatrophy
    p. pressure alveolar oxygen (PAO_2)
    p. pressure arterial oxygen (PaO_2)
    p. pressure of carbon dioxide
      (PCO_2)
    p. pressure of oxygen (PO_2)
    p. thromboplastin time (PTT)
partialis
    hypertrichosis p.
partial-thickness burn
particle
    Dane p.
    defective interfering p.
    DI p.
    signal recognition p. (SRP)
particulate matter
Partuss LA
parvilocular cyst
Parvoviridae
parvovirus
    p. B19
    human p. (HPV)
    human p. B19
parvum bovine Ig concentrate
PAS
    periodic acid-Schiff
    PAS stain
    PAS technique
P.A.S.
    P.A.S. Port catheter
    Sodium P.A.S.
Paschen body
Paser
PASI
    psoriasis area and severity index
Pasini epidermolysis bullosa

Pasini-Pierini
>P.-P. idiopathic atrophoderma
>P.-P. syndrome

passage
>blind p.
>percutaneous p.
>serial p.

passant
>en p.

passenger leukocyte
passion purpura
passive
>p. agglutination
>p. cutaneous anaphylactic reaction
>p. cutaneous anaphylaxis (PCA)
>p. cutaneous anaphylaxis test
>p. hemagglutination (PHA)
>p. immunity
>p. immunization
>p. immunoprophylaxis
>p. immunotherapy
>p. motion
>p. prophylaxis
>p. range of motion exercise
>p. transfer
>p. transference
>p. transfer test

Passy-Muir tracheostomy speaking valve
paste
>baking soda p.
>Camcreme ECG p.
>*Emplasterium urea* p.
>Lassar betanaphthol p.
>Lassar plain zinc p.
>Triple P.
>Unna p.
>Veiel p.
>zinc chloride p.

Pasteurella
>*P. aerogenes*
>*P. multocida*
>*P. pestis*
>*P. tularensis*

pasteurellosis
Pasteur vaccine
Pastia
>P. line
>P. sign

pastilles
>Mycostatin p.

patagium
>cervical p.

Patanol eye drops
patch
>butterfly p.
>Carrel p.
>cotton-wool p.
>eczematous p.
>herald p.
>moth p.
>mucous p.
>opaline p.
>peau d'orange p.
>PediaPatch Transdermal P.
>Peyer p.
>pruritic erythematous p.
>salmon p.
>shagreen p.
>smoker p.
>soldier p.
>p. stage
>p. test
>p. testing
>p. test interpretation
>Testoderm p.
>p. test scarring
>Transderm Scōp P.
>Trans-Plantar Transdermal P.
>Trans-Ver-Sal Transdermal P.
>Verukan solution

patchouli oil
patchy
>p. airspace consolidation
>p. infiltrate

Pate d'Unna
patellae
>chondromalacia p.

patellar
>p. tendinitis
>p. tendon-bearing orthosis

patellofemoral
>p. arthritis
>p. disease
>p. joint
>p. osteoarthritis
>p. pain syndrome

pathergy
pathoanatomy
Pathocil
pathoclisis
pathogen
>*Cunninghamella* p.
>opportunistic p.

NOTES

P

pathogenesis
  peripheral prion p.
pathogenetic
pathogenic blastomycetes
pathogenicity
pathognomic
pathognomonic
pathologically confirmed complete remission (PCR)
pathologic feature
pathology *pathology accession number*
  allograft p.
  Armed Forces Institutes of P. (AFIP)
  bite p.
pathometric
pathometry
pathophysiology
pathway
  arachidonic acid p.
  classical p. (CP)
  cross-priming p.
  cyclooxygenase p.
  effector p.
  endotoxin signaling p.
  Fas-based killing p.
  inositol triphosphate p.
  lectin p.
  lipoxygenase p.
  monooxygenase p.
  Notch signaling p.
  perforin killing p.
  perforin-mediated p.
  proinflammatory p.
  Raf/mitogen-activated protein kinase signaling p.
  Raper-Mason p.
  Vav/Rac p.
patient
  p. global assessment of disease activity
  hemophiliac p.
  nonhemophiliac p.
  p. patch test record sheet
Patois virus
patronymic
pattern
  apron p.
  ball-in-claw p.
  bimodal immunofluorescent p.
  cannonball p.
  Christmas tree p.
  church spire p.
  clock-face p.
  cockade p.
  differential expression p.
  p. of distribution
  fir-tree-like p.

  geographic p.
  ground-glass p.
  herringbone p.
  honeycomb staining p.
  p. of inheritance
  livedo p.
  lymphocutaneous p.
  Mercedes p.
  mulberry p.
  NBT mosaic p.
  netted p.
  N-linked p.
  nodular p.
  nuclear dot p.
  O-linked p.
  polycyclic p.
  polygenic inheritance p.
  restrictive ventilatory p.
  reticular p.
  rheumatoid p.
  serpiginous p.
  sporotricoid p.
  p. of staining
  starry-sky p.
  stellate p.
  webbed p.
  zosteriform p.
patterned
  p. alopecia
  p. leukoderma
pauciarthritis
pauciarticular
  p. juvenile chronic arthritis
  p. juvenile rheumatoid arthritis
  p. onset
  p. presentation
paucibacillary leprosy
pauciimmune glomerulonephritis
pauciinflammatory
paucimobilis
  Sphingomonas p.
Paul
  P. reaction
  P. test
paul
  Salmonella st. p.
Paul-Bunnell test
Paulo
  exanthematic typhus of São P.
Paulus criteria
paurometabolum
  Tsukamurella p.
Pautrier
  P. abscess
  P. microabscess
Paxene
Paxil
paxillin

Paxton disease
PBC
    primary biliary cirrhosis
PBL
    peripheral blood lymphocyte
pBluescript vector
PBMC
    peripheral blood mononuclear cell
PBMTx
    porcine bone marrow transplantation
PBPC
    peripheral blood progenitor cell
PBS
    phosphate-buffered saline
PBSC
    peripheral blood stem cell
PBSCT
    peripheral blood stem cell transplantation
PBV
    pulmonary blood volume
PBZ
    pyribenzamine
      PBZ-SR
PCA
    passive cutaneous anaphylaxis
      PCA test
PCB
    polychlorobiphenyl
PCE
    pseudocholinesterase
      PCE Oral
p-chloro-meta-xylenol (PCMX)
PCMX
    parachlorometaxylenol
    p-chloro-meta-xylenol
PCNA
    proliferating cell nuclear antigen
PCO_2
    partial pressure of carbon dioxide
PCP
    Pneumocystis carinii pneumonia
PCR
    pathologically confirmed complete
      remission
    polymerase chain reaction
      arbitrary primed PCR (AP-PCR)
      PCR assay
      PCR for HIV DNA
      mixed-linker PCR (ML-PCR)
      repetitive PCR (Rep-PCR)
      TB test by PCR
      PCR testing

PCT
    porphyria cutanea tarda
PD
      Bromfenex PD
      Iofed PD
      P and PD
        percussion and postural drainage
PDA
      Indocid PDA
PDAF
    platelet-derived angiogenesis factor
PDEGF
    platelet-derived epidermal growth factor
PDGF
    platelet-derived growth factor
PDGF-A
    isoform P.-A., -B
PDL
    pulsed-dye laser
    pulsed-dye laser therapy
PDS suture
PDT
    photodynamic therapy
PE
    phycoerythrin
      Guiatuss PE
      Halotussin PE
peach fuzz
peak
    biclonal p.
    p. expiratory flow (PEFR)
    p. expiratory flow rate
    p. flow meter
    p. flow sensitivity
    p. inspiratory ventilator pressure
    monoclonal p.
    p. nasal inspiratory flow (PNIF)
    p. serum level
    p. and trough
    widow's p.
peak-plateau response
peanut
pear
pearl
    collar of p.'s
    Epstein p.'s
    necklace of p.'s
    p. oyster shell pneumonitis
Pearson chi square test
peas
peau
    p. de chagrin

NOTES

P

peau *(continued)*
    p. d'orange
    p. d'orange patch
pecan tree
Peck-Joseph scissors
Pecquet
    P. cistern
    P. duct
    P. reservoir
pectoris
    pseudoangina p.
pectus excavatum
Pedameth
PediaCare Oral
Pediacof
PediaPatch Transdermal Patch
Pediapred Oral
Pedia-Profen
pediatric
    American Academy of P.'s (AAP)
    Cleocin P.
    p. dermogram
    Fedahist Expectorant p.
    p. infectious disease developmental screening test (PIDDST)
    p. scleroderma
Pediazole Oral
pedicellaria
    triple-jawed p.
pedicled flap
Pedi-Cort V topical
pediculation
pediculicide
Pediculoides ventricosus
pediculosis
    p. capillitii
    p. capitis
    p. corporis
    p. corporis vel vestimentorum
    p. palpebrarum
    p. pubis
    p. vestimenti
pediculous
Pediculus
    P. corporis
    P. humanus
    P. humanus capitis
    P. humanus capitis infestation
Pedi-Dri
Pedinol
Pediotic Otic
Pedi-Pro topical
pedis (*gen. of* pes)
Pedituss
pedrosoi
    compacta Jeanselmei p.
    Fonsecaea p.
    Hormodendron p.

peduncle
pedunculated
    p. fibroma
    p. seborrheic keratosis
peel
    chemical p.
    face p.
    familial continuous skin p.
    freshening p.
    Jessner's P.
    lunch-time p.
    phenol p.
    skin p.
peeling
    chemical p.
peeling-skin syndrome
PEEP
    positive end-expiratory pressure
Pefabloc SC
pefloxacin
PEFR
    peak expiratory flow
peg
    rete p.
pegademase
    p. bovine
pegylated
    p. interferon
    p. p55 TNF-R
PEH
    palmoplantar eccrine hidradenitis
pelade
pelage
pelidnoma
pelioma
peliosis hepatitis
pellagra
    glossitis of p.
    wet p.
pellagra-associated dermatitis
pellagrin
pellagroid
    p. dermatitis
    p. erythema
pellagrous
pellet
    chondrin p.
pelletieri
    Actinomadura p.
pellicle
    acquired p.
pellitory
    wall p.
Pelodera **dermatitis**
PELs
    permissible exposure limits
pelt

peltation
pelvic inflammatory disease (PID)
pemphigoid
    antiepiligrin cicatricial p. (AECP)
    benign mucosal p.
    Brunsting-Perry p.
    bullous p. (BP)
    cicatricial p. (CP)
    p. gestationis
    lichen planus p.
    mucous membrane p.
    ocular cicatricial p.
    p. syphilid
pemphigoides
pemphigosa
    variola p.
pemphigus
    p. acutus
    benign familial chronic p.
    Brazilian p.
    p. contagiosus
    p. erythematosus
    familial benign chronic p.
    foliaceous p.
    p. foliaceus (PF)
    p. gangrenosus
    p. hemorrhagicus
    herpetiform p. (HP)
    p. leprosus
    p. malignus
    p. neonatorum
    ocular p.
    old-man's p.
    paraneoplastic p. (PNP)
    p. syphiliticus
    p. vegetans
    p. vulgaris (PV)
pemphigus-like eruption
pen
    Pilot Spotlighter p.
penciclovir
pencil
    p. and cup deformity
    p. method
    solid carbon dioxide p.
    styptic p.
pendula
    cutis p.
pendulum
    fibroma p.
    molluscum p.

Penecort Topical
penetrans
    hyperkeratosis follicularis et
      parafollicularis in cutem p.
    Tunga p.
penetrant
Penetrex Oral
penicillamine
penicillin
    p. aqueous
    p. desensitization
    p. g benzathine
    p. g, benzathine and procaine,
      combined
    p. g procaine
    phenoxymethyl p.
    p. therapy
    unit of p.
    p. V potassium
    p. v suspension
penicillin-induced anaphylaxis
penicillin-penicilloyl human serum
  albumin (PPO-HSA)
penicillin-resistant *Streptococcus
  pneumoniae* (PRSP)
penicilliosis
Penicillium
    P. casseii
    P. marneffei
    P. notatum
penicilloyl
    p. G, G/V, V
penicilloyl-polylysine (PPL)
penile
    p. pearly papule
    p. sclerosing lymphangitis
penis
    Bowen disease of the glans p.
    glans p.
    induratio p. plastica
    kraurosis p.
    median raphe cyst of the p.
Pen-Kera lotion
Penlac nail lacquer
Pennsaid topical lotion
pensilis
    cutis p.
Pentacarinat injection
Pentacef
Pentam-300 Injection
pentamer

NOTES

P

pentamidine
  p. in aerosol form
  p. isethionate
Pentasa Oral
Pentastomida
Pentatrichomonas hominis
pentavalent gas gangrene antitoxin
pentazocine
penton antigen
pentosan
  p. polysulfate sodium
  sodium p.
pentoxifylline (PTX)
Pentrax
pentraxin protein family
Pen-Vee K Oral
People of Color Against AIDS Network (POCAAN)
PEP
  positive expiratory pressure
  postexposure prevention/postexposure
   prophylaxis
  PEP mask
Pepcid
  P. AC Acid Controller
  P. Oral
  P. RPD
peplomer
peplos
pepper
  betel p.
  black p.
  green p.
peppertree
  California p.
Pepscan study
pepsinogen-secreting zymogenic cell
peptide
  anaphylatoxin p.
  anionic neutrophil-activating p.
   (ANAP)
  p. antigen
  arthritogenic p.
  calcitonin gene-related p. (CGRP)
  chemotactic p.
  class II invariant chain-derived p.
   (CLIP)
  connective tissue-activating p.
   (CTAP)
  COOH-terminal p.
  cyclic citrullinated p.
  deamidated gliadin p.
  immunogenic p.
  p. ligand
  multiantigenic p. (MAP)
  procollagen type III
   aminoterminal p.
  signal p.

  substance P p.
  synovial antigenic p.
  thymic p.
  p. transporter protein
  vasoactive intestinal p. (VIP)
peptide-1
  monocyte chemotactic p. (MCP-1)
  neutrophil-activating p.
Peptide T
peptidoglycan
  bacterial p.
peptidoglycan-polysaccharide complex
Pepto-Bismol
Peptococcus niger
Peptol
Peptostreptococcus
  P. anaerobius
  P. asaccharolyticus
  P. magnus
  P. prevotii
  P. productus
  P. saccharolyticus
peracute
perambulating ulcer
percent reactive antibody/panel reactive antibody (PRA)
perch
perchlornaphthalin
perchloroethylene
Percogesic
percussion and postural drainage (P and PD)
percutaneous
  p. abscess and fluid drainage
   (PAFD)
  p. absorption
  p. conchotome biopsy technique
  p. passage
  p. test
peregrinum
  Mycobacterium p.
perenne
  Lolium p. (Lol p)
perennial
  p. allergic rhinitis
  p. rye
  p. rye grass
Perfectoderm Gel
perfloxacin
perfluoroalkylpolyether (PFAPE)
perfluorocarbon
perforans
  folliculitis nares p.
  mal p.
  malum p.
  scleromalacia p.
perforant
  mal p.

perforating
- p. calcific elastosis
- p. disease
- p. disease of hemodialysis
- p. disorder of uremia
- p. folliculitis
- p. granuloma annulare
- p. ulcer of foot

perforin
- p. killing pathway
- p. pore

perforin-mediated pathway

performance
- Western Ontario and McMaster Universities Osteoarthritis Index Physical Functioning subscale and chair-stand p. (WOMAC-PF)

perfosfamide

perfrigeration

perfume dermatitis

perfusion
- exsanguinous metabolic support p.
- extracorporeal liver p. (ECLP, ELP)
- ex-vivo liver p.
- hypothermic p.
- isolated limb p.

periacetabular osteotomy

Periactin

periadenitis mucosa necrotica recurrens

periadnexal dermis

perianal
- p. condylomata lata
- p. pruritus
- p. streptococcal cellulitis

perianth

periaortitis

periapical

periarteritis nodosa

periarthritis
- calcific p.
- shoulder p.

periarticular
- p. disorder
- p. ossification
- p. osteopenia
- p. osteoporosis
- p. syndrome

periauricular

peribronchial desquamation

peribronchiolar lymphocyte infiltration

péribuccale
- erythrose pigmentaire p.

pericarditis

pericardium

perichondrial implant

perichondritis
- auricular p.
- infectious p.

pericyte

periderm

perifollicular
- p. accentuation
- p. fibroma (PFF)
- p. fibrosis
- p. granuloma
- p. melanophage
- p. papulation

perifolliculitis
- p. capitis abscedens et suffodiens
- dissecting p.
- pustular p.
- superficial pustular p.

periglandular fibrosis

perigranulomatous fibrotic change

perihilar

perikarya

perimyocarditis
- rheumatic p.

perimyositis

perinatal
- p. gangrene of buttock
- p. septicemia

Perineal Skin Cleanser

perineural fibrosis

perinevic vitiligo

perinevoid vitiligo

perinuclear
- p. antineutrophil cytoplasmic antibody (P-ANCA)
- p. zone

periocular
- p. area
- p. dermatitis
- p. milia

period
- eclipse p.
- honeymoon p.
- incubation p. (IP)
- induction p.
- latent p.
- prepatent p.
- refractory p.

NOTES

P

periodic
- p. acid-Schiff (PAS)
- p. acid-Schiff-positive material
- p. acid-Schiff stain
- p. acid-Schiff technique
- p. edema
- p. fever syndrome
- p. leg movement
- p. peritonitis
- p. polyserositis

periodontitis-type Ehlers-Danlos syndrome

perionychia

perionyxis

perioral
- p. area
- p. dermatitis

periorbital
- p. area
- p. dermatitis
- p. erythema
- p. hyperpigmentation
- p. purpura

periorificial
- p. dermatitis
- p. lentiginosis

periosteal implant

periostosis
- idiopathic p.

peripheral
- p. airspace
- p. ameloblastoma
- p. anergy
- p. arthritis
- p. blood count
- p. blood eosinophilia
- p. blood lymphocyte (PBL)
- p. blood mononuclear cell (PBMC)
- p. blood progenitor cell (PBPC)
- p. blood stem cell (PBSC)
- p. blood stem cell rescue
- p. blood stem cell transplantation (PBSCT)
- p. fibrosis
- p. gangrene
- p. giant cell granuloma
- p. joint
- p. nerve
- p. nerve involvement
- p. nerve sheath tumor
- p. nervous system (PNS)
- p. neuritis
- p. neuromyopathy
- p. ossifying fibroma
- p. prion pathogenesis
- p. staining
- p. T-cell lymphoma
- p. type

periphlebitis

periplakin

periplasmic

periporate

periporitis

periporoma

Peri-Strips Dry

peritendinitis crepitans

peritonitis
- acute p.
- benign paroxysmal p.
- feline infectious p.
- periodic p.

periumbilical perforating pseudoxanthoma elasticum

periungual
- p. erythema
- p. fibroma
- p. telangiectasia
- p. wart

periungualis
- onychia p.

perivascular infiltrate

perivasculitis
- retinal p.

perlecan

perlèche

Perles
- Tessalon P.

PERM
- progressive encephalomyelitis with rigidity and myoclonus

permanent-press finish clothing dermatitis

permanganate
- potassium p.

Permapen injection

permeability
- vascular p.

permethrin

permissible exposure limits (PELs)

permissive
- p. hypercapnia
- p. MHC allele

Permitil

perna disease

pernicious anemia

pernio
- Besnier lupus p.
- p. cyanosis
- erythema p.
- lupus p.

perniosis

Pernox

peroneal
- p. nerve entrapment
- p. tendon

peroral intestinal biopsy

peroxidase
    p. cell marker
    eosinophil p.
    thyroid p. (TPO)
peroxidation
    lipid p.
peroxide
    benzoyl p.
    erythromycin and benzoyl p.
    hydrogen p.
Peroxin
    P. A5, A10
peroxisome proliferator-activated receptor-gamma (PPAR-gamma)
peroxynitrite
perphenazine
Persa-Gel
Persantine
Persian Gulf syndrome
persistence
    microbial p.
persistent
    p. acantholytic dermatosis
    p. edema
    p. generalized lymphadenopathy (PGL)
    p. light reaction
    p. light reactor
    p. pearly penile papule
    p. pyoderma
    p. light reactivity (PLR)
persister
Personal Best Peak Flowmeter
Persona ovulation predicting kit
perspiration
    insensible p.
    sensible p.
perspire
perstans
    acrodermatitis p.
    Dipetalonema p.
    erysipelas p.
    erythema dyschromicum p.
    erythema figuratum p.
    erythema gyratum p.
    hyperkeratosis lenticularis p.
    telangiectasia macularis eruptiva p. (TMEP)
    urticaria p.
    xanthoerythrodermia p.

persufflation
persulcatus
    Ixodes p.
persulfate salt
pertechnetate
    technetium p.
pertenue
    Treponema p.
Pert Plus
pertrichosis
pertussis
    p. agglutination test
    Bordetella p.
    p. immune globulin
    p. immunoglobulin
    p. vaccine
Peru
    balsam of P.
peruana
    verruca p.
    verruga p.
peruviana
    verruca p.
Peruvian wart
PERV
    porcine endogenous retrovirus
pes, gen. pedis
    p. anserinus bursa
    bicho dos p.
    dermatomycosis pedis
    dysesthesia pedis
    p. febricitans
    malum perforans pedis
    moccasin-type tinea pedis
    p. planus
    spina pedis
    tinea pedis
pest
    fowl p.
    swine p.
pesticemia
pestifer
    Salsola p.
pestiferous
pestilence
pestilential bubo
pestis
    Pasteurella p.
    Yersinia p.
Pestivirus

NOTES

P

PET
  positron emission tomography
  problem elicitation technique
petechia, pl. **petechiae**
  calcaneal p.
  linear p.
  Tardieu p.
petechial
  p. eruption
  p. hemorrhage
  p. typhus
petechiasis
P-E technique
petitgrain oil
Petriellidium boydii
petrolatum
  hydrated p.
  hydrophilic p.
  lanolin, cetyl alcohol, glycerin,
    and p.
  Liquid p.
  red veterinary p. (RVP)
  white p.
petroleum acne
Pette-Döring disease
Peutz-Jeghers syndrome
Peyer patch
Peyronie disease
PF
  pemphigus foliaceus
  pulmonary function
PF4
  platelet factor 4
PFAPE
  perfluoroalkylpolyether
PFB
  pseudofolliculitis barbae
Pfeiffer
  P. phenomenon
  P. syndrome
PFF
  perifollicular fibroma
PFGE
  pulsed field gel electrophoresis
Pfizerpen-AS injection
Pfizerpen injection
PFS
  Folex P.
  Tarabine P.
  Vincasar P.
PFT
  pulmonary function test
PFU
  plaque-forming unit

PG
  prostaglandin
  pyoderma gangrenosum
P/G
  Fulvicin P/G
PGD
  prostaglandin D
PGD$_2$
  prostaglandin D$_2$
PGE
  prostaglandin E
PGE$_1$
  prostaglandin E$_1$
PGE$_2$
  prostaglandin E$_2$
  purine-stimulated prostaglandin E$_2$
  PGE$_2$ synthase
PGF$_2$
  prostaglandin F2
  PGF$_2$ alpha
  PGF$_2$ synthase
PGH2
  prostaglandin H2
PGHS-1, -2 cDNA
PGI$_2$
  prostacyclin
  PGI$_2$ synthase
PGL
  persistent generalized lymphadenopathy
Ph
  Philadelphia chromosome
  Ph positive
pH
  blood p.
  low urine p.
  Propa p.
PHA
  passive hemagglutination
  phytohemagglutinin
phacoanaphylactic uveitis
phacoanaphylaxis
phacomatosis
Phadezym
  P. PRIST
  P. RAST
phaeohyphomycosis
phage
  beta p.
  defective p.
phagedena
  p. gangrenosa
  p. nosocomialis
  sloughing p.
  p. tropica

tropical p.
tropical sloughing p.
phagedenic ulcer
phagedenis
    Treponema p.
phagocyte
    p. dysfunction
    frustrated p.
    p. oxidative burst
    sinusoidal p.
phagocytic
    p. deficiency
    p. dysfunction disorders
      immunodeficiency
    p. dysfunction immunodeficiency
    p. function
    p. index
    p. thrombus
phagocytin
phagocytize
phagocytoblast
phagocytolysis
phagocytolytic
phagocytosable debris
phagocytose
phagocytosis
    frustrated p.
    induced p.
    spontaneous p.
phagocytotic
phagolysis
phagolysosome
phagolytic
phagosome
phagotype
phakoma
phakomatosis pigmentovascularis
phakomatous choristoma
phalanges
    proximal p.
phalloidin staining
phaneroscope
phanerozoite
phantom tumor
Pharmacia lancet
pharmacokinetic
    Dapsone P.'s
pharmacologic
    p. mediators of anaphylaxis
    p. therapy

pharyngeal
    p. gonorrhea
    p. pouch syndrome
pharyngitis
    arcanobacterial p.
    herpangina p.
    herpes p.
    streptococcal p.
pharyngoconjunctival
    p. fever
    p. fever virus
phase
    accelerated p. (AP)
    anagen growth p.
    catagen growth p.
    chronic
      myelocytic/myelogenous/myeloid
      leukemia accelerated p. (CML AP)
    chronic
      myelocytic/myelogenous/myeloid
      leukemia chronic p. (CML CP)
    eclipse p.
    growth p.
    horizontal growth p.
    p. I, II rheumatoid arthritis
    lag p.
    lichenoid p.
    logarithmic p.
    negative p.
    occlusive p.
    positive p.
    prepulseless p.
    presensitization p.
    pulseless p.
    resting p.
    stationary p.
    telogen p.
    vertical growth p.
Phazet lancet
Phemister triad
phenacetin
Phenameth Oral
Phenazine Injection
phenazopyridine
    sulfisoxazole and p.
Phendry Oral
Phenelzine
Phenerbel-S
Phenergan
    P. Injection
    P. Oral
    P. Rectal

NOTES

Phenetron Oral
phenindamine tartrate
pheniramine
    p., phenylpropanolamine, and
        pyrilamine
    phenyltoloxamine,
        phenylpropanolamine, pyrilamine,
        and p.
phenobarbital
    theophylline, ephedrine, and p.
phenol
    camphor, menthol and p.
    N-acetyl-4-S-cysteaminyl p.
    p. peel
phenolated disinfectant
phenolformaldehyde
phenology
phenolphthalein
phenol-preserved extract
phenomenon, pl. **phenomena**
    adhesion p.
    anaphylactoid p.
    angry back p.
    Arthus p.
    autoimmune p.
    Azzopardi p.
    booster p.
    Bordet-Gengou p.
    Chase-Sulzberger p.
    cheek p.
    Danysz p.
    Debré p.
    Denys-Leclef p.
    d'Herelle p.
    Ehrlich p.
    epitope-spreading p.
    erythrocyte adherence p.
    experimentally induced Köbner p.
        (KP-e)
    fall-and-rise p.
    gel p.
    generalized Shwartzman p.
    Gengou p.
    Gerhardt p.
    Gordon p.
    Hata p.
    Hecht p.
    Hektoen p.
    hunting p.
    immune adherence p.
    isomorphic p.
    jodbasedow p.
    Kasabach-Merritt p.
    Koch p.
    Koebner p.
    LE cell p.
    Leede-Rumpel p.
    Leichtenstern p.

    Liacopoulos p.
    Lucio leprosy p.
    lupus erythematosus p.
    Matuhasi-Ogata p.
    Mauserung p.
    Meirowsky p.
    Mills-Reincke p.
    Pfeiffer p.
    quellung p.
    Raynaud p.
    red cell adherence p.
    Rumpel-Leede p.
    Sanarelli p.
    Sanarelli-Shwartzman p.
    satellite p.
    Schultz-Charlton p.
    Shwartzman p.
    Splendore-Hoeppli p.
    spreading p.
    Sulzberger-Chase p.
    Theobald Smith p.
    Twort p.
    Twort-d'Herelle p.
    vacuum p.
phenothiazine
phenotype
    Bombay p.
    dominant p.
    Fairbanks arthritis p.
    McLeod p.
    PiZZ p.
    Ribbing arthritis p.
    Turner p.
    unexpected p.
    VanA p.
phenotypic mixing
Phenoxine
phenoxybenzamine hydrochloride
phenoxymethyl penicillin
phenylalanine metabolism
phenylbutazone
Phenyldrine
phenylephrine
    brompheniramine and p.
    chlorpheniramine, phenyltoloxamine,
        phenylpropanolamine, and p.
    guaifenesin, phenylpropanolamine,
        and p.
    p. hydrochloride
    isoproterenol and p.
    sodium sulfacetamide and p.
Phenylfenesin L.A.
phenylketonuria
phenylpropanolamine
    brompheniramine and p.
    chlorpheniramine, phenylephrine,
        and p.

chlorpheniramine, pyrilamine,
  phenylephrine, and p.
clemastine and p.
guaifenesin and p.
p. hydrochloride
phenylpyruvic oligophrenia
phenyltoloxamine
  acetaminophen and p.
  chlorpheniramine, phenylephrine,
    and p.
  p., phenylpropanolamine, and
    acetaminophen
  p., phenylpropanolamine, pyrilamine,
    and pheniramine
phenytoin
pheochromocytoma
pheohyphomycosis
pheomelanin
pheomycotic cyst
pheresis catheter
Phialophora
  P. richardsiae
  P. verruca
  P. verrucosa
Philadelphia
  P. chromosome (Ph)
  P. chromosome positive
Philip gland
philtrum
phimosis
pHisoDerm
pHisoHex
phi-X174
  bacteriophage p.-X.
phlebectasia
  congenital generalized p.
  corona p.
phlebectomy
phlebodissector
phlebography
phlebology
Phlebotomus
  Phlebotomus fever
  Phlebotomus fever virus
phlebotomy
Phlebovirus
phlegmasia
  p. alba
  p. alba dolens
  p. malabarica
phlegmon
  diffuse p.

phlegmonous
  p. abscess
  p. cellulitis
  p. erysipelas
  p. ulcer
phlei
  Mycobacterium p.
Phleum pratense
phlogistic
phlogosin
phlogotherapy
phloxine-tartrazine stain
phlyctaenodes
  herpes p.
phlyctena, pl. **phlyctenae**
phlyctenar
phlyctenoid
phlyctenosis
phlyctenous
phlyctenular
phlyctenule
phlyctenulosis
  allergic p.
  tuberculous p.
PHN
  postherpetic neuralgia
Phoma
  P. betae
  P. fungus
  P. species
phorbol ester
Phormia
phosophoinositol-3 (PI3)
phosphatase
  tartrate-resistant acid p. (TRAP)
phosphate
  antazoline p.
  Aralen phosphate with
    primaquine p.
  basic calcium p. (BCP)
  chloroquine p.
  Decadron P.
  dexamethasone sodium p.
  dihydroxyacetone p. (DHAP)
  Hexadrol p.
  histamine p.
  Hydrocortone P.
  nicotinamide adenine dinucleotide p.
    (NADPH)
  potassium titanyl p. (KTP)
  primaquine p.
phosphate-buffered saline (PBS)

NOTES

P

phosphatidylcholine-specific phospholipase C
phosphatidylinositol
phosphatidylserine
phosphatidylserine-prothrombin complex
phosphatidyl serine receptor
phospho-c-Jun
phosphodiester
phosphodiesterase isoenzyme inhibitor
phosphofructokinase
phosphoglycerolmutase
phosphoinositide
    p. 3 kinase
phospholipase
    p. A, A2, C
    p. enzyme
phospholipid
phosphonoformate
    trisodium p.
phosphorhidrosis
phosphoribosylaminoimidazole-carboxamide
phosphoribosyltransferase
    hypoxanthine-guanine p. (HGPRT)
phosphoridrosis
phosphorus
phosphorylase
    nucleoside p.
    purine nucleoside p. (PNP)
phosphorylated serine/arginine splicing
phosphorylation
    chondrocyte mitochondrial oxidative p.
    protein kinase A-dependent p.
    tyrosine p.
phosphotransferase deficiency
phossy jaw
photo
    p. aging
    p. epilation
    p. protection
photoacoustic injury
photoaging, photo aging
photoallergen
photoallergic
    p. contact dermatitis
    p. drug reaction
    p. sensitivity
photoallergy
    soap p.
photobiologic reaction
photobiology
photochemical
    p. reaction
    p. smog
photochemistry
photochemotherapy
    extracorporeal p.

    p. with oral methoxypsoralen therapy followed by UVA (PUVA)
photocontact dermatitis
photodamage
PhotoDerm
    P. filtered, flashlamp-pumped light source
    P. laser
    P. machine
    P. MultiLight system
    P. VL light source
photodermatitis
    contact p.
    drug-induced p.
photodermatosis
photodistribution
photodrug
    p. reaction
photodynamic
    p. sensitization
    p. therapy (PDT)
photoepilation
    flashlamp p.
photoerythema
Photofrin porfimer sodium
photogenica
    p. laser
    P. laser system
    urticaria p.
photoinactivation
photoingestant dermatitis
photology
photomechanical
photometry
    reflectance p.
photomicrography
photon absorptiometry
photoncia
photonosus
photoonycholysis
photo-patch test
photopathy
photopheresis
photophobia
photophoresis
    extracorporeal p.
photophytodermatitis
photoplethysmography (ppg)
photoradiation
photosensitive
    p. nonscarring dermatitis
    p. rash
photosensitivity
    p. dermatitis
    drug-induced bullous p.

p., ichthyosis, brittle hair, impaired intelligence, decreased fertility, and short stature (PIBIDS)

p., ichthyosis, brittle hair, impaired intelligence, decreased fertility, and short stature syndrome

p., ichthyosis, brittle hair, intellectual impairment

p., ichthyosis, brittle hair, intellectual impairment, decreased fertility, and short stature (PIBIDS)

p., ichthyosis, brittle hair, intellectual impairment, decreased fertility and short stature syndrome

p. reaction

photosensitization
contact p.

phototherapy
UVB p.

photothermolysis
selective p.

phototoxic
p. contact dermatitis
p. drug reaction
p. sensitivity
p. textile dermatitis

phototoxicity

phototoxis

PHP
pseudohypoparathyroidism

phragmospore

phrenic
p. nerve
p. nerve paralysis

phrynoderma

phthalate
butylbenzyl p. (BBP)

phthalic anhydride

phthiriasis

phthisicorum
chloasma p.

phycoerythrin (PE)

phycomycosis
subcutaneous p.

phycomycotic infection

phylacagogic

phylaxis

Phyllocontin Tablet

phylogenetic atavism

phyma, pl. **phymata**

phymatosis

physical
p. allergy
p. barrier
p. deconditioning
p. lobular panniculitis
p. stimulus
p. sunscreen
p. urticaria

physician global assessment of disease activity

physiologic
p. alopecia
p. test

physiological
p. dead space
p. dead space ventilation per minute

physiology
sleep p.

physostigmine

phytanic
p. acid
p. acid storage
p. acid storage disease

phytoagglutinin

phytodermatitis

Phytodolor

phytohemagglutinin (PHA)

phytomitogen

phytonadione

Phytophathoria infestans

phytophlyctodermatitis

phytophotodermatitis

phytophototoxic dermatitis

phytosterolemia

phytotoxic

phytotoxin

PI3
phosophoinositol-3

pian
p. bois
hemorrhagic p.

piannic
onychia p.

piano-key deformity

PIBF
progesterone-induced blocking factor

NOTES

P

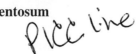

PIBIDS
    photosensitivity, ichthyosis, brittle hair, impaired intelligence, decreased fertility, and short stature
    photosensitivity, ichthyosis, brittle hair, intellectual impairment, decreased fertility, and short stature
        PIBIDS syndrome
picker's
    p. acne
    p. nodule
Pick and Go monitor
pickle weed pollen
pick-up maneuver
picomolar
Picornaviridae virus
picornavirus
picrate
    butamben p.
PID
    pelvic inflammatory disease
PIDDST
    pediatric infectious disease developmental screening test
PIE
    pulmonary infiltrate with eosinophilia
        PIE syndrome
piebald
    p. albinism
    p. skin
piebaldism
piebaldness
piece
    Fab p.
    Fc p.
piecemeal
    p. degranulation (PMD)
    p. necrosis
piechaudii
    Alcaligenes p.
pied
    mal perforant du p.
    p. rond rheumatism
piedra
    black p.
    p. nostras
    white p.
Piedraia hortae
Pierini
    atrophoderma of Pasini and P.
    idiopathic atrophoderma of Pasini and P.
    melanotic prurigo of P.
piesesthesia
piezogenic pedal papule
Piffard curette
pig
    p. aortic endothelial cell (PAEC)
    guinea p.
    mycoplasma pneumonia of p.
    p. skin
    virus pneumonia of p.
pigeon
    p. breeder's disease
    p. droppings
    p. feather
    p. serum protein (PSP)
pigment
    abnutzung p.
    age p.
    p. cell transplantation
    p. change
    incontinence of p.
    iron oxide p.
    melanotic p.
    minimal p. (MP)
pigmentaire
    Brocq erythrose peribuccale p.
pigmentary
    p. abnormality
    p. atopic dermatitis
    p. demarcation line
    p. syphilid
pigmentation
    Addison p.
    addisonian dermal p.
    amiodarone p.
    arsenic p.
    blue-gray p.
    epidermolysis bullosa simplex with mottled p.
    exogenous p.
pigmented
    p. ameloblastoma
    p. basal cell carcinoma
    p. hair epidermal nevus
    P. Lesion Study Group (PLSG)
    p. purpura
    p. purpuric lichenoid dermatitis
    p. purpuric lichenoid dermatitis of Gougerot
    p. purpuric lichenoid dermatosis
    p. spindle cell (PSC)
    p. villonodular synovitis (PVNS)
pigmenti
    incontinentia p.
pigmentolysin
pigmentosa
    familial urticaria p.
    morphea p.
    urticaria p.
pigmentosum
    morphea p.
    urticaria p.
    xeroderma p.

pigmentosus
    lichen planus p.
    nevus p.
pigmentovascularis
    phakomatosis p.
pig-to-primate model of xenotransplantation
pigweed
    redroot p.
    spiny p.
    p. weed pollen
pilar
    p. cyst
    p. neurocristic hamartoma
    p. sheath acanthoma
    p. tumor of scalp
pilaris
    favus p.
    juvenile pityriasis rubra p.
    keratosis p.
    lichen p.
    pityriasis rubra p.
pilar neurocristic hamartoma
pilary
pileous
pili (*pl. of* pilus)
piliferous
    p. cyst
piliform
pill
    Asiatic p.
    Doan's Backache P.
    Ge Jie Anti-asthma P.
    prom p.
pilocarpine
    p. iontophoresis sweat test
piloerection
piloid
piloleiomyoma
pilomatricoma
pilomatrix carcinoma
pilomatrixoma
    p. carcinoma
pilomotor reflex
pilonidal
    p. cyst
    p. fistula
    p. sinus
pilorum
    p. agenesis
    arrectores p.

    scissura p.
    vortices p.
pilose
pilosebaceous
    p. apparatus
    p. follicle
    p. ostium
    p. structure
    p. unit
pilosis
pilosus
    nevus p.
    nevus pigmentosus et p.
Pilot Spotlighter pen
pilus, pl. **pili**
    p. annulatus
    arrector p.
    p. bifurcatus
    F p.
    I p.
    p. incarnatus
    pili multigemini
    pili pseudoannulati
    R p.
    scapus pili
    p. tortus
    pili triangulati et canaliculi
    pili trianguli et canaliculi
Pima
pimozide
pimple
pincer
    p. jaw
    p. nail
pinch
    devil's p.
    p. graft
    pulp-to-pulp tip p.
    p. purpura
pincushioning
pine
    Australian p.
    loblolly p.
    lodgepole p.
    p. oil
    ponderosa p.
    p. resin
    p. resin-colophony
    slash p.
    p. tree pollen
    white p.
pineapple

NOTES

P

Pinellia
ping-pong
    p.-p. infestation
    p.-p. syphilis
pinhead-sized milia
pink
    p. disease
    p. salmon
    p. spot
pinkeye
Pinkus
    fibroepithelioma of P.
    P. tumor
pinna
pinocyte
pinocytosis
    active p.
pinosome
pinpoint electrocoagulation
pinpoint-sized milia
Pin-Rid
pinta treponematosis
pintids
pinto
    P. cannula
    mal del p.
pintoid
pintos
    mal de los p.
pinworm
Pin-X
pioglitazone HCl
PIP
    positive inspiratory pressure
    proximal interphalangeal
piperacillin sodium and tazobactam sodium
piperazine
    p. citrate
    p. hydrochloride
piper beetle
piperidine derivative
piperonal butoxide
Pipracil
pique
pirbuterol acetate
piriformis syndrome
Pirital virus
piritrexim isethionate
piroxicam
Pirquet
    P. reaction
    P. test
pistachio
pistillate
pit
    discrete p.
    ear p.

    Mantoux p.
    nail p.
    tooth p.
    p. viper bite
    p. viper snake
pitch wart
Pitrex
pitted
    p. keratolysis
    p. nail
pitting
    p. edema
    nail p.
    p. of nail
pituitary
    p. disorder
    p. snuff taker's lung
pityriasic alopecia
pityriasis
    p. alba
    p. alba atrophicans
    p. amiantacea
    p. capitis
    p. circinata
    p. folliculorum
    p. furfuracea
    Gibert p.
    Hebra p.
    p. lichenoid
    lichenoid acute p.
    p. lichenoides
    p. lichenoides chronica (PLC)
    p. lichenoides et varioliformis acuta (PLEVA)
    p. lingua
    p. maculata
    p. nigra
    p. rosea (PR)
    p. rosea-like eruption
    p. rotunda
    p. rubra
    p. rubra pilaris
    p. sicca
    p. simplex
    p. simplex faciei
    p. steatoides
    p. versicolor
pityriasis-type scale
pityrodes
    alopecia p.
pityroid
Pityrosporum
    P. orbiculare
    P. ovale
Pityrosporum **folliculitis**
pivalate
    clocortolone p.
pivampicillin

pivoxil
 cefditoren p.
Pixy321
Piz Buin
pizotifen
PiZZ phenotype
P-K
 Prausnitz-Kustner
  P-K antibody
  P-K reaction
  P-K test
PKA
 protein kinase A
PLA2 isoenzyme (types IIA, IV, V)
placebo
placebo-controlled oral challenge testing (DPOC)
placenta-eluted gamma globulin
placental
 p. sulfatase deficiency
 p. sulfatase deficiency syndrome
 p. syncytiotrophoblast
placentation
pladaroma
plague
 bubonic p.
 cattle p.
 duck p.
 fowl p.
 Pahvant Valley p.
 rabbit p.
 p. vaccine
 vector of p.
plain
 Citanest P.
 p. gut suture
 Ultraquin P.
PLA$_2$ isozyme
plakins
plakoglobin
plana
 verruca p.
planar xanthoma
planci
 Acanthaster p.
Planck's law
plane
 p. angioma
 diffuse p.
 Frankfort horizontal p.
 p. nevus

 p. wart
 p. xanthoma
planing
planopilaris
 lichen p. (LPP)
plant
 p. agglutinin
 p. antitoxin
 arum p.
 datura p.
 p. dermatitis
 p. oleoresin
 p. toxin
 p. virus
planta, pl. plantae
 verruca p.
plantain
 English p.
plantaire
 chromidroses p.
plantar
 p. dermatitis
 p. desquamation
 p. fascia
 p. hyperlinearity
 p. inoculum
 p. maceration
 p. nerve syndrome
 p. syphilid
 p. talalgia
 p. wart
plantare
 keratoma palmare et p.
plantaris
 epidermolytic keratosis palmaris et p.
 ichthyosis palmaris et p.
 keratoderma palmaris et p.
 keratosis palmaris et p.
 mycosis fungoides palmaris et p.
 pustulosis palmaris et p.
 tylosis palmaris et p.
 verruca palmaris et p.
plantibody
planum
 xanthoma p.
planus
 annular lichen p.
 atrophic lichen p.
 bullous lichen p.
 condyloma p.
 erosive lichen p.

NOTES

P

planus *(continued)*
    follicular lichen p.
    genital erosive lichen p.
    hepatitis-associated lichen p.
    hypertrophic lichen p.
    lichen ruber p.
    linear lichen p.
    oral condyloma p.
    oral (erosive) lichen p.
    pes p.
    ulcerative lichen p.
    zosteriform lichen p.

plaque
    annular erythematous p.
    atrophic p.
    attachment p.
    bacterial p.
    centrofacial p.
    cytoplasmic p.
    degenerative collagenous p.
    dental p.
    disseminées parapsoriasis en p.'s
    eczematoid pruritic p.
    erythematosquamous p.
    erythematous p.
    honeycomb p.
    p. index
    inflammatory p.
    lichenified p.
    milia en p.
    mucous p.
    parapsoriasis en p.
    p. psoriasis
    psoriatic p.
    red-purple p.
    shadow p.
    p. stage
    submucosal p.
    ulcerovegetating p.
    urticarial p.
    violaceous p.
    warty keratotic p.

plaque-forming unit (PFU)
plaque-like cutaneous mucinosis
Plaquenil
plaque-type psoriasis
plasma
    p. cell
    p. cell balanitis
    p. cell dyscrasia with
      polyneuropathy, organomegaly,
      endocrinopathy, monoclonal protein
    p. cell mucositis
    p. cell myeloma
    p. cell neoplasm
    p. cell pneumonia
    p. cellularis
    p. cell vulvitis

    p. fibronectin
    fresh frozen p.
    frozen p.
    p. kallikrein
    p. membrane
    poor platelet p. (PPP)
    p. protein autoantibody
    p. therapy
    zoster immune p. (ZIP)

plasmablasts
    rapidly dividing p.
plasmacellularis
    balanitis p.
plasmacyte
plasmacytoapheresis
plasmacytoma
plasmapheresis
    exchange p.
plasmid
    bacteriocinogenic p.
    conjugative p.
    F p.
    infectious p.
    nonconjugative p.
    R p.
    resistance p.
    transmissible p.
plasmin
plasminogen
    p. activator
    kringle 4 domain of p.
plasmoacanthoma
plasmodia
plasmodial meningitis
Plasmodium
    chloroquine-resistant *P. falciparum*
      (CRPF)
    P. falciparum
    P. malariae
    P. ovale
    P. vivax
plasmodium embolism
Plaster
    Mediplast P.
    Sal-Acid P.
Plastibase
plastic
    p. adhesive dressing
    p. iritis
    p. worker's lung
plastica
    induratio penis p.
plastid
Plastizote shoe
Plast-O-Fit thermoplastic bandage
   system
plate
    BioPress p.

Jaeger p.
lamellar p.
nail p.
V-type microtiter p.
white spots of the nail p.
plateau bronchodilation
platelet
p. activating/aggregating factor (PAF)
p. basic protein
p. concentrate
p. factor 4 (PF4)
hemolysis, elevated liver enzymes, low p. (HELLP)
p. neutralization procedure
p. neutralization test
washed maternal p.
platelet-activating
p.-a. factor (PAF)
p.-a. factor acetylhydrolase (PAF-AH)
platelet-aggregating factor (PAF)
platelet-derived
p.-d. angiogenesis factor (PDAF)
p.-d. epidermal growth factor (PDEGF)
p.-d. growth factor (PDGF)
plate-like crystal
Platelin, phospholipid platelet substitute
Platinol
Platinol-AQ
platinum
salt of p.
platonychia
platybasia
Platycodon
Platyhelminthes
platyonychia
platypnea
platysma
platyspondylia
Plaut-Vincent disease
PLC
pityriasis lichenoides chronica
pleckstrin homology domain
pledget
alcohol p.
pleiotropic cytokine
pleocytosis
pleomorphic
p. lipoma
p. lymphoma

Plesiomonas shigelloides
plethysmograph
plethysmography
pleura, pl. **pleurae**
pleural
p. abrasion
p. amyloidosis
p. friction rub
p. tag
pleurectomy
pleurisy
benign dry p.
diaphragmatic p.
epidemic benign dry p.
epidemic diaphragmatic p.
rheumatoid p.
tuberculous p.
pleuritic chest pain
pleuritis
pleurodesis
doxycycline p.
mechanical p.
pleurodynia
epidemic p.
pleuropericarditis
pleuro-pneumoniae-like organism (PPLO)
PLEVA
pityriasis lichenoides et varioliformis acuta
plexiform
p. angioma
p. neurofibroma
p. neuroma
p. spindle cell nevus (PSCN)
plexopathy
plexus
branchial p.
Kiesselbach p.
supragaleal p.
plica
p. neuropathica
p. polonica
p. syndrome
plicata
lingua p.
pachydermoperiostosis p.
plicatic acid
PLL
prolymphocytic leukemia
plombage
plot
Wu-Kabat p.

NOTES

435

PLR
    persistent light reactivity
PLSG
    Pigmented Lesion Study Group
PLSI
    Psoriasis Life Stress Inventory
plucked
       p. chicken papules appearance
       p. chicken skin
plug
       follicular p.
       keratotic p.
       laminated epithelial p.
       mucous p.
plugging
       mucous p.
plum
plume
       laser p.
Plummer nail
Plummer-Vinson syndrome
pluriorificialis
       ectodermosis erosiva p.
pluripotent
pluripotential cell
pluriresistant
plus
       Amvisc p.
       Clearasil B.P. p.
       Cold-Eezer P.
       Compound W p.
       Cutifilm P.
       Duramist p.
       Ionil-T p.
       Pert P.
       P & S p.
       P. Sinus
       Soluver p.
       p. strand
       Sustacal P.
PM
    polymyositis
       Midol PM
       PM 81 monoclonal antibody
P.M.
       Excedrin P.M.
PMA
    premenstrual exacerbation of asthma
PMD
    piecemeal degranulation
pMDI
    pressurized metered-dose inhaler
PML
    polymorphonuclear leukocyte
    progressive multifocal
      leukoencephalopathy
PMLE
    polymorphous light eruption
      eczematous PMLE
      familial PMLE
PMN
    polymorphonuclear neutrophil
PMR
    polymyalgia rheumatica
    proportionate morbidity ratio
PM-Scl
    polymyositis-scleroderma
      PM-Scl antigen
PMS-Cyproheptadine
PMS-Dexamethasone
PMS-Erythromycin
PMS-Ketoprofen
PMS-Lindane
PMS-Pseudoephedrine
PMS-Sodium Cromoglycate
PncCRM vaccine
PNCS
    primary neuroendocrine carcinoma of
      skin
PND
    postnasal drip
pneumatic otoscopy
Pneumatosis intestinalis
pneumococcal
      p. antigenuria
      p. C-polysaccharide (CPS)
      p. infection
      p. otitis media
      p. pneumolysin
      p. pneumonia
      p. polysaccharide
      p. polysaccharide/protein conjugate
       vaccine
      p. polysaccharide vaccine
      p. pyomyositis
      p. stain
pneumococcic abscess
pneumococcidal
pneumococcolysis
Pneumococcus
pneumoconiosis
Pneumocystis
      P. carinii
      P. carinii pneumonia (PCP)
pneumocystosis
    extrapulmonary p.
pneumocyte
    hydropic change in p.
    type II p.
pneumolysin
    pneumococcal p.
pneumomediastinum
pneumonia
    atypical p.
    bacterial pneumococcal p.

bronchiolitis obliterans with
    organizing p. (BOOP)
chronic eosinophilic p. (CEP)
community-acquired p. (CAP)
desquamative interstitial p. (DIP)
drug-induced p.
Eaton agent p.
eosinophilic p.
Friedländer p.
Hecht p.
idiopathic acute eosinophilic p.
lipoid p.
mycoplasmal p.
nosocomial p. (NP)
ovine progressive p.
plasma cell p.
pneumococcal p.
Pneumocystis carinii p. (PCP)
polymicrobial p.
primary atypical p.
progressive p.
recurrent bacterial p.
recurrent viral p.
usual interstitial p. (UIP)
ventilator-associated p.
viral p.
p. virus of mice
pneumoniae
    Chlamydia p.
    Klebsiella p.
    Mycoplasma p.
pneumonitis
    acute hypersensitivity p.
    acute lupus p.
    acute radiation p.
    chronic hypersensitivity p.
    desquamative interstitial p.
    hypersensitivity p. (HP)
    lymphocytic interstitial p. (LIP)
    pearl oyster shell p.
    radiation p.
    summer p.
    summer-type hypersensitivity p.
        (SHP)
    uremic p.
Pneumopent
pneumoperitoneum
pneumophila
    Legionella p.
Pneumo-Sleeve

pneumotachograph
pneumothorax, pl. **pneumothoraces**
    iatrogenic p.
Pneumovax 23
Pneumovirus
PNH
    paroxysmal nocturnal hemoglobinuria
PNIF
    peak nasal inspiratory flow
PNP
    paraneoplastic pemphigus
    purine nucleoside phosphorylase
PNS
    peripheral nervous system
PNU
    protein nitrogen unit
Pnu-Imune 23
PO$_2$
    partial pressure of oxygen
POA
    pancreatic oncofetal antigen
Poa pratensis
POCAAN
    People of Color Against AIDS Network
pock
pocket
        necrotic p.
        P. Scrubz
        P. SPO$_2$T
Pockethaler
        Vancenase P.
Pocketpeak peak flow meter
POCkit herpes test
pockmark
podagra
Pod-Ben-25
Podiatrix-TFM
Podiatrx-AF
podobromidrosis
Podocon-25
podofilox
Podofin
podophyllin and salicylic acid
podophyllum resin
PodoSpray nail drill system
Podoviridae
POEMS
        polyneuropathy, organomegaly,
        endocrinopathy, monoclonal
        gammopathy, and skin changes
        POEMS syndrome

NOTES

P

POF
premature ovarian failure
poikiloderma
acrokeratotic p.
p. atrophicans and cataract
p. atrophicans vasculare
p. of Civatte
Civatte p.
p. congenitale
crepey p.
hereditary sclerosing p. (HSP)
Jacobi p.
reticulated pigmented p.
p. vasculare atrophicans
p. vascularis atrophicans
poikilodermatomyositis
poikilodermatous parapsoriasis
point
Castellani p.
fibromyalgia trigger p.
Kienböck-Adamson p.
p. mutation
pointed
p. condyloma
p. wart
pointing
4-point Likert scale
5-point Likert scale
7-point Likert scale
6-point vitiligo disease activity scale
poison
p. bun sponge dermatitis
contact p.
corrosive p.
p. ivy
p. ivy dermatitis
p. oak
p. oak dermatitis
p. sumac
p. sumac dermatitis
poisoning
ciguatera p.
lead p.
mercury p.
scombroid fish p.
silver p.
strychnine p.
systemic p.
poisonous
Poisson-Pearson formula
pokeweed mitogen (PWM)
Poladex
polar
p. lepromatous
p. lepromatous leprosy
Polaramine
pol gene
polidocanol

poliglecaprone suture
polio
polioencephalitis infectiva
poliomyelitis
acute anterior p.
acute bulbar p.
chronic anterior p.
p. immune globulin (human)
p. immunoglobulin
Medin p.
mouse p.
p. vaccine
p. virus
poliosis
p. circumscripta
p. eccentrica
poliovirus
p. hominis
p. vaccine
p. vaccine, inactivated
p. vaccine, live, trivalent, oral
polish
nail p.
Polistes **sting**
polka-dot technique
polka fever
pollen
acacia tree p.
alder tree p.
alfalfa weed p.
p. antigen
ash tree p.
Bermuda grass p.
birch tree p.
black walnut tree p.
blue grass p.
box elder tree p.
brome grass p.
canary grass p.
cheat grass p.
cocklebur weed p.
cottonwood tree p.
curly dock weed p.
elm tree p.
English plantain weed p.
English walnut tree p.
eucalyptus tree p.
p. extract
false ragweed weed p.
goosefoot weed p.
grass p.
hazelnut tree p.
June grass p.
lamb's quarters weed p.
maple tree p.
mugwort weed p.
oak tree p.
olive tree p.

orchard grass p.
pickle weed p.
pigweed weed p.
pine tree p.
poplar tree p.
red top grass p.
Russian thistle weed p.
rye grass p.
sage weed p.
saltbush weed p.
salt grass p.
sheep sorrel weed p.
sweet vernal grass p.
tumbleweed weed p.
Western ragweed weed p.
wild oat grass p.
willow tree p.
windborne p.
pollen-induced allergic rhinitis
pollination
pollinosis, pollenosis
Cupressaceae p.
pollution
air p.
Polocaine injection
polonica
plica p.
poloxamer 188, 331
POL sclerosing solution
polyacrylamide
p. gel
p. gel electrophoresis (PAGE)
**polyacrylamide gel electrophoresis
(PAGE)**
polyacrylonitrile (PAN)
polyad
**poly (adenosine diphosphate-ribose)
polymerase (PADPRP)**
polyadenylylation
alternative p.
canonical p.
**poly(ADP-ribose)polymerase autoantibody
(PARP autoantibody)**
polyangiitis
microscopic p. (MPA)
p. overlap syndrome
polyarteritis
p. in childhood
p. nodosa (PAN)
p. nodosa syndrome

polyarthralgia
systemic p.
polyarthritis (PA)
asymmetric p.
cutaneous p.
epidemic p.
erosive p.
juvenile chronic p.
polyarticular
p. gonococcal arthritis
p. juvenile rheumatoid arthritis
p. septic arthritis
p. synovitis
polychemotherapy
polychlorobiphenyl (PCB)
polychlorodioxins
polychondritis
relapsing p.
polychotomous
polychromatic
Polycillin
Polycillin-N
Polycillin-PRB
polyclonal
p. activator
p. antibody
p. B cell
p. gammopathy
p. hypergammaglobulinemia
polycyclic
p. distribution of lesion
p. pattern
polycystic ovary disease
polycythemia vera
polydactylia
Polyderm foam dressing
polydioxanone suture (PDS suture)
polydysplastic epidermolysis
polydystrophy
pseudo-Hurler p.
polyene
polyethylene glycol precipitation assay
Polygam S/D
polygenic inheritance pattern
polyglactin 910 suture
**polyglandular autoimmune endocrine
disease**
polyglutamate
polyglycolic acid suture
polyglyconate suture
polygonal papule
polygonum

NOTES

P

polyhedral body
PolyHeme blood replacement product
polyhidrosis
Poly-Histine C, DM
Poly-Histine-D Capsule
polykaryon
polyleptic fever
polymastia
PolyMem
 P. alginate dressing
 P. alginate wound cover
 P. foam dressing
polymer
 collagen p.
 p. film dressing
 p. foam dressing
polymerase
 p. chain reaction (PCR, PRC)
 p. chain reaction assay
 p. chain reaction-based detection of
  hepatitis G virus
 p. chain reaction testing
 DNA p.
 poly (adenosine diphosphate-
  ribose) p. (PADPRP)
 RNA p.
 Taq p.
polymerization
 chondrocyte cytoskeletal actin p.
polymerized antigen
polymethyl methacrylate
polymicrobial
 p. arthritis
 p. bacteremia
 p. pneumonia
polymicrobic
polymorphe
 erythema p.
polymorphic
 p. eruption of pregnancy
 p. protein
 p. protoporphyria
 p. reticulosis
polymorphism
 allelic p.
 biallelic p.
 functional p.
 Hind III p.
 iatrogenic p.
 lipoprotein p.
 microsatellite p.
 nucleotide p.
 restriction fragment length p.
  (RFLP)
 single-strand conformation p.
  (SSCP)
 single-stranded conformational p.
  (SSCP)

polymorphonuclear
 p. cell
 p. leukocyte (PML)
 p. leukocyte collagenase
 p. leukocyte-dependent tissue
  destruction
 p. leukocyte elastase
 p. neutrophil (PMN)
polymorphous
 p. exanthema
 p. light eruption (PMLE)
 p. rash
Polymox
polymyalgia
 p. rheumatica (PMR)
 p. rheumatica syndrome
polymyositis (PM)
 juvenile dermatomyositis/p.
  (JDMS/PM)
polymyositis-scleroderma (PM-Scl)
 p.-s. antigen
polymyxa
 Bacillus p.
polymyxin
 bacitracin and p. b
 bacitracin, neomycin, and p. b
 p. b and hydrocortisone
 p. B-hydrocortisone suspension
 p. b sulfate
 neomycin and p. b
 oxytetracycline and p. b
polynesic
polyneuritiformis
 heredopathia atactica p.
polyneuritis
 acute idiopathic p.
 infectious p.
polyneuropathic amyloidosis
polyneuropathy
 familial amyloid p.
 familial amyloidotic p. (FAP)
 familial amyloidotic p. syndrome
 p., organomegaly, endocrinopathy,
  monoclonal gammopathy, and skin
  changes (POEMS)
polynucleosis
 neutrophil p.
polynucleotide antibody
polyolprepolymer
Polyomavirus
polyoma virus-associated interstitial
 nephritis
polyonychia
polyostotic fibrous dysplasia
polyp
 fibroepithelial p.
 intestinal p.
 nasal p.

polypapilloma
polypectomy
polypeptide
    CD4, human truncated-365 AA p.
    p. chain
    cyclic p.
    glutamine-rich p.
    p. hormone
    p. inhibitor
    islet amyloid p. (IAPP)
    proline-rich p.
polyphaga
    Acanthamoeba p.
polyphenol
    green tea p. (GTP)
Polyphenon E
polypi (*pl. of* polypus)
polyploid nevus
polypoid lesion
polypophyrin
polyposis
    chronic hyperplastic sinusitis with
      nasal p. (CHS/NP)
Poly-Pred Ophthalmic suspension
polypropylene suture
polypus, pl. **polypi**
polyquaternium-1
polyradiculoneuropathy
    chronic inflammatory
      demyelinating p. (CIDP)
polyradiculopathy
polysaccharide
    p. antigen
    pneumococcal p.
    specific soluble p.
polyserositis
    familial paroxysmal p.
    familial recurrent p.
    idiopathic p.
    periodic p.
    recurrent p.
    tuberculous p.
Polyskin
    P. II dressing
    P. II transparent film
    P. M.R. transparent film
polysomnograph
polysomnography (PSG)
Polysporin
    P. Ophthalmic
    P. Topical
polystichia

polystyrene latex
polysulfate
    calcium pentosan p.
Polytar
Polytec PI LaseAway
polytetrafluoroethylene
    expanded p. (ePTFE)
polythelia
polytomous
polytrichia
polytrichosis
Polytrim Ophthalmic
polyunguia
polyurethane film (PUF)
polyvalent
    p. allergy
    p. antiserum
    antivenin (*Crotalidae*) p.
    p. serum
    p. vaccine
polyvinyl chloride (PVC)
polyvinyldifluoride
PolyWic filler
POM
    pulse oximetry monitoring
pomade acne
Pompe disease
pomphoid
pompholyx
pomphus
Poncet
    P. disease
    P. rheumatism
ponderosa
    p. pine
    p. pine tree
Pondocillin
Ponds Prevent
Ponstel
Pontocaine
    P. injection
    P. topical
pool
    thapsigargin p.
pooled serum
poona
    Salmonella p.
poor
    p. marrow function
    p. platelet plasma (PPP)
poorly reversible asthma
Popeye sign

NOTES

P

popilliae
> *Paenibacillus p.*

poplar
> Lombardy p. tree
> p. tree
> p. tree pollen
> white p. tree

popliteal
> p. cyst
> p. fossa
> p. pterygium syndrome

popliteal-arcuate complex

POPP
> psoriatic onychopachydermoperiostitis

poppers' dermatitis

popsicle
> p. dermatitis
> p. panniculitis

population-based testing

porate

Porcelana Sunscreen

porcine
> p. bone marrow transplantation (PBMTx)
> p. endogenous retrovirus (PERV)
> p. hemagglutinating encephalomyelitis virus
> p. transmissible gastroenteritis

porcupine
> p. disease
> p. skin

pore
> dilated p.
> Kohn p.
> Oxy Deep P.
> perforin p.
> p. of Winer

Porges-Meier test

PORN
> progressive outer retinal necrosis

porocarcinoma

poroid hidradenoma

porokeratosis
> actinic p.
> disseminated superficial actinic p. (DSAP)
> linear p.
> Mibelli p.
> p. of Mibelli
> p. palmaris plantaris et disseminata
> p. plantaris discreta
> p. punctata

porokeratotic eccrine ostial

poroma
> apocrine p.
> eccrine p.
> follicular p.
> malignant eccrine p.

porphobilinogen

porphyria
> acute intermittent p. (AIP)
> ALA dehydratase deficiency p.
> congenital erythropoietic p. (CEP)
> p. cutanea tarda (PCT)
> erythropoietic p. (EPP)
> hepatic p.
> hepatoerythrocytic p. (HEP)
> hepatoerythropoietic p.
> mixed p.
> mixed hepatic p.
> South African genetic p.
> symptomatic p.
> p. variegata
> variegate p. (VP)

porphyric

porphyrin

porrigo
> p. decalvans
> p. favosa
> p. furfurans
> p. larvalis
> p. lupinosa
> p. scutulata

portal
> p. occlusion
> p. tract fibrosis
> p. venous and enteric drainage technique (P-E technique)

portoenterostomy
> hepatic p.

portopulmonary hypertension (PPHTN)

Portuguese
> P. jellyfish
> P. man-of-war
> P. man-of-war sting

port-wine
> p.-w. hemangioma
> p.-w. mark
> p.-w. nevus
> p.-w. stain (PWS)

Posada mycosis

Posada-Wernicke disease

position
> left side down-head up p.

positive
> p. anergy
> biologic false p. (BFP)
> CALLA p.
> common acute lymphocytic leukemia antigen p.
> p. end-expiratory pressure (PEEP)
> p. expiratory pressure (PEP)
> p. inspiratory pressure (PIP)
> p. patch test
> Ph p.
> p. phase

Philadelphia chromosome p.
p. predictive value (PPV)
p. reaction
p. rheumatoid factor
p. selection
positron emission tomography (PET)
posology
possible

minimal dose p.
postanesthetic effect
postbiopsy fistula
postcardiotomy syndrome
postdiphtheric paralysis
postencephalitic trophic ulcer
posterior

p. atlantodental interval (PADI)
p. interosseous nerve syndrome
p. interosseous neuropathy
p. scleritis
superior labrum anterior and p. (SLAP)
p. synechia formation
posteriores

limbi palpebrales p.
posteroanterior radiograph
postexertional microtrauma
postexposure prevention/postexposure prophylaxis (PEP)
postgrafting immunosuppression
postherpetic

p. erythema multiforme
p. neuralgia (PHN)
posthitis
post hoc analysis
postinfection lipoatrophy
postinfectious

p. encephalomyelitis syndrome
p. glomerulonephritis
p. steatorrhea
postinflammatory

p. hyperpigmentation
p. hypopigmentation
post-kala-azar dermal leishmanoid
postmastectomy lymphangiosarcoma
postmenopausal frontal fibrosing alopecia
postmiliarial hypohidrosis
postmortem

p. core protein degradation
p. pustule

p. tubercle
p. wart
postnasal drip (PND)
postnatal therapy
postoperative pressure alopecia
postosteotomy deformity
postpartum

p. alopecia
p. effect
p. thyroiditis (PPT)
postphlebitic syndrome
postprimary tuberculosis
postpyodermal acute glomerulonephritis
poststeroid panniculitis
poststreptococcal

p. glomerulonephritis (PSGN)
p. reactive arthritis (PSRA)
postsynaptic terminal
postthrombotic disease
posttransfusion

p. hepatitis (PST)
p. mononucleosis (PTM)
p. purpura
posttranslation
posttranslationally modified arginine residue
posttranslational protein modification
posttransplant

p. diabetes
p. erythrocytosis
p. lymphoproliferative disease (PTLD)
p. lymphoproliferative disorder (PTLD)
posttransplantation

p. lymphoproliferative disease (PTLD)
p. lymphoproliferative disorder (PTLD, PT-LPD)
posttraumatic

p. arthritis
p. pustular eruption
p. rheumatic meningitis
postulate

Ehrlich p.
Henle-Koch p.
Koch p.
postural drainage
postvaccinal encephalitis
postvenereal reactive arthritis
potassium

p. chloride stain (KOH)

NOTES

P

potassium *(continued)*
>   p. hydroxide (KOH)
>   p. hydroxide preparation
>   p. iodide
>   p. iodide enseals
>   penicillin V p.
>   p. permanganate
>   p. permanganate bath
>   p. permanganate crystal
>   p. permanganate solution
>   p. titanyl phosphate (KTP)
>   p. titanyl phosphate laser (KTP laser)

potato
>   sweet p.

potato-peeler method

potential
>   extravasation p.
>   mitochondrial membrane p.
>   sensory nerve action p. (SNAP)
>   stress-generated electric p.
>   zeta p.
>   zoonotic p.

potentially fatal asthma

potion
>   Donizetti p.
>   Wagner p.

Pott
>   P. gangrene
>   P. paralysis
>   P. puffy tumor

poultice

poultry handler's disease

poultryman's itch

poverty weed

povidone-iodine

Powassan
>   P. encephalitis
>   P. virus

powder
>   Absorbine Antifungal Foot p.
>   p. bed
>   facial p.
>   Flovent Rotadisk p.
>   full-coverage facial p.
>   Lotrimin AF Spray P.
>   transparent facial p.
>   Zeasorb-AF P.

power
>   P. Doppler ultrasonography
>   p. spectral analysis

powered air loss

pox
>   chicken p.
>   farmyard p.
>   Kaffir p.
>   zinc p.

poxviral mimicry

Poxviridae

poxvirus
>   p. officinalis

pp65(UL83) antigen

PPA
>   pyrophosphate arthritis-pseudogout
>   Guaifenex PPA 75

PPAR-gamma
>   peroxisome proliferator-activated receptor-gamma

PPD
>   purified protein derivative
>   purified protein derivative of tuberculin
>   PPD test

PPDA
>   paraphenylenediamine

pp′-DDE
>   pp′-dichlorodiphenyldichloroetene

pp′-dichlorodiphenyldichloroetene (pp′-DDE)

PPD-S
>   purified protein derivative-standard

ppg
>   photoplethysmography

PPH
>   primary pulmonary hypertension

p-phenylenediamine

PPHP
>   pseudopseudohypoparathyroidism

PPHTN
>   portopulmonary hypertension

PPi
>   pyrophosphate

PPIX
>   protoporphyrin IX

PPK
>   palmoplantar keratoderma

PPL
>   penicilloyl-polylysine
>   PPL skin test

PPLO
>   pleuro-pneumoniae-like organism

PPMS
>   primary-progressive multiple sclerosis

PPO-HSA
>   penicillin-penicilloyl human serum albumin

PPP
>   poor platelet plasma

PP-ribose-P

PPT
>   postpartum thyroiditis

PPV
>   positive predictive value

PR
>   pityriasis rosea

PR3
>   proteinase 3

PRA
  panel-reactive antibody
  percent reactive antibody/panel reactive
    antibody
  PRA testing
Practice
  Advisory Committee on
    Immunization P. (ACIP)
Prader-Willi syndrome
praecox
  icterus p.
  lymphedema p.
praepuffalis
  herpes p.
Pragmatar
prairie itch
PrameGel
Pramosone cream
pramoxine
  p. HCl
  p. hydrochloride
prasterone
pratense
  Phleum p.
pratensis
  dermatitis bullosa striata p.
  Poa p.
Pratt procedure
Prausnitz-Kustner (P-K)
  P.-K. antibody
  P.-K. reaction
  P.-K. syndrome
  P.-K. test
pravastatin
Prax
praziquantel
prazosin hydrochloride
PRC
  polymerase chain reaction
PRCA
  pure red cell aplasia
preauricular
  p. cyst
  p. sinus
pre-B
  p.-B. cell
  p.-B. cell expansion
precancer
precancerosa
  melanosis circumscripta p.
precancerous
  p. dermatitis

  p. lesion
  p. melanosis of Dubreuilh
  p. tumor
precipitate
  p. in gel
  p. in solution
precipitating antibody
precipitation
  double antibody p.
  hapten inhibition of p.
  immune p.
  p. test
precipitin
  p. assay
  p. reaction
  rheumatoid arthritis p. (RAP)
  serum p.
  p. test
precipitinogen
precipitinogenoid
precipitoid
precipitophore
Precise stapler
precision-point needle
precocious puberty
precursor
  mesenchymal p.
  p. molecule
Pred
  P. Forte Ophthalmic
  Liquid P.
  P. Mild Ophthalmic
Predaject injection
Predalone injection
Predcor injection
Pred-G Ophthalmic
Predicort-50 injection
predictive
  p. patch test
  p. testing
predispose
predisposition
  genetic p.
prednicarbate
Prednicen-M Oral
prednisolone
  chloramphenicol and p.
  p. and gentamicin
  neomycin, polymyxin b, and p.
  sodium sulfacetamide and p.
  p. tebutate
Prednisol TBA injection

NOTES

P

445

prednisone
    p. burst
    p. pulse
    p. taper
predominant
    p. DIP joint involvement
    p. distal interphalangeal joint
      involvement
    p. spondylitis
preemptive therapy
preeruptive
preexisting antibody
preformed
    p. antibody
    p. granule-associated mast cell
Prefrin Ophthalmic solution
Pregestimil
pregnancy
    p. alpha-2 glycoprotein (PAG)
    intrahepatic cholestasis of p.
    linea IgM dermatosis of p.
    mask of p.
    papular dermatitis of p.
    polymorphic eruption of p.
    pruritic folliculitis of p.
    pruritic inflammatory dermatosis
      of p.
    pruritic urticarial papules and
      plaques of p. (PUPPP)
pregnancy-associated glycoprotein
prehydration
preicteric fever
Preiser disease
preleukemia
Prelone Oral
premalignant tumor
prematura
    alopecia p.
premature
    p. aging
    p. alopecia
    p. ovarian failure (POF)
prematurity
    anetoderma of p.
premenstrual
    p. acne
    p. exacerbation of asthma (PMA)
Premier H. pylori assay
Premium stapler
premorbid
Premphase
premunition
premunitive
premycotic
prenatal therapy
preoperative anesthetic
preosteoblast
preosteoclast

prep
    touch p.
    xylol p.
preparation
    alum-precipitated p.
    hyperimmune gamma globulin p.
    KOH p.
    leukocyte-poor p.
    potassium hydroxide p.
    scabies p.
    Scholl Athlete's Foot P.
    Scholl Corn, Callus Plaster P.
    tar p.
    Tzanck p.
prepatellar bursitis
prepatent period
Pre-Pen
prepolypoid
prepriming effect
prepuce
prepulseless phase
preputiale
    sebum p.
Prescription Strength Desenex
presenile spontaneous gangrene
presenilis
    alopecia p.
presensitization phase
presentation
    pauciarticular p.
presenting clinical manifestation
preservation
    machine p. (MP)
    p. perfusion injury
    pulsatile p.
    p. reperfusion injury
preservative
    benzoate p.
    formaldehyde-releasing p. (FRP)
pressure
    p. alopecia
    ambulatory blood p. (ABP)
    bilevel positive airway p. (BiPAP)
    p. blister
    blood p.
    p. bulla
    casual blood p. (CBP)
    continuous positive airway p.
      (CPAP)
    expiratory positive airway p.
      (EPAP)
    p. gangrene
    inspiratory positive airway p.
      (IPAP)
    interstitial p.
    intracranial p. (ICP)
    intragraft p.
    peak inspiratory ventilator p.

positive end-expiratory p. (PEEP)
positive expiratory p. (PEP)
positive inspiratory p. (PIP)
pulmonary artery p.
p. sore
p. support ventilation (PSV)
p. ulcer
P. Ulcer Scale for Healing
  (PUSH)
P. Ulcer Scale for Healing tool
p. urticaria
zero end-expiratory p. (ZEEP)
**pressure-controlled inverse ratio
  ventilation**
pressure-induced urticaria
**pressure-regulated volume control
  ventilation**
**pressurized metered-dose inhaler
  (pMDI)**
PreSun lotion and gel
presynaptic terminal
prethrombotic
pretibial
p. fever
p. myxedema (PTM)
pretransplant donor blood transfusion
Pretz-D
Prevent
Gaviscon P.
Ponds P.
Prevention
Centers for Disease Control and P.
  (CDC)
preventive treatment
Preveon
Prevex
P. B
P. Diaper Rash cream
P. HC
Prevotella melaninogenica
prevotii
Peptostreptococcus p.
prezone
prick
p. puncture test
p. test concentration
p. testing
Pricker needle
prickle
p. cell
p. cell layer

prickle-cell
p.-c. carcinoma
p.-c. epithelioma
prickly heat
prick-prick test
prick-test method
prick-to-prick test
Prieur-Griscelli syndrome
prilocaine
lidocaine and p.
Primaderm dressing
Primapore absorptive wound dressing
primaquine
chloroquine and p.
p. phosphate
primary
p. adrenocortical failure
p. amyloid
p. amyloidotic arthropathy
p. angiitis of the central nervous
  system (PACNS)
p. areola
p. atypical pneumonia
p. biliary cirrhosis (PBC)
p. bubo
p. cell-mediated deficiency
p. complex
p. cutaneous adenoid cystic
  carcinoma
p. cutaneous amyloidosis
p. cutaneous aspergillosis
p. cutaneous B-cell lymphocytic
  leukemia
p. cutaneous B-cell lymphoma
p. cutaneous blastomycosis
p. cutaneous T-cell lymphoma
p. effusion lymphoma
p. epithelial germ
p. genital herpes simplex virus
p. herpes simplex infection
p. herpetic stomatitis
p. hyperaldosteronism
p. hyperhidrosis
p. hyperlipoproteinemia
p. hypogammaglobulinemia
p. idiopathic macular atrophy
p. immune response
p. immunodeficiency disorder
p. inoculation tuberculosis
p. irritant
p. irritant dermatitis
p. irritant reaction

NOTES

P

primary *(continued)*
 p. lesion
 p. localized amyloidosis
 p. lymphedema
 p. macular atrophy of skin
 p. neuroendocrine carcinoma
 p. neuroendocrine carcinoma of skin (PNCS)
 p. neuroendocrine tumor
 p. nonfunction (PRNF)
 p. pauciimmune necrotizing glomerulonephritis
 p. pulmonary histoplasmosis
 p. pulmonary hypertension (PPH)
 p. pulmonary parenchymal disease
 p. pyoderma
 p. rejection
 p. sclerosing cholangitis (PSC)
 p. Sjögren syndrome
 p. sore
 p. syphilis
 p. systemic amyloidosis
 p. systemic vasculitides (PSV)
 p. telangiectasia
primary-progressive multiple sclerosis (PPMS)
Primatene Mist
Primatized
Primaxin
prime-boost strategy
Primed cell
primer
 P. leg compression dressing
 sequence-specific p. (SSP)
primer-probe
 3 p.-p.
 OspA p.-p.
 OspB p.-p.
priming renal dialysis unit
Primula obconica
Principen
principle
 Castaneda p.
 diagnostic p.
Pringle disease
print
 scent p.
 tentacle p.
Prioderm
prion
 p. protein
 p. protein-origin amyloid deposit
prior drug exposure
priority
 law of p.
PRIST
 paper radioimmunosorbent test
 Phadezym PRIST

Pristine-100 allergy control product
private antigen
privet tree
PRNF
 primary nonfunction
Pro
 P. residue
 P. 2000 topical microbicide
proactivator
 C3 p.
Pro-Air
proalpha-chain
Pro-Amox
Proampacin
proapoptotic gene
probacteriophage
 defective p.
Probalan
proband
probe
 Acradinium-ester-labeled nucleic acid p.
 Arthro-BST arthroscopic p.
 cDNA p.
 door-knob p.
 IntraDop p.
 nucleic acid p.
 oligonucleotide p.
 radioactive p.
 viral p.
Proben-C
probenecid
 ampicillin and p.
 colchicine and p.
probiosis
probiotic
problem elicitation technique (PET)
problem-oriented
 p.-o. algorithm
 p.-o. diagnosis
procainamide
procaine
 p. hydrochloride
 penicillin g p.
procapsid
Procaryotae *(var. of* Prokaryotae*)*
procaryote *(var. of* prokaryote*)*
procaryotic *(var. of* prokaryotic*)*
procaterol
procedure
 Caldwell-Luc p.
 cheilectomy p.
 Darrach p.
 domino p.
 elimination p.
 fluorometric p.
 hemicallotasis p.
 Hoffman-Clayton p.

"Laser bra" p.
Microsporidia diagnostic p.
Mohs p.
olecranon p.
platelet neutralization p.
Pratt p.
Rotazyme diagnostic p.
Z-plasty p.

process
airspace p.
complement-mediated host defense p.
exocrinopathic p.
host-immune p.
nephritogenic p.
olecranon p.
recapitulation of ontogenesis p.
SoftLight laser/skin resurfacing p.

Pro-Clude
P.-C. transparent film
P.-C. transparent film wound dressing

procoagulant
procollagen
p. suicide
p. type II
p. type III aminoterminal peptide

Procort
Procrit
proctitis
pseudoinfectious p.

proctocolitis
ulcerative p.

Proctocort
procurement
regional organ p. (ROP)

Procuven solution
ProCyte
P. transparent adhesive film dressing
P. transparent film

Procytox
Pro-Depo injection
prodromal
p. stage
p. symptom

prodromon, pl. **prodroma**
Prodrox injection
product
AllerCare allergy control p.
Blue Peel skin health p.

cyclooxygenase p.
Exact skin p.
HLA-B27 gene p.
home cleaning p.
hypoallergenic p.
Lantiseptic skin care p.
lipoxygenase interaction p.
PolyHeme blood replacement p.
Pristine-100 allergy control p.
Refinity skin p.
Xcellerate T-cell p.

production
cytokine p.
p. of lymphokine
prostanoid p.
purulent sputum p.

productus
Peptostreptococcus p.

Proetz maneuver
Profen
P. II
P. LA

Profeta law
profile
angioedema p.
P. of Mood States Scale
relapsing-remitting p.
Western blot vaccine p.

Profore
P. 4-layer bandage
P. leg compression dressing
P. wound contact layer

profunda
miliaria p.
morphea p.
tinea p.

profundus
larva migrans p.
lupus erythematosus p.
nevus p.

profundus/panniculitis
lupus p.

profusa
lentiginosis p.

progenitalis
herpes p.

progenitor lymphoid cell
progeria
Hutchinson-Gilford p.
true p.

progeroid Ehlers-Danlos syndrome

NOTES

P

progesterone
progesterone-induced blocking factor (PIBF)
prognosis, pl. **prognoses**
prognostic
progonoma
melanotic p.
Prograf
Program
Childhood Asthma Management P. (CAMP)
National Asthma Education P. (NAEP)
National Immunization P. (NIP)
National Marrow Donor P. (NMDP)
Rush-Presbyterian St. Luke's Heart Failure and Transplant P.
progrediens
necrosis p.
progression
damaged joint p.
malignant p.
progressiva
acromelanosis p.
fibrodysplasia ossification p.
granulomatosis disciformis et p.
junctional epidermolysis bullosa p.
leukopathia symmetrica p.
progressive
p. acinar consolidation
p. azotemia
p. bacterial synergistic gangrene
p. disseminated histoplasmosis
p. encephalomyelitis with rigidity and myoclonus (PERM)
p. facial hemiatrophy
p. idiopathic atrophoderma
p. interstitial fibrosis
p. lipodystrophy
p. multifocal leukoencephalopathy (PML)
p. outer retinal necrosis (PORN)
p. pigmentary dermatosis
p. pneumonia
p. pneumonia virus
p. symmetrical verrucous erythrokeratodermia
p. symmetric erythrokeratodermia (PSEK)
p. symptom sclerosis (PSS)
p. synovial hypertrophy
p. systemic sclerosis (PSS)
p. vaccinia
proguanil
prohormone
Pro-Indo

proinflammatory
p. cytokine
p. cytokine response
p. effect
p. immunoreactant
p. pathway
Project
Rochester Epidemiology P. (REP)
Prokaryotae, Procaryotae
prokaryote, procaryote
prokaryotic, procaryotic
p. extracellular organism
prolactin
Prolastin
Prolene suture
Proleukin
prolidase deficiency
proliferans
angioendotheliomatosis p.
proliferating
p. cell nuclear antigen (PCNA)
p. pilar cyst
p. systematized angioendotheliomatosis
p. trichilemmal cyst
proliferation
acanthotic epidermal p.
p. disorder
endothelial cell p.
gliomatous p.
homeostasis-driven p.
intravascular endothelial p.
Masson intravascular endothelial p.
proliferation-associated antigen
proliferative
p. cell
p. dermatitis
p. fasciitis
p. glomerulonephritis
p. inflammatory disease
p. intimitis
p. lesion
p. synovitis
p. synovium
p. tenosynovitis
p. verrucous leukoplakia
prolificans
Scopulariopsis p.
ProLine endoscopic instrument
proline-rich polypeptide
prolixus
Rhodnius p.
prolongation
p. of expiration
expiratory p.
prolonged
p. diarrhea
p. pulmonary eosinophilia

Proloprim
prolyl
prolymphocytic leukemia (PLL)
Prometa
promethazine
    p. HCl
    p. hydrochloride
Prometh injection
Promit
promoter
    IL-10 gene p.
    neurofilament p.
promotor
    p. allele
    p. element
prom pill
pronator teres syndrome
Pronto Shampoo
Propaderm
Propadrine
Propagest
Propa pH
Propecia
properdin
    p. deficiency
    p. factor A, B, D, E
    p. system
prophage
    defective p.
prophylactic
    p. antibody
    p. treatment
prophylaxis
    active p.
    p. agent
    chemical p.
    malaria p.
    passive p.
    postexposure
      prevention/postexposure p. (PEP)
Prophyllin
propidium iodide
propionate
    clobetasol p.
    fluticasone p. (FP)
    halobetasol p.
propionate/salmeterol
    flucatisone p. (FP/Salm Combo)
Propionibacterium
    P. acnes
    P. propionicus

propionibacterium acne
propionicus
    Propionibacterium p.
Pro-Piroxicam
proportional assist ventilation
proportionate morbidity ratio (PMR)
propranolol hydrochloride
propria
    atrophia pilorum p.
    lamina p.
    miliaria p.
propylene
    p. glycol
    p. glycol allergy
    p. glycol dermatitis
propylthiouracil
proquazone
Prorex Injection
prosector's
    p. tubercle
    p. wart
prosodemic
Prosorba column device
prostacyclin (PGI$_2$)
    p. I3
    p. synthase
prostaglandin (PG)
    p. D (PGD)
    p. D$_2$ (PGD$_2$)
    p. E (PGE)
    p. E$_1$ (PGE$_1$)
    p. E$_2$ (PGE$_2$)
    p. H$_2$ (PGH$_2$)
    p. synthesis inhibition
prostanoid
    p. biosynthetic enzyme
    p. production
Prostaphlin
    P. injection
    P. Oral
ProstaScint monoclonal antibody
prostatitis
prosthesis, pl. **prostheses**
    silicone rubber p.
prosthetic joint
protease
    Hirudin-sensitive p.
    neutral p.
    p. nexin-1

NOTES

protease *(continued)*
    serine p.
    thiol p.
protease-activated receptor (PAR)
protease-antiprotease imbalance
proteasome
ProTec
Protectant
    LiquiShield-A Skin P.
protection
    photo p.
    Sundown Extra P.
    Sun Management Lip P.
    Sun Management Sensible P.
    p. test
    topical skin p. (TSP)
protective
    p. protein
    p. therapy
protector
    Heelbo decubitus p.
protein
    acetylation of cellular p.
    acetylation of serum p.
    actin-binding p.
    activator p. 1 (AP1)
    acute phase p.
    adhesion p.
    AL p.
        immunoglobulin light chain-origin
            amyloid deposit
    amyloid A p.
    amyloid fibril p.
    antibiotic p.
    p. antigen
    antiviral p. (AVP)
    arthritogenic p.
    Australian parrot p.
    azurophil granule p.
    B7 p.
    bactericidal-permeability-increasing p.
      (BPI protein)
    Bence Jones p.
    BPI p.
        bactericidal-permeability-
          increasing protein
    BvgS p.
    C p.
        complement protein
    p. C
    cartilage intermediate layer p.
      (CILP)
    cartilage matrix p.
    cartilage oligomeric matrix p.
      (COMP)
    CD28 p.
    p. C deficiency
    CD40 soluble p.

    cell adhesion p.
    p. C1 esterase inhibitor
    c-fos p.
    p. chip
    c-jun p.
    complement p. (C protein)
    complement control p. (CCP)
    p. contact dermatitis
    control p.
    C-reactive p. (CRP)
    CREB p.
    CTLA-4 soluble p.
    eosinophil cationic p. (ECP)
    eosinophil granule cationic p.
    eosinophil p. X
    ErbB-2 p.
    p. fever
    p. filaggrin
    F12-MABP fusion p.
    p. folding
    foreign p.
    freeze-dried p.
    G p.
    glucocorticoid-inducible p.
    glycosylphosphatidylinositol-
      anchored p.
    GP47, GP67 p.
    GPI-anchored p.
    haptenated p.
    heat-shock p. (HSP)
    heat-shock p. 70 (HSP-70)
    HEL p.
    hen egg lysozyme p.
    heterologous p.
    homeobox p.
    immune p.
    immunogenic p.
    220-kD p.
    38-kd P_o p.
    45-kilodalton p.
    p. kinase A (PKA)
    p. kinase A-dependent
      phosphorylation
    latex ELISA for antigen p.
      (LEAP)
    lipopolysaccharide binding p. (LBP)
    5-lipoxygenase-activating p. (FLAP)
    liver-specific p. (LSP)
    5-LO-activating p.
    M p.
    MacMARCKS p.
    macrophage inflammatory p. (MIP)
    major basic p. (MBP)
    major outer membrane p. (MOMP)
    maltose-binding p. (MABP, MBP)
    mannose-binding p.
    mitogen-activated p. (MAP)
    mitogen-activating p. (MAP)

monoclonal p.
monocyte chemoattractant p.
monocyte chemotactic p. (MCP)
mouse serum p. (MSP)
mouse urine p. (MUP)
myelin basic p. (MBP)
myeloblastic p.
Nef p.
neutrophil-activating p. (NAP)
NF-ATc p.
p. nitrogen unit (PNU)
nonhistone p.
nonspecific p.
Ontak p.
p. origin amyloid deposit
peptide transporter p.
pigeon serum p. (PSP)
plasma cell dyscrasia with
  polyneuropathy, organomegaly,
  endocrinopathy, monoclonal p.
platelet basic p.
polymorphic p.
prion p.
protective p.
ras p.
ras-mitogen-activated p.
rat serum p. (RSP)
rat urine p. (RUP)
Rb p.
receptor interacting p. (RIP)
recombinant LFA-3/IgG1 human
  fusion p.
retinoblastoma tumor suppressor p.
RFX-associated p. (RFXAP)
rhoGDI p.
p. S
SCA p.
secretory leukoprotease inhibitor p.
p. shock
p. shock therapy
single-chain antigen-binding p.
Sma- and Mad-related p. (SMAD)
Structural Classification of P.'s
  (SCOP)
Tamm-Horsfall p.
TAP1, TAP2 p.
TATA-binding p.
testis-specific binding p. (TSBP)
ToxR p.
p. transglutamination
variant amyloidogenic p.

Wiskott-Aldrich syndrome p.
  (WASP)
zinc finger p.
protein-1
  human monocyte chemoattractant p.
  monocyte chemoattractant p. (MCP-
  1)
proteinase
  p. 3 (PR3)
  aspartic p.
  connective tissue p.
  cysteine p.
  disintegrin p.
  ECM-degrading p.
  extracellular matrix-degrading p.
  p.-inhibitor
  lysosomal p.
  mast cell p.
  neutral p.
  serine p.
protein-energy malnutrition
protein-energy-related obesity
protein-losing
  p.-l. enteropathy
  p.-l. gastroenteropathy
proteinosis
  lipoid p.
proteinuria
  nephrotic-range p.
proteoglycan
  cartilage p.
  human stromelysin aggregated p.
  (H-SLAP)
  surface p.
proteolysis
proteolytic enzyme
proteomic map
Proteque SPS
Proteus
  P. mirabilis
  P. syndrome
  P. vulgaris
Prothazine
  P. injection
  P. Oral
protist
protistologist
protistology
protobe
protobiology
protocol
  2-day ultrarush p.

NOTES

P

protocol *(continued)*
    triple-drug therapy
       immunosuppression p.
Protoctista
proton
    p. leak
    p. magnetic resonance microscopy
protooncogene
    c-myc p.
    Fos p.
    Jun p.
protopianoma
Protopic
protoplast fusion
protoporphyria
    Besnier p.
    p. chronica multiformis
    erythropoietic p.
    p. estivalis
    p. ferox
    p. gestationis
    p. of Hebra
    Hutchinson summer p.
    melanotic p.
    p. mitis
    polymorphic p.
    p. prurigo agria
    p. simplex
    p. universalis
    winter p.
protoporphyrin
    p. IX (PPIX)
    zinc p. (ZPP)
protoporphyrinogen
Protostat Oral
Prototheca wickerhamii
protothecosis
Protovir
Protox
protozoa
    unicellular p.
protozoal
    p. abscess
    p. parasitic disease
protozoan infection
protracta
    Triatoma p.
Protropin II
protrusio acetabuli
protrusion
    infantile perianal pyramidal p.
protuberans
    dermatofibroma p.
    dermatofibrosarcoma p. (DFSP)
proud flesh
Provascar
Provatene
Pro-Vent arterial blood sampling kit

Proventil
    P. HFA
    P. Repetabs
Providence clamp
provirus
provocation
    bronchial p.
    p. typhoid
provocation-neutralization test
provocative
    p. dose testing
    p. use test (PUT)
Provocholine
Prowazek body
Prowazek-Greeff body
prowazekii
    Rickettsia p.
proxetil
    cefpodoxime p.
proximal
    p. bronchiectasis
    p. femoral osteotomy
    p. interphalangeal (PIP)
    p. nail matrix
    p. phalange
    p. pseudoarthrosis
Proximate
    P. II, III stapler
    P. RH stapler
prozone reaction
PRSP
    penicillin-resistant *Streptococcus*
    pneumoniae
Prudoxin cream
pruinosum
    Chrysosporium p.
prune
pruriginosus
    strophulus p.
pruriginous
prurigo
    actinic p.
    p. agria
    Besnier p.
    p. diathsique
    p. estivalis
    p. ferox
    p. gestationis
    p. gestationis of Besnier
    p. gravidarum
    Hebra p.
    p. hiemalis
    Hutchinson summer p.
    p. infantilis
    p. mitis
    p. nodularis
    p. papule
    p. simplex

p. simplex subacuta
summer p.
pruritic
p. dermatosis
p. erythematous patch
p. folliculitis of pregnancy
p. inflammatory dermatosis of
pregnancy
p. lesion
p. papule
p. urticarial papules and plaques
of pregnancy (PUPPP)
pruritica
puncta p.
pruritogenic
pruritus
p. ani
aquagenic p.
p. balnea
bath p.
biliary p.
brachioradial p.
central p.
Duhring p.
essential p.
p. estivalis
generalized p.
genital p.
p. hiemalis
paroxysmal p.
perianal p.
psychogenic p.
p. scroti
seasonal p.
senile p.
p. senilis
symptomatic p.
uremic p.
p. vulva
winter p.
psammoma
PSC
pigmented spindle cell
primary sclerosing cholangitis
PSCN
plexiform spindle cell nevus
PSE
Entex PSE
Guaifenex PSE
PSEK
progressive symmetric
erythrokeratodermia

P-selectin ligand
Pseudallescheria boydii
pseudallescheriasis
pseudarthrosis
Girdlestone p.
pseudoacanthosis nigricans
pseudoachondroplasia
pseudoagglutination
pseudoainhum
pseudoallergic reaction
pseudoalopecia areata
pseudoanaphylactic shock
pseudoanaphylaxis
pseudoaneurysm
ventricular p. (PVA)
pseudoangina pectoris
pseudoangiomatosis
eruptive p.
pseudoangiosarcoma
Masson p.
pseudoannulati
pili p.
pseudoarthrosis
proximal p.
pseudobacteremia
pseudobacteriuria
pseudocavitation
pseudochancre
p. redux
pseudocholinesterase (PCE)
pseudochromidrosis
pseudocolloid of lips
pseudocowpox virus
pseudocyst
digital mucinous p.
myxoid p.
pseudocystic rheumatoid arthritis
pseudodermachalasis
pseudodiphtheria
pseudodiphtheriticum
Bacillus p.
pseudodysentery
pseudoedema
pseudoemperipolesis
pseudoephedrine
acetaminophen, chlorpheniramine,
and p.
acrivastine and p.
brompheniramine and p.
carbinoxamine and p.
chlorpheniramine and p.
p. and dextromethorphan

NOTES

P

pseudoephedrine *(continued)*
    diphenhydramine and p.
    fexofenadine and p.
    guaifenesin and p.
    p. HCl
    p. and ibuprofen
    loratadine and p.
    terfenadine and p.
    triprolidine and p.
pseudoepitheliomatous
    p. hyperplasia
    p. keratotic and micaceous balanitis
pseudoerysipelas
pseudoexfoliation
pseudofolliculitis barbae (PFB)
pseudofracture
Pseudofrin
pseudogene
Pseudo-Gest Plus Tablet
pseudoglandular squamous cell carcinoma
pseudogout
pseudogynecomastia
pseudohorned cyst
pseudo-Hurler polydystrophy
pseudo-Hutchinson sign
pseudohyphae
pseudohypoparathyroidism (PHP)
pseudoicterus
pseudoinfection
pseudoinfectious proctitis
pseudojaundice
pseudo-Kaposi sarcoma
pseudolaxity
pseudolepromatous leishmaniasis
pseudoleukonychia
pseudolymphocytic choriomeningitis virus
pseudolymphoma
    B-cell p.
    cutaneous p.
    Spiegler-Fendt p.
    T-cell p.
pseudolysogenic
    p. strain
pseudolysogeny
pseudomalignant lymphoma
pseudomallei
    Burkholderia p.
    Malleomyces p.
    Pseudomonas p.
pseudomembrane
pseudomembranous colitis
pseudomeningitis
pseudomilium
    colloid p.
Pseudomonas
    P. aeruginosa
    P. aeruginosa bacteremia

    P. cepacia dermatitis
    P. elastase
    P. pseudomallei
    P. putida
pseudomonic acid
pseudomonilethrix
pseudoneuropathic joint
pseudonit
pseudoobstruction
    chronic intestinal p. (CIPO)
pseudoparalysis
    Parrot p.
pseudopelade
    Brocq p.
    p. of Brocq
pseudopelade-type alopecia
pseudophlegmon
    Hamilton p.
pseudophytophotodermatitis
pseudopilus, pl. **pseudopili**
    p. annulatus
pseudopneumonia
pseudopod
pseudopodagra
pseudoporphyria
pseudoproteinuria
pseudopseudohypoparathyroidism (PPHP)
pseudopseudothrombophlebitis
pseudorabies virus
pseudoradicular syndrome
pseudoreaction
pseudorecidive
pseudoreplica
pseudorheumatism
pseudorheumatoid
pseudorubella
pseudosarcomatous fasciitis
pseudoscar
    spontaneous p.
    stellate p.
pseudoscarlatina
pseudoseptic arthritis
pseudosmallpox
pseudosyndactyly
pseudotattooing
pseudothrombophlebitis
pseudotrichinosis
pseudotuberculosis
    Yersinia p.
pseudotumor
    p. cerebri
    orbital p.
pseudotumoral mediastinal amyloidosis
pseudo-Turner syndrome
pseudovariola
Pseudovent PED capsule
pseudoxanthoma elasticum (PXE)
pseudoxanthomatous mastocytosis

PSG
  polysomnography
PSGN
  poststreptococcal glomerulonephritis
psilate
psilosis
psilostachya
  Ambrosia p.
psilothin
psilotic
psittaci
  Chlamydia p.
psittacosis
  p. inclusion body
  p. virus
psoas
PsoE
  erythrodermic psoriasis
psora
psoralen
  p. compound
  p. ultraviolet A (PUVA)
  p. ultraviolet A-range (PUVA)
  p. ultraviolet A regimen/therapy
Psorcon
  P. topical
  P. topical steroid
psorelcosis
psoriasic
psoriasiform
  p. dermatitis
  p. epidermal hyperplasia
  p. eruption
psoriasiformis
  parakeratosis p.
psoriasis
  p. annularis
  p. annulata
  anti-CD11a humanized monoclonal
    antibody for p.
  p. area and severity index (PASI)
  p. arthropathica
  p. arthropica
  Barber p.
  p. buccalis
  p. circinata
  circinate p.
  p. diffusa
  p. discoidea
  p. discoides
  drop-like p.
  erythrodermic p. (PsoE)

exfoliative p.
p. figurata
figurate p.
flexural p.
generalized pustular p.
genital p.
p. geographica
geriatric p.
p. guttata
guttate p.
p. gyrata
gyrate p.
Ingram regimen for p.
intertriginous p.
intraepidermal microabscess of p.
inverse p.
p. inveterata
P. Life Stress Inventory (PLSI)
p. lingua
localized pustular p.
microabscess of p.
napkin p.
p. nummularis
p. orbicularis
ostraceous p.
p. ostreacea
palmar p.
plaque p.
plaque-type p.
p. punctata
pustular p.
rupioid p.
p. rupioides
p. spondylitica
treatment of p.
p. universalis
volar p.
von Zumbusch pustular p.
psoriatic
  p. arthritis
  p. arthritis mutilans
  p. arthritis with spinal involvement
  p. arthropathy
  p. onychopachydermoperiostitis
    (POPP)
  p. plaque
  p. sacroiliitis
  p. spondylitis
psoriatica
  arthropathia p.
psoriatic-type scale

NOTES

P

psoriaticum
    erythroderma p.
psoric
psoriGel
Psorion
    P. Cream
    P. Topical
psoroid
psorophthalmia
psoroptic acariasis
psorous
PSP
    pigeon serum protein
PSRA
    poststreptococcal reactive arthritis
PSS
    progressive symptom sclerosis
    progressive systemic sclerosis
P&S Shampoo
PST
    posttransfusion hepatitis
PSV
    pressure support ventilation
    primary systemic vasculitis
    primary systemic vasculitides
    Quantum PSV
psychocutaneous disease
Psychodidae
psychogalvanic
psychogalvanometer
psychogenic
    p. factor
    p. pain syndrome
    p. pruritus
    p. purpura
    p. reaction
psychoitchical
psychological stimulus
psycho-neuro-immuno-endocrine axis
psychoneuroimmunology
psychophysiologic disorder
psychosis
psychosocial intervention
psychotropic
    p. agent
    p. agent therapy
psyllium seed
4-p syndrome
PTA
    pancreas transplant alone
PTDM
pteronyssinus
    Dermatophagoides p.
pterygium
    p. colli
    p. inversum unguis
pthiriasis
    p. capitis

    p. corporis
    p. pubis
Pthirus
    P. pubis
    P. pubis infestation
PTLD
    posttransplantation lymphoproliferative
    disease
    posttransplantation lymphoproliferative
    disorder
    posttransplant lymphoproliferative
    disease
    posttransplant lymphoproliferative
    disorder
PT-LPD
    posttransplantation lymphoproliferative
    disorder
PTM
    posttransfusion mononucleosis
    pretibial myxedema
ptosis
PTT
    partial thromboplastin time
PTX
    pentoxifylline
puberty
    precocious p.
pubes
pubescence
pubic
    p. baldness
    p. louse
pubis
    osteitis p.
    pediculosis p.
    pthiriasis p.
    Pthirus p.
public antigen
pubomadesis
pudenda (*pl. of* pudendum)
pudendal ulcer
pudendi
    granuloma p.
pudendum, pl. pudenda
    ulcerating granuloma of p.
pudicitiae
    erythema p.
pudore
    erythema a p.
pudoris
    erythema p.
puellaris
    erythrocyanosis crurum p.
puellarum
    erythrocyanosis frigida crurum p.
Puente disease
puerorum
    hydroa p.

puerperal
  p. bacteremia
  p. fever
puerperium
PUF
  polyurethane film
puff
  buff p.
Pulex irritans
pulicans
  purpura p.
pulicicide
pulicide
pulicosa
  purpura p.
pulicosis
pulicosistungiasis
pull cell
pulling boat hand
pullulans
  Aureobasidium p.
Pullularia
Pulmanex
Pulmicort Turbuhaler
Pulmo-Aide
  P.-A. nebulizer
  P.-A. Traveler
pulmonale
  cor p.
pulmonary
  p. adenomatosis of sheep
  p. agenesis
  p. amyloidosis
  p. artery pressure
  p. aspergillosis
  p. blood volume (PBV)
  p. capillary hemangiomatosis
  p. disease anemia syndrome
  p. embolism
  p. flushing
  p. function (PF)
  p. function test (PFT)
  p. hemorrhage
  p. hemosiderosis
  p. hypertension
  p. infiltrate with eosinophilia (PIE)
  p. lesion
  p. lymphoma
  p. mycosis
  p. necrobiotic nodule
  p. nodulosis
  p. occlusive vasculopathy

  p. sarcoidosis
  p. sling syndrome
  p. surfactant
  p. toilet
  p. vascular resistance (PVR)
  p. venoocclusive disease (PVOD)
Pulmonet spirometer
pulmonic valve closure sound
PulmoSonic
pulmowrap
Pulmozyme
pulp abscess
pulpal abscess
pulposus
  nucleus p.
pulp-to-pulp tip pinch
pulsatile preservation
pulse
  p. dosing
  p. methylprednisolone
  p. oximetry device
  p. oximetry monitoring (POM)
  paradoxical p.
  P. Peel
  prednisone p.
  p. rate
  spin-echo p.
  steroid p.
  p. test
pulsed-dye
  p.-d. laser (PDL)
  p.-d. laser therapy (PDL)
pulsed field gel electrophoresis (PFGE)
PulseDose oxygen delivery technology
pulseless
  p. disease
  p. phase
pulsus paradoxus
pultaceous
Pulvules
  Cinobac P.
  Co-Pyronil 2 P.
  Ilosone P.
  Seromycin P.
pumice stone
pumilus
  Bacillus p.
pump
  Alpha 1 p.
  continuous subcutaneous insulin
    infusion p. (CSIIP)
  elastomeric p.

NOTES

P

pump *(continued)*
    Klein p.
    Na$^+$-K$^+$ ATPase p.
    sodium-potassium ATPase p.
    Wells Johnson p.
pumpkin
punch
    Accuderm p.
    Australian p.
    Baker-Cummings p.
    p. biopsy
    Dyonics suction p.
    Keyes p.
    Loo p.
    Orentreich p.
    skin p.
    upcurved p.
punched-out erosion
puncta pruritica
punctata
    acne p.
    chondrodysplasia p.
    keratosis palmoplantaris p.
    onychia p.
    porokeratosis p.
    psoriasis p.
punctate
    p. area of increased signal (PAIS)
    p. bleeding
    erythema p.
    p. hemorrhage
    p. keratoderma
    p. porokeratotic keratoderma
punctated metalloproteinase
punctatum
    erythema p.
    keratoderma p.
punctum
puncture
puncture wound
pupate
pupil
    Adie tonic p.
    Argyll Robertson p.
PUPPP
    pruritic urticarial papules and plaques of
    pregnancy
pura *(pl. of* pus)
Puralube Tears solution
pure
    p. neural leprosy
    p. red cell aplasia (PRCA)
purging
    tumor cell p.
    in vitro p.
Puri-Clens wound cleanser
purified
    p. protein derivative (PPD)

    p. protein derivative-standard (PPD-S)
    p. protein derivative test
    p. protein derivative of tuberculin (PPD)
    p. talc
purine
    p. analog
    p. metabolism
    p. nucleoside phosphorylase (PNP)
    p. nucleoside phosphorylase deficiency
    p. nucleotide adenosine triphosphate
    p. nucleotide cycle
    p. ribonucleotide
    p. ring
purine-stimulated prostaglandin E$_2$ (PGE$_2$)
purinoceptor
Purinol
purple-red papule
purple sail dermatitis
Purpose cleanser
purpura
    actinic p.
    acute idiopathic thrombocytopenic p.
    acute vascular p.
    allergic nonthrombocytopenic p.
    anaphylactoid p.
    p. angioneurotica
    p. annularis telangiectodes
    p. annularis telangiectodes of Majocchi
    autoimmune p.
    autoimmune thrombocytopenic p.
    Bateman p.
    p. bullosa
    p. cachectica
    chronic idiopathic thrombocytopenic p.
    p. cryoglobulinemia
    cutaneous p.
    drug-induced p.
    Ducas and Kapetanakis pigmented p.
    dysproteinemic p.
    p. en cocarde avec oedema
    essential thrombocytopenic p.
    factitious p.
    fibrinolytic p.
    p. fulminans
    Gardner-Diamond p.
    p. hemorrhagica
    Henoch p.
    Henoch-Schönlein p. (HSP)
    hypergammaglobulinemic p.
    hyperglobulinemic p.

idiopathic thrombocytopenic p.
  (ITP)
p. iodica
itching p.
Landouzy p.
macular p.
p. maculosa
Majocchi p.
p. nervosa
nonblanching p.
nonpalpable p.
nonthrombocytopenic p.
obstructive p.
orthostatic p.
palpable p.
passion p.
periorbital p.
pigmented p.
p. pigmentosa chronica
pinch p.
posttransfusion p.
psychogenic p.
p. pulicans
p. pulicosa
p. rheumatica
Schamberg p.
Schönlein p.
scorbutic p.
senile p.
p. senilis
p. simplex
skin p.
solar p.
stasis p.
steroid p.
p. symptomatica
thrombocytopenic p.
thrombotic thrombocytopenic p.
  (TTP)
traumatic p.
p. urticans
p. variolosa
Waldenström p.
Werlhof p.
purpurascens
  Epicoccum p.
purpureum
  Trichophyton p.
purpuric
  p. halo
  p. lesion

p. phototherapy-induced eruption
p. pigmented lichenoid dermatitis
pursed lips breathing
purse-string mouth
purulent
  p. arthritis
  p. sputum
  p. sputum production
puruloid
pus, pl. **pura**
  p. tube
Pusey emulsion
PUSH
  Pressure Ulcer Scale for Healing
    PUSH tool
puss
  p. caterpillar
  p. caterpillar sting
pustula, pl. **pustulae**
  p. maligna
pustulant
pustular
  p. acne
  p. acrodermatitis
  p. bacterid
  p. dermatosis
  p. eruption
  p. folliculitis
  p. lesion
  p. melanosis
  p. miliaria
  p. patch-test reaction
  p. perifolliculitis
  p. psoriasis
  p. psoriasis of the palms and
    soles of Barber
  superficial p.
  p. syphilid
pustulation
pustule
  follicular p.
  Kogoj p.
  malignant p.
  postmortem p.
  spongiform p.
  sterile p.
pustuliform
pustulocrustaceous
pustulosa
  acne p.
  acrodermatitis p.
  miliaria p.

NOTES

P

461

pustulosa *(continued)*
>parakeratosis p.
>trichomycosis p.
>varicella inoculata p.

pustulosis
>acute generalized exanthematous p. (AGEP)
>p. palmaris et plantaris
>palmoplantar p.
>p. palmoplantaris
>sterile eosinophilic p.
>p. vacciniformis acuta

pustulosum
>eczema p.
>erysipelas p.

pustulotic arthrosteitis
PUT
>provocative use test

putative oxidative cleavage site
putida
>*Pseudomonas p.*

putrescentiae
>*Tyrophagus p.*

Puumala virus
PUVA
>oral administration of psoralen and subsequent exposure to long wavelength ultraviolet light
>photochemotherapy with oral methoxypsoralen therapy followed by UVA
>psoralen ultraviolet A
>psoralen ultraviolet A-range
>>foil bath PUVA
>>PUVA regimen/therapy
>>topical PUVA

PUVA-induced lentigo
PV
>pemphigus vulgaris

PVA
>ventricular pseudoaneurysm

PVC
>polyvinyl chloride

PVM virus
PVNS
>pigmented villonodular synovitis

PVOD
>pulmonary venoocclusive disease

PVR
>pulmonary vascular resistance

PWM
>pokeweed mitogen

PWS
>port-wine stain

PXE
>pseudoxanthoma elasticum

pycnidia
pycnidium

pyemia
pyemic abscess
Pyemotes ventricosus
pyknodysostosis
pyknosis
pyknotic cell
pylori
>*Campylobacter p.*
>*Helicobacter p.*

Pym fever
Pyocidin-Otic
pyocin
pyocyanine
pyocyanolysin
pyoderma
>blastomycosis-like p.
>chancriform p.
>p. chancriforme faciei
>p. faciale
>p. gangrenosum (PG)
>granulomatous p.
>intractable p.
>malignant p.
>persistent p.
>primary p.
>secondary p.
>superficial follicular p.
>superficial granulomatous p.
>p. ulcerosum tropicalum
>p. vegetans
>p. verrucosum

pyodermatitis
pyodermatosis
pyodermatous
>p. infection
>p. skin lesion

pyodermia
>p. facialis
>p. gangrenosa

pyogenes
>*Streptococcus p.*

pyogenic
>p. abscess
>p. arthritis
>p. bacterium
>p. fever
>p. granuloma
>p. infection
>p. osteomyelitis
>p. sacroiliitis
>p. sterile arthritis, pyoderma gangrenosum and acne (PAPA)

pyogenicum
>granuloma p.

pyohemia
pyomyositis
>pneumococcal p.
>tropical p.

pyosis
  Corlett p.
  Manson p.
  p. palmaris
  p. tropica
pyostomatitis vegetans
Pyradone
Pyral
  Jaa P.
pyrantel pamoate
pyrazinamide (PZA)
  rifampin, isoniazid, and p.
pyrethrin
  p.'s and piperonyl butoxide
pyrethroid
  synthetic p.
pyrethrum
pyrexia
  tick p.
pyribenzamine (PBZ)
pyridinoline crosslink
pyridoxine deficiency
pyridoxol deficiency
pyriformis syndrome
pyrilamine
  pheniramine, phenylpropanolamine,
    and p.
pyrimethamine
  sulfadoxine and p.
pyrimidine
  fluorinated p.

Pyrinate
  A-200 P.
pyrindinyl imidazole
Pyrinex Pediculicide Shampoo
Pyrinyl
  P. II
  P. II Liquid
  P. Plus Shampoo
pyrithione
  zinc p.
  p. zinc
Pyrobombus **sting**
pyrogen
  endogenous p.
pyroglobulin
pyroglyphid mite
pyrophosphate (PPi)
  alkaline phosphatase and p.
  p. arthritis-pseudogout (PPA)
  p. arthropathy
pyrophosphohydrolase
  nucleoside triphosphate p. (NTPPH,
    NTPPPH)
pyrotoxin
pyruvate kinase deficiency
pyruvic acid
PZA
  pyrazinamide

NOTES

P

Q
    Q albumin
    Q fever
6q
    chromosome 6q
QA antigen
QALY
    quality-adjusted life-year
Q-angle
QCT
    quantitative computed tomography
1q duplication
QIE
    quantitative immunoelectrophoresis
QOL
    quality of life
QPCR
    quantitative polymerase chain reaction
    QPCR assay
(q23q31)
    trisomy of chromosome II, dup(1)
    (q23q31)
QSRL
    Q-switched ruby laser
Q-switched
    Q.-s. alexandrite laser
    Q.-s. Nd:YAG laser
    Q.-s. neodymium:YAG laser
    (QSYAG)
    Q.-s. ruby laser (QSRL)
QSYAG
    Q-switched neodymium:YAG laser
Quad-A-Hist
Quadrinal
quadroma
quail bronchitis virus
quality
    q. of life (QOL)
    Q. of Life score
quality-adjusted life-year (QALY)
Quant broth
Quantikine ELISA kit
quantitation of B cell
quantitative
    q. complement assay
    q. computed tomography (QCT)
    q. HCV RNA
    q. immunoassay for urine
    myoglobin
    q. immunoelectrophoresis (QIE)
    q. immunoglobulin analysis
    q. polymerase chain reaction
    (QPCR)
    q. polymerase chain reaction assay
    q. precipitin reaction

Quanti-Test System
Quantum PSV
Quaranfil virus
quarantine
quarter
    lamb's q.
quarter-evil
quarter-ill
quartz-iodine lamp
quartz lamp
quasicontinuous-wave laser
quaternary
    q. ammonium
    q. syphilis
quaternium-15
quaternium-18 bentonite
queen
    q. palm
    q. palm tree
Queensland tick typhus
quellung
    q. phenomenon
    q. reaction
    q. test
quenching
    fluorescence q.
Quest
    Tranquility Q.
questionnaire
    Childhood Health Assessment Q.
    (CHAQ)
    Clinical Health Assessment Q.
    (CLINHAQ)
    EQ-5D EuroQol q.
    Fibromyalgia Impact Q. (FIQ)
    Health Assessment Q. (HAQ)
    Modified Health Assessment Q.
    (MHAQ)
    revised Skindex q.
    rhinoconjunctivitis-specific quality of
    life q. (RQLQ)
    Skindex q.
    Stanford Health Assessment Q.
    (HAQ)
QUEST study
Queyrat
    erythroplasia of Q.
Quibron-T, -T/SR
Quickscreen assay
QuickVue One-Step Allergen Screen
Quiess
quinacrine
Quincke
    Q. disease

Quincke *(continued)*
    Q. edema
    Q. I syndrome
quinidine
quinine
    q. fever
    q. sulfate
quinolizidine
quinolones
Quinquaud disease

Quinsana Plus topical
quintana
    Bartonella q.
    Rochalimaea q.
quinti
    adductor digiti q.
quinupristin/dalfopristin
Quotidian fever
QUS-2 calcaneal ultrasonometer
QVAR

R

R antigen
R&C Shampoo
R factor
R gene
R pilus
R plasmid
r24 antibody
RA
rheumatoid arthritis
rhinocerebral aspergillosis
RA synoviocyte line
rabbit
r. antithymocyte globulin (RATG)
r. antithymocyte globulin polyclonal antibody
r. bush
r. epithelium
r. fibroma
fibromatosis virus of r.
r. fibroma virus
r. myxoma virus
r. plague
virus III of r.
rabbitpox
r. virus
rabid
rabies
r. immune globulin, human
r. immunoglobulin
r. vaccine, Flury strain egg-passage
r. virus
r. virus, Flury strain
r. virus, Kelev strain
r. virus vaccine
Rabson-Mendenhall syndrome
raccoon eyes
racemosa
livedo r.
racemosus
Mucor r.
Racet Topical
racial melanoderma
racket nail
RAD 001
radial
r. immunodiffusion (RID)
r. nerve
r. scar
radiation
r. burn
cold quartz r.
r. dermatitis
r. dermatosis
dopa r.

electromagnetic r.
r. erythema
foreign body r.
ionizing r.
Jones-Mote r.
Mitsuda r.
r. pneumonitis
r. spectrum
r. therapy
ultraviolet r.
wheal and erythema r.
radical
free r.
r. mastectomy
oxygen free r.
radicans
Rhus r.
Toxicodendron r.
radiciform
radicular nerve root
radiculitis
radiculoganglionitis
radiculopathy
radioactive probe
radioallergosorbent test (RAST)
radioassay
C1qR r.
radiobacter
Agrobacterium r.
radiocarpal joint
radiocontrast
radiodermatitis
acute r.
chronic r.
r. emulsion (RE)
radiodurans
Deinococcus r.
radioepidermitis
radioepithelitis
radiograph
posteroanterior r.
radiographic
r. contrast media (RCM)
r. erosion
radioimmunoassay (RIA)
Raji cell r.
radioimmunodiffusion
radioimmunoelectrophoresis
radioimmunoprecipitation assay (RIPA)
radioimmunosorbent test (RIST)
radiolabeled iodine
radioligand assay
radiologic osteoarthritis (ROA)
radiolunate
radiometric resin system

R

radiometry
> BACTEC r.

radionuclide ventriculography
radioreceptor assay
radiosensitivity
radiotherapy (RT)
> eosinophilic, polymorphic, and pruritic eruption associated with r.

radium necrosis
RADS
> reactive airways dysfunction syndrome

RAEB
> refractory anemia with excess blasts

RAEB-t
> refractory anemia with excess blasts in transformation

Raf/mitogen-activated protein kinase signaling pathway
Ragnell scissors
RAG1, RAG2 gene
ragweed (RW)
> canyon r.
> desert r.
> false r.
> giant r.
> r. oil dermatitis
> slender r.
> Western r.

ragwort
rail
> Railguard bed r.

Railguard bed rail
railroad tracking
Rainbow vacuum
rain splash
raised border
raisin
Raji
> R. cell
> R. cell radioimmune assay
> R. cell radioimmunoassay

Rajka and Langeland scoring system
rake
rale
> coarse r.

raloxifene
Raman shifting
Ramelet phlebectomy hook
Ramirez
> ashy dermatosis of R.

Ramos B-cell line
Ramsay Hunt syndrome
ram's horn nail
Ranawat triangle method
random breeding
range
> interquartile r. (IQR)

Ranikhet disease
ranitidine hydrochloride
RANKL
> receptor activator of nuclear factor kappa B ligand

RANTES
> regulated upon activation, normal T-cell expressed and secreted

ranula
RAP
> rheumatoid arthritis precipitin

Rapamune
rapamycin
Raper-Mason pathway
rapid
> r. canities
> r. cooling
> r. eye movement (REM)
> r. eye movement sleep
> r. eye movement sleep-related hypoxemia
> r. plasma reagin (RPR)
> r. whole blood test (RWBT)

Rapide
> Voltaren R.

rapidly
> r. dividing plasmablasts
> r. progressive necrotizing glomerulonephritis (RPGN)

Rappaport classification
Rapp-Hodgkin ectodermal dysplasia
raquette
> ongles en r.

rare
> r. mycosis
> r. system reaction

rarefaction
> mottled r.

rash
> ammonia r.
> antitoxin r.
> astacoid r.
> atopic dermatitis r.
> black currant r.
> brown-tail r.
> butterfly r.
> cable r.
> caterpillar r.
> crystal r.
> diaper r.
> drug r.
> ecchymotic r.
> generalized maculopapular r.
> gum r.
> heat r.
> heliotrope r.
> hemorrhagic r.
> hydatid r.

R

juvenile rheumatoid arthritis r.
lupus erythematous-like r.
macular r.
maculopapular r.
malar butterfly r.
mulberry r.
Murray Valley r.
napkin r.
nettle r.
papulovesicular r.
photosensitive r.
polymorphous r.
red r.
rose r.
serum r.
skin r.
slapped-cheek r.
summer r.
sunburn-like r.
tooth r.
violaceous shawl pattern r.
violaceous V neck pattern r.
wandering r.
wildfire r.

ras-mitogen-activated protein
raspberry
r. lesion
r. nevus
r. tongue

ras protein
RAST
radioallergosorbent test
Phadezym RAST

rat
r. flea bite
r. mite dermatitis
r. serum protein (RSP)
r. urine protein (RUP)
Wistar r.

rat-bite fever
rate
erythrocyte sedimentation r. (ESR)
glomerular filtration r. (GFR)
graft survival r.
low absolute glomerular filtration r.
low flow r.
moisture vapor transmission r.
 (MVTR)
peak expiratory flow r.
pulse r.
respiratory r.

Westergren sedimentation r.
zeta sedimentation r.

RATG
rabbit antithymocyte globulin
RATG polyclonal antibody

ratio
carpal to metacarpal r.
CD4/CD8 r.
dead space:tidal volume r.
graft-to-recipient weight r. (GRWR)
helper-suppressor cell r.
inspiratory to expiratory r. (I:E)
International Normalization R.
 (INR)
Mantel-Haenszel weighted odds r.
proportionate morbidity r. (PMR)
residual volume to total lung
 capacity r. (RV/TLC)
risk r. (RR)
standardized incidence r. (SIR)
Standard Morbidity R. (SMR)
therapeutic r.
ventilation/perfusion r.
zinc protoporphyrin:heme r.

rattlesnake bite
Rauscher leukemia virus
rauwolfia drug
RAV
Rous-associated virus

ray
grenz r.

Rayer disease
Rayleigh scattering
Raynaud
R. disease
R. phenomenon
R. syndrome

RBC
red blood cell
RBC surface

Rb protein
RCA
reactive cutaneous
angioendotheliomatosis

rCD4
CD4, human recombinant soluble r.

RCE
renal cholesterol embolization

RCM
radiographic contrast media

RCR
replication-competent retrovirus

NOTES

RCR *(continued)*
    RCR assay
    RCR testing
RD
    rhabdomyosarcoma
        human RD
RDEB
    recessive dystrophic epidermolysis
      bullosa
RDS
    respiratory distress syndrome
rDsg
    recombinant desmoglein
RE
    radiodermatitis emulsion
        Biafine RE
ReA
    reactive arthritis
reacher
    long-handled dressing r.
reactant
    acute phase r. (APR)
Reactine
reaction
    absent r.
    accelerated r.
    acute anaphylactic r.
    acute phase r.
    acute pulmonary r.
    acute transfusion r.
    adverse drug r.
    adverse drug-induced r. (ADR)
    allergic r.
    anamnestic r.
    anaphylactic hypersensitivity r.
    anaphylactoid r.
    angry back r.
    antigen-antibody r.
    Arthus r.
    Arthus-type r.
    Ascoli r.
    associative r.
    autoimmune type of r.
    autologous mixed leukocyte r.
    Bloch r.
    bullous drug r.
    capsular precipitation r.
    Casoni r.
    cell-mediated immunologic drug r.
    Chantemesse r.
    cholera-red r.
    cocarde r.
    complement-fixation r.
    constitutional r.
    cross r.
    cutaneous graft-versus-host r.
    cytotoxic immunologic drug r.
    Dale r.

    delayed hypersensitivity
      immunologic drug r.
    delayed systemic r.
    delayed transfusion r.
    demarcated r.
    depot r.
    dermatophytid r.
    dermotuberculin r.
    Dick r.
    diffuse histiocytic r.
    dopa r.
    drug r.
    early r.
    early-phase r. (EPR)
    eczematous r.
    endotoxic r.
    epicutaneous r.
    false-negative r.
    false-positive r.
    Fernandez r.
    fixation r.
    fixed drug r.
    flocculation r.
    focal r.
    foreign-body r.
    Forssman antigen-antibody r.
    Frei-Hoffmann r.
    fungal id r.
    gel diffusion r.
    Gell and Coombs r.
    Gerhardt r.
    graft-versus-host r.
    granulomatous inflammatory r.
    group r.
    Gruber r.
    Gruber-Widal r.
    Haber-Weiss r.
    Hapten-type r.
    hematologic r.
    Herxheimer r.
    homocytotropic r.
    homograft r.
    hunting r.
    hypersensitivity r.
    hysterical r.
    id r.
    idiosyncratic drug r.
    IgE-dependent immunologic drug r.
    immediate hypersensitivity r.
    immediate phase r. (IPR)
    immediate transfusion r.
    immediate wheal r.
    immune complex immunologic
      drug r.
    immune complex-mediated drug r.
    immunologic drug r.
    incompatible blood transfusion r.
    inflammation r.

R

insulin r.
intracutaneous r.
intradermal r.
irritant patch-test r.
Janus r.
Jarisch-Herxheimer r.
Jones-Mote r.
Koebner r.
late-phase r. (LPR)
late-phase allergic r.
late-phase cutaneous r. (LPCR)
latex fixation r.
lepromatous r.
lepromin r.
ligase chain r.
local r.
Loewenthal r.
marked localized r.
Mazzotti r.
miostagmin r.
miscellaneous r.
Mitsuda r.
mixed agglutination r.
mixed lymphocyte culture r.
Montenegro r.
negative r.
Neufeld r.
neutrophil antibody and
  transfusion r.
nitritoid r.
nonanaphylactic r. (NAR)
nondrug-related r.
r. of nonidentity
nonimmediate-type immunologic
  drug r.
nonimmunologic drug r.
r. of partial identity
passive cutaneous anaphylactic r.
Paul r.
persistent light r.
photoallergic drug r.
photobiologic r.
photochemical r.
photodrug r.
photosensitivity r.
phototoxic drug r.
Pirquet r.
P-K r.
polymerase chain r. (PCR, PRC)
positive r.
Prausnitz-Kustner r.
precipitin r.

primary irritant r.
prozone r.
pseudoallergic r.
psychogenic r.
pustular patch-test r.
quantitative polymerase chain r.
  (QPCR)
quantitative precipitin r.
quellung r.
rare system r.
reversed Prausnitz-Küstner r.
reverse transcriptase-polymerase
  chain r. (RT-PCR)
reverse transcription polymerase
  chain r. (RT-PCR)
ribonucleic acid-polymerase chain r.
  (RNA-PCR)
Roger r.
Schultz-Charlton r.
Schultz-Dale r.
self-limited allergic r.
serum r.
severe acute allergic r.
severe immediate r.
severe systemic r.
Shwartzman r.
skin r.
specific r.
suprasternal r.
symptomatic r.
systemic r.
thiuram-alcohol r.
toxic systemic r.
transfusion r.
Treponema pallidum
  immobilization r.
two-stage r.
type I–III hypersensitivity r.
type III immune complex drug r.
type I–IV immunologic drug r.
type IV delayed hypersensitivity r.
vaccinoid r.
vascular r.
vasomotor r.
vasovagal r.
in vivo r.
Wassermann r. (W.r.)
Weil-Felix r.
Weinberg r.
well-demarcated skin r.
wheal-and-erythema r.
wheal-and-flare r.

NOTES

reaction *(continued)*
 whitegraft r.
 Widal r.
 zonal type r.
reactional leprosy
reactiva
 meningitis necrotoxica r.
reactivate
reactivation
 sunburn r.
reactive
 r. airways disease
 r. airways dysfunction syndrome
 (RADS)
 r. arthritis (ReA)
 r. cutaneous angioendotheliomatosis
 (RCA)
 r. lysis
 r. oxygen intermediate (ROI)
 r. oxygen species (ROS)
 r. perforating collagenosis (RPC)
 r. postinfectious synovitis
 r. salpingitis
reactivity
 airway r.
 antihost r.
 immediate skin r.
 persistent light r. (PLR)
 specific alteration in
 immunologic r.
reactor
 persistent light r.
reading
 delayed patch test r.
reading-frame-shift mutation
reagent
 Melzer r.
 TriZol r.
reagin
 atopic r.
 rapid plasma r. (RPR)
 r. screen test (RST)
 unheated serum r. (USR)
reaginic
 r. antibody
 r. hypersensitivity
REAL
 Revised European-American
 Classification of Lymphoid Neoplasms
 Revised European-American Lymphoma
 REAL classification
Rea-Lo
rearrangement
 immunoglobulin gene r.
Reatine
Rebetron
rebound dermatitis

Rebuck
 R. skin window
 R. skin window technique
recalcitrant wart
recall
 Dermatology Education by R.
 (DERM)
 ultraviolet r.
 r. urticaria (RU)
recapitulation of ontogenesis process
Receptin
receptor
 r. activator of nuclear factor kappa
 B ligand (RANKL)
 antigenic binding r.
 antimuscarinic acetylcholine r.
 B-cell antigen r.
 bone morphogenetic protein r.
 brush border r.
 C3b r.
 C4b r.
 C5b-9 r.
 C3bBb r.
 C3/C4 r.
 C3dg r.
 CD44 Hyaluronic acid r.
 CD26/vitronectin r.
 complement r. 1–4 (CR (1–4))
 costimulatory r.
 C1q r.
 Fc r.
 Fc gamma r. III
 fibronectin r.
 G-protein-coupled r.
 homing r.
 IL-1 r.
 r. interacting protein (RIP)
 killer cell inhibitory r. (KIR)
 lymphocyte homing r.
 natural cytotoxicity r.
 nicotinic acetylcholine r.
 opsonic r.
 phosphatidyl serine r.
 protease-activated r. (PAR)
 r. site
 soluble r.
 surface r.
 T-cell r. (TCR)
 T-cell antigen r.
 thyroid-stimulating hormone r.
 (TSH-R)
 Toll r.
 transmembrane r.
 TSH r. (TSH-R)
 tumor necrosis factor r.
receptor-gamma
 peroxisome proliferator-activated r.-
 g. (PPAR-gamma)

receptor-ligand interaction
recessive
> autosomal r.
> r. dystrophic epidermolysis bullosa (RDEB)
> r. trait
> r. X-linked ichthyosis

recidivans
> leishmaniasis r.
> r. leishmaniasis (RL)

recidive
> chancre r.

recipient
> crossmatch-positive r.
> elective low-risk r.
> high-risk r. (HRR)
> renal transplant r. (RTR)
> single-lung transplant r.
> SLT r.

recipient-donor pairs
reciprocal transfusion
recirculation
> lymphocyte r.

Recklinghausen
> R. disease
> R. disease type I

reclusa
> *Loxosceles* r.

Reclus disease
recognition
> cognate r.
> r. factor

recoil
> elastic r.

recombinant
> r. allergen
> r. desmoglein (rDsg)
> r. gamma interferon
> r. human interleukin-1 receptor antagonist
> r. human relaxin
> r. human tissue factor pathway inhibitor (r-hT-FPI)
> r. immunoblot assay (RIBA)
> r. LFA-3/IgG1 human fusion protein
> r. strain
> r. vector

recombinase-activating gene
recombination
> genetic r.
> high frequency of r.

recombinational activity
recombinatorial
Recombivax HB
recommended exposure level (REL)
reconstitution
> hematopoietic r.
> multilineage r.

reconstruction
> lymphatic r. (LR)

recorder
> sensory nerve action potential sleep r.
> SNAP sleep r.

recovery
> short tau inversion r. (STIR)

recrudescent
> r. typhus
> r. typhus fever

recruitment
> host-generated neutrophils r.

rectal
> r. gonorrhea
> Phenergan R.
> Rowasa R.
> r. ulceration

rectus abdominis syndrome
recurrens
> herpes simplex r.
> periadenitis mucosa necrotica r.

recurrent
> r. aspiration
> r. bacterial pneumonia
> r. cutaneous abscess
> r. erythema multiforme minor
> r. genital herpes simplex virus
> r. infection
> r. infundibulofolliculitis
> r. intraoral herpes simplex virus
> r. labial herpes simplex virus
> r. palmoplantar hidradenitis
> r. polyserositis
> r. respiratory laryngeal papillomatosis
> r. ulcer
> r. urticaria
> r. viral pneumonia

recurrentis
> *Borrelia* r.

red
> r. albinism
> r. alder
> r. alder tree

NOTES

red *(continued)*
    r. balls
    basic r. 46
    r. birch
    r. blood cell (RBC)
    r. blood cell surface
    r. bug bite
    r. cedar
    r. cedar tree
    r. cell adherence phenomenon
    r. cell adherence test
    r. cell antigen
    r. cell membrane alteration
    r. eye
    r. feed dermatitis
    r. granulation
    r. half-moon
    r. halo
    r. imported fire ant
    r. imported fire ant sting
    r. lunula
    r. man syndrome
    r. maple
    r. maple tree
    r. moss dermatitis
    r. mulberry
    r. mulberry tree
    r. neuralgia
    r. papule
    r. papule and nodule
    r. rash
    r. sponge dermatitis
    r. sweat
    r. tide dermatitis
    r. top
    r. top grass pollen
    r. veterinary petrolatum (RVP)
reddening
    r. of oropharyngeal mucosa
    r. of palm
    r. of soles of feet
RediTabs
    Claritin R.'s
"red man" syndrome
redox stress
red-purple plaque
redroot pigweed
redtop A grass
reduced
    r. cold ischemic time
    r. joint survey (RJS)
    r. liver transplant (RLT)
reduced-size
    r.-s. liver transplant (RSLT)
    r.-s. liver transplantation (RSLT)
reducing substance

reductase
    5 alpha r.
    thioredoxin r. (TR)
reduction
    leukotriene r.
    Palomar E2000 ruby laser hair r.
Redutemp
Reduviidae
redux
    chancre r.
    pseudochancre r.
redwood tree
reed
    r. canary
    common r.
Reed-Sternberg cell
reedy nail
reenameling
Reenstierna antiserum
reepithelialization
Reese
    R. dermatome
    R. Pinworm Medicine
Refinity
    R. Coblation system
    R. skin care solution
    R. skin product
reflectance-guidance laser selection
reflectance photometry
reflex
    r. cough
    nasobronchial r.
    pilomotor r.
    stretch r.
    submersion r.
    r. sympathetic dystrophy (RSD)
    r. sympathetic dystrophy syndrome
reflux
    gastroesophageal r. (GER)
refractoriness
    exercise-induced r.
refractory
    r. anemia with excess blasts (RAEB)
    r. anemia with excess blasts in transformation (RAEB-t)
    r. period
Refresh Plus Ophthalmic solution
Refsum
    R. disease
    R. syndrome
regimen
    Goeckerman r.
    immunomodulating drug r.
    nonmyeloablative conditioning r.
    steroid-sparing r.

regimen/therapy
>psoralen ultraviolet A r.
>PUVA r.

region
>complementarity-determining r.
>(CDR)
>constant r.
>hinge r.
>hypervariable r.
>I r.
>intertriginous r.
>paratracheal r.
>ringworm of genitocrural r.
>switch r.
>upstream regulatory r. (URR)
>variable r.

regional
>r. granulomatous lymphadenitis
>r. organ procurement (ROP)
>R. Organ Procurement Agency
>(ROPA)

Register
>Norfolk Arthritis R. (NOAR)

Registry
>Cord Blood R.
>International Pancreas Transplant R.
>(IPTR)
>R. of the International Society for
>Heart and Lung Transplantation

Regranex

regressing atypical histiocytosis

regression
>Cox r.
>multivariate logistic r.
>spontaneous r.

regular
>r. Aveeno
>Esoterica R.
>Iodex R.

regulated upon activation, normal T-cell expressed and secreted (RANTES)

regulation
>leukotriene r.
>tolerance through r.

regulator
>cystic fibrosis-transmembrane
>conductance r. (CFTR)
>lysosome trafficking r. (LYST)

regulatory CD4+ T cell

regulon
>BvgAS r.

reinfection
>graft r.
>r. tuberculosis

reinoculation

Reiter
>R. disease
>R. syndrome
>R. test

rejection
>accelerated r.
>acute cellular xenograft r.
>acute humoral r. (AHR)
>acute vascular xenograft r. (AVXR)
>allograft r.
>cardiac r.
>r. cascade
>cellular xenograft r.
>chronic allograft r.
>delayed xenograft r. (DXR)
>ductopenic r.
>first-set r.
>graft r.
>hyperacute organ r.
>islet allograft r.
>primary r.
>second set r.
>steroid-resistant acute r.
>xenograft r.

REL
>recommended exposure level

Relafen

relapsing
>r. febrile nodular nonsuppurative
>panniculitis
>r. fever
>r. polychondritis

relapsing-remitting
>r.-r. multiple sclerosis (RRMS)
>r.-r. profile

related transplant

relation
>opposition-versus-pressure r.

relationship
>temporal r.

relative
>r. immunity
>immunochemical r.
>r. risk

relaxation
>smooth muscle r.

Relaxed Skin Tension Line (RSTL)

NOTES

relaxin
> recombinant human r.

relaxometry

release
> allergen-induced mediator r.
> delayed anagen r.
> delayed telogen r.
> immediate antigen r.
> immediate telogen r.
> leukocyte histamine r.
> myoglobin r.
> sustained r.

releaser
> direct histamine r.

releasing factor (RF)

relevant sting history

Reliable Change Index

Relief
> Allergy R.
> DayQuil Sinus with Pain R.
> Mini Thin Asthma R.
> Nasal & Sinus R.
> R. Ophthalmic solution
> Vicks DayQuil Sinus Pressure & Congestion R.

Reliever
> Arthritis Foundation Pain R.

Relpal algorithm

REM
> rapid eye movement
> reticular erythematous mucinosis
> REM sleep
> REM sleep-related hypoxemia
> REM syndrome

Remak sign

Remedy
> Scholl 2-Drop Corn R.

Remicade

remission
> brief metabolic r.
> metabolic r.
> pathologically confirmed complete r. (PCR)

remitting
> r. necrotizing acrocyanosis
> r. seronegative symmetrical synovitis
> r. seronegative symmetric synovitis with pitting edema (RS3PE)

remnant
> cervicothymic r.

remodeling
> extracellular matrix r.
> tissue r.

removal
> excisional r.
> Lasertrolysis hair r.

LightSheer diode laser system for permanent hair r.

remover
> Histofreezer cryosurgical wart r.
> Mosco callus and corn r.
> Scholl Wart R.
> Wart R.

renal
> r. biopsy
> r. cholesterol embolization (RCE)
> r. cyst
> r. failure
> r. involvement
> r. transplant
> r. transplant recipient (RTR)

Rendu-Osler-Weber
> R.-O.-W. disease
> R.-O.-W. syndrome

Renova cream

REO
> respiratory enteric orphan
> REO virus

ReoPro monoclonal antibody

Reoviridae

Reovirus

Reovirus-like agent

REP
> Rochester Epidemiology Project

repair
> abnormal DNA r.
> DNA r.
> Lich-Gregoire r.
> staged abdominal r. (STAR)
> tissue r.

repeat
> r. open-application testing (ROAT)
> r. open reaction application test
> short consensus r.'s
> tetratricopeptide r.
> variable numbers of tandem r.'s (VNTR)

repeated
> r. exposure
> r. respiratory infection

repellent
> Cutter insect r.
> dimethyl carbate butopyropoxyl insect r.
> dimethyl phthalate insect r.
> UltraThon insect r.

repens
> dermatitis r.
> erythema gyratum r.

reperfusion
> hepatic ischemia and r. (HIR)
> r. injury

Repetabs
>Proventil R.

repetitive PCR (Rep-PCR)

Repifermin

repigmentation

replacement
>enzyme r.
>r. therapy

replica

RepliCare
>R. hydrocolloid
>R. hydrocolloid dressing

replicase

replicate

replication

replication-competent
>r.-c. retrovirus (RCR)
>r.-c. retrovirus assay

replicative
>r. form (RF)
>r. senescence

replicator

repository therapy

Rep-PCR
>repetitive PCR

Re-PUVA
>combination retinoid and PUVA therapy

requirement
>immunization r.

RES
>reticuloendothelial system

Rescriptor

rescue
>peripheral blood stem cell r.

Resectisol Irrigation solution

reserve
>bone marrow r.
>breathing r. (BR)
>coronary flow r. (CFR)
>heart rate r. (HRR)

reservoir
>r. host
>r. of infection
>Ommaya r.
>Pecquet r.

ResiDerm

residual
>r. thermal damage (RTD)
>r. volume
>r. volume to total lung capacity ratio (RV/TLC)

residue
>aliphatic r.
>posttranslationally modified arginine r.
>Pro r.

resin
>epoxy r.
>ethyleneurea melamine formaldehyde r.
>formaldehyde r.
>pine r.
>podophyllum r.
>thermosetting r.

resin-colophony
>pine r.-c.

resistance
>airway r.
>bacteriophage r.
>r. factor
>insulin r.
>r. plasmid
>pulmonary vascular r. (PVR)

resistance-inducing factor

resistance-transfer factor

resistance-transferring episome

resistant bacterium

resistentiae
>locus minoris r.

Resorcin

resorcinol

resorption
>Weichselbaum lacunar r.

resorptive arthropathy

Respaire-120 SR

Respaire-60 SR

Respa-1st

Respbid

RespiGam

Respihaler
>Decadron Phosphate R.

Respinol-G

respiration
>Cheyne-Stokes r.

respirator
>BABYbird r.

respiratory
>r. acidosis
>r. burst
>r. change
>r. distress
>r. distress syndrome (RDS)
>r. enteric orphan (REO)

NOTES

respiratory *(continued)*
  r. enteric orphan virus
  r. failure
  r. rate
  r. syncytial virus (RSV)
  r. syncytial virus immune globulin intravenous (RSV-IGIV)
  r. syncytial virus IV immune globulin
Respirgard II nebulizer
Respitrace machine
responder T cell
response
  anamnestic r.
  antigen-specific immune r.
  autoimmune r.
  biphasic r.
  booster r.
  bronchoconstrictor r.
  cholinergic r.
  delayed-type hypersensitivity r.
  early-phase r.
  endogenous immune r.
  exaggerated bronchoconstrictor r.
  graft-versus-host r. (GVHR)
  histiocytic r.
  host r.
  humoral immune r.
  IgE-mediated r.
  immune r. (Ir)
  immunologic r.
  irritant patch-test r.
  isomeric r.
  isomorphic r.
  late-phase r.
  Lewis triple r.
  nephropathic immune r.
  peak-plateau r.
  primary immune r.
  proinflammatory cytokine r.
  secondary immune r.
  seroconversion r.
  somatosensory evoked r.
  sympathoneural r.
  T-dependent r.
  Th-1 mediated immune r.
  T-independent r.
  transferred immune r.
  triple r.
  in vitro proliferative lymphocyte r.
  white line r.
  xenogeneic cellular immune r.
responsiveness
  airway r.
rest
  r. hypoxemia
  r., ice, compresses, elevation (RICE)

restaurant syndrome
resting
  r. nevus
  r. phase
  r. splint
restitope
Reston
  R. foam
  R. foam wound dressing
  R. hydrocolloid dressing
  R. subtype
restorative sleep
Restore
  R. alginate dressing
  R. alginate wound cover
  R. hydrocolloid
  R. hydrocolloid dressing
  R. hydrogel dressing
  R. impregnated gauze
  R. wound cleanser
restriction
  r. fragment length
  r. fragment length polymorphism (RFLP)
  major histocompatibility complex r.
  MHC r.
restrictive
  r. cardiomyopathy
  r. dermopathy
  r. functional impairment
  r. lung disease
  r. ventilatory pattern
restrictus
  Aspergillus r.
resurfacing
  cosmetic skin r. (CSR)
  laser skin r. (LSR)
  Skinlight erbium:YAG laser system for skin r.
resuscitation
  cardiopulmonary r.
retardation
  growth r.
rete
  r. peg
  r. ridge
  r. ridge hyperplasia
retention
  bromsulfophthalein r.
  r. cyst
  r. triad
reticular
  r. degeneration
  r. dermis
  r. dysgenesis
  r. erythematous mucinosis (REM)
  r. erythematous mucinosis syndrome

r. lesion
r. pattern
reticularis
acropigmentatio r.
angiitis livedo r.
dermatopathia pigmentosa r.
idiopathic livedo r.
livedo r.
pars r.
zona r.
reticulata
folliculitis ulerythema r.
folliculitis ulerythematosa r.
reticulate
r. array
r. body
r. hyperpigmentation
r. hypopigmentation
r. pigmented anomaly
reticulated
r. black solar lentigo
r. papillomatosis
r. pigmented poikiloderma
reticulatum
atrophoderma r.
reticule
reticulin fiber
reticulocyte count
reticuloendothelial
r. blockade
r. cell
r. hyperplasia
r. system (RES)
reticuloendothelioma
reticuloendotheliosis
avian r.
familial r.
leukemic r.
reticuloendothelium
reticulogranuloma
reticulohistiocytic granuloma
reticulohistiocytoma
reticulohistiocytosis
congenital self-healing r.
r. disease
multicentric r. (MR)
self-healing r.
reticuloid
actinic r.
reticulosis
benign inoculation r.
disseminated pagetoid r.

epidermotropic r.
histiocytic medullary r.
lipomelanic r.
localized pagetoid r.
medullary r.
pagetoid r.
polymorphic r.
Sézary r.
reticulum
r. cell carcinoma
endoplasmic r.
r. fiber
reticulum-cell sarcoma
retiform
r. erythema
r. hemangioendothelioma
parapsoriasis r.
r. parapsoriasis
Retin-A
R.-A. Micro
R.-A. Micro Topical
retina
retinacula of ankle
retinal
r. examination
r. exudate
r. hemorrhage
r. perivasculitis
r. pigment epithelial cell (RPE)
r. thrombophlebitis
retinitis
cytomegalovirus r.
varicella-zoster virus r.
VZV r.
retinoblastoma tumor suppressor protein
retinochoroidopathy
birdshot r.
retinoic acid
retinoid
gold r.
r. therapy
Retinol-A
retinyl acetate-induced arthritis
retractor
Desmarres r.
Langenbeck r.
Parker r.
Roux r.
Upper Hands self-retaining r.
retransplantation (Re-Tx)
retroelement
retroperitoneal fibrosis

NOTES

R

retropharyngeal
Retrovir
    R. injection
    R. Oral
retroviral vector
Retroviridae
retrovirus
    r. group
    lymphotropic r.
    MFG-IRAP r.
    porcine endogenous r. (PERV)
    replication-competent r. (RCR)
retrovirus-associated lymphoma
Re-Tx
    retransplantation
Reu curette
Rev
revaccination
reverse
    r. cutting needle
    r. endocytosis
    r. passive hemagglutination
    r. tetracycline transactivator
    r. transcriptase
    r. transcriptase-polymerase chain reaction (RT-PCR)
    r. transcription polymerase chain reaction (RT-PCR)
reversed
    r. passive anaphylaxis
    r. passive latex agglutination
    r. Prausnitz-Küstner reaction
reversible posterior leukoencephalopathy (RPLS)
reversion
Reversionex
revertant
Revised
    R. European-American Classification of Lymphoid Neoplasms (REAL)
    R. European-American Lymphoma (REAL)
    R. European-American Lymphoma classification
revised Skindex questionnaire
Rev-responsive element (RRE)
revulsion
Reye syndrome
Rezine
RF
    releasing factor
    replicative form
    rheumatoid factor
    IgG RF
        immunoglobulin G rheumatoid factor
    IgM RF
        immunoglobulin M rheumatoid factor
    RF test
RFLA
    rheumatoid factor-like activity
RFLP
    restriction fragment length polymorphism
RFXAP
    RFX-associated protein
RFX-associated protein (RFXAP)
R-Gel
RH
    rheumatoid
Rh
    rhesus
    Rh antigen
    Rh blocking test
    Rh factor
    Rh immune globulin intravenous (RhIGIV)
    Rh isoantigen
rhabditic dermatitis
rhabdomyolysis syndrome
rhabdomyoma
rhabdomyosarcoma (RD)
    human r.
Rhabdoviridae
rhabdovirus
rhacoma
rhagades
rhagadiform
rhagas
$RH_o(D)$
    R. globulin
    R. immunoglobulin
rheometer
    Haake r.
rheophoresis
rheostat
    ceramide-S1P r.
rhesus (Rh)
    r. factor
    r. rotavirus (RRV)
    r. theta defensin 1 (RTD-1)
rheum
    salt r.
Rheumatex
    R. test
    R. test for rheumatoid factor
rheumatic
    r. erythema
    r. fever
    r. perimyocarditis
rheumatica
    polymyalgia r. (PMR)
    purpura r.
    scarlatina r.

rheumaticum
  erythema annulare r.
rheumatism
  European League Against R.
    (EULAR)
  palindromic r.
  pied rond r.
  Poncet r.
  tuberculous r.
rheumatocelis
rheumatoid (RH)
  r. arthritis (RA)
  r. arthritis precipitin (RAP)
  r. arthritis vaccine
  r. atlantoaxial subluxation
  r. cachexia
  r. clawing
  r. disease
  r. episcleritis
  r. factor (RF)
  r. factor-like activity (RFLA)
  r. factor test
  r. factor titer
  r. nodule
  r. nodulosis
  r. pachymeningitis
  r. pannus
  r. pattern
  r. pleurisy
  r. rheumatic vasculitis
  r. scleritis
  r. synovial fibroblast
  r. synovial macrophage-like/dendritic
    cell
rheumatologist
rheumatology
  American College of R. (ACR)
  World Health
    Organization/International League
    of Associations for R.
    (WHO/ILAR)
Rheumaton
  R. test
  R. test for rheumatoid factor
Rheumatrex
RhIGIV
  Rh immune globulin intravenous
Rhinalar
Rhinaris-F
rhinitis
  acute r.
  allergic r.

endocrine r.
foreign body r.
granulomatosis r.
gustatory r.
infectious r.
r. medicamentosa
r. nervosa
perennial allergic r.
pollen-induced allergic r.
seasonal allergic r. (SAR)
vasomotor r. (VMR)
rhinobronchitis
  allergic r.
rhinocerebral
  r. aspergillosis (RA)
  r. infection
Rhinocladiella aquaspera
rhinoconjunctivitis
  allergic r.
  Parietaria-induced r.
**rhinoconjunctivitis-specific quality of life
  questionnaire (RQLQ)**
Rhinocort
rhinomanometry
rhinometry
  acoustic r. (AR)
rhinophyma
rhinopneumonitis
  equine r.
rhinoprobe
rhinorrhea
  cerebrospinal r.
rhinoscleroma
rhinoscleromatis
  Klebsiella r.
rhinoscopy
rhinosinusitis
rhinosporidiosis
Rhinosporidium seeberi
Rhinosyn Liquid
Rhinosyn-PD Liquid
rhinotracheitis
  feline viral r.
  infectious bovine r. (IBR)
Rhinovirus
rhinovirus
  bovine r.'s
  r. challenge test
  equine r.'s
Rhizopus
  R. arrhizus

R

NOTES

Rhizopus *(continued)*
    R. nigricans
    R. oryzae
Rhodacine
rhodamine isothiocyanate
Rhodis
Rhodis-EC
Rhodnius prolixus
Rhodococcus
    R. equi
    R. erythropolis
rhodopsin-type coupling
Rhodotorula rubra
Rhodurea
rhoGDI protein
Rholosone
rhombic flap
rhomboencephalitis
rhomboid
    r. glossitis
    r. swelling
rhonchus, pl. rhonchi
rhopheocytosis
Rhoprolene
Rhoprosone
Rhovail
r-hT-FPI
    recombinant human tissue factor pathway
    inhibitor
rhus
    r. dermatitis
    R. diversiloba
    R. radicans
    R. toxicodendron
    R. toxicodendron antigen
    R. venenata
    R. venenata antigen
    R. vernix
rhusiopathiae
    Erysipelothrix r.
rhyparia
rhysodes
    Acanthamoeba r.
RHYTHM
    Froben-SINUS R.
rhythmical dermatosis
rhytide rhytia / rhytides
rhytidectomy
    cervicofacial r.
rhytidoplasty
RIA
    radioimmunoassay
RIBA
    recombinant immunoblot assay
    HCV by RIBA
    RIBA HCV
    RIBA II antibody testing

Ribas-Torres disease
ribavirin
Ribbing arthritis phenotype
riboflavin deficiency
ribonuclease protection assay (RPA)
ribonucleic
    r. acid (RNA)
    r. acid-polymerase chain reaction
    (RNA-PCR)
ribonucleoprotein (RNP)
    r. antigen
    small nuclear r. (snRNP)
    U3 small nuclear r.
ribonucleotide
    purine r.
ribosomal
ribosome
ribosylated
ribotide
    aminoimidazole carboxamide r.
    (AICAR)
ribovirus
ribozyme
RICE
    rest, ice, compresses, elevation
rice
    r. body
    r. itch
richardsiae
    Phialophora r.
Richner-Hanhart
    R.-H. keratoderma
    R.-H. syndrome
richteria
    Solenopsis saevissima r.
Richter syndrome
ricin
    R. A
    anti-B4 blocked r.
    B4 blocked r.
ricinus
    Ixodes r.
rickets
Rickettsia
    R. akari
    R. australis
    R. conorii
    R. prowazekii
    R. rickettsii
    R. tsutsugamushi
    R. typhi
rickettsia
    r. vaccine, attenuated
rickettsial infection
rickettsialpox
rickettsii
    Rickettsia r.

rickettsiosis
    Eastern tick-borne r.
rickettsiostatic
Ricobid
Ricord chancre
RID
    radial immunodiffusion
    RID Mousse
    RID Shampoo
Ridaura
Rida virus
Ridenol
ridge
    broad-based rete r.
    interpapillary r.
    rete r.
ridged wart
Ridley classification
RIE
    rocket immunoelectrophoresis
Riedel struma
Rieger anomaly
Riehl
    R. melanoderma
    R. melanosis
rifabutin
Rifadin
    R. Injection
    R. Oral
Rifamate
rifampin
    r. and isoniazid
    r., isoniazid, and pyrazinamide
rifampin-isoniazid-streptomycin-
    ethambutol (RISE)
rifampin-isoniazid-streptomycin-
    ethambutol-resistant tuberculosis
rifamycin
rifapentine
Rifater
rifaximin
Rift
    R. Valley fever
    R. Valley fever virus
Right
    Breathe R.
rigid thoracoscope
rigor
Riley-Day syndrome
Riley-Smith syndrome
Rilutek
riluzole

Rimactane Oral
rimantadine hydrochloride
rimexolone
rinderpest virus
ring
    Kayser-Fleischer r.
    r. precipitin test
    purine r.
    r. shadow
    r. ulcer
    Walsh pressure r.
    Wessely r.
    Woronoff r.
ringed hair
ringhook method of Feuerstein
ringworm
    r. of axilla
    r. of beard
    black-dot r.
    r. of body
    crusted r.
    r. of the face
    r. of foot
    r. of genitocrural region
    gray-patch r.
    r. of the groin
    r. of the hand
    honeycomb r.
    hypertrophic r.
    r. of nail
    Oriental r.
    r. of the scalp
    scaly r.
    Tokelau r.
    r. yaw
Rinkel serial endpoint titration
Rinkle testing
Rinne test
RinoFlow nasal wash and sinus system
Rinse
    Nix Creme R.
Rio rosewood
RIP
    receptor interacting protein
RIPA
    radioimmunoprecipitation assay
ripe lesion
rippling muscle disease
Risdon incision
RISE
    rifampin-isoniazid-streptomycin-
    ethambutol

NOTES

risedronate
RISE-resistant tuberculosis
risk
  r. ratio (RR)
  relative r.
RIST
  radioimmunosorbent test
Ritchie articular index
ritonavir
  lopinavir and r.
Ritter disease
Rituxan monoclonal antibody
rituximab
Rivasone
river
  r. birch
  r. blindness
RJS
  reduced joint survey
RL
  recidivans leishmaniasis
RLT
  reduced liver transplant
RNA
  ribonucleic acid
    antisense RNA
    RNA glycosidase toxin
    HAV RNA
    HCV RNA
    messenger RNA (mRNA)
    RNA polymerase
    quantitative HCV RNA
    RNA tumor virus
RNA-PCR
  ribonucleic acid-polymerase chain
  reaction
Rnase P
RNeasy mini kit
RNP
  ribonucleoprotein
    RNP antigen
ROA
  radiologic osteoarthritis
road burn
Ro antigen
ROAT
  repeat open-application testing
RoBathol oil
Robaxin
robe
  Hunter r.
Robicillin VK Oral
Robidrine
Robinson disease
Robinul Forte
Robitet Oral
Robitussin-PE
Robitussin Severe Congestion Liqui-Gels

Robles disease
Robomol
robustus
  arthritis r.
Rocaltrol
Rocephin
Rochalimaea
  R. henselae
  R. quintana
Rocha-Lima inclusion
Roche Amplicor CMV DNA assay
Rochester Epidemiology Project (REP)
rocket immunoelectrophoresis (RIE)
Rockwool dermatitis
Rocky
  R. Mountain spotted fever
  R. Mountain spotted fever vaccine
  R. Mountain tick
rod
  Gram-negative r.
  Gram-positive r.
rodent ulcer
rodhaini
  Babesia r.
Rodnan skin thickness score
rodonalgia
Roederer ecchymosis
roentgen alopecia
roentgenogram
roentgen-ray dermatitis
roetheln
RO-Eye drops
RO-Eyewash
RoEzIt skin moisturizer
Rofact
rofecoxib
Roferon-A
Rogaine Topical
Roger
  R. reaction
  R. symptom
Roho mattress
ROI
  reactive oxygen intermediate
Roitter disease
Rokitansky-Aschoff sinus
rolipram
roll
  banana r.
rolled shoulder lesion
Rollet chancre
rolling neutrophil
Romaña sign
Romanus lesion
Romberg
  R. hemiatrophy
  R. sign
  R. syndrome

R

Rombo syndrome
Römer test
Rondec
    R. drops
    R. Filmtab
    R. Syrup
Rondec-TR
Rondo inhaler
ronds
    corps r.
room temperature
root
    nail r.
    orris r.
    radicular nerve r.
ROP
    regional organ procurement
ROPA
    Regional Organ Procurement Agency
rope
    r. burn
    r. sign
RO-Predphate
roquinimex
ROS
    reactive oxygen species
rosacea
    acne r.
    corticosteroid r.
    granulomatous r.
    hypertrophic r.
    keratitis r.
    tuberculoid r.
rosaceaform dermatitis
rosacea-like
    r.-l. tuberculid
    r.-l. tuberculid of Lewandowski
Rosai-Dorfman
    R.-D. disease
    R.-D. syndrome
rose
    r. Bengal staining
    r. cold
    r. fever
    r. rash
    r. spot
    r. water ointment
rosea
    atypical pityriasis r.
    inverse pityriasis r.
    pityriasis r. (PR)
rose-bengal stain

Rosenbach
    R. disease
    erysipeloid of R.
    R. erysipeloid
Rosen papular eruption
Rosenthal-French dosimeter
roseola
    epidemic r.
    idiopathic r.
    r. infantilis
    r. infantum
    syphilitic r.
    r. vaccinia
roseola-like illness
roseolous
rosette
    r.'s of cell
    E r.
    EAC r.
    T-cell r.
    r. test
rosette-forming cell
Rose-Waaler test
rosewood
    Rio r.
rosin
Ross
    R. River fever
    R. River virus
RoSSA/RoSSB antibody test
rostratum
    Exserohilum r.
rosuvastatin
rot
    Barcoo r.
    jungle r.
Rotacaps
    Ventolin R.
Rotahaler inhaler
Rotamune vaccine
RotaShield vaccine
rotating
    r. air impactor
    r. arm impactor
    r. wire brush
rotation
    r. flap
    timed intermittent r.
rotator cuff
rotavirus
    r. gastroenteritis

NOTES

rotavirus *(continued)*
    group C r.
    rhesus r. (RRV)
Rotazyme diagnostic procedure
röteln
Roth-Bernhardt disease
Rothia dentocariosa
Rothmann-Makai syndrome
Rothmund syndrome
Rothmund-Thomson syndrome
Roth spot
Rotorod sampler
rotoslide
rotunda
    pityriasis r.
rouge
    homme r.
    L'Homme r.
rough marsh elder
Roujeau
    DRESS syndrome of Bocquet
      and R.
    drug rash with eosinophil and
      systemic symptoms of Bocquet
      and R.
rouleaux
round
    r. body
    r. facies
    r. fingerpad sign
roundworm
Rous
    R. sarcoma
    R. sarcoma virus (RSV)
    R. sarcoma virus immune globulin
      intravenous (RSV-IGIV)
    R. tumor
Rous-associated virus (RAV)
Roux
    R. retractor
    R. spatula
Roux-en-Y hepaticojejunostomy
Roux-Y loop
Rovighi sign
Rowasa Rectal
Rowe elimination diet for food allergies
Rowell syndrome
roxithromycin
Royl-Derm wound hydrogel dressing
RPA
    ribonuclease protection assay
RPC
    reactive perforating collagenosis
RPD
    Pepcid RPD
RPE
    retinal pigment epithelial cell

RPGN
    rapidly progressive necrotizing
      glomerulonephritis
RPLS
    reversible posterior leukoencephalopathy
RPR
    rapid plasma reagin
      RPR circle card test
RQLQ
    rhinoconjunctivitis-specific quality of life
      questionnaire
RR
    risk ratio
RRE
    Rev-responsive element
RRMS
    relapsing-remitting multiple sclerosis
RRV
    rhesus rotavirus
RSD
    reflex sympathetic dystrophy
      RSD syndrome
RSLT
    reduced-size liver transplant
    reduced-size liver transplantation
RSP
    rat serum protein
RS3PE
    remitting seronegative symmetric
      synovitis with pitting edema
RST
    reagin screen test
RSTL
    Relaxed Skin Tension Line
RSV
    respiratory syncytial virus
    Rous sarcoma virus
RSV-IGIV
    respiratory syncytial virus immune
      globulin intravenous
    Rous sarcoma virus immune globulin
      intravenous
Rs virus
RT
    radiotherapy
RTD
    residual thermal damage
RTD-1
    rhesus theta defensin 1
RT-PCR
    reverse transcriptase-polymerase chain
      reaction
    reverse transcription polymerase chain
      reaction
RTR
    renal transplant recipient
RU
    recall urticaria

rub
    pleural friction r.
    tendon friction r.
    r. test
Rubarth
    R. disease
    R. disease virus
rubber
    r. additive dermatitis
    Brazilian r.
    2-L r. bag
    r. man syndrome
rubedo
rubefacient
rubefaction
rubella
    r. arthritis
    congenital r.
    r. HI test
    r. IgG ELISA test
    r. and mumps vaccines, combined
    r. vaccine virus
    r. virus vaccine, live
rubelliform
rubeola virus
rubeosis
ruber
    lichen r.
ruberous
rubescent
Rubinstein-Taybi syndrome
Rubivirus
rubor
    skin r.
rubra
    keratosis pilaris r.
    miliaria r.
    pityriasis r.
    Rhodotorula r.
    stria r.
    trichomycosis r.
rubricytes
rubrifacient
rubrum
    eczema r.
    tinea r.
    Trichophyton r.
ruby
    r. laser
    r. spot

rudiment
    calcaneal r.
    hair r.
rudimentary
    r. cephalocele
    r. meningocele
    r. supernumerary digit
Rud syndrome
ruffling
    membrane r.
rufous
    r. oculocutaneous albinism
ruga, pl. **rugae**
Rugger-jersey spine
rugosa
    Candida r.
rugose
rugous
rule
    nines r.
    r. of nines
Rumalon
ruminantium
    Cowdria r.
Rumpel-Leede
    R.-L. phenomenon
    R.-L. sign
    R.-L. test
running
    r. intradermal stitch
    r. simple stitch
runt disease
runting syndrome
Runyon classification
RUP
    rat urine protein
rupia escharotica
rupial syphilid
rupioides
    psoriasis r.
rupioid psoriasis
rural cutaneous leishmaniasis
rush immunotherapy
Rush-Presbyterian St. Luke's Heart Failure and Transplant Program
Russell
    R. body
    R. viper venom time
Russian
    R. autumn encephalitis
    R. autumn encephalitis virus
    R. olive

R

NOTES

Russian *(continued)*
    R. olive tree
    R. spring-summer encephalitis
    R. spring-summer encephalitis
      Eastern subtype
    R. spring-summer encephalitis virus
    R. spring-summer encephalitis
      Western subtype
    R. thistle
    R. thistle weed pollen
    R. tick-borne encephalitis
Rust
    R. disease
    R. syndrome
rusting
Ru-Tuss
    R.-T. DE
Ruvalcaba-Myhre-Smith syndrome
Ru-Vert-M
RVP
    red veterinary petrolatum
RVPaba

RVPaque
RV/TLC
    residual volume to total lung capacity
    ratio
RW
    ragweed
RWBT
    rapid whole blood test
RWJ 57504
rye
    R. classification
    r. grass pollen
    r. meal
    perennial r.
    wild r.
Rymed
Rymed-TR
Rynacrom
Ryna Liquid
Rynatan
Rynatuss

S

S antigen
Bel-Phen-Ergot S
S unit of streptomycin

SA

salicylic acid
Sinutab SA
Targel SA

SAA

severe aplastic anemia

Saalfield expressor

SAARD

slow-acting antirheumatic drug

saber shin

Sabin-Feldman dye test

Sabin vaccine

Sabouraud

S. agar
S. medium

sabre

coup de s.
en coup de s.

SAC

seasonal allergic conjunctivitis

sacbrood

sacchari

Fusarium s.

saccharide

O-linked s.

saccharolyticus

Peptostreptococcus s.

Saccharomyces

S. cerevisiae
S. neoformans

sacer ignis

sac fungus

Sachs-Georgi test

sacral

s. agenesis type 1 syndrome
s. root sheath ectasia
s. spot

sacroiliitis

psoriatic s.
pyogenic s.

sacrospinalis muscle

Sactimed-I-Sinald disinfectant

SAD

specific antibody deficiency

SADBE

squaric acid dibutylester

saddle

s. nose
s. nose deformity

saddleback

s. caterpillar

s. caterpillar sting
s. fever

Saenger macula

SAF-Clens wound cleanser

Safe Tussin

safety-pin appearance

Saf-Gel hydrogel dressing

Safranin O stain

sage

coast s.
s. weed pollen

sagebrush

saginata

Taenia s.

sailor's

s. neck
s. skin

saimiri

Herpesvirus s.
herpesvirus s. (HVS)

Saint

S. Anthony's fire
S. Ignatius itch

Saizen

Sakaguchi-Kauppi method

SAL

salicylic acid-lactic acid
SAL paint

Sal

Salac

Salacid Ointment

Sal-Acid Plaster

Salagen Oral

Salazopyrin

salbutamol

Saleto-200, -400

Saleto-CF

Salflex

Salgesic

salicylanilides

halogenated s.

salicylate

choline s.
glucuronidation s.
magnesium s.
methyl s.
nonacetylated s.

salicylic

s. acid (SA)
s. acid collodion
s. acid and lactic acid
s. acid-lactic acid (SAL)
s. acid-lactic acid paint
s. acid and propylene glycol

salicylism

S

saligenin compound
saligna
    eucalyptus s.
salina
    Artemisia s.
saline
    s. agglutinin
    Broncho S.
    s. isohemagglutinin
    phosphate-buffered s. (PBS)
    s. sodium citrate (SSC)
    Tris-buffered s. (TBS)
Salisbury common cold virus
saliva
    enzymatic s.
    s. substitute
Salivart
salivary
    s. gland
    s. gland virus
    s. gland virus disease
    s. scintigraphy
Salk vaccine
salmeterol xinafoate
salmincola
    Nanophyetus s.
salmon
    s. calcitonin
    s. patch
    pink s.
Salmonella
    S. arizonae
    S. arthritis
    S. bredeney
    S. choleraesuis
    S. enteritidis
    S. montevideo
    S. panama
    S. paratyphi
    S. poona
    S. st. paul
    S. typhi
    S. typhimurium
salmonella
    s. osteomyelitis
salmonellosis
salmonicolor
    Sporobolomyces s.
salpingitis
    reactive s.
salsalate
Salseb
Salsitab
Salsola pestifer
SALT
    skin-associated lymphoid tissue
salt
    aluminum s.

    s. cedar
    s. cedar tree
    Epsom s.'s
    gold s.'s
    s. grass
    s. grass pollen
    s. and pepper lesion
    persulfate s.
    s. of platinum
    s. rheum
    s. sensitivity
    silver s.'s
    sodium s.
    s. solution
    theophylline s.
    s. water boil
saltbush weed pollen
saltwater catfish
saltwort
salute
    allergic s.
salvage therapy
Salve
    Callus S.
    Scholl Corn S.
sampler
    Anderson s.
    gravitational s.
    impaction s.
    inertial suction s.
    Rotorod s.
    Sartorious air s.
    suction s.
Samter syndrome
San
    S. Joaquin Valley fever
    S. Miguel sea lion virus
Sanarelli phenomenon
Sanarelli-Shwartzman phenomenon
sand
    s. flea
    s. flea bite
sandal
    keratodermic s.
    s. strap dermatitis
sandfly
    s. bite
    s. fever
    s. fever virus
Sandimmune (SIM)
    S. injection
    S. Oral
Sandoglobulin
sandpaper dermabrader
sandwich assay
sandworm disease

Sanfilippo
  S. mucopolysaccharidosis
  S. syndrome
SangCya oral solution
sanguineus
  Allodermanyssus s.
  nevus s.
  sudor s.
sanguisuga
  Triatoma s.
Sanochrysin
Sansert
Santyl
  S. enzymatic debrider
  S. enzymatic debriding agent
SAP-1
  stress-activated protein 1
saphenous nerve entrapment
SAPHO
  synovitis, acne, pustulosis, hyperostosis,
    osteitis
  SAPHO syndrome
saponin
Sapporo criteria
saprophytic
  s. disease
  s. flora
  s. fungi
saquinavir mesylate
SAR
  seasonal allergic rhinitis
SARA
  sexually acquired reactive arthritis
Saran Wrap therapy
sarcoid
  s. arthritis
  Boeck s.
  Darier-Roussy s.
  s. granuloma
  miliary s.
  morpheaform s.
  papular s.
  Spiegler-Fendt s.
sarcoidal
sarcoid-like granulomatous myopathy
sarcoidosis
  Boeck s.
  cardiac s.
  cutaneous s.
  Danielssen-Boeck s.
  extraocular s.
  extrapulmonary s.

  ichthyosiform s.
  ocular s.
  pulmonary s.
sarcolemma
sarcoma
  Abernethy s.
  African cutaneous Kaposi s.
  African lymphadenopathic Kaposi s.
  African-variety Kaposi s.
  avian s.
  disseminated Kaposi s.
  epithelioid s.
  Kaposi s. (KS)
  melanotic s.
  multiple idiopathic hemorrhagic s.
  pseudo-Kaposi s.
  reticulum-cell s.
  Rous s.
sarcomatosis cutis
sarcomatous
sarcomere
Sarcophaga
sarcophagi fly
Sarcopsylla
Sarcoptes
  S. hominis
  S. scabiei
sarcoptic
  s. acariasis
  s. mange
sarcosepsis
sarcosis
sarcosporidiosis
sardine
sargassum
  Japanese s.
sargramostim
Sarna HC
Sartorious air sampler
SAS
  statistical analysis system
SASSAD
  Six-Area, Six-Sign Atopic Dermatitis
  SASSAD severity index
**SAStid Plain Therapeutic Shampoo and
  Acne Wash**
satellite
  s. buboes
  s. cell
  s. erythematous papule
  s. lesion
  s. phenomenon

S

NOTES

satellitosis
Satinique Anti-Dandruff
saturated solution of potassium iodide
  (SSKI)
saturation analysis
saturnine gout
saucerization technique
sauna suit
Saunders-Zwilling hypothesis
sauriasis
sauriderma
saurine
sauriosis
sauroderma
    ichthyosis s.
sausage
    s. digit
    s. finger
    s. toe
sausage-shaped bulla
savitum
    Helminthosporium s.
sawtooth strategy
saxitoxin
SBE
    subacute bacterial endocarditis
SBM
    subbasement membrane
    subepithelial basement membrane
SBTx
    small bowel transplantation
SC
    stratum corneum
        LightSheer SC
        Pefabloc SC
sc
    subcutaneous
SCA
    single-chain antigen-binding
        SCA protein
scab
scabby mouth
Scabene
    S. Lotion
    S. Shampoo
scabetic
scabicidal
scabicide
scabiei
    Sarcoptes s.
scabies
    animal s.
    Boeck s.
    crusted s.
    environmental s.
    hair follicle mite s.
    hyperkeratotic s.

s. incognito
keratotic s.
nodular s.
Norwegian s.
s. preparation
scabietic
    s. mite
scabieticide
scabious
scabrities unguium
scaffold
    knottin s.
scald
scalded skin syndrome
scale
    aluminum density step s.
    arthritis impact measurement s.
      (AIMS)
    Borg s.
    branny s.
    carpet-tack s.
    Childhood Myositis Assessment S.
      (CMAS)
    Chisolm s.
    expanded disability status s.
      (EDSS)   *Hamilton s.*
    Greenspan s.   *(chair)*
    illness attitude s. (IAS)
    lamellar s.
    lichen-type s.   *Ludwg s.*
    Likert s.
    Lund-Browder burn s.   *hair density*
    Mankin histologic/histochemical s.
    micaceous s.
    ostraceous s.
    Outerbridge s.
    pityriasis-type s.
    4-point Likert s.
    5-point Likert s.
    7-point Likert s.
    6-point vitiligo disease activity s.
    Profile of Mood States S.
    psoriatic-type s.
    Sessing pressure ulcer
      assessment s.
    Shea pressure ulcer assessment s.
    Shea s. (stages I-IV)
    silver-white s.
    silver-white-colored s.
    silvery s.
    Tarply s.
    visual analog s. (VAS)
    Ways of Coping S.
    WOMAC stiffness s.
scaling skin-colored lesion
scall
    milk s.

scalp
- dissecting cellulitis of s.
- dissection cellulitis of s.
- s. folliculitis
- hair and s.
- s. infection
- s. louse
- pilar tumor of s.
- ringworm of the s.
- scurfy s.
- seborrheic dermatitis of the s.

scalpel
- Shaw hemostatic s.
- s. skimming

Scalpicin Topical

scaly
- s. ringworm
- s. tetter

scan
- high-resolution computed tomography s.
- HRCT s.
- indium chloride s.
- single-photon emission computed tomography s.
- SPECT s.
- Tc polyphosphate s.
- technetium s.
- ventilation/perfusion lung s. (V/Q lung scan)
- V/Q lung s.
  - ventilation/perfusion lung scan

scanner
- SilkTouch CO$_2$ Flash S.
- Softscan laser s.

scanning
- indium-labeled s.

Scanpor
- S. acrylate adhesive
- S. tape

scapi (*pl. of* scapus)

scapularis
- *Ixodes s.*

scapulocostal syndrome

scapulothoracic
- s. articulation
- s. syndrome

scapus, pl. **scapi**
- s. pili

scar
- atrophic white s.
- cigarette-paper s.

- s. formation
- hypertrophic s.
- ice-pick type s.
- keloidal type s.
- paper-thin s.
- papyraceous s.
- radial s.
- shilling s.
- white s.

scarf nevus

scarification test

scarificator

scarifier
- Berkeley s.

scarify

scarlatina
- anginose s.
- s. hemorrhagica
- s. latens
- s. maligna
- s. rheumatica
- s. simplex

scarlatinal nephritis

scarlatinella

scarlatiniform
- s. eruption
- erythema s.
- s. erythema

scarlatiniforme
- erythema s.

scarlatinoid

scarlet
- s. fever
- s. fever antitoxin
- s. fever erythrogenic toxin

scarring
- cigarette-paper s.
- keloidal s.
- patch test s.
- s. vertex alopecia

SCAS
- Self Care Assessment Schedule

SCAT
- short-contact treatment

scattering
- Rayleigh s.
- Thomson s.

scavenger
- s. cell
- s. macrophage

SCB
- DuoDerm S.

NOTES

S

493

SCC
squamous cell carcinoma
SCD
sickle cell disease
Scedosporium apiospermum
scent print
SCF
stem cell factor
Schfifer syndrome
Schafer-Branauer syndrome
Schäfer syndrome
Schamberg
S. comedo extractor
S. dermatitis
S. disease
S. expressor
S. fever
S. progressive pigmented purpuric dermatosis
S. purpura
Schaumann
S. benign lymphogranulomatosis
S. body
Schedule
Self Care Assessment S. (SCAS)
Scheie
S. mucopolysaccharidosis
S. syndrome
Scheinpharm Triamcine-A
scheme
Kauffmann-White s.
Schenck disease
schenckii
Sporothrix s.
Sporotrichum s.
Scheuermann disease
Schick
S. method
S. sign
S. test
S. test toxin
Schiff
periodic acid-S. (PAS)
Schilder disease
Schimmelpenning syndrome
Schirmer test
schistocyte
Schistosoma
S. haematobium
S. japonicum
S. mansoni
S. mekongi
schistosomal
s. dermatitis
s. granuloma of scrotum
schistosome
s. cercarial dermatitis
s. granuloma

schistosomiasis
ectopic cutaneous s.
hepatosplenic s.
Manson s.
visceral s.
schizonychia
schizotrichia
Schmidt syndrome
Schmorl node
Schnitzler syndrome
Schober
S. test
S. test for spondylitis
schoenleinii
Achorion s.
Trichophyton s.
Scholl
S. Athlete's Foot Preparation
S. Corn, Callus Plaster Preparation
S. Corn Salve
S. 2-Drop Corn Remedy
S. Wart Remover
S. Zino
Schönlein
S. disease
S. purpura
Schönlein-Henoch syndrome
Schopf syndrome
Schridde cancer hair
Schuco 2000 nebulizer
Schüller-Christian syndrome
Schultz-Charlton
S.-C. phenomenon
S.-C. reaction
Schultz-Dale reaction
Schultze acroparesthesia
Schultze-type acroparesthesia
Schwann cell
schwannoma
granular cell s.
Schweninger-Buzzi
anetoderma of S.-B.
S.-B. anetoderma
sciatic
s. nerve
s. nerve entrapment
SCID
severe combined immune deficiency
severe combined immunodeficiency
severe combined immunodeficiency disease
severe combined immunodeficiency disorder
SCID mice
SCIDA
Athabascan type of severe combined immunodeficiency disease

SCIG
  subcutaneous immunoglobulin
scintigraphy
  salivary s.
  Tc-human serum albumin s.
scintillation counter
scintiscan
scissors
  s. biopsy
  blepharoplasty s.
  dissecting s.
  Gibbs-Gradle s.
  Gorney-Freeman straight facelift s.
  Gorney straight facelift s.
  Gradle s.
  Kaye s.
  LaGrange s.
  Lahey s.
  Laschal s.
  Lister s.
  Littauer s.
  Malis s.
  Matarasso facelift s.
  Metzenbaum s.
  Northbent s.
  O'Brien s.
  Peck-Joseph s.
  Ragnell s.
  Shortbent s.
  Spencer s.
  Stevens tenotomy s.
  utility s.
scissura pilorum
sc-kit
  soluble c-kit
Scl-70 antibody
Sclavo serum
SCLE
  subacute cutaneous lupus erythematosus
sclera
  donor s.
scleradenitis
scleral defect
scleredema
  s. adultorum
  Buschke s.
  s. diutinum
  s. neonatorum
sclerema
  s. adiposum
  s. neonatorum
scleriasis

scleritis
  diffuse s.
  nodular s.
  nonrheumatoid s.
  posterior s.
  rheumatoid s.
scleroatrophy, sclerotylosis
  anetoderma s.
  atrophoderma s.
  lichen sclerosus s.
  striae s.
sclerodactylia annularis ainhumoides
sclerodactyly
scleroderma
  adultorum s.
  s. autoantigen CENP-B
  Buchscher s.
  diffuse s.
  environmental s.
  linear s.
  localized s.
  pediatric s.
  s. renal crisis (SRC)
  sclerosis sine s.
  s. septal panniculitis
  systemic sclerosis sine s. (ssSSc)
scleroderma-like
  s.-l. eruption
  s.-l. skin thickening
sclerodermatitis
sclerodermatomyositis
sclerodermatous
sclerodermiformis
  hypodermitis s.
sclerodermitis
sclerodermoid
Sclerodex
ScleroLaser
scleromalacia perforans
scleromyxedema
scleronychia
ScleroPLUS flashlamp-pumped pulsed tunable dye laser
sclerosed
sclerosing
  s. agent
  s. cholangitis
  s. hemangioma
  s. lipogranuloma
  s. lymphangitis
  s. lymphosarcoma

S

NOTES

sclerosing *(continued)*
    s. panniculitis
    s. sweat duct carcinoma
sclerosis
    amyotrophic lateral s. (ALS)
    Baló concentric s.
    s. corii
    s. cutanea
    diffuse progressive systemic s.
    drug-induced progressive
      symptom s.
    environment progressive symptom s.
    limited progressive systemic s.
    linear progressive systemic s.
    localized progressive systemic s.
    lupoid s.
    multiple s.
    primary-progressive multiple s.
      (PPMS)
    progressive symptom s. (PSS)
    progressive systemic s. (PSS)
    relapsing-remitting multiple s.
      (RRMS)
    s. sine scleroderma
    systemic s. (SSc)
    tuberous s. (TSC)
sclerostenosis
sclerosus
    genital lichen s.
    lichen s.
    s. lichen
sclerotherapy
sclerothrix
sclerotic body
sclerotrichia
sclerotylosis *(var. of* scleroatrophy)
scoliosis
    dolorimeter s.
Scolopendra
    S. heres
    S. heres bite
scombroid
    s. dermatitis
    s. fish poisoning
SCOP
    Structural Classification of Proteins
scopolamine
Scopulariopsis
    S. brevicaulis
    S. brumptii
    S. inflatum
    S. prolificans
SCORAD
    Severity Scoring of Atopic Dermatitis
    SCORAD index
scorbutic
    s. dysentery
    s. purpura

score
    APACHE II s.
    Beck Depression Inventory s.
    Birmingham Vasculitis Activity S.
      (BVAS)
    Borg s.
    Brasfield chest radiograph s.
    Child-Pugh s.
    Child-Turcotte-Pugh s.
    damage index s.
    Fitzpatrick wrinkle s.
    five-factor s. (FFS)
    Karnofsky s.
    Kellgren s.
    Leicester s.
    modified Rodman skin thickness s.
    nasal congestion s. (NCS)
    nasal symptom s. (NSS)
    Quality of Life s.
    Rodnan skin thickness s.
    Sharp s.
    Shwachman clinical s.
    Skin Intensity S. (SIS)
    skin thickness s.
    SSS s.
    t s.
    total skin s.
    UNOS 3, 4 s.
    vitiligo disease activity s.
    WOMAC pain s.
    z s.
scorpion
    bark s.
    common striped s.
    s. fish
    s. sting
Scotch Tape test
sCR1
    soluble complement receptor type 1
scrapie
    sheep s.
scraping
    fungal s.
    KOH s.
    nasal s.
Scraple disease
scratch
    s. chamber test
    s. testing
screen
    AlaTOP inhalant allergy s.
    QuickVue One-Step Allergen S.
    s. test
    TORCH viral s.
    toxoplasmosis, other, rubella,
      cytomegalovirus, and herpes
      viral s.

screening
    s. audiometry
    S. Patch Test Kit
    spirometric s.
    systematic polymorphism s.
screw-worm fly
scrofula
scrofuloderma, scrofulodermia
    eczema s.
    s. gummosa
    papular s.
    verrucous s.
scrofulosis
    lichen s.
scrofulosorum
    acne s.
    lichen s.
scrofulous
    lichen s.
scrotalis
    lingua s.
scrotal tongue
scroti
    pruritus s.
scrotum
    schistosomal granuloma of s.
scrub
    Exidine S.
    Techni-Care surgical s.
    s. typhus
Scrubz
    Pocket S.
    Travel S.
scruff
SCT
    stem cell transplant
sculpturatus
    Centruroides s.
sculptured nail
scurf
scurfy scalp
scurvy
scute
scutular
scutularis
    parakeratosis s.
scutulata
    ichthyosis s.
    porrigo s.
scutulum

Scytalidium
    S. dimidiatum
    S. hyalinum
SD
    standard deviation
    WinRho SD
S/D
    Gammagard S/D
    Polygam S/D
SDF-1
    stromal-cell-derived factor-1
SDKT
    simultaneous double kidney
    transplantation
SDS-PAGE
    sodium dodecyl sulfate-polyacrylamide
    gel electrophoresis
SDZ ASM 981
SE
    surgical excision
SEA
    seronegativity, enthesopathy, arthropathy
sea
    s. anemone
    s. anemone dermatitis
    s. anemone sting
    s. bathers' eruption
    s. boot foot
    s. cucumber
    s. cucumber dermatitis
    s. cucumber sting
    s. louse dermatitis
    s. nettle dermatitis
    s. snake
    s. snake bite
    s. urchin
    s. urchin dermatitis
    s. urchin granuloma
    s. urchin sting
    s. water boil
sea-blue
    s.-b. histiocyte syndrome
    s.-b. histiocytosis
Sea-Clens wound cleanser
sealant
    fibrin s.
    Tisseel fibrin s.
seal finger
seams
    tetracycline s.
Searl ulcer

S

NOTES

season
> growing s.

seasonal
> s. allergic conjunctivitis (SAC)
> s. allergic rhinitis (SAR)
> s. allergy
> s. pruritus

SeaSorb
> S. alginate dressing
> S. alginate wound cover

seatworm infection

seaweed dermatitis

sebacea
> ichthyosis s.

sebaceous, sebaceus
> s. adenocarcinoma
> s. adenoma
> s. carcinoma
> s. cyst
> s. epithelioma
> s. gland (SG)
> s. horn
> lupus s.
> s. miliaria
> nevus s.
> s. nevus
> s. nevus of Jadassohn
> s. senile hyperplasia
> s. trichofolliculoma
> s. tubercle
> s. tumor

sebaceum
> adenoma s.
> molluscum s.
> tuberculum s.

sebaceus
> lupus s.
> nevus s.

Seba-Nil

Sebasorb lotion

Sebcur

Sebcur/T

sebolith

sebopsoriasis

seborrhea
> s. adiposa
> s. capitis
> s. cerea
> concrete s.
> s. corporis
> eczematoid s.
> s. faciei
> s. furfuracea
> s. generalis
> s. nigra
> s. oleosa
> s. sicca
> s. squamosa neonatorum

seborrheic
> s. blepharitis
> s. dermatitis
> s. dermatitis-like condition
> s. dermatitis of the scalp
> s. dermatosis
> s. eczema
> s. keratosis
> s. verruca
> s. wart

seborrheica
> acanthoma verrucosa s.
> acanthosis s.
> acne s.
> alopecia s.
> corona s.
> dermatitis s.

seborrhiasis

seborrhoeicum
> eczema s.

Sebulex

Sebulon

sebum
> s. cutaneum
> s. preputiale

Sebutone

second
> forced expiratory volume in 1 s. (FEV$_1$)
> s. set rejection

secondary
> s. adrenocortical failure
> s. agammaglobulinemia
> s. amyloid
> s. antibody deficiency
> s. cataract
> s. cutaneous B-cell lymphocytic leukemia
> s. cutaneous B-cell lymphoma
> s. disease
> s. effect
> s. encephalitis
> s. hyperlipoproteinemia
> s. hyperparathyroidism
> s. hypogammaglobulinemia
> s. immune response
> s. immunodeficiency
> s. infection
> s. lesion
> s. lymphatic tissue (SLT)
> s. lymphedema
> s. panhypopituitarism
> s. psychiatric disorder
> s. pyoderma
> s. Sjögren syndrome
> s. smoke
> s. syphilid
> s. syphilis

s. systemic amyloidosis
s. telangiectasia
s. tuberculosis
s. tumor-associated cutaneous amyloidosis
second-degree burn
second-line drug (SLD)
Secrétan syndrome
secrete
secreted
regulated upon activation, normal T-cell expressed and s. (RANTES)
secretion
C-peptide s.
excessive s.
secretor
s. factor
secretory
s. antibody study
s. coil
s. component
s. component deficiency
s. immunoglobulin
s. immunoglobulin A
s. leukoprotease inhibitor
s. leukoprotease inhibitor protein
s. otitis media
s. PLA_2 enzyme
s. vesicle function
section
horizontal s.
snap-frozen s.
vertical s.
SED
spondyloepiphyseal dysplasia
sedative therapy
Sedi-Stain
seeberi
Rhinosporidium s.
seed
s. corn
millet s.
psyllium s.
sesame s.
s. tick
s. wart
seglycin CS/DS
segment
apicoposterior s.
N s.

segmental
s. hyalinizing vasculitis
s. neurofibromatosis
s. nevus
s. vitiligo
segmentectomy
Segond fracture
Seidlmayer syndrome
Seip-Lawrence syndrome
seizure
Seldane-D
selectins
selection
negative s.
positive s.
reflectance-guidance laser s.
tumor cell negative s.
selective
s. antipolysaccharide antibody deficiency (SPAD)
s. estrogen receptor modulator (SERM)
s. mesentericography
s. photothermolysis
Selects
Coppertone Skin S.
selenium
s. deficiency
s. sulfide
Selestoject
self-antigen
muscle s.-a.
Self Care Assessment Schedule (SCAS)
self-healing reticulohistiocytosis
self-infection
self-injecting epinephrine
self-limited allergic reaction
self-nonself discrimination
Self-Perception Profile for children
Selsun
S. Blue
S. Blue Shampoo
S. Gold
S. Gold for Women
selvagem
endemic fogo s.
fogo s. (FS)
semelincident
semicircular
s. lipoatrophy
s. lipotrophy
semiimpermeable membrane

NOTES

S

semimembranosus complex
semipermeable dressing
semiquantitative
    s. disease extent index
semisynthetic analog
Semken forceps
Semliki Forest virus
Semmes-Weinstein test
Semple vaccine
Semprex
Semprex-D
Sendai virus
Senear-Usher
    S.-U. disease
    S.-U. syndrome
Seneca snakeroot
senescence
    replicative s.
senescent arthritis
senile
    s. alopecia
    s. angioma
    s. atrophoderma
    s. ectasia
    s. elastosis
    s. fibroma
    s. gangrene
    s. hemangioma
    s. ichthyosis
    s. keratoderma
    keratoma s.
    s. keratoma
    s. keratosis
    s. lentigo
    s. melanoderma
    s. pruritus
    s. purpura
    s. sebaceous hyperplasia
    s. skin
    s. wart
senilis
    alopecia s.
    keratosis s.
    lentigo s.
    malum coxae s.
    pruritus s.
    purpura s.
    verruca plana s.
senior synonym
sennetsu
    Ehrlichia s.
sense nucleotide
sensible perspiration
sensitiva
    trichosis s.
sensitive
    temperature s. (TS)

sensitivity
    acquired s.
    allergic s.
    animal dander s.
    antibiotic s.
    aspirin s.
    atopic s.
    autoerythrocyte s.
    earlobe sign of nickel s.
    idiosyncratic s.
    induced s.
    multiple chemical s.
    nickel s.
    peak flow s.
    photoallergic s.
    phototoxic s.
    salt s.
sensitization
    active s.
    aerosol s. (AS)
    autoerythrocyte s.
    cross s.
    photodynamic s.
sensitize
sensitized
    s. antigen
    s. cell
    s. lymphocyte
sensitizer
sensitizing
    s. dose
    s. injection
    s. substance
sensor
    ClipTip reusable s.
    Cross Top replacement oxygen s.
    Infinity s.
    SpiroSense flow s.
Sensorcaine-MPF
sensorineural dysfunction
sensory
    s. ganglion
    s. nerve action potential (SNAP)
    s. nerve action potential sleep
      recorder
sensu stricto
Sential
sentinel
    s. animal
    s. lymph node (SLN)
    s. tag
sentrin
sentrinization
seositis
seotonin
SEPA dermal absorption enhancer
SEPA/minoxidil

separation
 epidermal-dermal s.
 eschar s.
Sephadex Bead
Sepracor
Seprafilm bioresorbable membrane
sepsis, pl. **sepses**
 group JK *Corynebacterium* s.
sepsis-induced
 s.-i. DIC
 s.-i. disseminated intravascular
 coagulation
 s.-i. thrombocytopenia
septa
 interlobular s.
 S. Topical Ointment
septal
 s. embolus
 s. panniculitis
septic
 s. arthritis
 s. dactylitis
 s. embolus
 s. shock
 s. shock syndrome
SeptiCare wound cleanser
septicemia
 Aeromonas s.
 bacterial s.
 Bruce s.
 Candida s.
 DF2 s.
 gonococcal s.
 perinatal s.
 streptococcal s.
 typhoid s.
Septisol
septoplasty
 graft s.
Septra DS
sequela of influenza
sequence
 Aertemia Salinas s.
 chi s.
 complement s.
 consensus s.
 immunostimulatory DNA s. (ISS)
 long terminal repeat s. (LTR)
 mitochondrial targeting s. (MTS)
 Shine-Dalgarno s.
 signal s.

sequence-specific
 s.-s. oligonucleotide probe
 hybridization (SSOP)
 s.-s. primer (SSP)
sequencing
 direct s.
sequential
 s. determinant
 s. probability ratio test (SPRT)
sequestration
 s. cyst
 s. dermoid
sequestrum, pl. **sequestra**
sequoiosis
sera (*pl. of* serum)
Serax
Seretide
Serevent
Sergent white line
serial
 s. dilutional intradermal skin test
 s. passage
series
 20-allergen Hermal screening s.
serine
 s. esterase
 s. protease
 s. proteinase
serine-threonine kinase
serivumab
SERM
 selective estrogen receptor modulator
sermorelin acetate
seroconversion response
serodiagnosis
seroepidemiology
serofast
serologic test for syphilis (S.T.S.)
serology
seroma
Seromycin Pulvules
seronegative
 s. oligoarthritis
 s. rheumatoid arthritis
 s. rheumatoid syndrome
 s. spondyloarthropathy
seronegativity, enthesopathy, arthropathy (SEA)
seropositive
 anti-HCV s.
 antihepatitis C virus s.

NOTES

S

seropositive *(continued)*
    s. disease
    s. rheumatoid arthritis
seroprevalence
seropurulent
serosal fibrosis
serosanguineous
serositis, pl. **serositides**
    adhesive s.
    multiple s.
serotaxis
serotherapy
serotonergic
serotonin
serotype
    heterologous s.
    homologous s.
serotyping
serovaccination
serovar
SERPACWA
    skin exposure reduction paste against
    chemical warfare agents
serpentina
    ichthyosis s.
serpentine
serpiginosa
    elastosis perforans s. (EPS)
    zona s.
serpiginosum
    angioma s.
    s. angioma
serpiginosus
    lupus s.
serpiginous
    s. pattern
    s. ulcer
serpigo
serpin
Serratia marcescens
Serrefine clamp
sertraline
    s. HCl
    s. hydrochloride
serum, pl. **sera**
    s. accident
    active s.
    s. agglutinin
    s. alpha-antitrypsin
    s. amyloid A, P component
    antianthrax s.
    antibotulinus s.
    anticholera s.
    anticomplementary s.
    anticrotalus s.
    antiepithelial s.
    s. antiglomerular-basement-membrane
      antibody

antilymphocyte s. (ALS)
antimeningococcus s.
antipneumococcus s.
antirabies s.
antireticular cytotoxic s.
antisnakebite s.
antitoxic s.
bacteriolytic s.
Behring s.
B fraction s.
blister s.
blood s.
s. C3
s. C4
C fraction s.
s. complement C1–C9
s. complement level
convalescence s.
convalescent s.
Coombs s.
despeciated s.
s. disease
dried human s.
s. eruption
foreign s.
s. hepatitis (SH)
s. hepatitis virus
heterologous s.
homologous s.
horse s.
human measles immune s.
human pertussis immune s.
human scarlet fever immune s.
hyperimmune s.
s. IgA
s. IgM
immune s. (IS)
s. immunofixation electrophoresis
  (SIFE)
inactivated s.
liquid human s.
lymphatolytic s.
s. marker
measles convalescent s.
mouse s.
s. nephritis
s. neutralization
nonimmune s.
normal horse s.
North American antisnakebite s.
polyvalent s.
pooled s.
s. precipitin
s. protein electrophoresis (SPEP)
s. protein electrophoretic finding
s. protein electrophoretogram (SPE)
s. rash
s. reaction

Sclavo s.
s. shock
s. sickness
specific s.
s. therapy
thyrotoxic s.
s. uric acid
serumal
serum-fast
serum-opsonized
sesame seed
sesquioleate
sorbitan s. (SS)
sessile
Sessing pressure ulcer assessment scale
set
s. of idiotopes
SinoJect puncture s.
seta, pl. **setae**
setosa
trichosis s.
seven-year itch
severe
s. acute allergic reaction
s. aplastic anemia (SAA)
s. chronic allergic condition
s. combined immune deficiency (SCID)
s. combined immune deficiency syndrome
s. combined immunodeficiency (SCID)
s. combined immunodeficiency disease (SCID)
s. combined immunodeficiency disorder (SCID)
s. combined immunodeficient mice
s. deforming osteogenesis imperfecta
s. immediate reaction
s. obstruction
s. respiratory failure
s. systemic reaction
severity
s. of allergy symptom
Dermatology Index of Disease S. (DIDS)
S. Scoring of Atopic Dermatitis (SCORAD)
Sevin
sewer fly
sex factor

sexine
sexually
s. acquired reactive arthritis (SARA)
s. transmitted disease (STD)
Sézary
S. cell
S. erythroderma
S. reticulosis
S. syndrome
SF
stimulating factor
synovial fluid
sFas
soluble Fas
SG
sebaceous gland
stratum granulosum
SGF
simulated gastric fluid
SGS
silicone gel sheeting
SH
serum hepatitis
sinus histiocytosis
Shade
S. UvaGuard sunscreen
S. UvaGuard sunscreen lotion
shadow
nodular s.
s. plaque
ring s.
shaft
hair s.
shagbark
s. hickory
s. hickory tree
shaggy thick wall
shagreen
s. patch
s. skin
shaking of walnuts
Shaklee
S. Dandruff Control
S. Sunscreen
Sham
S. TENS
S. transcutaneous electrical nerve stimulator
shampoo
A-200 S.
Anti-Dandruff S.

NOTES

shampoo *(continued)*
    Avant Garde S.
    bifonazole s.
    Carmol S.
    Dandruff Treatment S.
    Exsel S.
    G-well S.
    Head & Shoulders S.
    Keep Clear Anti-Dandruff S.
    Kwell S.
    Lice-Enz S.
    Nizoral A-D S.
    Pronto S.
    P&S S.
    Pyrinex Pediculicide S.
    Pyrinyl Plus S.
    R&C S.
    RID S.
    Scabene S.
    Selsun Blue S.
    Tisit S.
    T/SA S.
    T/Sal S.
    Zincon S.
Shampooing Anti-Pelliculaire
Shapiro-Wilke W test
shared epitope
Sharing
    United Network for Organ S.
    (UNOS)
shark skin
sharp
    s. dissection
    S. score
    s. spoon
Sharplan SilkTouch flashscan surgical
  laser
sharply circumscribed nodule
shave
    s. biopsy
    s. technique
shaver
    MicroPlaner soft tissue s.
Shaw hemostatic scalpel
shawl distribution
Shea
    S. pressure ulcer assessment scale
    S. scale (stages I-IV)
sheath
    s. cell
    cuticle of inner root s.
    fibrous s.
    giant cell tumor of tendon s.
    (GCTTS)
    inner root s.
    nerve s.
    outer root s.
    tendon s.

shedding
    nail s.
    virus s.
Sheehan syndrome
sheep
    contagious ecthyma (pustular
     dermatitis) virus of s.
    s. epithelium
    pulmonary adenomatosis of s.
    s. scrapie
    s. sorrel
    s. sorrel weed pollen
    s. wool
sheep-pox virus
sheet
    AcryDerm hydrogel s.
    Aquasorb hydrogel s.
    beta-pleated s.
    ClearSite hydrogel s.
    Conformant contact layer s.
    Curagel Hydrogel s.
    Derma-Gel hydrogel s.
    Dermanet contact layer s.
    Elasto-Gel hydrogel s.
    Flexderm hydrogel s.
    keratinous s.
    material safety data s. (MSDS)
    Mepitel contact layer s.
    2nd Skin hydrogel s.
    s.'s of nevus cells
    N-Terface contact layer s.
    Nu-Gel hydrogel s.
    patient patch test record s.
    Silastic s.
    Silk Skin s.
    Tegagel hydrogel s.
    Tegapore contact-layer s.
    Telfa Clear contact layer s.
    THINSite hydrogel s.
    Transorbent hydrogel s.
    Vigilon hydrogel s.
sheeting
    Cica-Care topical gel s.
    DermaSof gel s.
    New Beginnings topical gel s.
    occlusive s.
    silicone gel s. (SGS)
    Topigel occlusive s.
shellfish
shell nail
shelter foot
shield
    Sof-Gel palm s.
shift
    antigenic s.
shifting
    Raman s.
Shiga-like toxin

Shigella
>*S. flexneri*
>*S. flexneri dysenteriae*
>*S. infection*
>*S. sonnei*

shigelloides
>*Aeromonas s.*
>*Plesiomonas s.*

shigellosis
Shiley tracheostomy tube
shilling scar
shimamushi disease
shin
>saber s.
>s. splint
>s. spot
>toasted s.

Shine-Dalgarno sequence
shiner
>allergic s.

Shingles Relief Pak
ship fever
shipping
>s. fever
>s. fever virus

Shiseido Sunblock
shock
>anaphylactic s.
>anaphylactoid s.
>s. antigen
>endotoxin s.
>histamine s.
>hypovolemic s.
>osmotic s.
>protein s.
>pseudoanaphylactic s.
>septic s.
>serum s.
>thermal s.

shocking dose
shoe
>Ambulator s.
>s. dye dermatitis
>Plastizote s.

shoe-leather dermatitis
Shohl solution
Shope
>S. fibroma
>S. fibroma virus
>S. papilloma
>S. papilloma virus

shop typhus

short
>s. anagen telogen effluvium
>s. bowel syndrome
>s. consensus repeats
>s. incubation hepatitis
>s. tau inversion recovery (STIR)

Shortbent scissors
short-chain type X collagen
short-contact
>s.-c. therapy
>s.-c. treatment (SCAT)

short-course
>directly observed therapy s.-c.
>(DOTS)

short-haired breed
short-term immunotherapy (STI)
shoulder
>cuff-tear arthropathy s.
>frozen s.
>s. girdle
>Head & S.'s
>Milwaukee s.
>s. periarthritis

shoulder-hand syndrome
showerhead infiltrator
SHP
>summer-type hypersensitivity
>pneumonitis

shrimp
shrinking lung syndrome
Shuco-Myst nebulizer
Shulman syndrome
shunt
>arteriovenous s.
>distal splenorenal s. (DSRS)
>Gott s.
>hexose monophosphate s. (HMS)
>side-to-side portacaval s.
>ventriculoperitoneal s. (VP)

shunting
>venoarterial s.

Shur-Clens wound cleanser
Shwachman clinical score
Shwartzman
>S. phenomenon
>S. reaction

SI
>syncytium-inhibiting

SIADH
>syndrome of inappropriate excretion of
>antidiuretic hormone

NOTES

S

sialadenitis
    myoepithelial s.
sialectasia
sialidase
sialidosis
sialoglycoprotein antigen
sialography
    parotid s.
sialometaplasia
    necrotizing s.
sialomucin
sialoprotein
    bone s. (BSP)
Sibine
    S. *stimulea*
    S. *stimulea* sting
sibling bone marrow transplantation
sicca
    cholera s.
    s. feature
    keratoconjunctivitis s.
    onychia s.
    pityriasis s.
    seborrhea s.
    s. symptom
    s. syndrome
siccation
    electrode s.
siccum
    eczema s.
sick
    s. building syndrome
    s. euthyroid
sickle
    s. cell anemia
    s. cell disease (SCD)
    s. cell trait
    s. cell ulcer
sickling
    hepatic s.
sickness
    African horse s.
    motion s.
    serum s.
    spotted s.
side-chain theory
side effect
sideroderma
sideropenic
    canities segmentata s.
side-to-side portacaval shunt
SIDS
    sudden infant death syndrome
Siemens
    ichthyosis bullosa of S. (IBS)
SIF
    simulated intestinal fluid

SIFE
    serum immunofixation electrophoresis
sign
    ABCD s.
    Albright s.
    Albright dimpling s.
    Asboe-Hansen s.
    Auspitz s.
    Babinski s.
    bandage s.
    Biederman s.
    Biernacki s.
    Blatin s.
    Borsieri s.
    Brunati s.
    bulge s.
    Bunnell s.
    Buschke-Ollendorf s.
    butterfly s.
    clavicular s.
    closed accordion s.
    Comby s.
    contralateral s.
    Crowe s.
    Cullen s.
    cutaneous s.
    Darier s.
    Dawbarn s.
    daylight s.
    Demarquay s.
    Dennie s.
    Dennie-Morgan s.
    Dew s.
    dimple s.
    Dubois s.
    echo s.
    Elliot s.
    Ewart s.
    Faget s.
    Filipovitch s.
    flag s.
    floating-tooth s.
    Forchheimer s.
    Goggia s.
    Gottron s.
    Grisolle s.
    groove s.
    hair collar s.
    Hamman s.
    Hatchcock s.
    headlight s.
    Hertoghe s.
    Higouménaki s.
    Hoffman s.
    Hoover s.
    Hoyne s.
    Hutchinson s.
    impingement s.

Krisovski s.
Lasègue s.
Lennhoff s.
Leser-Trélat s.
Lhermitte s.
Lovibond profile s.
matchbox s.
McMurray s.
melanoma warning s.
Milian s.
Mirchamp s.
Muehrcke s.
Nikolsky s.
oil drop s.
Osler s.
Parrot s.
Pastia s.
Popeye s.
pseudo-Hutchinson s.
Remak s.
Romaña s.
Romberg s.
rope s.
round fingerpad s.
Rovighi s.
Rumpel-Leede s.
Schick s.
Silex s.
Sisto s.
Spurling s.
Steinberg thumb s.
tail s.
Thomson s.
Tresilian s.
trolley-track s.
Vaughn-Jackson s.
Vierra s.
Walker-Murdoch s.
Wimberger s.
Winterbottom s.
Yergason supination s.

SignaDress
S. Sterile hydrocolloid
S. Sterile hydrocolloid dressing

signal
nuclear localization s. (NLS)
s. peptide
punctate area of increased s. (PAIS)
s. recognition particle (SRP)
s. sequence
"stop" s.

s. transducer and activator of transcription (STAT)
s. transduction
s. transduction and activator of transcription (STAT)

signet ring lymphoma

significance
granulomatous lesions of unknown s. (GLUS)
McNemar test of s.
monoclonal gammopathy of unknown s. (MGUS)

SIL
squamous intraepithelial lesion

Siladryl Oral

Silafed Syrup

Silaminic Expectorant

Silastic
S. sheet
S. tubing

Sildicon-E

silencer of death domain (SODD)

"silent" chest

silent lupus nephritis

Silex sign

Silfedrine
Children's S.

silica
s. dust exposure
s. granuloma

silicone
s. breast augmentation
s. deposition
s. gel
s. gel sheeting (SGS)
s. grease
s. oil
s. particle disease
s. rubber prosthesis
s. sheeting therapy
s. synovitis

silicosis

siliquosa
variola s.

siliquose desquamation

silk
S. Laser
S. Skin sheet
s. suture

SilkLaser
2040 erbium S.

NOTES

507

SilkTouch
S. CO$_2$ Flash Scanner
S. laser
Sillence type II–IV osteogenesis imperfecta
Silon wound dressing
Siloskin dressing
Silphen Cough
sIL-1R
Silvadene
silver
Grocott methenamine s. (GMS)
s. impregnation
s. nitrate
s. poisoning
s. protein, mild
s. salts
s. stain (IFA)
s. sulfadiazine
Silverlon wound packing strip
silver-methenamine stain
silver-white-colored scale
silver-white scale
silvery
s. scale
s. scaly lesion
SIM
Sandimmune
Simbu virus
simiae
herpesvirus s.
simian
s. vacuolating virus No. 40 (SV40)
s. virus (SV)
Simmond syndrome
Simplastin Excel
Simple
S. Scoring System (SSS)
simple
s. allotype
s. drug
s. lentigo
s. pulmonary eosinophilia
s. stitch
simplex
acne s.
angioma s.
Anisakis s.
dermatitis s.
disseminated herpes s.
EB s.
epidermolysis bullosa s.
Epstein-Barr s.
erythema s.
exulceratio s.
generalized epidermolysis bullosa s.

herpes s.
hidroacanthoma s.
hypertrophicum s.
ichthyosis s.
impetigo s.
lentigo s.
lichen chronicus s.
localized epidermolysis bullosa s.
lymphangioma superficium s.
ocular herpes s.
orofacial herpes s.
pityriasis s.
protoporphyria s.
prurigo s.
purpura s.
scarlatina s.
steatocystoma s.
toxoplasmosis, other infections, rubella, cytomegalovirus infection, and herpes s. (TORCH)
s. variant
verruca s.
Simpson dysmorphia syndrome
simulated
s. gastric fluid (SGF)
s. intestinal fluid (SIF)
Simulect
Simulium
simultaneous
s. double kidney transplantation (SDKT)
s. kidney-pancreas transplantation (SKPT)
s. pancreas-kidney transplant (SPK)
simvastatin
Sinarest 12 Hour Nasal solution
Sindbis
S. fever
S. virus
Sine-Aid IB
sinensis
Cloncorchis s.
Sinequan
Sinex
S. Long-Acting
Vicks S.
Singh index
single
s. (gel) diffusion precipitin test in one dimension
s. photon emission computed tomography (SPECT)
s. radial immunodiffusion (SRID)
s. spike
single-breath nitrogen washout test
single-cell ion imaging system

single-chain
  s.-c. antigen-binding (SCA)
  s.-c. antigen-binding protein
single-hit kinetics
single-hook Frazier skin hook
single-lung
  s.-l. transplant (SLT)
  s.-l. transplant recipient
single-peak pork insulin
single-photon emission computed tomography scan
single-strand conformation polymorphism (SSCP)
single-stranded
  s.-s. anti-DNA antibody
  s.-s. conformational polymorphism (SSCP)
  s.-s. DNA
Singulair
sinobronchial
SinoJect puncture set
sinopulmonary disease
Sinubid
Sinufed Timecelles
Sinulin
sinus
  barber pilonidal s.
  cutaneous s.
  dental s.
  s. histiocytosis (SH)
  Motrin IB S.
  pilonidal s.
  Plus S.
  preauricular s.
  Rokitansky-Aschoff s.
  s. tract
  transillumination of s.
sinusitis
  acute paranasal s.
  allergic fungal s. (AFC)
  chronic paranasal s.
  ethmoid s.
sinusoid
  cavernous s.
sinusoidal
  s. blood flow
  s. cell
  s. lining cell injury
  s. phagocyte
sinusoidalization

Sinutab
  S. SA
  S. Tablet
sinuvertebral nerve
Siphonaptera
Siphoviridae
Sippy diet
Sips distribution
SIR
  standardized incidence ratio
siro
  Acarus s.
  Tyroglyphus s.
sirolimus
SIRS
  systemic inflammatory response syndrome
SIS
  Skin Intensity Score
sisal
Sister Mary Joseph nodule
Sisto sign
SIT
  specific injection immunotherapy
site
  antibody combining s.
  antigen-binding s.
  antigen-combining s.
  combining s.
  immune privileged s.
  immunologically privileged s.
  putative oxidative cleavage s.
  receptor s.
SiteGuard MVP transparent adhesive film dressing
sitophila
  Neurospora s.
sitostanol
situ
  carcinoma in s.
  in s.
  malignant melanoma in s.
situs inversus
SITx
  small intestinal transplantation
Six-Area, Six-Sign Atopic Dermatitis (SASSAD)
sixth venereal disease
size
  lesion s.
SJ441 antibody

NOTES

S

Sjögren
   S. disease
   S. syndrome (SS)
   S. syndrome A (SS-A)
   S. syndrome B (SS-B)
Sjögren-Larsson syndrome
SJS
   Stevens-Johnson syndrome
SkareKare silicon gel-filled cushion
Skeele curette
skeletal abnormality
skiagraphica
   dermatitis s.
skimming
   scalpel s.
skin
   acid s.
   alligator s.
   Apligraf tissue-engineered s.
   artificial s.
   s. atrophy
   s. bends dermatitis
   blistering s.
   bronzed s.
   s. cancer
   citrine s.
   combination s.
   composite cultured s. (CCS)
   congenital absence of s. (CLAS)
   crocodile s.
   deciduous s.
   diamond s.
   s. disease syndrome
   s. dissemination
   dry s.
   elastic s.
   elephant s.
   enamel paint s.
   s. eruption
   S. Exposure Reduction Paste
     Against Chemical Warfare
   s. exposure reduction paste against
     chemical warfare agents
     (SERPACWA)
   farmer's s.
   Favre-Racouchot s.
   fish s.
   for s. (FS)
   freeze-dried s.
   glabrous s.
   glossy s.
   golfer's s.
   granulomatous slack s.
   hanging s.
   hidden nail s.
   s. hook
   hyperextensible s. type I–VIII
   hyperirritable s.

India rubber s.
infantile acute hemorrhagic edema
  of the s.
Integra artificial s.
S. Intensity Score (SIS)
s. involvement
knobby s.
lackluster s.
lax s.
leopard s.
s. lesion
lizard s.
loose s.
s. lubrication
s. lubrication therapy
lymphocytic infiltration of the s.
marble s.
Milian citrine s.
mixed tumor of s.
monoclonal protein, s.
mosaic s.
nail s.
2nd S. hydrogel sheet
Oxy-5 Advanced Formula for
  Sensitive S.
Oxy-10 Advanced Formula for
  Sensitive S.
parchment s.
s. peel
piebald s.
pig s.
plucked chicken s.
porcupine s.
s. prick test (SPT)
primary macular atrophy of s.
primary neuroendocrine carcinoma
  of s. (PNCS)
s. punch
s. purpura
s. rash
s. reaction
s. rubor
sailor's s.
senile s.
shagreen s.
shark s.
slack s.
s. stone
striate atrophy of s.
sulci of s.
s. tag
S. Temp collagen
s. test antigens, multiple
s. testing
s. test unit (STU)
thickened s.
s. thickness score
toad s.

s. trephine
true s.
tuberculosis of s.
s. type
s. typing I–VI
s. ulcer
volar s.
waxy s.
s. wheal
white spots of s.
s. window technique
s. writing
yellow s.
skin-associated lymphoid tissue (SALT)
skin-based assay
skinbound disease
Skin-Cap spray
skin-colored
s.-c. lesion
Skindex questionnaire
SkinLaser system
Skinlight
S. erbium:YAG laser
S. erbium:YAG laser system for
skin resurfacing
skin-limited histiocytosis
skin-puncture test
Skinscan device
skin-sensitizing antibody
Skin-So-Soft
Avon S.-S.-S.
skin-specific histocompatibility antigen
SkinTech medical tattooing device
SkinTegrity
S. hydrogel dressing
S. impregnated gauze
S. wound cleanser
Skinvisible lotion
Sklowsky symptom
SKPT
simultaneous kidney-pancreas
transplantation
SK-SD
streptokinase-streptodornase
skull
hot-cross-bun s.
natiform s.
sky-blue spot
SLA
soluble liver antigen
slack skin

SLAM
Systemic Lupus Activity Measure
SLAP
superior labrum anterior and posterior
slapped-cheek
s.-c. appearance
s.-c. rash
slapped-face appearance
slash
s. pine
s. pine tree
SLC
synovial lining cell
SLD
second-line drug
SLE
systemic lupus erythematosus
SLE Disease Activity Index
(SLEDAI)
SLEDAI
SLE Disease Activity Index
sleep
S. Aid
alpha-nonrapid eye movement s.
alpha-NREM s.
s. anomaly
s. apnea
s. apnea/hypopnea syndrome
s. apnea syndrome
delta s.
desynchronized s.
s. efficiency
nonREM s.
nonrestorative s.
paradoxical s.
s. physiology
rapid eye movement s.
REM s.
restorative s.
slow wave s.
stage 1, 4 s.
stage 4 s.
s. study
sleep-disordered breathing
Sleep-Eze D
Sleep-eze 3 Oral
Sleepinal
Sleepwell 2-nite
SLE-like syndrome
slender ragweed

NOTES

S

Sleuth
    CO S.
    ETO S.
    HBT S.
SLICC
    Systemic Lupus International
    Collaborating Clinics
sliding-bucket mucosal flap
slippery
    s. elm
    s. elm tree
SLJM
    syndrome of limited joint mobility
SLN
    sentinel lymph node
Sloan liniment
Slo-bid
Slo-Niacin
slope-shouldered lesion
Slo-Phyllin GG
slough
sloughed bronchial epithelium
sloughing
    mucosal s.
    s. phagedena
    s. ulcer
slow
    s. fever
    s. virus
    s. virus disease
    s. vital capacity (SVC)
    s. wave sleep
slow-acting antirheumatic drug
  (SAARD)
slow-reacting
    s.-r. factor of anaphylaxis (SRF-A)
    s.-r. substance (SRS)
    s.-r. substance of anaphylaxis
    (SRS-A)
slow-twitch morphology of muscle fiber
SLP1000 diode laser system
SLT
    secondary lymphatic tissue
    single-lung transplant
    split-liver transplantation
    SLT recipient
slurry
    talc s.
slush
    dry-ice s.
Sly
    S. mucopolysaccharidosis
    S. syndrome
SMAD
    Sma- and Mad-related protein
small
    s. airways dysfunction
    s. bowel transplantation (SBTx)

    s. intestinal transplantation (SITx)
    s. noncleaved cell (SNC)
    s. nuclear ribonucleoprotein
    (snRNP)
    s. plaque parapsoriasis
    s. tonsil
    s. vessel vasculitis
small-plaque
    parapsoriasis s.-p.
smallpox
    fulminating s.
    s. handler's lung
    hemorrhagic s.
    malignant s.
    modified s.
    s. vaccine
    s. virus
    West Indian s.
Sma- and Mad-related protein (SMAD)
Sm antigen
SMART
    S. anti-CD3
Smart Trigger
SMAS
    superficial musculoaponeurotic system
smear
    darkfield examination of tissue s.
    nasal s.
    Tzanck s.
    wet s.
    Ziehl-Neelsen s.
smegmatis
    Mycobacterium s.
Smith antigen
Smith-Pedersen mold
Smith-Riley syndrome
smog
    industrial s.
    photochemical s.
smoke
    cigarette s.
    s. inhalation
    secondary s.
    tobacco s.
smoker
    s. keratosis
    s. patch
smooth
    s. jawed needle holder
    s. leprosy
    s. muscle hamartoma
    s. muscle relaxation
    s. skin-colored lesion
    s. stinger
smotherweed
SMR
    Standard Morbidity Ratio

SMS
  stiff-man syndrome
smut
  Bermuda s.
  corn s.
  cultivated barley s.
  cultivated corn s.
  cultivated oat s.
  cultivated rye s.
  cultivated wheat s.
  Johnson s.
snail-track ulcer
snake
  Arizona coral s.
  s. bite
  copperhead s.
  coral s.
  cottonmouth s.
  Eastern coral s.
  pit viper s.
  sea s.
  terrestrial s.
  Texas coral s.
  s. venom
  venomous s.
  water moccasin s.
snakebite
snakeroot
  Seneca s.
SNAP
  sensory nerve action potential
  SNAP sleep recorder
snap-frozen section
Snaplets-EX
Snaplets-FR granule
snapping
  s. finger
  s. hip
SNC
  small noncleaved cell
Sneddon syndrome
Sneddon-Wilkinson disease
sneezeweed
sneezing
  paroxysmal s.
SnET2
snowball aggregate
snowbank aggregate
snowshoe hare virus
snRNP
  small nuclear ribonucleoprotein
  U3 snRNP

snuffles
SNV
  systemic necrotizing vasculitis
SO$_2$
  sulfur dioxide
soak therapy
soap
  Alpha-Keri s.
  Ayndet moisturizing s.
  Baby Magic s.
  Basis s.
  Clinique Antiacne S.
  Derma S.
  s. dermatitis
  Derm-Vi S.
  Dial s.
  Dove s.
  hard-milled s.
  Mazon Medicated S.
  s. photoallergy
  syndet-based bar s.
soapfish dermatitis
sobria
  Aeromonas s.
soccer toe
SODD
  silencer of death domain
sodium
  actinoquinol s.
  alendronate s.
  aminosalicylate s.
  Ampicin S.
  s. aurothioglucose
  s. aurothiomalate
  s. bicarbonate
  Brequinar s.
  carboxymethylcellulose s.
  cefazolin s.
  cefmetazole s.
  cefonicid s.
  cefoperazone s.
  cefotaxime s.
  cefoxitin s.
  ceftizoxime s.
  ceftriaxone s.
  cephalothin s.
  cephapirin s.
  s. citrate and citric acid
  cloxacillin s.
  colistimethate s.
  s. cromoglycate
  cromolyn s.

NOTES

S

sodium *(continued)*
    diclofenac s.
    dicloxacillin s.
    Diphenylan S.
    s. dodecyl sulfate-polyacrylamide gel electrophoresis (SDS-PAGE)
    s. dodecyl sulfate-polyacrylamide gradient slab gel
    s. etidronate
    foscarnet s.
    s. hyaluronate
    s. hydroxide
    s. hypochlorite solution
    s. hyposulfite
    intravesical oxychlorosene s.
    s. lauryl sulfate
    Lescol fluvastatin s.
    levothyroxine s.
    meclofenamate s.
    2-mercaptoethane sulphonate s. (mesna)
    methicillin s.
    mezlocillin s.
    s. morrhuate
    nafcillin s.
    naproxen s.
    nedocromil s.
    olsalazine s.
    oxacillin s.
    oxychlorosene s.
    paraaminosalicylate s.
    S. P.A.S.
    s. pentosan
    pentosan polysulfate s.
    Photofrin porfimer s.
    piperacillin sodium and tazobactam s.
    s. salt
    stibogluconate s.
    S. Sulamyd Ophthalmic
    s. sulfacetamide
    s. sulfacetamide and fluorometholone
    s. sulfacetamide and phenylephrine
    s. sulfacetamide and prednisolone
    s. tetradecyl sulfate
    s. thiosulfate
    tolmetin s.
    s. versenate solution
    warfarin s.
sodium-PCA
    lactic acid and s.-P.
sodium-potassium (Na$^+$-K$^+$)
    s.-p. ATPase pump
Sofban orthopedic padding wool
Sof-Cil
Sof-Gel palm shield
SofSorb absorptive dressing

soft
    s. chancre
    s. corn
    s. keratin
    s. lesion
    S. N Dry Merocel sponge
    s. nevus
    s. papilloma
    s. sore
    s. tick
    s. tissue
    s. tissue calcification
    s. ulcer
    s. wart
SoftCloth absorptive dressing
Softech endotracheal tube
SoftForm facial implant
Softgels
    Vita-Plus E S.
SoftLight
    S. laser hair removal system
    S. laser/skin resurfacing process
Softscan laser scanner
Sof-Wick dressing
Solage Topical solution
solani
    Fusarium s.
    Stemphylium s.
Solaquin
    S. Forte
    S. Forte cream
solar
    s. cheilitis
    s. comedo
    s. dermatitis
    s. elastosis
    s. fever
    s. ink-spot lentigo
    s. keratosis
    s. purpura
    s. urticaria
Solarase topical gel
solare
    eczema s.
    erythema s.
solaris
    dermatitis s.
    macula s.
    s. urticaria
Solatene
Solbar sunscreen
soldering
    s. flux
    s. fumes
soldier patch
sole
    diffuse hyperkeratosis of palms and s.'s

S

s. dyshidrosis
symmetric lividity of the s.'s
solenonychia
Solenopsis
    S. geminata
    S. invecta
    S. invecta sting
    S. richteri sting
    S. saevissima richteria
Solganal
solid
    s. carbon dioxide
    s. carbon dioxide pencil
    s. hidradenoma
    s. organ transplantation (SOT)
    s. phase immunoassay (SPIA)
solid-phase C1q-binding assay
solid-state dye laser
solid-tumor marker
solitary
    s. angiokeratoma
    s. keratoacanthoma
    s. mastocytoma
    s. simple lymphangioma
solium
    Taenia s.
SoloSite
    S. hydrogel dressing
    S. wound gel
soluble
    s. cell adhesion molecule
    s. c-kit (sc-kit)
    s. complement receptor type 1
    (sCR1)
    s. co-stimulatory factor
    s. Fas (sFas)
    s. liver antigen (SLA)
    s. receptor
    s. specific substance (SSS)
    S. T4
    s. tumor necrosis factor-a receptor
    type I (sTNF-RI)
Solu-Cortef
Solugel
Solumbra sunscreen clothing
Solu-Medrol Injection
solum unguis
Solurex L.A.
Soluspan
    Celestone S.
solution
    Adsorbotear Ophthalmic s.

Afrin Nasal S.
AK-Dilate Ophthalmic s.
AK-Nefrin Ophthalmic s.
Akwa Tears s.
Alibour s.
Allerest 12 Hour Nasal S.
aluminum chloride s.
Anti-Sept bactericidal scrub s.
AquaSite Ophthalmic s.
aqueous s.
Atrovent Inhalation S.
azelastine hydrochloride
    ophthalmic s.
B5 s.
Belzer s.
Bion Tears s.
Bluboro s.
Bouin s.
Burow s.
carbol-fuchsin s.
Chlorphed-LA Nasal S.
ciclopirox topical s.
Collins s.
Comfort Tears s.
Crolom Ophthalmic s.
Dakrina Ophthalmic s.
Dey-Drop Ophthalmic s.
Dristan Long Lasting Nasal s.
Dry Eyes s.
Dry Eye Therapy s.
DuoFilm S.
Duration Nasal s.
Dwelle Ophthalmic s.
EC s.
Euro-Collins s.
Exidine s.
extracellular crystalloid s.
Eye-Lube-A s.
flunisolide nasal s.
Fowler s.
Freezone s.
Fungoid AF Topical s.
Hanks balanced salt s. (HBSS)
HypoTears PF s.
hypotonic s.
Intal Nebulizer s.
intracellular crystalloid s.
I-Phrine Ophthalmic s.
Isopto Frin Ophthalmic s.
Isopto Plain s.
Isopto Tears s.
Just Tears s.

NOTES

solution *(continued)*
>Kaletra oral s.
>Lacril Ophthalmic s.
>Liquifilm Forte s.
>Liquifilm Tears s.
>lopinavir/ritonavir oral s.
>Lotrimin AF S.
>LubriTears s.
>Melanex s.
>Michel s.
>Monsel s.
>Murine s.
>Murocel Ophthalmic s.
>Mydfrin Ophthalmic s.
>Nasalcrom Nasal s.
>Nature's Tears s.
>Neosporin Ophthalmic S.
>Neo-Synephrine 12 Hour Nasal s.
>Neo-Synephrine Ophthalmic s.
>NTZ Long Acting Nasal S.
>Nu-Tears II s.
>OcuCoat PF Ophthalmic s.
>POL sclerosing s.
>potassium permanganate s.
>precipitate in s.
>Prefrin Ophthalmic s.
>Procuven s.
>Puralube Tears s.
>Refinity skin care s.
>Refresh Plus Ophthalmic s.
>Relief Ophthalmic s.
>Resectisol Irrigation s.
>salt s.
>SangCya oral s.
>Shohl s.
>Sinarest 12 Hour Nasal s.
>sodium hypochlorite s.
>sodium versenate s.
>Solage Topical s.
>STS sclerosing s.
>St. Thomas s.
>Tear Drop s.
>TearGard Ophthalmic s.
>Teargen Ophthalmic s.
>Tearisol s.
>Tears Naturale Free s.
>Tears Naturale II s.
>Tears Plus s.
>Tears Renewed s.
>TRIS-buffered saline s. (TBS)
>trivalent oral poliovirus s.
>Tween-TRIS-buffered saline s. (TTBS)
>Twice-A-Day Nasal s.
>Ultra Tears s.
>University of Wisconsin s. (UW solution)
>UV s.

>UW s.
>>University of Wisconsin solution
>Verukan s.
>Vicks Sinex Long-Acting Nasal s.
>vinegar s.
>Viva-Drops s.
>Vleminckx s.
>4-Way Long Acting Nasal S.

Soluver plus
solvent-based mascara
somaliensis
>*Streptomyces s.*

somatic
>s. agglutinin
>s. antigen
>s. hypermutation
>s. mutation

SomatoKine
somatomedin C
somatosensory evoked response
somatotype
>body s.

somatropin
Sominex Oral
sommeil
>maladie du s.

SomnoStar apnea testing device
soni
>*Moniliformis s.*

sonicate
Sonne dysentery
sonnei
>*Shigella s.*

Sony VHS HQ Digital Picture video
Soothe-N-Seal
soot wart
SorbaView wound dressing
sorbitan sesquioleate (SS)
Sorbsan
>S. alginate dressing
>S. alginate wound cover
>S. wound dressing

sordes
sore
>bay s.
>bed s.
>canker s.
>chrome s.
>Cochin s.
>cold s.
>Delhi s.
>desert s.
>diphtheric desert s.
>fever s.
>fungating s.
>Gallipoli s.
>hard s.
>Kandahar s.

Lahore s.
mixed s.
s. mouth
Naga s.
Oriental s.
pressure s.
primary s.
soft s.
summer s.
tropical s.
Umballa s.
veldt s.
venereal s.
water s.
soremouth virus
soremuzzle
soreness
sor gene
sorghum grass
Soriatane
sorivudine
sorrel
sheep s.
sorter
fluorescence-activated cell s.
(FACS)
sorting
fluorescence-activated cell s.
(FACS)
fluorescent-activated cell s. (FACS)
SOT
solid organ transplantation
Soto syndrome
Sotradecol
souffle
sound
coarse breath s.
diminished breath s.
pulmonic valve closure s.
source
intense pulsed light s. (IPLS)
monochromatic light s.
PhotoDerm filtered, flashlamp-
pumped light s.
PhotoDerm VL light s.
South
S. African genetic porphyria
S. African hemorrhagic fever
S. African tick fever
S. American blastomycosis
S. American trypanosomiasis
Southeast Asian fever

Southern blot
sowdah
Soyalac
soybean
s. flour
s. grain dust mite
s. meal
soy milk
SP
Cordran S.
Sp-100
SP-10 spirometer
SP90 miniblade
SpA
spondyloarthropathy
space
blood-filled slit-like s.
intercellular s.
marrow s.
medial hemijoint articular s.
physiological dead s.
subgaleal s.
Tenon s.
space-occupying lesion
spacer
Ellipse compact s.
SPAD
selective antipolysaccharide antibody
deficiency
spade finger
**spaghetti and meatballs appearance of
spores and hyphae**
Spanish
S. fly
S. fly sting
S. influenza
S. toxic oil syndrome
Spanlang-Tappeiner syndrome
spanner
multimembrane s.
sparfloxacin
sparganosis
sparing
island of s.
spark-gap apparatus
SPART analyzer
spasm
epidemic transient diaphragmatic s.
spasmogen
SpaTouch PhotoEpilation system
spatula
Roux s.

S

NOTES

SPE
serum protein electrophoretogram
streptococcal pyrogenic exotoxin
Spearman rank test
specialized transduction
special lesion
species
Phoma s.
reactive oxygen s. (ROS)
species-specific antigen
specific
s. active immunity
s. alteration in immunologic
reactivity
s. anergy
s. antibody deficiency (SAD)
s. antigen
s. antiserum
s. bactericide
s. capsular substance
s. disease
s. hemolysin
s. IgE antibody level
s. immune globulin (human)
s. injection immunotherapy (SIT)
s. opsonin
s. passive immunity
s. reaction
s. serum
s. soluble polysaccharide
s. soluble sugar
s. transduction
specificity
speck finger
speckled
s. lentiginous nevus
s. staining
speckled-pattern
s.-p. ANA
s.-p. antinuclear antibody
SPECT
single photon emission computed
tomography
SPECT scan
Spectam injection
Spectazole topical
spectinomycin hydrochloride
spectra (*pl. of* spectrum)
Spectracef
spectral analysis
spectratyping
Spectrobid
spectrofluorometer
spectrofluorometry
spectrophotometer
spectrophotometry

spectroscopy
diffuse reflectance s. (DRS)
flame emission s. (FES)
Spectro Tar
spectrum, pl. **spectra**
antimicrobial s.
broad s.
S. Designs facial implant
radiation s.
S. ruby laser
toxin s.
wide s.
speech apraxia
Spencer scissors
Spengler fragment
SPEP
serum protein electrophoresis
SPEP test
spermatolysin
spermatolysis
spermatolytic
spermatoxin
spermine
spermolysis
spermotoxin
Spexil
SPF
sun protection factor
sphacelation
sphaceloderma
sphaericus
Bacillus s.
sphenoethmoidectomy
sphenoid dysplasia
spherocytosis
hereditary s.
Spherulin
sphigosine kinase
Sphingobacterium
sphingolipid
sphingolipidosis
Sphingomonas paucimobilis
sphingomyelinase-D
SPI
Standards for Pediatric Immunization
SPIA
solid phase immunoassay
spica cast
spicule
hyperkeratotic s.
spider
s. angioma
arterial s.
s. bite
black widow s.
brown recluse s.
s. ectasia
fiddle-back s.

s. hemangioma
s. mole
s. nevus
s. telangiectasia
s. telangiectasis
s. venom
violin-back s.
spider-burst
Spiegler-Fendt
S.-F. pseudolymphoma
S.-F. sarcoid
Spiegler tumor
spike
s. formation
single s.
spiloma
spiloplaxia
spilus
nevus s.
spina
s. bifida-associated latex allergy
s. pedis
spinach
spinal
s. accessory nerve palsy
s. dysraphism
s. fluid test
spinale
tache s.
spindle
s. cell
s. cell carcinoma
s. cell hemangioendothelioma
s. cell lipoma
s. cell melanoma
s. and epithelioid cell nevus
spindle-shaped cell
spine
bamboo s.
horny s.
Rugger-jersey s.
venom-bearing s.
spin-echo pulse
Spinhaler inhaler
spinigerum
Gnathostoma s.
spinipalpis
Ixodes s.
spinosa
ichthyosis s.
spinosum
stratum s.

spinous layer
spinulosa
trichostasis s.
spinulosus
folliculitis decalvans et lichen s.
lichen pilaris seu s.
spiny
s. pigweed
s. structure
spiradenitis
spiradenoma
eccrine s.
malignant eccrine s.
spiral
Curschmann s.
Herxheimer s.
spiralis
Trichina s.
Trichinella s.
spiramycin
spirillar
s. abscess
s. dysentery
Spirillum minus
Spirochaeta pallida
spirochetal disease
spirochete
corkscrew s.
s. infection
spirochetemia
spirochetolysis
spirochetosis
spirogram
forced expiratory s. (FES)
spirometer
Flash portable s.
MicroPlus s.
Pulmonet s.
SP-10 s.
Spirovit SP-1 portable s.
spirometric screening
spirometry
incentive s.
Tri-Flow incentive s.
spironolactone
Spiroplasma apis
SpiroSense flow sensor
Spirovit SP-1 portable spirometer
spiruroid larva migrans
Spitz
S. nevus
S. tumor

S

NOTES

spitzoid malignant melanoma
SPK
    simultaneous pancreas-kidney transplant
splash
    rain s.
    wave s.
splatter
    fountain-spray s.
spleen
    synergic s.
splendens
    lamina s.
Splendore-Hoeppli phenomenon
splenectomy (Splx)
splenic index
splenomegaly
splenotoxin
spliceosomal component
splicing
    phosphorylated serine/arginine s.
splint
    hindfoot s.
    resting s.
    shin s.
splinter
    s. forceps
    s. hemorrhage
split
    s. adjuvant technique
    s. papule
    s. tolerance
split-liver transplantation (SLT)
split-thickness skin graft (STSG)
splitting nail
split-virus vaccine
Splx
    splenectomy
spodogenous
spodophorous
Spondweni virus
spondylitica
    psoriasis s.
spondylitide
spondylitis
    ankylosing s. (AS)
    Bekhterev-Strümpell s.
    juvenile ankylosing s. (JAS)
    s. ossificans ligamentosa
    predominant s.
    psoriatic s.
    Schober test for s.
spondyloarthropathy (SpA)
    seronegative s.
    undifferentiated s.
spondylodiscitis
spondyloepiphyseal dysplasia (SED)
spondylolisthesis
    isthmic s.

spondylolysis
spondylometry
spondylosis
    s. deformans
    s. hyperostotica
    ochronotic s.
sponge
    chondrocyte s.
    s. diver disease
    s. fisherman disease
    Helistat collagen matrix s.
    Instat collagen matrix s.
    Soft N Dry Merocel s.
    s. spicule dermatitis
spongiform
    s. pustule
    s. pustule of Kogoj
spongiosis
    eosinophilic s.
spongiotic vesicle
spontanea
    dactylolysis s.
spontaneous
    s. agglutination
    s. allergy
    s. gangrene of newborn
    s. phagocytosis
    s. pseudoscar
    s. regression
    s. spinal epidural hematoma
    (SSEH)
spoon
    s. nail
    sharp s.
spora
    air s.
sporadic
    s. atypical mole-melanoma
    syndrome
    s. dysentery
    s. typhus
sporangiospore
sporangium
Sporanox Oral
spore
    airborne s.
    mold s.
Sporidin-G
sporoagglutination
Sporobolomyces salmonicolor
Sporothrix schenckii
sporotrichosis
    cutaneous s.
    disseminated s.
    fixed cutaneous s.

mucocutaneous s.
visceral s.
sporotrichositic chancre
sporotrichotic chancre
Sporotrichum schenckii
sporotricoid pattern
sporotriquin test
sporozoite
sporozooid
Sport
Coppertone S.
Fruit of the Earth Moisturizing
Aloe S.
London Drugs S.
S. Wipes
sports medicine
SPO₂T
Pocket S.
spot
antimony s.
ash leaf s.
Bier s.
Bitot s.
blue s.
café-au-lait s.
Campbell-De Morgan s.
cayenne pepper s.
cherry s.
Christopher s.
cinnabar red s.
cotton-wool s.
De Morgan s.
Filatov s.
Forchheimer s.
Fordyce s.
gift s.
Horder s.
Koplik s.
liver s.
mongolian s.
mulberry s.
pain s.
pink s.
rose s.
Roth s.
ruby s.
sacral s.
shin s.
sky-blue s.
temperature s.
s. test
Trousseau s.

typhoid s.
warm s.
s. weld
SpotCheck+ handheld pulse oximeter
spotted
s. fever
s. leprosy
s. lunula
s. sickness
spotted-fever tick
spray
aerosol s.
Astelin Nasal S.
azelastine hydrochloride nasal s.
budesonide aqueous nasal s.
(BANS)
CaldeCort Anti-Itch Topical S.
Clear Caladryl S.
Decongestant Nasal S.
Fluori-Methane Topical S.
Nasarel Nasal S.
Ony-Clear S.
Skin-Cap s.
Tri-Nasal S.
vapocoolant s.
spreading phenomenon
spring
s. dermatosis
s. ophthalmia
spring-assisted knee extension orthosis
sprout
Brussels s.
SPRT
sequential probability ratio test
spruce tree
sprue
celiac s.
nontropical s.
SPS
Proteque SPS
SPT
skin prick test
SPTL
subcutaneous panniculitis-like T-cell
lymphoma
Spumavirinae
Spumavirus
spun-glass hair
spur
bony s.
calcaneal s.
heel s.

S

NOTES

Spurling sign
sputum, pl. **sputa**
    copious s.
    purulent s.
    s. viscosity and elasticity
SQ
    subcutaneous
squama
squamate
squame
squamosum
    eczema s.
    erythroderma s.
squamous
    s. cell
    s. cell carcinoma (SCC)
    s. cell epithelioma
    s. cell layer
    s. cell lung tumor
    s. intraepithelial lesion (SIL)
square-shouldered lesion
squaric acid dibutylester (SADBE)
squarrose
squash
squeeze effect
SR
    Aerolate SR
    Deconamine SR
    Respaire-120 SR
    Respaire-60 SR
    Surgam SR
SR-31747
Sr
    Congess Sr
SRC
    scleroderma renal crisis
SRF-A
    slow-reacting factor of anaphylaxis
SRID
    single radial immunodiffusion
SRM
    standardized response mean
SRP
    signal recognition particle
SRS
    slow-reacting substance
SRS-A
    slow-reacting substance of anaphylaxis
SS
    Sjögren syndrome
    sorbitan sesquioleate
    SS hemoglobin disease
    Uroplus SS
S.S.
    Argyrol S.S.
SS-A
    Sjögren syndrome A

SS-B
    Sjögren syndrome B
SSC
    saline sodium citrate
    suprascapular nerve compression
SSc
    systemic sclerosis
SSCP
    single-strand conformation polymorphism
    single-stranded conformational
      polymorphism
SSD
    SSD AF
    SSD Cream
SSEH
    spontaneous spinal epidural hematoma
S-shaped closure
SSKI
    saturated solution of potassium iodide
SSM
    superficial spreading melanoma
SSOP
    sequence-specific oligonucleotide probe
      hybridization
SSP
    sequence-specific primer
SSPE
    subacute sclerosing panencephalitis
SSS
    Simple Scoring System
    soluble specific substance
    SSS score
SSSS
    staphylococcal scalded skin syndrome
ssSSc
    systemic sclerosis sine scleroderma
SSZ
    sulfasalazine
S-T
    S.-T. Cort
    S.-T. Cort Topical
ST
    surrogate tolerogenesis
St.
    St. Anthony fire
    St. Joseph Adult Chewable Aspirin
    St. Louis encephalitis
    St. Louis encephalitis virus
    St. Thomas solution
stabilate
stable
    s. fly
    s. fly bite
    s. knob trimer
Stachybotrys atra
stacking
    epidermal s.

stadiometry
stadium, pl. **stadia**
  s. acmes
  s. augmenti
  s. caloris
  s. decrementi
  s. defervescentiae
  s. fluorescentiae
  s. frigoris
  s. incrementi
  s. invasionis
  s. sudoris
stage
  algid s.
  cold s.
  convalescent s.
  defervescent s.
  incubative s.
  s. of invasion
  Kellgren-Lawrence s.
  latent s.
  meningeal s.
  patch s.
  plaque s.
  prodromal s.
  s. 1, 4 sleep
  s. 4 sleep
  Tanner pubertal s.
  tumor s.
staged abdominal repair (STAR)
staging
  Ann Arbor s.
  Breslow thickness in melanoma s.
  s. classification for Hodgkin
    disease
  TNM s.
  tumor, node, metastasis s.
stain
  acid Schiff s.
  ACIS immunohistochemical s.
  Alcian blue s.
  aldehyde-fuchsin s. (AFS)
  alizarin red S s.
  Automated Cellular Imaging System
    immunohistochemical s.
  Bodian s.
  bovine rotavirus s.
  Brown-Brenn s.
  Brown and Brenn s.
  calcofluor s.
  Clay-Adams s.
  Congo red s.

cytotoxin-positive s.
Dieterle s.
Diff-Quik s.
elastic fibers s.
eosin s.
Evans blue s.
Fite s.
fluorescent antibody s. (FA)
Giemsa s.
Gram s.
hematoxylin and eosin s. (H&E)
Hotchkiss-McManus s.
immunofluorescent s.
Kinyoun s.
levodopa s.
Masson trichrome s.
MPO bone marrow s.
    myeloperoxidase bone marrow
    stain
mucicarmine s.
myeloperoxidase bone marrow s.
  (MPO bone marrow stain)
neuron-specific enolase s.
nonspecific esterase s.
NSE s.
PAS s.
periodic acid-Schiff s.
phloxine-tartrazine s.
pneumococcal s.
port-wine s. (PWS)
potassium chloride s. (KOH)
rose-bengal s.
Safranin O s.
silver s. (IFA)
silver-methenamine s.
Swartz-Lamkins s.
Swartz-Medrik s.
Verhoeff-van Gieson s.
walnut-juice s.
Warthin-Starry s.
Wright s.
Ziehl-Neelsen s.
staining
  avidin-biotin-peroxidase s.
  diffuse s.
  Hoechst s.
  nucleolar s.
  pattern of s.
  peripheral s.
  phalloidin s.
  rose Bengal s.
  speckled s.

S

NOTES

Stallerkit
Stallerpointe needle
staminate
standard
    s. deviation (SD)
    S. Morbidity Ratio (SMR)
standardized
    s. incidence ratio (SIR)
    s. response mean (SRM)
Standards
    National Committee for Clinical
      Laboratory S. (NCCLS)
    S. for Pediatric Immunization (SPI)
standing cutaneous cone defect
Stanford Health Assessment
  Questionnaire (HAQ)
stanozolol
Stanton disease
Staphcillin
Staph. protein A column therapy
StaphVAX
staphylococcal
    s. abscess
    s. blepharitis
    s. enterotoxin
    s. protein A binding assay
    s. scalded skin syndrome (SSSS)
    s. toxic shock syndrome
staphylococcal-binding assay
staphylococcolysin
staphylococcolysis
Staphylococcus
    S. *albus*
    S. *aureus*
    S. *aureus* arthritis
    S. *aureus* vaccine
    S. *epidermidis*
    S. *hominis*
    S. *lugdunensis*
    methicillin-resistant S. *aureus*
      (MRSA)
staphylococcus
    s. antitoxin
staphyloderma
staphylodermatitis
staphylogenes
    impetigo s.
    sycosis s.
staphylohemolysin
staphylolysin
staphylotoxin
stapler
    Auto Suture SFS s.
    Precise s.
    Premium s.
    Proximate II, III s.
    Proximate RH s.
    USSC s.

stapling
    bleb s.
STAR
    staged abdominal repair
star
    S. Sync
    venous s.
Starcam large field of view gamma
  camera
starch bath
starch-iodine test
starfish
    s. dermatitis
    s. sting
starry-sky pattern
startle disease
starvation syndrome
stasis
    dermatitis s.
    s. dermatitis
    eczema s.
    s. eczema
    s. purpura
    s. vascular ulcer
STAT
    signal transducer and activator of
      transcription
    signal transduction and activator of
      transcription
state
    anaphylactic s.
    carrier s.
    excited s.
    hypercoagulable s.
    hyperimmune s.
static gangrene
Staticin topical
stationary phase
statistical analysis system (SAS)
Statistics
    National Center for Health S.
      (NCHS)
stature
    brittle hair, intellectual impairment,
      decreased fertility, short s.
      (BIDS)
    decreased fertility, short s.
    ichthyosis plus brittle hair,
      intellectual impairment, decreased
      fertility, short s. (IBIDS)
    impairment, decreased fertility,
      short s.
    photosensitivity, ichthyosis, brittle
      hair, impaired intelligence,
      decreased fertility, and short s.
      (PIBIDS)
    photosensitivity, ichthyosis, brittle
      hair, intellectual impairment,

decreased fertility, and short s. (PIBIDS)

status
- s. asthmaticus
- s. cosmeticus
- s. criticus
- s. epilepticus

staurosporine

stavudine

STD
sexually transmitted disease

STD-E Pads

steal effect

stealthing gene

Stealth virus

stearalkonium ammonium chloride

stearic acid

stearothermophilus
Bacillus s.

steatocystoma
- multiplex s.
- s. multiplex
- s. simplex

steatohepatitis

steatoides
- pityriasis s.

steatoma

steatorrhea
- postinfectious s.

steatosis
- macrovesicular s.
- microvesicular s.

steel
- S. Bars high protein nutrition bar
- s. factor

Stegman-Tromovitch bandage

Steinberg
- S. test
- S. thumb sign

Steinbrocker
- S. classification
- S. criteria

Stein-Leventhal syndrome

stellar nevus

stellate
- s. abscess
- s. angioma
- s. ganglion block
- s. ganglion blockade
- s. hair
- s. morphology
- s. pattern

- s. patterned disease
- s. pseudoscar
- s. telangiectasis

stem
- s. cell
- s. cell factor (SCF)
- s. cell transplant (SCT)
- s. cell transplantation

Stemex

Stemphylium
- *S. botryosum*
- *S. solani*

stenosing tenosynovitis

stenosis, pl. **stenoses**
- bronchial s.
- cicatricial s.
- subglottic tracheal s.
- tracheal s.

stenothermal

Stenotrophomonas maltophilia

stent
- T-Y s.

stenting
- ureteric s.

Stephania tetranda

Stephanurus dentatus

Sterapred Oral

stercoralis
- *Strongyloides s.*

sterile
- s. abscess
- s. eosinophilic pustulosis
- s. pustule
- s. technique

sterilisans
- therapia magna s.

sterility

sterilization
- discontinuous s.
- fractional s.
- intermittent s.

sterilize

sterilizer

Steri-Strips

Sterneedle tuberculin test

sternoclavicular
- s. articulation
- s. disease
- s. hyperostosis
- s. joint
- s. joint degeneration

sternocleidomastoid muscle

NOTES

S

sternocostal joint
sternocostoclavicular hyperostosis
sternomastoid
steroid
    s. acne
    anabolic s.
    s. burst
    s. chalk
    s. fever
    group 5 topical s.
    s. myopathy
    Psorcon topical s.
    s. pulse
    s. purpura
    s. sulfatase deficiency
    systemic s.
    s. taper
    topical s.
    s. ulcer
steroid-dependent asthma
steroidogenic enzyme
steroid-resistant acute rejection
steroid-sparing
    s.-s. regimen
    s.-s. treatment
sterol
stethoscope dermatitis
Stevens-Johnson syndrome (SJS)
Stevens tenotomy scissors
Stewart-Treves syndrome
STI
    short-term immunotherapy
stibogluconate sodium
Sticker disease
Stickler
    S. syndrome
    S. syndrome, type I, II, III
Stieva-A Forte
Stifcore
stiff-hand syndrome
stiff-man syndrome (SMS)
stiffness
    morning s.
stiff-person syndrome
stiff-skin syndrome
stigma, pl. stigmata
stigmatic
stilbestrol
Still disease
stimulating factor (SF)
stimulation
    alpha adrenergic s.
    beta adrenergic s.
    juxtacrine s.
    transcutaneous electrical nerve s.
      (TENS)
stimulator
    long-acting thyroid s. (LATS)

    Sham transcutaneous electrical
      nerve s.
    transcutaneous electrical
      neuromuscular s. (TENS)
stimulea
    Sibine s.
stimulus, pl. stimuli
    chemical s.
    extrauterine environmental s.
    physical s.
    psychological s.
sting
    Africanized honeybee s.
    ant s.
    Apis mellifera s.
    arthropod s.
    ashgray blister beetle s.
    bark scorpion s.
    bee s.
    blister beetle s.
    blue bottle s.
    Bombus s.
    box jellyfish s.
    brown moth larvae s.
    brown-tail moth s.
    bumblebee s.
    caterpillar s.
    catfish s.
    Centruroides exilicauda s.
    Centruroides sculpturatus s.
    Centruroides vittatus s.
    Chironex fleckeri s.
    coelenterate s.
    common striped scorpion s.
    Dolichorespula s.
    Epicauta fabricii s.
    Epicauta vitlata s.
    Euproctis chrysorrhoea s.
    European blister beetle s.
    fire ant s.
    fire coral s.
    gypsy moth larva s.
    honeybee s.
    hornet s.
    Hymenoptera s.
    insect s.
    Io moth larva s.
    jellyfish s.
    Lymantria dispar s.
    Lytta vesicata s.
    marine animal s.
    Megabombus s.
    Megalopyge opercularis s.
    millipede s.
    Paederus gemellus s.
    Paederus limnophilus s.
    Paravespula s.
    Polistes s.

Portuguese man-of-war s.
puss caterpillar s.
Pyrobombus s.
red imported fire ant s.
saddleback caterpillar s.
scorpion s.
sea anemone s.
sea cucumber s.
sea urchin s.
Sibine stimulea s.
Solenopsis invecta s.
Solenopsis richteri s.
Spanish fly s.
starfish s.
sting ray s.
striped blister beetle s.
Vespula s.
wasp s.
yellow jacket s.

stinger
barbed s.
imbedded s.
smooth s.

stinging
s. caterpillar
s. coral dermatitis
s. water dermatitis

stingray hickey
stink gland
stinkweed
stippled nail
STIR
short tau inversion recovery

stitch
buried subcutaneous s.
corner s.
half-buried mattress s.
horizontal mattress s.
running intradermal s.
running simple s.
simple s.
tip s.
vertical mattress s.

STM
streptomycin

sTNFR gene
sTNF-RI
soluble tumor necrosis factor-a receptor
type I

Stobo antigen
stochastic methylation

stock
s. strain
s. vaccine

stocking
s. nevus
Venodyne compression s.
Zipzoc s.

Stockman nodule
stoichiometry
Stokoguard outdoor cream
stomach
watermelon s.

stomal dermatitis
stomatitis
allergic contact s.
angular s.
aphthous s.
bovine papular s.
cotton roll s.
denture s.
fusospirochetal s.
gangrenous s.
gonococcal s.
lead s.
s. medicamentosa
mercurial s.
nicotine s.
s. papulosa
primary herpetic s.
ulcerative s.
vesicular s.

stomatodynia
stomatomalacia
stomatomycosis
stomatonecrosis
stomatonoma
stomatopyrosis
Stomoxys bite
stone
pumice s.
skin s.

stool
s. culture
mucous s.

stool-step maneuver
stop bath
"stop" signal
storage
cold s. (CS)
ex vivo organ s.
neutral lipid s.
phytanic acid s.

NOTES

S

store and forward images
stork-bite lesion
Stoxil
straight hair nevus
straight-leg
    s.-l. duration maneuver
    s.-l. lift maneuver
strain
    BORSA s.
    carrier s.
    cell s.
    0157-H7 s.
    hypothetical mean s. (HMS)
    lysogenic s.
    modified vaccinia virus Ankara s.
    pseudolysogenic s.
    rabies virus, Flury s.
    rabies virus, Kelev s.
    recombinant s.
    stock s.
    type s.
strand
    AcryDerm S.'s
    complementary s.
    homology of s.
    plus s.
    viral s.
S-transferase
    glutathione S.-t. (GST)
strata (pl. of stratum)
StrataSorb composite wound dressing
strategy
    prime-boost s.
    sawtooth s.
stratification
stratum, pl. strata
    s. basale
    central s.
    s. compactum
    s. corneum (SC)
    s. corneum epidermidis
    s. corneum unguis
    s. disjunctum
    s. germinativum
    s. granulosum (SG)
    s. lucidum
    s. malpighii
    s. mucosum
    s. spinosum
strawberry
    s. angioma
    s. birthmark
    s. hemangioma
    s. hypertrophicum
    s. mark
    s. nevus
    s. tongue
straw itch

streak
    angioid s.
    meningitic s.
streaking
    s. leukocyte factor
    linear s.
street virus
Strength
    Allerest Maximum S.
    Aspirin Free Anacin Maximum S.
    Bayer Low Adult S.
    Clearasil Maximum S.
    Clocort Maximum S.
    Cortaid Maximum S.
    Vanceril Double S.
streptobacillary fever
Streptobacillus moniliformis
streptocerca
    Dipetalonema s.
    Mansonella s.
streptococcal
    s. balanoposthitis
    s. cellulitis
    s. M1
    s. M3
    s. M antigen
    s. nephritis
    s. pharyngitis
    s. pyrogenic exotoxin (SPE)
    s. septicemia
    s. tonsillitis
    s. toxic shock syndrome
Streptococcus
    S. agalactiae
    S. faecalis
    S. infection
    S. intermedius
    S. M antigen
    penicillin-resistant *S. pneumoniae* (PRSP)
    S. pyogenes
    S. viridans
streptococcus, pl. streptococci
    beta-hemolytic s.
    s. erythrogenic toxin
    group A s. (GAS)
    group A beta-hemolytic s. (GABHS)
    group B s. (GBS)
    hemolytic s.
streptoderma
streptodermatitis
streptogenes
    erythema s.
streptogramin
streptokinase-streptodornase (SK-SD)
streptolysin O

Streptomyces
  S. *somaliensis*
  S. *toyocaensis*
  S. *tsukubaensis*
streptomycin (STM)
  G unit of s.
  L unit of s.
  s. sulfate
  S unit of s.
  s. unit
streptozyme (STZ)
  s. agglutination test
  s. titer
stress
  electrophilic s. (ES)
  emotional s.
  s. fracture
  intrapsychic s.
  oxidative s. (OS)
  redox s.
stress-activated protein 1 (SAP-1)
stress-generated electric potential
stretch
  s. mark
  s. reflex
stria, pl. **striae**
  s. alba
  s. albicans
  atrophic s.
  s. atrophica
  striae cutis distensae
  elastotic s.
  striae gravidarum
  s. nasi transversa
  s. rubra
  striae scleroatrophy
  Wickham s.
striata
  dermatitis pratensis s.
  leukonychia s.
  melanonychia s.
striatal
striate atrophy of skin
striatum
  atrophoderma s.
striatus
  lichen s.
stricto
  sensu s.
stridor

string
  s. bean
  s. of pearls configuration
strip
  Breathe Right nasal s.
  Cover-Strip wound closure s.
  Nu-Hope skin barrier s.
  Silverlon wound packing s.
stripe
  Mees s.
  s. technique
striped
  s. blister beetle
  s. blister beetle sting
stripper
  Fischer s.
  Oesch perforation invagination s.
stroke volume (SV)
stromal cell
stromal-cell-derived factor-1 (SDF-1)
stromatolysis
stromelysin
Strongyloides
  S. *stercoralis*
  S. *venezuelensis*
strongyloidiasis
  disseminated s.
Strongylus
strontium sulfide
strophulosus
  lichen s.
strophulus
  s. candidus
  s. intertinctus
  s. pruriginosus
Strother acrochordonectomy
Structural Classification of Proteins (SCOP)
structure
  amyloid s.
  fibril s.
  gene s.
  hair-like s.
  osmiophilic crystal s.
  pilosebaceous s.
  spiny s.
  tertiary s.
struma, pl. **strumae**
  Riedel s.
strumosa
  dactylitis s.

S

NOTES

strumous
    s. abscess
    s. bubo
Strümpell disease
Struthers
    ligament of S.
strychnine poisoning
Stryker
    S. arthroscope
    S. microshaver
Stryker-Halbeisen syndrome
S.T.S.
    serologic test for syphilis
STSG
    split-thickness skin graft
STS sclerosing solution
STU
    skin test unit
stucco keratosis
stuck-on appearance
study
    aerometric s.
    case control s.
    cohort s.
    Collaboration Transplant S.
    European Anti-ICAM Renal
      Transplant S. (EARTS)
    S. of Left Ventricular Dysfunction
    meglumine diatrizoate enema s.
    metabolic s.
    NASTRA s.
    nerve conduction s. (NCS)
    North American Pediatric Renal
      Transplant Cooperative S.
      (NAPRTCS)
    North American Study of
      Treatment for Refractory
      Ascites s.
    North American Study of
      Treatment for Refractory Ascites
      (NASTRA)
    Pepscan s.
    QUEST s.
    secretory antibody s.
    sleep s.
    tagged white blood cell s.
    T1-weighted s.
    T2-weighted s.
    UCF s.
    urinary free cortisol s.
stupe
Sturge-Weber
    S.-W. encephalotrigeminal
      angiomatosis
    S.-W. syndrome
sty, stye
Styloviridae

styptic
    s. collodion
    s. pencil
STZ
    streptozyme
    STZ titer
Su antigen
subacromial bursitis
subacuta
    prurigo simplex s.
subacute
    s. bacterial endocarditis (SBE)
    s. cutaneous lupus erythematosus
      (SCLE)
    s. inclusion body encephalitis
    s. nodular migratory panniculitis
    s. phase shoulder impairment
    s. sclerosing leukoencephalitis
    s. sclerosing panencephalitis (SSPE)
    s. spongiform encephalopathy
subaponeurotic hemorrhage
subaxial listhesis
subbasement
    s. membrane (SBM)
    s. membrane thickening
subcalcaneal pain syndrome
subchondral
    s. cyst
    s. erosion
subclass
    immunoglobulin s.
subclinical
    s. asthma
    s. leprosy
subconfluent keratinocyte
subcorneal
    s. blister
    s. pustular dermatitis
    s. pustular dermatosis
subcutanea
    lipogranulomatosis s.
    urticaria s.
subcutaneous (sc, SQ)
    s. calcification
    s. dirofilariasis
    s. emphysema
    s. epinephrine
    s. fat necrosis
    s. fat necrosis of newborn
    s. felon
    s. fungal infection
    s. fungus
    s. granuloma annulare
    s. granulomatous nodule
    s. immunoglobulin (SCIG)
    s. injection
    s. morphea
    s. mycosis

s. myiasis
s. necrotizing infection
s. nevus
s. panniculitis-like T-cell lymphoma (SPTL)
s. phycomycosis
s. pseudosarcomatous fibromatosis
s. rheumatoid nodule
s. T-cell lymphoma
subcuticular felon
subcutis
subdeltoid bursitis
subdermal
subdermic
subepidermal
s. abscess
s. calcified nodule
s. nodular fibrosis
s. vesiculation
subepithelia
subepithelial
s. basement membrane (SBM)
s. fibrosis
subepithelium
suberosis
subfecundity
subgaleal space
subgallate
bismuth s.
subglottic tracheal stenosis
subglottis
subinfection
subinhibitory
subintegumental
subitum
exanthema s.
subjective synonym
sublamina densa
sublingual-swallow immunotherapy
subluxation
atlantoaxial s.
dorsoradial s.
metacarpophalangeal joint s.
palmar s.
rheumatoid atlantoaxial s.
submersion reflex
submitogenic
submucosa
submucosal
s. gland hypertrophy
s. plaque
subpapular

subperiosteal felon
subplasmalemmal F-actin
subpolar lepromatous leprosy
subsalicylate
bismuth s.
subscale
WOMAC Physical Function s.
subsegmental bronchus
subsensitivity
bronchoprotective s.
subset
CD4 T cell s.
CD4+ T cell s.
CD8 T cell s.
substance
amorphous s.
bacteriotropic s.
blood group s.
bone-seeking s.
exogenous s.
ground s.
nonirritating test s.
s. P
s. P peptide
reducing s.
sensitizing s.
slow-reacting s. (SRS)
soluble specific s. (SSS)
specific capsular s.
thiobarbituric acid-reactive s.
substitute
Apligraf skin s.
Biobrane/HF skin s.
Biobrane synthetic skin s.
Dermagraft-TC skin s.
Platelin, phospholipid platelet s.
saliva s.
TransCyte skin s.
substrate solution additive
subsulfate
ferric s.
subsynovium
subtalar joint
subtegumental
subtilis
Bacillus s.
subtraction
differential gene s.
subtrochanteric
subtropical
subtype
Reston s.

NOTES

S

subtype *(continued)*

    Russian spring-summer encephalitis Eastern s.

    Russian spring-summer encephalitis Western s.

    Sudan s.

    tickborne encephalitis Central European s.

    tickborne encephalitis Eastern s.

    Zaire s.

subungual

    s. abscess

    s. exostosis

    s. hematoma

    s. hyperkeratosis

    s. melanoma

    s. wart

subungualis

    hyperkeratosis s.

subunit vaccine

succinate

    hydrocortisone sodium s.

    lithium s.

    sumatriptan s.

succinyl

succinylcholine

succulence

sucking

    s. blister

    s. louse

Sucquet-Hoyer canal

sucralfate

suction

    Bowins s.

    s. loose body forceps

    s. sampler

suction-socket prosthetic dermatitis

Sudafed

    S. 12 Hour

    S. Plus Liquid

    S. Plus Tablet

sudamen

sudamina

sudaminal

Sudan

    S. black

    S. cell marker

    S. subtype

sudation

sudden

    s. infant death syndrome (SIDS)

    s. unexpected death in infants (SUDI)

    s. unexplained death in infants (SUDI)

Sudex

SUDI

    sudden unexpected death in infants

    sudden unexplained death in infants

Sudodrin

sudomotor

sudor

    s. sanguineus

    s. urinosus

sudoral

sudoresis

sudoriferous

    s. abscess

    nevus s.

sudorific

sudorikeratosis

sudoriparous

    s. abscess

    s. angioma

sudoris

    stadium s.

sudorometer

sudorrhea

Suds

    Murex S.

SUDS HIV-1 diagnostic testing

Sufedrin

sufentanil

suffodiens

    folliculitis et perifolliculitis abscedens et s.

    perifolliculitis capitis abscedens et s.

sugar

    s. beet

    s. maple

    s. maple tree

    specific soluble s.

sugarcane ear

suggillation

suicide

    s. cell

    s. gene

    procollagen s.

suid herpesvirus

suis

    Actinobacillus s.

    Haemophilus s.

suit

    sauna s.

sukhapakla

sulbactam

    ampicillin and s.

sulcatum

    keratoderma plantare s.

    keratolysis plantare s.

    keratoma plantare s.

sulci (*pl. of* sulcus)

sulconazole
    s. nitrate
Sulcosyn topical
sulcus, pl. **sulci**
    s. chancre
    sulci cutis
    s. of matrix of nail
    sulci of skin
Sulf-10 Ophthalmic
sulfacetamide
    sodium s.
    s. sodium scalp treatment lotion
    sulfur and sodium s.
Sulfacet-R topical
sulfadiazine
    silver s.
    s., sulfamethazine, and
      sulfamerazine
sulfadoxine and pyrimethamine
sulfa drug
Sulfair Ophthalmic
sulfamerazine
    sulfadiazine, sulfamethazine, and s.
Sulfamethoprim
sulfamethoxazole
Sulfamylon topical
sulfapyridine
sulfasalazine (SSZ)
sulfate
    amikacin s.
    aminosidine s.
    atropine s.
    bleomycin s.
    Capastat s.
    capreomycin s.
    chondroitin s.
    chondroitin s. B
    chondroitin sulfate/dermatan s.
      (CS/DS)
    colistin s.
    dehydroepiandrosterone s. (DHEAS)
    ephedrine s.
    gentamicin s.
    heparin s.
    hydroxychloroquine s.
    hydroxyquinoline s.
    indinavir s.
    kanamycin s.
    magnesium s.
    metaproterenol s.
    morphine s.
    neomycin s.

    netilmicin s.
    nickel s.
    paromomycin s.
    polymyxin b s.
    quinine s.
    sodium lauryl s.
    sodium tetradecyl s.
    streptomycin s.
    terbutaline s.
    trospectomycin s.
    vinblastine s.
    zinc s.
sulfation
Sulfatrim DS
sulfhydryl compound
sulfide
    barium s.
    selenium s.
    strontium s.
Sulfimycin
sulfinpyrazone
sulfisoxazole
    erythromycin and s.
    s. and phenazopyridine
sulfites
sulfonamide
    alpha-amino-p-toluene s.
    toluene s.
sulfonate
sulfonylurea
sulfosalicylate
    meclocycline s.
sulfoxide
    albendazole s.
    dimethyl s. (DMSO)
Sulfoxyl
sulfur
    s. dioxide (SO_2)
    s. flake
    s. granule
    s. and salicylic acid
    s. and sodium sulfacetamide
sulfureum
    Trichophyton s.
sulfuric acid
sulindac
Sulsal
Sulzberger-Bloch syndrome
Sulzberger-Chase phenomenon
Sulzberger-Garbe
    S.-G. disease
    S.-G. syndrome

NOTES

533

sumac, sumach
    poison s.
    swamp s.
sumatriptan succinate
summer
    s. acne
    s. asthma
    s. dermatosis
    s. eruption
    s. itch
    s. pneumonitis
    s. prurigo
    s. rash
    s. sore
summer-type hypersensitivity
  pneumonitis (SHP)
Sumycin Oral
sun
    s. and chemical combination
      damage
    S. Defense Lip Block
    S. Defense Sunscreen
    s. exposure
    S. Management Lip Protection
    S. Management Sensible Protection
    s. protection factor (SPF)
Sunblock
    Coppertone Waterproof S.
    London Drugs S.
    Marcelle S.
    Shiseido S.
sunburn
    s. reactivation
sunburn-like rash
Sundown Extra Protection
sunflower
sunscreen
    chemical s.
    s. clothing
    Coppertone S.
    DuraScreen s.
    Esoterica S.
    London Drugs S.
    NO-AD S.
    Ombrelle s.
    Parsol 1789 s.
    physical s.
    Porcelana S.
    Shade UvaGuard s.
    Shaklee S.
    Solbar s.
    Sun Defense S.
    Umbrelle s.
Sunseekers
sunset glow
Supartz injection
Supasa

super
    S. Ebonettes flock-lined glove
    s. long-pulse diode laser system
superantigen syndrome
superaspirin
superciliorum
    heterotrichosis s.
superfamily
    immunoglobulin s.
superfatted synthetic detergent
superficial
    s. angioma
    s. basal cell carcinoma
    s. basal cell epithelioma
    s. burn
    s. corium
    s. follicular pyoderma
    s. folliculitis
    s. granulomatous pyoderma
    s. hemangioma
    s. infection
    s. malignant melanoma
    s. migratory thrombophlebitis
    s. musculoaponeurotic system
      (SMAS)
    s. pustular
    s. pustular perifolliculitis
    s. spreading melanoma (SSM)
superficialis
    esophagitis dissecans s.
    lupus s.
    nevus lipomatodes s.
    nevus lipomatosus cutaneus s.
superinduce
superinfection
superior labrum anterior and posterior
  (SLAP)
supernatant
    concanavalin A-stimulated T^H cell
    line s.
supernate
supernumerary digit
superoxide anion
superpigmentation
supine-to-prone maneuver
supine-to-sit maneuver
supisotype
suppedanium
supplemental oxygen
support
    s. group
    volume-assured pressure s. (VAPS)
supportive therapy
suppository
    Anucort HC s.
    Anuprep HC s.
    Anusol-HC s.

AVC s.
Truphylline s.
suppression
allotype s.
linked s.
T-cell s.
transferable T-cell s.
suppressor
s. cell
immune s. (Is)
suppressor-sensitive mutant
suppuration
suppurativa
genital hidradenitis s.
hidradenitis s.
suppurative arthritis
suprabasal clefting
suprabasilar acantholysis
supracondylar nonunions
suprafollicularis
keratosis s.
supragaleal plexus
supramalleolaris
erythrocyanosis s.
Supramid suture
suprascapular
s. nerve compression (SSC)
s. nerve entrapment
s. nerve palsy
supraspinatus tendon
suprasternal reaction
Suprax
suprofen
sural nerve entrapment
suramin keratosis
SureCell Strep A test
Sure-Closure skin stretching system
SurePress leg compression dressing
SureSite transparent film
surface
s. antigen
dorsal s.
extensor s.
flexor s.
s. freezing
hepatitis B s. (HB$_s$)
s. Ig-expressing B cell
s. microscopy
s. proteoglycan
RBC s.
s. receptor
red blood cell s.

surface-targeted plasmin inhibitor
surfactant
hydrolysis of s.
pulmonary s.
surfer's knot
Surgam SR
Surgeons
American Society of Transplant S.
(ASTS)
surgery
acne s.
collimated bema handpiece (CBH-1)
for laser s.
continuous-wave dye laser s.
laser s.
microscopically controlled s.
Mohs micrographic s. (MMS)
video-assisted thoracic s. (VATS)
surgical
s. erysipelas
s. excision (SE)
s. therapy
s. thrombectomy
s. tuberculosis
Surgilene suture
SurgiPulse XJ laser
Surgitron
Ellman S.
Surgitube tubing
surrogate
s. marker
s. tolerogenesis (ST)
sursanure
surveillance
immune s.
immunological s.
survey
environmental s.
Health and Activity Limitation S.
(HALS)
human immune status s. (HISS)
Papworth heart donor s.
reduced joint s. (RJS)
survival
failure-free s. (FFS)
susceptibility cassette
suspectum
Heloderma s.
suspension
AK-Spore H.C. Ophthalmic s.
amoxicillin/clavulanate s.
AMX/CL s.

S

NOTES

suspension *(continued)*
    Aristocort Intralesional S.
    betamethasone sodium phosphate
        and acetate s.
    cefuroxime axetil s. (CAE)
    Children's Advil S.
    Children's Motrin S.
    Cortisporin Ophthalmic S.
    FML-S Ophthalmic s.
    penicillin v s.
    polymyxin B-hydrocortisone s.
    Poly-Pred Ophthalmic s.
    Terra-Cortril Ophthalmic S.
    Vexol Ophthalmic s.
Sus-Phrine
Sustacal Plus
sustained release
Sustaire
Sustiva
sutilains
Sutton
    S. disease
    S. nevus
    S. ulcer
suture
    chromic gut s.
    Dexon s.
    Ethicon s.
    Ethilon s.
    Maxon s.
    Novafil s.
    nylon s.
    PDS s.
        polydioxanone suture
    plain gut s.
    poliglecaprone s.
    polydioxanone s. (PDS suture)
    polyglactin 910 s.
    polyglycolic acid s.
    polyglyconate s.
    polypropylene s.
    Prolene s.
    silk s.
    Supramid s.
    Surgilene s.
    Vicryl s.
SV
    simian virus
    stroke volume
SV40
    simian vacuolating virus No. 40
SV40-adenovirus hybrid
SVC
    slow vital capacity
swamp
    s. fever
    s. fever virus

    s. itch
    s. sumac
Swann antigen
swan-neck deformity
Sw^a antigen
swarming
Swartz-Lamkins stain
Swartz-Medrik stain
sweat
    s. bee
    black s.
    s. chloride
    s. chloride elimination
    colliquative s.
    fetid s.
    s. gland
    s. gland carcinoma
    insensitive s.
    malodorous s.
    red s.
sweating
    excessive s.
sweat-retention syndrome
sweaty
    s. feet syndrome
    s. sock dermatitis
    s. sock syndrome
Swedish old tuberculin
Sween Cream
sweet
    s. clover
    S. disease
    s. potato
    S. syndrome
    s. vernal
    s. vernal grass
    s. vernal grass pollen
sweetgum tree
swelling
    boggy s.
    Calabar s.
    cervical lymph node s.
    fugitive s.
    joint s.
    Neufeld capsular s.
    nodules, eosinophilia, rheumatism,
        dermatitis, and s. (NERDS)
    rhomboid s.
    tropical s.
Swift disease
Swim-Ear Otic
swimmer's
    s. dermatitis
    s. itch
swimming pool granuloma
swine
    atrophic rhinitis of s.
    s. encephalitis virus

s. epithelium
s. fever
s. fever virus
s. influenza
s. influenza virus
s. pest
transmissible gastroenteritis virus of s.
s. vesicular disease
swinepox virus
Swiss
S. chard
S. cheese appearance
S. mouse leukemia virus
S. 3T3 fibroblast
S. Therapy eye mask
S. type agammaglobulinemia
switch
class s.
s. region
switching
immunoglobulin class s.
sycamore tree
sycoma
sycondroses
sycosiforme
ulerythema s.
sycosiform fungous infection
sycosis
bacillogenic s.
s. barbae
Brocq lupoid s.
coccogenic s.
s. contagiosa
s. frambesiformis
s. framboesia
s. framboesiaeformis
herpetic s.
hyphomycotic s.
lupoid s.
nonparasitic s.
s. nuchae
s. nuchae necrotisans
parasitic s.
s. staphylogenes
tinea s.
s. vulgaris
Sydenham chorea
sydowi
Aspergillus s.
Syllamalt
Sylvest disease

Symadine
Symmers pipe-stem fibrosis
Symmetrel
symmetric
s. keratoderma
s. lividity of the soles
s. progressive leukopathy
s. reticulonodular x-ray change
symmetrica
dyschromatosis s.
erythrokeratodermia progressive s.
keratoderma s.
leukopathia punctata reticularis s.
symmetrical gangrene
symmetricum faciei
symmetry
axis of s.
sympathectomy
digital s.
sympathetic
s. nervous system
s. ophthalmia
s. synovitis
sympathica
meningitis s.
sympathomimetic
sympathoneural response
symphalangism
Symphony patient monitoring system
symphysis
symptom
asthma-like s.
classic allergy s.
coincidental s.
drug rash with eosinophil and systemic s. (DRESS)
frequency of allergy s.
gastrointestinal s.
Haenel s.
neuropsychiatric s.
prodromal s.
Roger s.
severity of allergy s.
sicca s.
Sklowsky s.
Wartenberg s.
symptomatic
s. erythema
s. fever
s. porphyria
s. pruritus
s. reaction

NOTES

S

symptomatic *(continued)*
s. therapy
s. ulcer
symptomatica
alopecia s.
livedo reticularis s.
purpura s.
Synacort Topical
Synagis
Synalar-HP Topical
Synalar Topical
synanthem
synapsin I
synaptophysin
synarthroses
Sync
Star S.
synchronized intermittent mechanical ventilation
synchronous
s. intermittent mandatory ventilation
s. tissue lesion
syncopal attack
syncope
syncytia
syncytial virus
syncytioblast
syncytiotrophoblast
placental s.
syncytium-inhibiting (SI)
syndactylia
syndactyly
syndecan
syndesmophyte formation
syndesmophytosis
syndesmosis, pl. **syndesmoses**
syndet
synthetic detergent
syndet-based bar soap
syndrome
Aarskog-Scott s.
Achard-Thiers s.
Achenbach s.
acquired hyperostosis s. (AHYS)
acquired immune deficiency s. (AIDS)
acquired immunodeficiency s. (AIDS)
actinic reticuloid s.
acute retroviral s.
acute seroconversion s.
Adamantiades-Behçet s.
Adams-Oliver s.
addicted scrotum s.
adulterated rapeseed oil-associated toxic oil s.
adult respiratory distress s. (ARDS)
AEC s.

Alagille s.
Albright s.
Aldrich s.
Alezzandrini s.
Alibert-Bazin s.
Alström s.
aminopterin s.
amyloid s.
anaphylactic s.
androgen-dependent s.
Angelman s.
angioedema-urticaria-eosinophilia s.
angry back s.
ANOTHER s.
anterior spinal artery s.
antibody-deficient s. (ADS)
anticardiolipin antibody s.
antiphospholipid antibody s. (APS)
antisynthetase s.
aortic arch s.
APECED s.
Apert s.
Arndt-Gottron s.
arterial-ecchymotic type Ehlers-Danlos s.
arthrochalasia-type Ehlers-Danlos s.
arthrogryposis congenita, distal, type I, II s.
Ascher s.
ataxia telangiectasia s.
atypical mole s.
auriculotemporal s.
autoerythrocyte sensitization s.
autoimmune lymphoproliferative s. (ALPS)
autoimmune paraneoplastic s.
autoimmune polyglandular s. (APS)
autonomic imbalance s.
autosomal-dominant periodic fever s.
Babinski s.
Babinski-Vaquez s.
baboon s.
Bäfverstedt s.
Baló concentric s.
Bannayan-Riley-Ruvalcaba s.
Bannwarth s.
Banti s.
Bardet-Biedl 1–5 s.
bare lymphocyte s.
Barraquer-Simons s.
Bart s.
Barth s.
Bart-Pumphrey s.
basal cell nevus s.
Basan s.
Bateman s.
Bazex s.

Bearn-Kunkel s.
Bearn-Kunkel-Slater s.
Bechterew s.
Behçet s.
Beradinelli-Seip s.
Bernard-Soulier s.
bicipital s.
BIDS s.
bird egg s.
Birt-Hogg-Dubé s. (BHD)
Björnstad s.
Blatin s.
bleached rubber s.
blind loop s.
Blizzard s.
Bloch-Siemens-Sulzberger s.
Bloch-Sulzberger s.
Bloom s.
Bloom-Torre-Machacek s.
blue rubber-bleb nevus s.
blue-toe s.
Bockenheimer s.
Böök s.
Bourneville s.
Bourneville-Pringle s.
bowel bypass s.
brachio-oto-renal s.
brachydactyly, mental retardation s.
brachydactyly, type B1, C, E s.
Brett s.
brittle hair, intellectual impairment,
  decreased fertility, short stature s.
brittle nail s.
bronchiolitis obliterans s. (BOS)
Brooke-Spiegler s.
brown-spot s.
Bruck s.
Brugsch s.
Bruns s.
B-thalassemia s.
Buckley s.
Budd-Chiari s.
burning mouth s.
burning vulva s.
Buschke-Ollendorf s.
bypass arthritis-dermatitis s.
C s.
cachexia s.
café coronary s.
Cairns s.

calcinosis cutis, osteoma cutis,
  poikiloderma, and skeletal
  abnormalities s.
calcinosis cutis, Raynaud
  phenomenon, esophageal motility
  disorder, sclerodactyly, and
  telangiectasia s.
Caldwell s.
Canada-Cronkhite s.
Canale-Smith s.
Caner-Decker s.
Caplan s.
carcinoid s.
cardiocutaneous s.
cardio-facio-cutaneous s.
Carney s.
carpal tunnel s. (CTS)
cauda equina s.
cellular immune deficiency s.
  (CIDS)
cellular immunity deficiency s.
cervical acceleration-deceleration s.
Chanarin-Dorfman s.
chancriform s.
Charlin s.
Chauffard s.
Chauffard-Still s.
Chediak-Higashi s. (CHS)
chemical hypersensitivity s.
CHILD s.
CHIME s.
Chinese restaurant s.
chondrodysplasia punctata s.
chorda tympani s.
Christ-Siemens-Touraine s.
chronic fatigue s.
chronic fatigue immune
  deficiency s. (CFIDS)
chronic fatigue and immune
  dysfunction s. (CFIDS)
chronic infantile neurological
  cutaneous and auricular s.
chronic mucocutaneous
  candidiasis s.
chronic pain s.
Churg-Strauss s. (CSS)
CINCA s.
classic type Ehlers-Danlos s.
Clouston s.
CMC s.
Cobb s.
Cockayne s.

S

NOTES

539

syndrome *(continued)*

Coffin-Lowry s.
Coffin-Siris s.
Cogan s.
coloboma, heart anomaly, ichthyosis, mental retardation, and ear abnormality s.
combined immunodeficiency s.
complex regional pain s. (CRPS)
congenital hemidysplasia with ichthyosiform erythroderma and limb defects s.
congenital rubella s.
Conradi-Hünermann s.
COPS s.
cosmetic intolerance s.
Costello s.
Crandall s.
craniocarpotarsal s.
craniosynostosis Adelaide type s.
craniosynostosis type 1, 2 s.
CREST s.
Crigler-Najjar s.
Cronkhite-Canada s.
Cross-McKusick-Breen s.
Crouzon s.
Crowe-Dickermann s.
Crow-Fukase s.
crowned dens s.
cubital tunnel s.
Cushing s.
DaCosta s.
Danbolt-Closs s.
defibrination s.
Degos s.
Degos-Delort-Tricot s.
dengue shock s.
Dennie-Marfan s.
denture-sore-mouth s.
de Quervain s.
dermatitis-arthritis-tenosynovitis s.
De Sanctis-Cacchione s.
Devic s.
diabetic hand s.
diabetic stiff-hand s.
diffuse infiltrative lymphocytosis s.
DiGeorge s.
disease s.
distal intestinal obstruction s.
Donath-Landsteiner s.
Dorfman-Chanarin s.
double-crush s.
Down s.
drug-induced delayed multiorgan hypersensitivity s. (DIDMOS)
drug-induced SLE s.
Duncan s.
Dunnigan s.
dyskinetic cilia s.
dysplastic nevus s.
easy bruising s.
Eaton-Lambert s.
ectrodactyly-ectodermal dysplasia-clefting s.
EEC s.
effort s.
Ehlers-Danlos s.
Elejalde s. (ES)
Ellis-van Creveld s.
empty sella s.
eosinophilia-myalgia s. (EMS)
eosinophilic fasciitis s.
eosinophilic myalgia s.
eosinophilic pulmonary s.
erythrodysesthesia s.
euthyroid sick s.
excited skin s. (ESS)
exercise-induced respiratory distress s. (EIRDS)
Fabry s.
familial amyloidotic polyneuropathy s.
familial articular hypermobility s.
familial atypical multiple mole melanoma s. (FAMMM)
familial cholestasis s.
familial hypermobility s.
familial nephropathic amyloidosis s.
Fanconi s.
fasciitis-panniculitis s.
favid Favre-Racouchot s.
Favre-Racouchot s.
Fegeler s.
Felty s.
female pseudo-Turner s.
fetal alcohol s.
fetal hydantoin s.
fibromyalgia s. (FMS)
fibronectin-deficient type Ehlers-Danlos s.
fibrosing s.
Fiessinger-Leroy s.
Fiessinger-Leroy-Reiter s.
Fiessinger-Rendu s.
Fisher s.
Fitz-Hugh and Curtis s.
Fleischner s.
Flynn-Aird s.
follicular degeneration s.
Fong s.
Franceschetti-Jadassohn s.
Franceschetti-Klein s.
Freeman-Sheldon s.
Frey s.
Gardner s.
Gardner-Diamond s.

genital Reiter s.
Gerstmann-Straussler-Scheinker s.
Gianotti-Crosti s.
giant cell arteritis s.
Gilbert s.
Giroux-Barbeau s.
gloves and socks s. (GSS)
glucagonoma s.
glucocorticoid withdrawal s.
GLUS s.
Gold Schnapps s.
Goltz s.
Goltz-Gorlin s.
Goodpasture s.
Gopalan s.
Gorlin s.
Gorlin-Chaudhry-Moss s.
Gorlin-Goltz s.
Gorman s.
Gottron s.
Gougerot s.
Gougerot-Blum s.
Gougerot-Carteaud s.
Graham Little s.
Graham-Little-Piccardi-Lasseur s.
Gravis-type Ehlers-Danlos s.
green nail s.
Greither s.
Griscelli s. (GS)
Grönblad-Strandberg s.
Guillain-Barré s.
Gulf War s. (GWS)
Günther s.
Haber s.
HAIR-AN s.
Hallermann-Streiff s.
Hallopeau-Siemens s.
Hamman-Rich s.
hand-and-foot s.
Happle s.
Harada s.
Harter s.
Hawes-Pallister-Landor s.
Hay-Wells s.
Heck s.
Heerfordt s.
Heiner s.
HELLP s.
Helweg-Larssen s.
hemangioma-thrombocytopenia s.
hematopoietic failure s.

hemolysis, elevated liver enzymes, and low platelet s.
hemolytic uremic s. (HUS)
hemophagocytic s.
hemorrhagic fever with renal s. (HFRS)
Henoch-Schönlein s. (HSS)
hepatopulmonary s. (HPS)
hereditary periodic fever s.
Herlitz s.
Hermansky-Pudlak s.
Hermansky-Pudlak s. type IV, VI
Hirschowitz s.
Hitzig s.
Holmes-Adie s.
Holt-Oram s.
Horner s.
Howell-Evans s.
human dermatosparaxis type Ehlers-Danlos s.
Hunt s.
Hunter s.
Hunter-Thompson s.
Huriez s.
Hurler s.
Hurler-Scheie s.
Hutchinson-Gilford s.
hydralazine s.
hydralazine-associated lupus-like s.
hypereosinophilic s. (HES)
hyper-IgE s.
hyper-IgM s. (HIM)
hyperimmunoglobulinemia s. (HID)
hyperimmunoglobulinemia D, E s.
hypermobile-type Ehlers-Danlos s.
hypermobility s.
hyperostotic s.
hyperventilation s. (HVS)
hyperviscosity s.
hypocomplementemic urticarial vasculitis s. (HUVS)
hypocomplementemic vasculitis urticarial s.
iatrogenic Cushing s.
IBIDS s.
ichthyosis plus brittle hair, intellectual impairment, decreased fertility, short stature s.
idiopathic hypereosinophilic s. (IHES)
idiopathic nephrotic s.
iliotibial band s.

NOTES

S

syndrome *(continued)*
immunodeficiency s.
impingement s.
s. of inappropriate excretion of
 antidiuretic hormone (SIADH)
inflammatory bowel s. (IBS)
inherited complement deficiency s.
irritable bowel s. (IBS)
Isaacs s.
Jackson-Lawler s.
Jackson-Sertoli s.
Jackson-Weiss s.
Jacobsen s.
Jadassohn-Lewandowsky s.
Jaffe-Campanacci s.
Jessner s.
Job s.
Kabuki s.
Kartagener s.
Kasabach-Merritt s.
Kawasaki s.
Kelley-Seegmiller s.
keratitis-ichthyosis-deafness s.
Kettle s.
Keutel s.
KID s.
Kindler s.
kinky-hair s.
Klauder s.
Klein-Waardenburg s.
Klinefelter s.
Klippel-Feil s.
Klippel-Trenaunay s.
Klippel-Trenaunay-Parkes-Weber s.
Klippel-Trenaunay-Weber s.
Kobberling-Dunnigan s.
Kostmann s.
Kuru s.
kyphoscoliosis type Ehlers-Danlos s.
LAMB s.
Lambert-Eaton s.
Lambert-Eaton myasthenic s.
 (LEMS)
Landry s.
Landry-Guillain-Barré s.
Langer-Giedion s.
Larsen s.
late respiratory systemic s. (LRSS)
latex-fruit s.
Laugier-Hunziger s.
Lawrence-Seip s.
lazy leukocyte s. (LLS)
Ledderhose s.
lentigines, atrial myxoma, and blue
 nevi s.
Lenz-Majewski s.
LEOPARD s.
Lépine-Froin s.

Leredde s.
Leri-Weill s.
Lesch-Nyhan s.
Lewis-Summer s.
Libman-Sacks s.
lichen planus overlap s.
Liddle s.
limb-mammary s.
s. of limited joint mobility (SLJM)
Löffler s.
Lofgren s.
loose anagen hair s.
Louis-Bar s.
lupus s.
lupus-like s.
lupus-scleroderma overlap s.
Lyell s.
lymphedema-distichiasis s.
lymphocytosis s.
Maffucci s.
malignant mole s.
malignant neuroleptic s.
marfamoid hypermobility s.
Marfan s.
marfanoid hypermobility s.
Marie-Bamberger s.
Marinesco-Sjögren s.
Maroteaux-Lamy s.
marrow failure s.
Marshall s.
Marshall-White s.
MASS s.
mastocytosis s.
Mauriac s.
McCune-Albright s.
McKusick s.
McKusick-Kaufman s.
megacystic microcolon s.
Meischer s.
Melkersson s.
Melkersson-Rosenthal s.
Melnick-Fraser s.
MEN s.
Mendelson s.
Menkes kinky hair s.
Mibelli s.
Milian s.
Milwaukee knee s.
Milwaukee shoulder s.
Mitis-type Ehlers-Danlos s.
mitochondrial DNA s.
mitral valve prolapse, aortic
 anomalies, skeletal changes, and
 skin changes s.
modified varicella-like s. (MVLS)
MORFAN s.
Morquio s.
Moynahan s.

Mucha-Habermann s.
Muckle-Wells s.
mucocutaneous lymph node s.
  (MLNS)
Muir-Torre s.
multiple drug allergy s.
multiple hamartoma s.
multiple lentigines s.
multiple mucosal neuroma s.
multiple sulfatase deficiency s.
Munchausen s.
Muscle-Wells s.
musician's overuse s.
myasthenia gravis s.
myelodysplastic s. (MDS)
myofascial pain s. (MPS)
myonecrosis s.
Naegeli s.
Naegeli-Franceschetti-Jadassohn s.
nail-patella s.
nail-patella-elbow s.
NAME s.
Nelson s.
nephrotic s.
NERDS s.
nerve compression-degeneration s.
nerve entrapment s.
Netherton s. (NS)
neurocutaneous s.
neurofibromatosis, type 1 s.
nevi, atrial myxoma, myxoid
  neurofibroma, and ephelides s.
nevoid basal cell carcinoma s.
  (NBCCS)
Nezelof s.
Nicolau s.
Nieden s.
nodules, eosinophilia, rheumatism,
  dermatitis, and swelling s.
nonallergic rhinitis with
  eosinophilia s. (NARES)
nonarticular s.
Nonne-Milroy-Meige s.
Noonan s.
occipital horn s.
occuloglandular s.
occupation-related s.
ocular-mucous membrane s.
ocular-scoliotic type Ehlers-
  Danlos s.
oculo-oral-genital s.
odonto-tricho-ungual-digital-palmar s.

Ollendorf s.
Olmsted s.
Omenn s.
one hand-two foot s.
oral allergy s. (OAS)
oral-ocular-genital s.
organic dust toxic s. (ODTS)
Osler s. II
Osler-Weber-Rendu s.
OSMED s.
osteogenesis imperfecta s.
overlap s.
overuse s.
4-p s.
Paget abscess s.
painful-bruising s.
Pallister-Hall s.
Pallister mosaic aneuploid s.
palmar fasciitis and polyarthritis s.
palmoplantar erythrodysesthesia s.
pants paresthesia s.
PAPA s.
Papillon-Lèfevre s.
papular-purpuric gloves and
  socks s.
papular-purpuric stocking and
  glove s.
papulovesicular acrolocated s.
paraneoplastic s.
Parinaud oculoglandular s.
Parrot s.
Parry-Romberg s.
Pasini-Pierini s.
patellofemoral pain s.
peeling-skin s.
periarticular s.
periodic fever s.
periodontitis-type Ehlers-Danlos s.
Persian Gulf s.
Peutz-Jeghers s.
Pfeiffer s.
pharyngeal pouch s.
photosensitivity, ichthyosis, brittle
  hair, impaired intelligence,
  decreased fertility, and short
  stature s.
photosensitivity, ichthyosis, brittle
  hair, intellectual impairment,
  decreased fertility and short
  stature s.
PIBIDS s.

S

NOTES

543

syndrome *(continued)*
    PIE s.
    piriformis s.
    placental sulfatase deficiency s.
    plantar nerve s.
    plica s.
    Plummer-Vinson s.
    POEMS s.
    polyangiitis overlap s.
    polyarteritis nodosa s.
    polymyalgia rheumatica s.
    popliteal pterygium s.
    postcardiotomy s.
    posterior interosseous nerve s.
    postinfectious encephalomyelitis s.
    postphlebitic s.
    Prader-Willi s.
    Prausnitz-Kustner s.
    Prieur-Griscelli s.
    primary Sjögren s.
    progeroid Ehlers-Danlos s.
    pronator teres s.
    Proteus s.
    pseudoradicular s.
    pseudo-Turner s.
    psychogenic pain s.
    pulmonary disease anemia s.
    pulmonary sling s.
    pyriformis s.
    Quincke I s.
    Rabson-Mendenhall s.
    Ramsay Hunt s.
    Raynaud s.
    reactive airways dysfunction s.
     (RADS)
    rectus abdominis s.
    "red man" s.
    reflex sympathetic dystrophy s.
    Refsum s.
    Reiter s.
    REM s.
    Rendu-Osler-Weber s.
    respiratory distress s. (RDS)
    restaurant s.
    reticular erythematous mucinosis s.
    Reye s.
    rhabdomyolysis s.
    Richner-Hanhart s.
    Richter s.
    Riley-Day s.
    Riley-Smith s.
    Romberg s.
    Rombo s.
    Rosai-Dorfman s.
    Rothmann-Makai s.
    Rothmund s.
    Rothmund-Thomson s.
    Rowell s.

    RSD s.
    rubber man s.
    Rubinstein-Taybi s.
    Rud s.
    runting s.
    Rust s.
    Ruvalcaba-Myhre-Smith s.
    sacral agenesis type 1 s.
    Samter s.
    Sanfilippo s.
    SAPHO s.
     synovitis, acne, pustulosis,
      hyperostosis, osteitis
    scalded skin s.
    scapulocostal s.
    scapulothoracic s.
    Schfifer s.
    Schäfer s.
    Schafer-Branauer s.
    Scheie s.
    Schimmelpenning s.
    Schmidt s.
    Schnitzler s.
    Schönlein-Henoch s.
    Schopf s.
    Schüller-Christian s.
    sea-blue histiocyte s.
    secondary Sjögren s.
    Secrétan s.
    Seidlmayer s.
    Seip-Lawrence s.
    Senear-Usher s.
    septic shock s.
    seronegative rheumatoid s.
    severe combined immune
     deficiency s.
    Sézary s.
    Sheehan s.
    short bowel s.
    shoulder-hand s.
    shrinking lung s.
    Shulman s.
    sicca s.
    sick building s.
    Simmond s.
    Simpson dysmorphia s.
    Sjögren s. (SS)
    Sjögren s. A (SS-A)
    Sjögren s. B (SS-B)
    Sjögren-Larsson s.
    skin disease s.
    sleep apnea s.
    sleep apnea/hypopnea s.
    SLE-like s.
    Sly s.
    Smith-Riley s.
    Sneddon s.

Soto s.
Spanish toxic oil s.
Spanlang-Tappeiner s.
sporadic atypical mole-melanoma s.
staphylococcal scalded skin s.
  (SSSS)
staphylococcal toxic shock s.
starvation s.
Stein-Leventhal s.
Stevens-Johnson s. (SJS)
Stewart-Treves s.
Stickler s.
Stickler s., type I, II, III
stiff-hand s.
stiff-man s. (SMS)
stiff-person s.
stiff-skin s.
streptococcal toxic shock s.
Stryker-Halbeisen s.
Sturge-Weber s.
subcalcaneal pain s.
sudden infant death s. (SIDS)
Sulzberger-Bloch s.
Sulzberger-Garbe s.
superantigen s.
sweat-retention s.
sweaty feet s.
sweaty sock s.
Sweet s.
synostosis s.
synovitis, acne, pustulosis,
  hyperostosis, osteitis s.
systemic inflammatory response s.
  (SIRS)
systemic lupus erythematosus-like s.
TAR s.
    thrombocytopenia-absent-radius
      syndrome
tarsal tunnel s.
TASS s.
    thyroiditis, Addison disease,
      Sjögren syndrome, sarcoidosis
      syndrome
Tay s.
tendonitis-fascitis s.
thalassemia s.
Thibierge-Weissenbach s.
third and fourth pharyngeal
  pouch s.
Thompson s.
thoracic outlet s.

thrombocytopenia-absent-radius s.
  (TAR syndrome)
thrombocytopenic purpura/hemolytic
  uremic s. (TTP-HUS)
thyroiditis, Addison disease, Sjögren
  syndrome, sarcoidosis s. (TASS
  syndrome)
Tietze s.
tight building s.
toasted skin s.
TORCH s.
Torre s.
total allergy s.
Touraine s.
Touraine-Solente-Golé s.
Townes-Brock s.
toxic oil s. (TOS)
toxic shock s. (TSS)
toxic shock-like s. (TSLS)
toxoplasmosis, other infections,
  rubella, cytomegalovirus infection,
  and herpes simplex s.
Treacher Collins s.
tricho-rhino-phalangeal s.
trichothiodystrophy s.
trigeminal trophic s.
trisomy 20 s.
trophic s.
Trousseau s.
tumor-lysis s.
tumor necrosis factor receptor-
  associated periodic s. (TRAPS)
Turner s.
Turner-Kieser s.
two feet-one hand s.
Ullrich-Turner s.
uncombable hair s.
undifferentiated autoimmune s.
  (UAS)
undifferentiated connective tissue s.
  (UCTS)
Unna-Thost s.
unusual lupus erythematosus-like s.
Urbach-Wiethe s.
Van Lohuizen s.
vascular type Ehlers-Danlos s.
velocardiofacial s.
Verner s.
Vogt-Koyanagi s.
Vogt-Koyanagi-Harada s. (VKHS)
Vohwinkel s.
von Hippel-Landau s.

S

NOTES

syndrome *(continued)*
    vulvar vestibulitis s.
    Waardenburg s.
    Waardenburg-Shah s.
    Waldenström s.
    wasting s.
    Waterhouse-Friderichsen s.
    Weber-Cockayne s.
    Wegener granulomatosus s.
    Weill-Marchesani s.
    Weissenbach s.
    Weissenbach-Zweymuller s.
    Well s.
    Wells s.
    Werner s.
    Wernicke-Korsakoff s.
    whistling face s.
    Widal s.
    Windmill-Vane-Hand s.
    Wiskott-Aldrich s. (WAS)
    Wissler s.
    Wissler-Fanconi s.
    Wyburn-Mason s.
    X-linked Ehlers-Danlos s.
    X-linked lymphoproliferative s.
    XYY s.
    yellow nail s.
    Young s.
    Zimmerman-Laband s.
    Zinsser-Cole-Engman s.
    Zinsser-Engman-Cole s.
syndromic
Synemol topical
Synercid
synergic spleen
synergistic
synergistic gangrene
Synflex
Syn-Flunisolide
Syngamus trachea
syngeneic
    s. cell
    s. graft
    s. heart transplant
    s. transplantation
syngenesioplasty
syngenesiotransplantation
syngenic
syngraft
Syn-Minocycline
synonym
    objective s.
    senior s.
    subjective s.
synophrys
synostosis, pl. **synostoses**
    s. syndrome
synovectomy

synovial
    s. antigenic peptide
    s. biopsy
    s. capillary
    s. cyst
    s. fibroblast
    s. fluid (SF)
    s. fluid change
    s. hemangioma
    s. hemosiderosis
    s. hyperplasia
    s. hypoxia
    s. lining
    s. lining cell (SLC)
    s. lining cell type A
    s. lipoma
    s. membrane
    s. membrane tophus
    s. mesenchyme
    s. tissue
synovia T cell
synoviocyte
    fibroblast-like s. (FLS)
    fibroblast lineage s.
    fibroblast-shaped s.
    macrophage-like s.
    type A s.
synovioma
    benign giant cell s.
synoviorthosis
synovitis
    s., acne, pustulosis, hyperostosis,
      osteitis (SAPHO, SAPHO
      syndrome)
    s., acne, pustulosis, hyperostosis,
      osteitis syndrome
    asymptomatic cricoarytenoid s.
    discrete s.
    eosinophilic s.
    glenohumeral s.
    nodular s.
    pigmented villonodular s. (PVNS)
    polyarticular s.
    proliferative s.
    reactive postinfectious s.
    remitting seronegative
      symmetrical s.
    silicone s.
    sympathetic s.
    tuberculous s.
    villonodular s.
synovium
    fibrous s. (FS)
    hyperplastic s. (HS)
    proliferative s.
Syn-Rx
syntenic group
Synthaderm wound dressing

synthase
    brain PGD_2 s.
    citrate s.
    endoperoxide s.
    hematopoietic PGD_2 s.
    inducible nitric oxide s.
    LTC_4 s.
    oligoadenylate s.
    PGE_2 s.
    PGF_2 s.
    PGI_2 s.
    prostacyclin s.
    thromboxane s.
synthesis, pl. **syntheses**
    cellular immunodeficiency with abnormal immunoglobulin s.
    chondrocyte proteoglycan s.
    de novo pyrimidine s.
    s. inhibitor
    matrix s.
    melanin s.
    vitamin D s.
synthetase
    adenylosuccinic acid s.
    alanyl-transfer ribonucleic acid s.
    alanyl-tRNA s.
    aminoacyl-tRNA s.
    glycyl-transfer ribonucleic acid s.
    glycyl-tRNA s.
    histidyl-tRNA s.
    isoleucyl-tRNA s.
    threonyl-tRNA s.
    tRNA s.
synthetic
    s. antigen
    s. depot corticosteroid
    s. detergent (syndet)
    s. pyrethroid
Synvisc
syphilid
    acneform s.
    acuminate papular s.
    annular s.
    bullous s.
    corymbose s.
    ecthymatous s.
    erythematous s.
    flat papular s.
    follicular s.
    frambesiform s.
    gummatous s.
    impetiginous s.

    lenticular s.
    macular s.
    miliary papular s.
    nodular s.
    nummular s.
    palmar s.
    papular s.
    papulosquamous s.
    pemphigoid s.
    pigmentary s.
    plantar s.
    pustular s.
    rupial s.
    secondary s.
    tertiary s.
    varioliform s.
syphilide
syphilionthus
syphilis
    Captia test for s.
    s. chancre
    congenital s.
    s. d'emblée
    early congenital s.
    early latent s.
    endemic s.
    gumma of tertiary s.
    gummatous s.
    s. hereditaria tarda
    s. of iris
    late benign s.
    late cardiovascular s.
    late congenital s.
    late latent s.
    latent s.
    late osseous s.
    noduloulcerative s.
    noduloulcerative tertiary s.
    nonvenereal s.
    osseous s.
    parenchymatous s.
    ping-pong s.
    primary s.
    quaternary s.
    secondary s.
    serologic test for s. (S.T.S.)
    tertiary cutaneous s.
    tertiary noduloulcerative s.
    tubercular tertiary s.
    visceral s.
syphilitic
    s. alopecia

S

NOTES

syphilitic *(continued)*
  s. dactylitis
  s. fever
  s. inguinal adenitis
  s. leukoderma
  s. onychia
  s. roseola
  s. spastic spinal paralysis
  s. spinal muscular atrophy
  s. ulcer
syphilitica
  acne s.
  alopecia s.
  impetigo s.
syphiliticum
  erythema nodosum s.
  tuberculum s.
syphiliticus
  clavus s.
  lichen s.
  pemphigus s.
  tophus s.
syphiloderm
syphiloderma
  papular s.
syphilologist
syphilology
syphiloma
  Fournier s.
syphilomatous
syphilophobia
syringadenoma
syringe
  Luer-Lok s.
syringe-assisted liposuction
syringoacanthoma
syringoadenoma
  s. papilliferum
syringocystadenoma papilliferum
syringofibroadenoma
  eccrine s.
syringoid carcinoma
syringoma
  chondroid s.
  clear cell s.
  eruptive s.
  malignant chondroid s.
syringometaplasia
  eccrine squamous s.
syringomyelia
syrup
  Actagen S.
  albuterol sulfate S.
  Allerfrin S.
  Allerphed S.
  Anamine S.
  Aprodine S.
  S. of Aristocort

Benylin Cough S.
Bromfed S.
Bydramine Cough S.
Carbodec S.
Cardec-S S.
Decofed S.
Deconamine S.
Drixoral S.
Histalet S.
Hydramyn S.
Kenacort S.
Naldecon-EX Children's S.
Rondec S.
Silafed S.
Triofed S.
Triposed S.
Tusstat S.
Uni-Bent Cough S.
Sysmex SE-9500 machine
system
  Aastrom Replicell S.
  Accents s.
  AccuProbe s.
  Accu-set S.
  Acusyst-Xcell monoclonal antibody
    culturing s.
  Aladdin infant flow s.
  AlaSTAT allergy immunoassay s.
  Allerderm Protective Glove S.
  APACHE II s.
  arch-loop-whorl s. (ALW)
  Aria CPAP s.
  Aura Laser s.
  Automated Cellular Imaging S.
    (ACIS)
  automated cytochemical s.
  autonomic nervous s.
  BacT/Alert Microbial Detection S.
  BACTEC s.
  Basic Clinical Scoring S. (BCSS)
  Bionicare 1000 stimulator s.
  blood group s.
  Brasfield scoring s.
  carbon dioxide laser scanner s.
  Cardiovit AT-10 ECG/spirometry
    combination s.
  central nervous s. (CNS)
  Circulaire aerosol drug delivery s.
  CMS AccuProbe 450 s.
  Coleman microinfiltration s.
  Companion 314 nasal CPAP s.
  complement s.
  Costa's Simple Scoring S.
  DAR breathing s.
  dermal s.
  Derma 20 laser s.
  DermMaster s.
  DNA-anti-DNA s.

DPAP interactive airway management s.
drug-induced depression of immune s.
Dyna-Care pressure pad s.
Dyonics Dyosite office arthroscopy s.
Dyonics InteliJet fluid management s.
EpiLaser laser-based hair removal s.
EpiLight hair removal s.
EpiStar diode laser s.
Finger Phantom pulse oximeter testing s.
Gell and Coombs classification s.
genetic depression of immune s.
GentleLASE Plus laser s.
GentlePeel skin exfoliation s.
Haversian s.
hematopoietic s.
Hunstad tumescent liposuction s.
hypothalamic-pituitary-adrenal s.
HY-TEC automated allergy diagnostic s.
immune s.
indicator s.
integumentary s.
Kaplan PenduLaser 115 laser s.
kinin s.
Larsen grading s.
Levulin PDT s.
LightSheer SC laser hair removal s.
LPI excimer laser s.
lymphoreticular s. (LRS)
Lyra laser s.
s. of macrophage
Medi-Facts s.
monocyte-macrophage s.
mononuclear phagocyte s. (MPS)
MultiLight s.
MultiPulse laser s.
myeloperoxidase-hydrogen peroxide halide s.
NADPH oxidase s.
nervous s.
Norwood classification s.
Nu-Derm S.
Nu-Trake Weiss emergency airway s.
Nuvolase 660 laser s.

Orbasone s.
organ transplantation s.
Ortho-Ice Multipaks s.
Oxyfil oxygen refilling s.
Panasol II home phototherapy s.
Para-Pak Ultra Ecofix s.
peripheral nervous s. (PNS)
PhotoDerm MultiLight s.
PhotoGenica laser s.
Plast-O-Fit thermoplastic bandage s.
PodoSpray nail drill s.
primary angiitis of the central nervous s. (PACNS)
properdin s.
Quanti-Test S.
radiometric resin s.
Rajka and Langeland scoring s.
Refinity Coblation s.
reticuloendothelial s. (RES)
RinoFlow nasal wash and sinus s.
Simple Scoring S. (SSS)
single-cell ion imaging s.
SkinLaser s.
SLP1000 diode laser s.
SoftLight laser hair removal s.
SpaTouch PhotoEpilation s.
statistical analysis s. (SAS)
superficial musculoaponeurotic s. (SMAS)
super long-pulse diode laser s.
Sure-Closure skin stretching s.
sympathetic nervous s.
Symphony patient monitoring s.
ThAIRapy vest airway clearance s.
Therakos UVAR s.
TheraPEP positive expiratory pressure therapy s.
transdermal therapeutic s. (TTS)
TruPulse CO2 laser s.
Uganda Cancer Institute staging s.
UltraFine erbium laser s.
United States Renal Data S. (USRDS)
Vaccine Adverse Events Reporting S. (VAERS)
Vbeam pulse dye laser s.
Vornado Air Quality S.
Wound Stick measuring s.
YagLazr s.
Zimmer Pulsavac wound debridement s.

systematic polymorphism screening

S

NOTES

systematized nevus

systemic

    s. acne

    s. amyloid

    s. anaphylaxis

    s. antibacterial therapy

    s. antifungal therapy

    s. autoaggression

    s. autoimmune disease

    s. candidiasis

    s. corticosteroid

    s. febrile disease

    s. fungal infection

    s. hyalinosis

    s. hypersensitivity angiitis

    s. inflammatory response syndrome (SIRS)

    s. juvenile rheumatoid arthritis

    S. Lupus Activity Measure (SLAM)

    s. lupus erythematosus (SLE)

    s. lupus erythematosus-like syndrome

    S. Lupus International Collaborating Clinics (SLICC)

    s. malignancy

    s. mastocytosis

    s. necrotizing vasculitis (SNV)

    s. poisoning

    s. polyarteritis nodosa

    s. polyarthralgia

    s. proliferating angioendotheliomatosis

    s. reaction

    s. sclerosis (SSc)

    s. sclerosis sine scleroderma (ssSSc)

    s. steroid

    s. visceral amyloidosis

T
time
T agglutinogen
T antigen
T cell
T cell-B cell collaboration
T cell fibroblast
chloramine T
Cleocin T
T cytotoxic cell (Tc)
Dalacin T
T gel
T locus
T lymphocyte
Ortho-Kung T (OKT)
T tubule
T zone
T zone complexion
T3
triiodothyronine
T4
thyroxine
Soluble T4
t
t score
T1-weighted study
T2-weighted study
TAA
triamcinolone acetonide
TA-AIDS
transfusion-associated AIDS
TAB
temporal artery biopsy
T.A.B.
typhoid A&B
T.A.B. vaccine
Tabanidae
tabes dorsalis
tabetic
t. facies
t. neurosyphilis
t. osteoarthropathy
tablet
Actagen T.
Actifed Allergy T.
Afrin T.
Allercon T.
Allerfrin T.
allergy t.
Aprodine T.
Aristocort T.
Benadryl Decongestant Allergy T.
BQ T.
Bromfed T.
Bromphen T.

Carbiset T.
Carbiset-TR T.
Cenafed Plus T.
Chlor-Trimeton 4 Hour Relief T.
Deconamine T.
decongestant t.
Dimaphen T.
Dimetapp T.
Ditropan XL oxybutynin chloride
extended-release t.
Fedahist T.
Genac T.
headache t.
Histalet Forte T.
Hista-Vadrin T.
Kenacort T.
Klerist-D T.
Lamisil T.
meloxicam t.
Mobic T.
Phyllocontin T.
Pseudo-Gest Plus T.
Sinutab T.
Sudafed Plus T.
terbinafine hydrochloride t.
Triposed T.
Tylenol Cold Effervescent
Medication t.
Veltane T.
Vicks DayQuil Allergy Relief 4
Hour t.
Tabs
Apo-Doxy T.
Travel T.
TAC
tacrolimus
transiently amplifying cell
triamcinolone cream
Tacalciol
Tac antigen
Tacaribe complex of virus
Tacaryl
TACE
transarterial chemoembolization
tache
t. bleuâtres
t. cérébrale
t. méningéale
t. noire
t. spinale
tachetic
tachyarrhythmia
tachycardia
tachyphylaxis
tachypnea

Tac-3, -40 Injection
tacrolimus (FK506, TAC)
    t. hydrate
    t. ointment
tacrolimus-associated
    t.-a. diabetes
    t.-a. mutism
tactile cell of Merkel-Ranvier
tactiles
    toruli t.
TAD
    transient acantholytic dermatosis
TAE
    total abdominal evisceration
Taenia
    T. saginata
    T. solium
taeniacide
tag
    cutaneous t.
    identification t.
    pleural t.
    sentinel t.
    skin t.
Tagamet-HB
tagged white blood cell study
Tahyna virus
TAI
    thoracoabdominal irradiation
tail sign
Takahara disease
Takayasu
    T. arteriopathy
    T. arteritis
    T. disease
TAL
    triamcinolone lotion
talalgia
    plantar t.
talc
    t. lotion
    purified t.
    t. slurry
    zinc oxide, cod liver oil, and t.
Talcum
tall dock
talon noir
Tamine
Tamm-Horsfall protein
tamoxifen
Tanafed
tangential
    t. biopsy
    t. excision
tangent-to-circle excision
Tangier disease
tanned red cell

tanner
    T. mesher device
    T. pubertal stage
    t. ulcer
Tanner-Vandeput mesh dermatome
tanning
    t. bed
    delayed t.
    immediate t.
Tantafed
TAO
    thromboangiitis obliterans
    thyroid-associated ophthalmopathy
    triamcinolone ointment
tapasin
tape
    Cath-Secure t.
    ColorZone t.
    Cordran t.
    Deknatel wound t.
    Dermicel t.
    Elastikon elastic t.
    Micropore t.
    Scanpor t.
taper
    prednisone t.
    steroid t.
tapeworm
    dog t.
TAP1, TAP2 protein
TaqMan assay
Taq polymerase
tar
    t. acne
    t. bath
    coal t.
    DHS T.
    T. Distillate
    T. Doak
    juniper t.
    t. keratosis
    t. melanosis
    ointment of t.
    t. preparation
    Spectro T.
    wood t.
Tarabine PFS
Taractan
TARC
    thymus and activation-regulated
      chemokine
tarda
    familial spondyloepiphyseal
      dysplasia t.
    lues t.
    osteogenesis imperfecta t.
    porphyria cutanea t. (PCT)
    syphilis hereditaria t.

Tardan
Tardieu petechia
tardus
    nevus spilus t.
Targel SA
target
    t. cell
    t. lesion
    t. of rapamycin inhibitor (TOR
    inhibitor)
targetoid hemosiderotic hemangioma
(THH)
Targretin
Taro-Desoximetasone
Taro-Sone
Tarply scale
tarsal tunnel syndrome
tarsi
    acne t.
    tinea t.
TAR syndrome
tartaric acid
Tart cell
tartrate
    belladonna, phenobarbital, and
    ergotamine t.
    phenindamine t.
    trimeprazine t.
tartrate-resistant
    t.-r. acid phosphatase (TRAP)
    t.-r. acid phosphatase positive cell
tartrazine
Tarui disease
TASS syndrome
TAT
    thrombin-antithrombin III
Tat
TATA
    tumor-associated transplantation antigen
TATA-binding protein
tat gene
tattoo
    amalgam t.
    eyeline t.
    oral t.
tattooing effect
Tau-Cl
tau-globulin
taurine chloramine
tautology
Tavist
Tavist-1, -D

tax
    viral protein t.
taxa
Taxol
taxon
taxonomic
taxonomy
    numerical t.
Taylor disease
Tay-Sachs disease
Tay syndrome
tazarotene topical gel
Tazicef
Tazidime
tazobactam
Tazorac
TB
    tuberculosis
        TB test by PCR
TBAB
    thyroid-blocking antibody
T- and B-cell severe combined
immunodeficiency disease
TBI
    total body irradiation
    tumor burden index
TBII
    thyroid-binding inhibitory
    immunoglobulin
    thyrotropin-binding inhibitory
    immunoglobulin
TBS
    Tris-buffered saline
    TRIS-buffered saline solution
TBSA
    total body surface area
3TC
Tc
    T cytotoxic cell
    technetium
        Tc polyphosphate scan
TCA
    trichloroacetic acid
TCB
    total counts bound
Tc-dimercaptosuccinic acid (DMSA)
T-cell
    T.-c. antibody labeling
    T.-c. antigen receptor
    T.-c. counter-receptor interaction
    T.-c. defect
    T.-c. erythroderma

NOTES

T-cell *(continued)*
T.-c. growth factor (TCGF)
T.-c. growth factor-1
T.-c. growth factor-2
T.-c. involvement
T.-c. large granuloma lymphocyte leukemia
T.-c. leukemia virus type 1
T.-c. lymphocytic leukemia
T.-c. lymphocytoma cutis
T.-c. lymphoma
T.-c. marker
T.-c. pseudolymphoma
T.-c. receptor (TCR)
T.-c. replacing factor
T.-c. rosette
T.-c. suppression
T.-c. xenorecognition
T-cell-mediated
T.-c.-m. autoimmune disease
T.-c.-m. delayed type hypersensitivity dermatitis
TCGF
T-cell growth factor
⁹⁹ᵐTc-HMPAO
TCHT
traditional Chinese herbal therapy
Tc-human serum albumin scintigraphy
TCN
tetracycline
TCR
T-cell receptor
Tc1, Tc2 cell
TD
trichodiscoma
T.D.
Diamine T.D.
Td
tetanus-diphtheria
TDD
thoracic duct drainage
T-dependent
T.-d. antigen
T.-d. response
T/Derm
Neutrogena T.
TDI
isocyanate TDI
T1DM
type 1 diabetes mellitus
T2DM
type 2 diabetes mellitus
TDT
transmission disequilibrium testing
TDTH cell
TdT-positive
TE
trichoepithelioma

tea
Mexican t.
tear
artificial t.'s
T. Drop solution
t. lysozyme
TearGard Ophthalmic solution
Teargen Ophthalmic solution
Tearisol solution
Tears
Liquifilm T.
T. Naturale
T. Naturale Free solution
T. Naturale II solution
T. Plus solution
T. Renewed solution
tebutate
prednisolone t.
Tec family of cytoplasmic protein tyrosine kinase
technetium (Tc)
t. diphosphonate
t. pertechnetate
t. scan
technetium-99m hexamethylpropylene amine oxime-single-photon-emission computed tomography (HMPAO-SPECT)
Techni-Care
T.-C. surgical scrub
T.-C. wound cleanser
technique
aseptic t.
Blenderm patch t.
Boyden chamber t.
cognitive-behavioral t.
cytogenic t.
dipstick t.
enzyme-multiplied immunoassay t. (EMIT)
Fegan t.
fluorescent antibody t.
freehand t.
Hotchkiss-McManus t.
immunodiffusion t.
immunofluorescence t.
immunometric t.
Ingram t.
interval mapping t.
Jerne t.
joint protection t.
laser-assisted internal fabrication t.
Lich t.
LIFT t.
light scatter t.
lymphoablative t.
Mancini t.
Mohs fresh-tissue t.

Ouchterlony double diffusion t.
PAS t.
P-E t.
    portal venous and enteric drainage
    technique
percutaneous conchotome biopsy t.
periodic acid-Schiff t.
polka-dot t.
portal venous and enteric
  drainage t. (P-E technique)
problem elicitation t. (PET)
Rebuck skin window t.
saucerization t.
shave t.
skin window t.
split adjuvant t.
sterile t.
stripe t.
thermal quenching t.
trichloroacetic acid-tape t.
tumescent t.
volumetric t.
whole-body antibody t. (IMX)
technology
    gene-knockout t.
    PulseDose oxygen delivery t.
tecogalan
tectate
Tectiviridae
Tedral
Teejel
teeth (*pl. of* tooth)
Tegaderm
    T. HP transparent film
    T. semipermeable dressing
    T. transparent dressing
    T. transparent dressing with
    absorbent pad
Tegagel
    T. dressing/sheet
    T. hydrogel
    T. hydrogel dressing
    T. hydrogel sheet
Tegagen
    T. HG alginate wound dressing
    T. HG, HI alginate wound cover
    T. HI alginate dressing
Tegapore
    T. contact-layer sheet
    T. contact-layer wound dressing
Tegasorb
    T. synthetic dressing

    T. Thin hydrocolloid
    T. Thin hydrocolloid dressing
Tega-Vert Oral
Tegison
Tegopen
Tegretol
Tegrin
Tegrin-HC Topical
tegument
tegumentary epithelium
tegumentum
TEH
    theophylline, ephedrine, and hydroxyzine
teicoplanin
Telachlor Oral
Teladar Topical
telangiectasia
    ataxia t.
    calcinosis cutis, Raynaud
      phenomenon, esophageal motility
      disorder, sclerodactyly, t.
      (CREST)
    cephalooculocutaneous t.
    dermatomal superficial t.
    essential t.
    hemorrhagic t.
    hereditary hemorrhagic t. (HHT)
    t. macularis eruptiva perstans
      (TMEP)
    nevoid t.
    oculocutaneous t.
    periungual t.
    primary t.
    secondary t.
    spider t.
    unilateral dermatomal superficial t.
    unilateral nevoid t.
    t. verrucosa
    wire-loop shaped t.
telangiectasis, pl. **telangiectases**
    hereditary hemorrhagic t.
    linear t.
    multiple hereditary hemorrhagic t.
    spider t.
    stellate t.
    tortuous t.
telangiectatic
    t. erythema
    t. mat
    t. matting (TM)
    t. systemic mastocytosis
    t. wart

T

NOTES

telangiectatica
  livedo t.
telangiectaticum
  granuloma t.
telangiectodes
  acne t.
  elephantiasis t.
  purpura annularis t.
telar
Teldrin Oral
telemetry
  home-based t. (HBT)
  multiple parameter t. (MPT)
teletactor
teleutospore
Telfa
  T. Clear contact layer sheet
  T. composite dressing
Telfamax absorptive dressing
Teline Oral
teliospore
telmisartan
telogen
  t. effluvium
  t. hair
  t. phase
telomeric
telopeptide
TEM
  transmission electron microscopy
  triethylenemelamine
temafloxacin
Temaril
Temovate topical
temperate
  t. bacteriophage
  t. virus
temperature
  maximum t.
  minimum t.
  optimum t.
  room t.
  t. sensitive (TS)
  t. spot
temperature-dependent dermatosis
temperature-sensitive
  t.-s. mutant
  t.-s. oculocutaneous albinism
template
  Dermal Regeneration T.
  t. theory
temporal
  t. artery biopsy (TAB)
  t. canthus
  t. giant cell arteritis
  t. relationship

temporomandibular
  t. dysfunction (TMD)
  t. joint
Tempra
TEN
  toxic epidermal necrolysis
tenascin
Tendersorb ABD absorptive dressing
Tenderwrap leg compression dressing
tendinitis
  bicipital t.
  t. bursitis
  calcific t.
  patellar t.
tendinopathy
  degenerative t.
tendinosis
tendinosum
  xanthoma t.
tendinous xanthoma
tendon
  Achilles t.
  t. friction rub
  peroneal t.
  t. sheath
  supraspinatus t.
  t. xanthoma
tendonesis effect
tendonitis-fascitis syndrome
tenesmus
teniposide
ten-nail dystrophy
tennis
  t. elbow
  t. shoe foot
  t. toe
Tenon
  T. capsule
  T. space
Ten-O-Six
tenosynovectomy
tenosynovitis
  de Quervain stenosing t.
  dorsal wrist t.
  flexed t.
  gonococcic t.
  gonorrheal t.
  proliferative t.
  stenosing t.
  tenosynovium t.
tenosynovium tenosynovitis
tenoxicam acid
TENS
  transcutaneous electrical nerve
    stimulation
  transcutaneous electrical neuromuscular
    stimulator
  Sham TENS

tensile strength of osteoarthritic
    cartilage
tension-time index
tentacle print
tenuis
    Alternaria t.
    Nocardia t.
Tequin
Terak Ophthalmic Ointment
teratogenic effect on pregnant women
Terazol
terbinafine
    t. hydrochloride
    t. hydrochloride cream
    t. hydrochloride tablet
terbutaline sulfate
terconazole
terebrans
    basiloma t.
terfenadine and pseudoephedrine
Terfonyl
Terinacei
terminal
    t. cascade
    t. hair
    postsynaptic t.
    presynaptic t.
    visual display t. (VDT)
terminator
    DNA-chain t.
terpine anhydride
Terra-Cortril Ophthalmic Suspension
Terramycin
    T. IM injection
    T. Oral
    T. w/Polymyxin B Ophthalmic
        Ointment
terrestrial snake
terreus
    Aspergillus t.
Terry nail
Tersa-Tar
tertiary
    t. cutaneous syphilis
    t. follicle
    t. granule
    t. noduloulcerative syphilis
    t. structure
    t. syphilid
    t. yaw
tertile

Teschen
    T. disease
    T. disease virus
Tessalon Perles
TEST
    T.R.U.E. T.
test
    A1 t.
    ACADERM patch t.
    acid-Schiff t.
    adhesion t.
    Adson t.
    AlaSTAT latex allergy t.
    alkali patch t.
    allergen inhalation challenge t.
    Amplicor viral load t.
    Amplified Mycobacterium
        Tuberculosis Direct T.
    analysis of variance t.
    Ana-Sal HIV t.
    ANOVA t.
    antibiotic sensitivity t.
    antigenemia t.
    antigliadin IgG, IgA t.
    antiglobulin t.
    antihuman globulin t.
    antinuclear antibody screening t.
    antistreptolysin-O t.
    Ascoli t.
    ASO t.
    atopy patch t. (APT)
    augmented histamine t.
    bacterial phagocytosis t.
    basophil degranulation t.
    BCR/abl gene re-arrangement t.
    bentonite flocculation t.
    Bioclot t.
    blood coagulation t.
    bronchial inhalation challenge t.
    bronchial provocation t.
    broth t.
    Brucella card t.
    Buhler t.
    C3 t.
    C4 t.
    Calmette t.
    Candida skin t.
    capillary fragility t.
    capillary resistance t.
    Captia t.
    Casoni intradermal t.
    Casoni skin t.

T

NOTES

557

test *(continued)*
    CF t.
    challenge t.
    chamber-scarification t.
    Chiron bDNA viral load t.
    chi-square t.
    chloride sweat t.
    Christmas tree t.
    chrome patch t.
    closed patch t.
    Clostridium difficile t. (CLOtest)
    Coamatic protein C t.
    Cobas Amplicor CMV Monitor t.
    coccidioidin skin t.
    Cochran-Mantel-Haenszel t.
    collagen vascular serologic t.
    colony-stimulating factor fluorescent
      treponemal antibody-absorption t.
      (CSF-FTA-ABS)
    colony-stimulating factor
      microhemagglutination-*Treponema*
      pallidum t. (CSF-MHA-TP)
    color allergy screening t. (CAST)
    Combi t.
    combion t.
    complement t.
    complement-fixation t.
    Confide HIV t.
    conjunctival provocation t. (CPT)
    Coombs t.
    cosmetic allergy t.
    Coulter ICD-Prep t.
    Cox-Mantel t.
    Crithidia luciliae indirect
      immunofluorescence t. (CLIFT)
    CSD skin t.
    cutaneous tuberculin t.
    cutireaction t.
    cystic fibrosis t.
    cytotoxic t.
    cytotropic antibody t.
    DA pregnancy t.
    Davidsohn differential t.
    dexamethasone suppression t. (DST)
    DFA t.
    diagnostic t.
    Dick t.
    dimethylgloxime nickel spot t.
    direct agglutination t.
    direct Coombs t.
    direct fluorescent antibody t.
    DNA-binding t.
    DNA hybridization t.
    DNA probe t.
    double immunodiffusion in agarose
      gels t.
    Draize Repeat Insult patch t.
    Ducrey t.

    Dunnett multiple comparison t.
    EBNA IgG ELISA t.
    EB nuclear antigen t.
    EB-specific IgM t.
    EB viral capsid antigen t.
    electrotransfer t.
    ELISA t.
    ELISPOT t.
    Envacor t.
    enzyme allergosorbent t. (EAST)
    enzyme-linked immunosorbent
      assay t.
    epicutaneous t.
    epsilometric t.
    Epstein-Barr nuclear antigen t.
    Epstein-Barr-specific immunoglobulin
      M t.
    Epstein-Barr virus t.
    erythrocyte adherence t.
    false-negative patch t.
    false-positive patch t.
    false-positive syphilis t.
    Farr t.
    Finkelstein t.
    First Check rapid diagnostic t.
    Fisher two-tailed exact t.
    flocculation t.
    fluorescein-conjugated monoclonal
      antibody immunofluorescent t.
    fluorescein-tagged monoclonal
      antibody immunofluorescent t.
    fluorescent treponemal antibody-
      absorption t.
    forearm ischemic exercise t.
    Formo-Test t.
    Foshay t.
    Frei t.
    Freund complete adjuvant t.
    FTA-ABS t.
    gel diffusion precipitin t.
    Gen-Probe rapid tuberculosis t.
    Gerhardt t.
    glove-powder inhalation t.
    glove-use t.
    goodness-of-fit chi-square t.
    Göthlin t.
    grind t.
    guinea pig maximization t.
      (GPMT)
    Hair dressing screening tray t.
    Ham t.
    Hamilton t.
    HBV DNA probe t.
    head compression t.
    head distraction t.
    Heaf t.
    Helisal rapid blood t.
    hemadsorption virus t.

hemagglutination t.
Hess t.
Hinton t.
histoplasmin-latex t.
HIV DNA PCR t.
H-SLAP t.
human stromelysin aggregated proteoglycan t.
hybridization t.
Hycor rheumatoid factor IgA ELISA autoimmune t.
hydrogen breath t.
hyperventilation provocation t. (HVPT)
ice cube t.
IgE radioallergosorbent t.
IgG avidity t.
immune adhesion t.
ImmunoCard STAT! Rotavirus t.
immunologic pregnancy t.
indirect agglutination t.
indirect Coombs t.
indirect fluorescent antibody t.
indirect hemagglutination t.
INR clotting t.
    international normalized ratio clotting test
insulin skin t.
international normalized ratio clotting t. (INR clotting test)
intracutaneous t.
intradermal skin t.
intraperitoneal glucose tolerance t. (IPGTT)
intravenous glucose tolerance t. (IVGTT)
Ito-Reenstierna t.
Jadassohn-Bloch t.
Keller ultraviolet t.
killing t.
k82 ImmunoCap t.
Kolmer t.
Kolmogorov-Smirnov t.
Kruskal-Wallis t.
Kveim t.
Lachman t.
latex agglutination t.
latex allergy t.
latex fixation t.
leishmania t.
leishmanin t.

Leishman-Montenegro-Donovan intradermal t.
lepromin t.
leukocyte esterase t. (LET)
leukocyte histamine release t.
Liatest C4b-BP t.
lignocaine monoethylglycine xylidine excretion t.
liver function t. (LFT)
lupus band t. (LBT)
lupus erythematosus cell t.
lymphogranuloma venereum complement fixation t. (LGV-CFT)
macrophage migration inhibition t.
macroscopic agglutination t.
Mann-Whitney U t.
Mantel-Haenszel t.
Mantoux t.
mast cell degranulation t.
t. material
Maurer optimization t.
Mazzotti t.
McKenzie t.
McNemar t.
McNemar t. of significance
Mecholyl skin t.
Meinicke t.
methacholine chloride skin t.
MHA-TP t.
microhemagglutination-*Treponema pallidum* t.
microimmunofluorescence t. (MIF)
microlymphocytotoxicity t.
microscopic agglutination t.
midpoint skin t.
migration inhibition t.
migration inhibitory factor t.
Minor iodine-starch t.
Mitsuda t.
mixed agglutination t.
mixed lymphocyte culture t.
MLC t.
modified Draize t.
Moloney t.
monoLISA t.
Mono-Vac t.
Montenegro t.
MTD T.
mucin clot t.
multiple puncture t. (MPT)
multiple puncture tuberculin t.

NOTES

T

test *(continued)*
    Multitest t.
    mumps sensitivity t.
    Murray t.
    Mycobacterium tuberculosis
     Direct T.
    nasal antigen challenge t.
    nasal provocation t.
    negative control t.
    negative patch t.
    negative schick t.
    neutralization t.
    Newman-Keuls t.
    nitroblue tetrazolium t.
    nontreponemal flocculation t.
    N-telopeptide urine t.
    occlusive patch t.
    t. for O&P
    open application t.
    open epicutaneous t. (OET)
    open patch t.
    OsteoGram bone density t.
    Osteomark urine-based t.
    Ouchterlony t.
    OX-2, -19 t.
    oxacillin disk diffusion t.
    Pap t.
      Papanicolaou test
    Papanicolaou t. (Pap test)
    paper radioimmunosorbent t.
     (PRIST)
    paracoccidioidin skin t.
    passive cutaneous anaphylaxis t.
    passive transfer t.
    patch t.
    Paul t.
    Paul-Bunnell t.
    PCA t.
    Pearson chi square t.
    pediatric infectious disease
     developmental screening t.
     (PIDDST)
    percutaneous t.
    pertussis agglutination t.
    photo-patch t.
    physiologic t.
    pilocarpine iontophoresis sweat t.
    Pirquet t.
    P-K t.
    platelet neutralization t.
    POCkit herpes t.
    Porges-Meier t.
    positive patch t.
    PPD t.
    PPL skin t.
    Prausnitz-Kustner t.
    precipitation t.
    precipitin t.

    predictive patch t.
    prick-prick t.
    prick puncture t.
    prick-to-prick t.
    protection t.
    provocation-neutralization t.
    provocative use t. (PUT)
    pulmonary function t. (PFT)
    pulse t.
    purified protein derivative t.
    quellung t.
    radioallergosorbent t. (RAST)
    radioimmunosorbent t. (RIST)
    rapid whole blood t. (RWBT)
    reagin screen t. (RST)
    red cell adherence t.
    Reiter t.
    repeat open reaction application t.
    RF t.
    Rh blocking t.
    Rheumatex t.
    rheumatoid factor t.
    Rheumaton t.
    rhinovirus challenge t.
    ring precipitin t.
    Rinne t.
    Römer t.
    rosette t.
    Rose-Waaler t.
    RoSSA/RoSSB antibody t.
    RPR circle card t.
    rub t.
    rubella HI t.
    rubella IgG ELISA t.
    Rumpel-Leede t.
    Sabin-Feldman dye t.
    Sachs-Georgi t.
    scarification t.
    Schick t.
    Schirmer t.
    Schober t.
    Scotch Tape t.
    scratch chamber t.
    screen t.
    Semmes-Weinstein t.
    sequential probability ratio t.
     (SPRT)
    serial dilutional intradermal skin t.
    Shapiro-Wilke W t.
    single-breath nitrogen washout t.
    skin prick t. (SPT)
    skin-puncture t.
    Spearman rank t.
    SPEP t.
    spinal fluid t.
    sporotriquin t.
    spot t.
    starch-iodine t.

Steinberg t.
Sterneedle tuberculin t.
streptozyme agglutination t.
SureCell Strep A t.
TheoFAST t.
thermostable opsonin t.
tine t.
tourniquet t.
TPHA t.
TPI t.
transfer t.
Trendelenburg t.
treponemal t.
Treponema pallidum
  hemagglutination t.
Treponema pallidum
  immobilization t.
Trichophyton skin t.
Trolab wool alcohol t.
T.R.U.E. allergy patch t.
tube precipitin t.
tuberculin skin t.
tuberculin tine t.
tuberculin titer t.
Tukey standardized range t.
Tzanck t.
urea breath t. (UBT)
use t.
VDRL t.
virus neutralization t.
vitamin C t.
in vitro t.
Vollmer t.
volume t.
Wassermann fast t.
Weber t.
Weil-Felix t.
Western blot electrotransfer t.
Whiff t.
Widal serum t.
Wilcoxon rank sum t.
Winn t.
x-square t.
Yates corrected chi square t.
testacea
  cutis t.
testerma
  Jadassohn t.
testing
  antimicrobiology susceptibility t.
  battery patch t.

conjunctival t.
delayed hypersensitivity skin t.
electrodermal t.
epidermal t.
genotypic antiretroviral resistance t.
  (GART)
histocompatibility t.
human immunodeficiency virus
  antigen t.
hypersensitivity skin t.
John Dory fish prick t.
panel-reactive antibody t.
p24 antigen t.
patch t.
PCR t.
placebo-controlled oral challenge t.
  (DPOC)
polymerase chain reaction t.
population-based t.
PRA t.
predictive t.
prick t.
provocative dose t.
RCR t.
repeat open-application t. (ROAT)
RIBA II antibody t.
Rinkle t.
scratch t.
skin t.
SUDS HIV-1 diagnostic t.
transmission disequilibrium t. (TDT)
venom t.
testis-specific binding protein (TSBP)
Testoderm patch
testosterone
test/score
  MEGX t.
TET
  tetracycline
tetanolysin
tetanospasmin
tetanotoxin
tetanus
  t. antitoxin
  t. antitoxin unit
  t. immune globulin
  t. immune globulin, human
  t. immunoglobulin
  t. toxin
  t. toxoid
  t. toxoid, adsorbed

NOTES

T

561

tetanus *(continued)*
 t. toxoid, fluid
 t. vaccine
tetanus-diphtheria (Td)
tetanus-perfringens antitoxin
Tete virus
tetra-acetate
tetracaine
 t. hydrochloride
 t. with dextrose
Tetracap Oral
tetracycline (TCN, TET)
 t. seams
 t. transactivator
tetracycline-resistant *Neisseria*
 gonorrhoeae **(TRNG)**
Tetracyn
tetrad
 acne t.
tetrahydrozoline hydrochloride
Tetralan
 acetyl ethyl tetramethyl T. (AETT)
 T. Oral
tetramethylthiuram dermatitis
Tetram Oral
Tetramune fish food
tetranda
 Stephania t.
Tetrasine Extra Ophthalmic
tetratricopeptide repeat
tetrazolium
 nitroblue t. (NBT)
tetrodotoxin
tetter
 branny t.
 brawny t.
 crusted t.
 dry t.
 foot t.
 honeycomb t.
 humid t.
 milk t.
 moist t.
 scaly t.
 wet t.
Texacort Topical
Texas
 T. coral snake
 T. coral snake bite
textile dermatitis
texture
 coarse t.
textus, pl. **textus**
TF
 tissue factor
TFCC
 triangular fibrocartilage complex

TFI
 tumor of the follicular infundibulum
TFPI
 tissue factor pathway inhibitor
TG
 thyroglobulin
Tg cell
TGE
 transmissible gastroenteritis virus
  TGE virus
T/Gel
 Neutrogena T.
 T. Neutrogena
TGF
 transforming growth factor
 trypanosome growth factor
TGF-alpha
 transforming growth factor-alpha
TGFB
 transforming growth factor-beta
TGF-B
 transforming growth factor-B
TGF-beta
 transforming growth factor-beta
TGF-induced immunosuppression
TGV
 trapped gas volume
TH2
 T-helper-2 lymphocyte
Th
 T-helper cell
 thyroid
Th2
 T-helper type 2 cell
  Th2 cell
Th3
 T-helper type 3 cell
TH1 cytokine
Th-1 mediated immune response
ThAIRapy vest airway clearance system
thalassemia
 alpha t.
 Bart t.
 t. major
 t. syndrome
thalidomide
Thalimune
thallus
Thalomid
thanatophobic
thanatophoric diastrophic
 chondrodysplasia
thapsigargin pool
Thayer-Martin medium
Th1 cell
thecal felon
Theiler
 T. disease

T. mouse encephalomyelitis virus
T. original strain of mouse
   encephalomyelitis virus (TO)
Thelazia
thelerethism
thelium, pl. **thelia**
T-helper
   T.-h. cell (Th)
   T.-h. type 2 cell (Th2)
   T.-h. type 3 cell (Th3)
T-helper-2 lymphocyte (TH2)
Theo-24
Theobald Smith phenomenon
Theobid
Theochron
Theoclear L.A.
Theo-Dur
TheoFAST test
Theo-G
Theolair
Theolate
theophylline
   anhydrous t.
   dihydroxypropyl t.
   t., ephedrine, and hydroxyzine
      (TEH)
   t., ephedrine, and phenobarbital
   t. and guaifenesin
   t. salt
theophylline-induced convulsion
theorem
   binomial t.
theory, pl. **theories**
   Arrhenius-Madsen t.
   cellular immune t.
   clonal deletion t.
   clonal selection t.
   Ehrlich side-chain t.
   Fisher-Race t.
   forbidden-clone t.
   germ t.
   immune t.
   instructive t.
   Metchnikoff t.
   neural t.
   side-chain t.
   template t.
Theospan-SR
Theovent
Theo-X
thèque

Thera-Boot leg compression dressing
TheraCys
Therafectin
Therakos UVAR system
Theramin Expectorant
TheraPEP positive expiratory pressure
   therapy system
therapeutic
   t. immunology
   t. interferon
   t. irradiation
   t. malaria
   t. ratio
therapia magna sterilisans
Theraplex Z
therapy
   ACTH t.
   adrenocorticosteroid t.
   adrenocorticotropic hormone t.
   alkylating t.
   alternate-day t.
   antibacterial t.
   antibody-directed enzyme prodrug t.
      (ADEPT)
   antifungal t.
   anti-IIb-IIIA mAB t.
   antiinflammatory t.
   antipruritic t.
   antituberculous t.
   antiviral t.
   around-the-clock oral maintenance
      bronchodilator t.
   5 ATGAM antilymphocyte t.
   augmentation t.
   autoserum t.
   BAL t.
      British Anti-Lewisite therapy
   biomagnetic t.
   blood transfusion t.
   British Anti-Lewisite t. (BAL
      therapy)
   calcipotriene t.
   Candida t.
   chloroquine t.
   coherence t.
   combination retinoid and PUVA t.
      (Re-PUVA)
   conventional asthma t. (CAT)
   cyclosporine maintenance t.
   cytotoxic immunosuppressive t.
   Diabetic Skin T.

NOTES

T

therapy *(continued)*
    diagnostic surgical t.
    dressing t.
    empiric t.
    estrogen replacement t. (ERT)
    factor replacement t.
    fever t.
    fluid t.
    fluorinated corticosteroid-occlusive t.
    foreign protein t.
    gene t.
    gold t.
    grenz ray t.
    heat t.
    heparinoid t.
    heterovaccine t.
    high-dose immunosuppressive t.
      (HDIT)
    highly active antiretroviral t.
      (HAART)
    HSV-thymidine kinase ex-vivo
      cell t.
    hydroxychloroquine t.
    hyperbaric oxygen t.
    immunocompetent tissue t.
    immunoglobulin replacement t.
    immunosuppressive t. (IST)
    interferon t.
    intralesional corticosteroid t.
    Levulan photodynamic t.
    MAb t.
        monoclonal antibody therapy
    maggot t.
    malarial t.
    medical t.
    monoclonal antibody t. (MAb
      therapy)
    multidrug t. (MDT)
    Neova Eye T.
    nonspecific t.
    NTBC t.
        2-(2-nitro-4-
          trifluoromethylbenzoyl)-3-
          cyclohexanedione
    occlusive t.
    occupational t. (OT)
    5 OKT3 antilymphocyte t.
    oral iron t.
    orthomolecular t.
    penicillin t.
    pharmacologic t.
    photodynamic t. (PDT)
    plasma t.
    postnatal t.
    preemptive t.
    prenatal t.
    protective t.
    protein shock t.

    psychotropic agent t.
    pulsed-dye laser t. (PDL)
    radiation t.
    replacement t.
    repository t.
    retinoid t.
    salvage t.
    Saran Wrap t.
    sedative t.
    serum t.
    short-contact t.
    silicone sheeting t.
    skin lubrication t.
    soak t.
    Staph. protein A column t.
    supportive t.
    surgical t.
    symptomatic t.
    systemic antibacterial t.
    systemic antifungal t.
    toothpaste swish t.
    topical antibacterial t.
    topical antifungal t.
    topical cytotoxic t.
    traditional Chinese herbal t.
      (TCHT)
    triple t.
    vaccine t.
    Vaseline Lip T.
    VIMRxyn light-activated t.
    vitamin B t.
    vitamin K t.
TheraSnore oral appliance
Theratope-STn vaccine
thermal
    t. anhidrosis
    t. burn
    t. cycler
    t. elastosis
    t. flushing
    t. hyperalgia
    t. quenching technique
    t. relaxation time
    t. shock
Thermazene
thermescent skin treatment
***Thermoactinomyces* vulgaris**
thermoduric
thermogenic anhidrosis
thermolabile opsonin
thermolamp
thermophile
thermophilic
thermophylic
thermoplastic elastomer (TPE)
thermoregulation
thermoresistable
        Mycobacterium t.

thermosetting resin
thermostabile
thermostable
    t. opsonin
    t. opsonin test
thermotolerant
Theroxide Wash
thesaurismosis
thesaurosis
theta antigen
THH
    targetoid hemosiderotic hemangioma
thiabendazole
thiacetazone
thiamine deficiency
thiazide
Thibierge-Weissenbach syndrome
thick
    t. and sticky mucus
    t. tongue
thickened skin
thickening
    disciform t.
    fibrous intimal t. (FIT)
    scleroderma-like skin t.
    subbasement membrane t.
thickness
    Breslow t.
    carotid intima-media wall t.
Thiemann disease
thienamycin
Thiersch graft
thimerosal
thin-layer immunoassay
thin-section CT
THINSite
    T. hydrogel sheet
    T. with BioFilm hydrogel topical
      wound dressing
thiobarbituric acid-reactive substance
thioglucose
    gold sodium t. (GSTG)
Thioglycollate
thioguanine
thiol protease
thiomalate
    gold sodium t. (GSTM)
Thiomersal
thiopronine

thiopropanolsulphonate
    gold t.
thioredoxin (TRX)
    t. reductase (TR)
thioridazine
thiosulfate
    gold t.
    sodium t.
thiourea
third
    t. disease
    t. and fourth pharyngeal pouch
      syndrome
third-degree burn
third-generation cephalosporin
thistle
    Russian t.
thiuram-alcohol reaction
thiuram mix
Thomas needle
Thompson
    T. dermatoplasty
    T. syndrome
Thomsen antibody
Thomson
    T. poikiloderma congenitale
    T. scattering
    T. sign
thoracentesis
thoracic
    t. duct drainage (TDD)
    t. organ transplant
    t. outlet syndrome
thoracoabdominal
    t. dyssynchrony
    t. irradiation (TAI)
    t. paradox
thoracocardiography
thoraco-lumbar-sacral orthosis
thoracoplasty
thoracoscope
    rigid t.
thoracoscopy
thoracostomy
    tube t.
Thoratec ventricular assist device
Thorazine
three-day
    t.-d. fever
    t.-d. measles
threonyl-tRNA synthetase

NOTES

T

thresher's lung
threshold
    acoustic reflex t.
    t. audiometry
    erythema t.
    t. limit value (TLV)
    minimum elicitation t. (MET)
thrill
thrive
    failure to t.
thrix annulata
throat
    itchy t.
thrombasthenia
    Glanzmann t.
thrombectomy
    surgical t.
thrombi (pl. of thrombus)
thrombin-antithrombin III (TAT)
thromboangiitis obliterans (TAO)
thrombocytopenia
    amegakaryocytic t. (AT)
    autoimmune t. (AITP)
    autoimmune neonatal t.
    drug-induced t.
    familial t.
    immune t.
    isoimmune neonatal t.
    sepsis-induced t.
thrombocytopenia-absent-radius syndrome
  (TAR syndrome)
thrombocytopenic
    t. hemangiomatosis
    t. purpura
    t. purpura/hemolytic uremic
      syndrome (TTP-HUS)
thrombogenesis
thrombolytic
thrombomodulin
thrombophilia
    lupus t.
thrombophlebitis
    retinal t.
    superficial migratory t.
thrombopoietin (TPO)
thrombosis, pl. thromboses
    cerebral venous sinus t. (CVST)
    dural sinus t.
    graft t.
thrombospondin (TSP)
thrombotic
    t. gangrene
    t. thrombocytopenic purpura (TTP)
thromboxane synthase
thrombus, pl. thrombi
    intramural t.
    phagocytic t.
throwing act

thrush
    oral t.
thumb
    t. forceps
    gamekeeper's t.
Thunder God vine
thylacitis
thymectomy
thymi (pl. of thymus)
thymic
    t. alymphoplasia
    t. dysplasia
    t. epithelial cell
    t. hormone
    t. hypoplasia
    t. irradiation (TI)
    t. lymphopoietic factor
    t. peptide
    t. transplantation
thymidine
    hypoxanthine, aminopterin and t.
      (HAT)
thymin
thymine
thymocyte
Thymoglobulin
Thymol
thymoma
    murine t.
thymopathy
thymopentin
thymopoietin
thymosin
thymus, pl. thymi, thymuses
    t. and activation-regulated
      chemokine (TARC)
    congenital aplasia of t.
    t. nurse cell
thymus-derived leukemia
thymus-independent antigen
thymus-replacing factor
Thyro-Block
thyroglobulin (TG)
thyroglossal cyst
thyroid (Th)
    t. acropachy
    t. disorder
    t. peroxidase (TPO)
thyroid-associated ophthalmopathy
  (TAO)
thyroid-binding inhibitory
  immunoglobulin (TBII)
thyroid-blocking antibody (TBAB)
thyroiditis
    t., Addison disease, Sjögren
      syndrome, sarcoidosis syndrome
      (TASS syndrome)
    chronic autoimmune t.

Hashimoto t.
immune-mediated t.
painless t.
postpartum t. (PPT)
thyroid-stimulating
    t.-s. antibody (TSAb)
    t.-s. hormone (TSH)
    t.-s. hormone-displacing antibody
    t.-s. hormone receptor (TSH-R)
    t.-s. hormone receptor antibody
thyroperoxidase antibody
thyrotoxic
    t. complement-fixation factor
    t. serum
thyrotoxicosis
thyrotoxin
thyrotropin-binding inhibitory
  immunoglobulin (TBII)
thyroxine (T4)
Thysanosoma actinoides
thysanotrichica
    ichthyosis t.
TI
    thymic irradiation
TI-23 cytomegalovirus monoclonal
  antibody
Tiacid
Tiamol
tiaprofenic acid
tibial nerve
Ticar
ticarcillin
    t. and clavulanic acid
    t. disodium
tic douloureux
TICE
    TICE Bacillus Calmette-Guérin
    Live
    TICE Bacillus Calmette-Guérin live
    (TICE BCG)
    TICE BCG
tick
    t. bite
    t. bite alopecia
    black-legged t.
    California black-legged t.
    deer t.
    t. fever
    hard t.
    Ixodes dammini t.
    Ixodes pacificus t.
    Ixodes ricinus wood t.

Lone Star t.
Pacific t.
t. paralysis
t. pyrexia
Rocky Mountain t.
seed t.
soft t.
spotted-fever t.
t. typhus
western black-legged t.
wood t.
tickborne
    t. encephalitis Central European
      subtype
    t. encephalitis Eastern subtype
    t. encephalitis virus
    t. relapsing fever
TI-CMV
    tissue-invasive cytomegalovirus
      TI-CMV disease
tidal
    t. irrigation
    t. volume
Tieche nevus
Tielle absorptive dressing
tie-over bolster dressing
Tietze syndrome
TIF
    tropic immersion foot
tiger snake antivenom
tight
    t. asthmatic
    t. building syndrome
tightness
    Bunnell intrinsic t.
TIL
    tumor-infiltrating lymphocyte
      TIL cell
      TIL cell assay
Tilade Inhalation Aerosol
Tilcotil
tilorone
tiludronate
time (T)
    activated partial thromboplastin t.
      (APTT)
    cold ischemia t.
    dilute Russell viper venom t.
    generation t.
    germinative t.
    kaolin clotting t.
    lead t.

T

NOTES

time (*continued*)
    median survival t. (MST)
    partial thromboplastin t. (PTT)
    reduced cold ischemic t.
    Russell viper venom t.
    thermal relaxation t.
    transit t.
Timecelles
    Sinufed T.
timed intermittent rotation
Timentin
timolol
Timoptic Ophthalmic
Timoptic-XE Ophthalmic
timori
    Brugia t.
timorian filariasis
timothy grass
TIMP
    tissue inhibitor of metalloproteinase
TIN
    tubulointerstitial nephritis
Tinactin
TINA monitor
TinBen
TinCoBen
tinctorial change
tincture
    Arning t.
    Fungoid t.
    Green soap t.
Tindall effect
T-independent response
tinea
    t. amiantacea
    t. axillaris
    t. barbae
    black dot t.
    t. capitis
    t. ciliorum
    t. circinata
    t. conus
    t. corporis
    t. cruris
    t. decalvans
    t. dermatitis
    t. faciei
    t. favosa
    t. furfuracea
    t. glabrosa
    t. imbricata
    t. incognito
    t. inguinalis
    t. kerion
    t. manuum
    t. nigra
    t. nodosa
    t. pedis

    t. pedis et manus
    t. profunda
    t. rubrum
    t. sycosis
    t. tarsi
    t. tonsurans
    t. tropicalis
    t. unguium
    t. versicolor
tine test
tingible body
Tinidazole
Tinted
    Oxy-5 T.
Tinver Lotion
tinzaparin sodium injectable
tip
    doorknob spray t.
    t. stitch
tire-patch appearance
Ti-Screen
Tisit
    T. Blue Gel
    T. Liquid
    T. Shampoo
Tisseel fibrin sealant
tissue
    acellular pannus t.
    autodigestion of connective t.
    bronchus-associated lymphoid t.
    (BALT)
    t. confirmation
    connective t.
    cynomolgus macaque t.
    decidual t.
    t. detritus
    elastic t.
    extraarticular t.
    t. factor (TF)
    t. factor pathway inhibitor (TFPI)
    fibroblastic t.
    t. fluke
    granulation t.
    gut-associated lymphoid t. (GALT)
    hemangiomatous t.
    t. inhibitor of metalloproteinase
    (TIMP)
    mesenchymal t.
    mucosa-associated lymphoid t.
    (MALT)
    necrotic t.
    neural t.
    organ-cultured corneal t.
    t. remodeling
    t. repair
    secondary lymphatic t. (SLT)
    skin-associated lymphoid t. (SALT)
    soft t.

synovial t.
t. transglutaminase (Ttg)
tissue-activated fibroblast
tissue-invasive cytomegalovirus (TI-CMV)
tissue-specific antigen
Tissue-Tek OCT medium
titanium dioxide
titanium:sapphire laser
titer
antinuclear antibody t.
antirotavirus IgA t.
antistreptolysin-O t.
ASLO t.
ASO t.
C-ANCA t.
geometric mean t. (GMT)
IgG t.
indirect Coombs t.
mycoplasma IgM t.
P-ANCA t.
rheumatoid factor t.
streptozyme t.
STZ t.
titin
titration
Rinkel serial endpoint t.
Ti-U-Lac HC
Ti-UVA-B
tixocortol-21-pivalate
Tj antigen
TLC
total lung capacity
TLI
total lymphoid irradiation
TLV
threshold limit value
T-lymphocyte
TM
telangiectatic matting
tympanic membrane
Tm cell
TMD
temporomandibular dysfunction
TMEP
telangiectasia macularis eruptiva perstans
TMP
trimethyl psoralen
TMP-SMX
trimethoprim-sulfamethoxazole
TNF
tumor necrosis factor
TNF inhibitor

TNF mRNA cytokine
TNF receptor II gene
TNF-alpha
tumor necrosis factor-alpha
TNF-R
pegylated p55 T.-R.
TNM
tumor, node, metastasis
TNM staging
TO
Theiler original strain of mouse
encephalomyelitis virus
TO virus
toad skin
toasted
t. shin
t. skin syndrome
tobacco
t. leaf extract
t. smoke
wild t.
TobraDex Ophthalmic
tobramycin and dexamethasone
Tobrex Ophthalmic
tocopherol deficiency
Todd-Hewitt broth
toe
black t.
hammer t.
Hong Kong t.
t. itch
jogger t.
mallet t.
sausage t.
soccer t.
tennis t.
toeweb
Tofranil
Togaviridae virus
togavirus
toilet
bronchial t.
pulmonary t.
Tokelau ringworm
tolbutamide
Tolectin DS
tolerance
acquired intrathymic t.
donor-specific t.
high dose t.
immune t.
immunological t.

NOTES

anti-TNF
Enbrel
etanercept

tolerance *(continued)*
    immunologic high dose t.
    impaired glucose t. (IGT)
    nonresponder t.
    oral t.
    organ-specific t.
    split t.
    t. through deletion
    t. through regulation
tolerization
tolerize
tolerogen
tolerogenesis
    surrogate t. (ST)
tolerogenic
tolerogenicity
Toll receptor
tolmetin sodium
tolnaftate
tolu
    balsam of t.
toluene
    t. sulfonamide
tomato tumor
tombstoning
tomodensitometry
    computerized t.
tomography
    cine computed t.
    computed t. (CT)
    fluorine-18 2-fluoro-2-deoxy-D-
      glucose-positron emission t.
      (FDG-PET)
    high-resolution computed t. (HRCT)
    optical coherent t.
    positron emission t. (PET)
    quantitative computed t. (QCT)
    single photon emission computed t.
      (SPECT)
    technetium-99m hexamethylpropylene
      amine oxime-single-photon-emission
      computed t. (HMPAO-SPECT)
tone
    Ambi Skin T.
    bronchial smooth muscle t.
tongue
    baked t.
    black hairy t.
    burning t.
    caviar t.
    claudication of t.
    coated t.
    fissured t.
    furrowed t.
    geographic t.
    glossy t.
    grooved t.
    hobnail t.

    osseous choristoma of the t.
    painful t.
    raspberry t.
    scrotal t.
    strawberry t.
    thick t.
    transitory benign plaque of t.
    white strawberry t.
tonofibril
tonofilament
tonofilament-cytoplasmic plaque linker
tonsil
    absent t.
    hypertrophic t.
    small t.
tonsillectomy
tonsillitis
    streptococcal t.
tonsillopharyngitis
tonsurans
    herpes t.
    tinea t.
    Trichophyton t.
tool
    Pressure Ulcer Scale for Healing t.
    PUSH t.
tooth, pl. **teeth**
    Hutchinson teeth
    Micro-Adson forceps with teeth
    t. pit
    t. rash
toothpaste swish therapy
top
    red t.
Topactin
Top-Count microplate scintillation
  counter
tophaceous gout
tophus, pl. **tophi**
    intraarticular t.
    synovial membrane t.
    t. syphiliticus
topical
    Achromycin t.
    Aclovate t.
    Acticort t.
    Actinex t.
    Aeroseb-HC t.
    Akne-Mycin t.
    Ala-Cort t.
    Ala-Quin t.
    Ala-Scalp t.
    Alphatrex t.
    t. anesthetic
    t. antibacterial therapy
    t. antifungal therapy
    t. antipruritic
    Anusol HC-1 t.

Anusol HC-2.5% t.
Aquacare t.
Aquaphor Antibiotic t.
Aristocort A t.
A/T/S t.
Baciguent t.
BactoShield t.
Bactroban t.
t. BCNU
Benadryl t.
Betalene t.
Betatrex t.
Beta-Val t.
Borofax t.
CaldeCort t.
Caldesene t.
Carmol t.
Carmol-HC t.
Cetacort t.
Cleocin T t.
Clinda-Derm t.
Cloderm t.
Cordran SP t.
Corque t.
CortaGel t.
Cortaid Maximum Strength t.
Cortaid with Aloe t.
Cort-Dome t.
Cortef Feminine Itch t.
t. corticosteroid
Cortin t.
Cortizone-5 t.
Cortizone-10 t.
Cruex t.
Cutivate t.
Cyclocort t.
t. cytotoxic therapy
Debrisan t.
t. decongestant
Delcort t.
Del-Mycin t.
Delta-Tritex t.
Dermacomb t.
Dermacort t.
Dermarest Dricort t.
Derma-Smoothe/FS t.
Dermolate t.
Dermtex HC with Aloe t.
Desitin t.
DesOwen t.
Diprolene AF t.
Diprosone t.

Dyna-Hex t.
t. eczema
Efudex t.
Elase t.
Elase-Chloromycetin t.
Eldecort t.
Elocon t.
Emgel t.
EMLA t.
Erycette t.
EryDerm T.
Erygel T.
Erymax t.
erythromycin t.
E-Solve-2 t.
ETS-2% t.
Eurax t.
Exelderm t.
Florone E t.
Fluonex t.
Fluonid t.
Fluoroplex t.
Flurosyn t.
Flutex t.
FS Shampoo t.
Furacin t.
Garamycin T.
G-myticin t.
Gynecort t.
Halog t.
Halog-E t.
Halotex t.
t. hemostatic agent
Hibiclens t.
Hibistat t.
Hi-Cor-1.0 t.
Hi-Cor-2.5 t.
Hycort t.
Hydrocort t.
Hydro-Tex t.
Hysone t.
Hytone t.
Kenalog t.
Kenonel t.
t. khellin
LactiCare-HC t.
Lamisil t.
Lanaphilic T.
Lanvisone t.
Lida-Mantle HC t.
Lidex t.
Lidex-E t.

T

NOTES

topical *(continued)*
    Locoid t.
    Maxiflor t.
    Maxivate t.
    Meclan t.
    Merlenate t.
    MetroGel t.
    Micatin T.
    t. moisturizer
    Monistat-Derm t.
    Mycifradin Sulfate T.
    Mycitracin T.
    Mycogen II T.
    Mycolog-II T.
    Myconel T.
    Mycostatin t.
    Mytrex F t.
    Naftin t.
    Neo-Cortef T.
    Neomixin t.
    N.G.T. T.
    Nilstat t.
    t. nitrogen mustard (NH2)
    Nizoral T.
    Novacet t.
    Nutracort t.
    Nutraplus T.
    Nystex t.
    Nyst-Olone II t.
    t. ophthalmic vasoconstrictor
    Orabase HCA t.
    Ovide t.
    Oxistat t.
    Oxsoralen t.
    Pedi-Cort V t.
    Pedi-Pro t.
    Penecort t.
    Polysporin T.
    Pontocaine t.
    Psorcon t.
    Psorion t.
    t. PUVA
    Quinsana Plus t.
    Racet T.
    Retin-A Micro t.
    Rogaine t.
    Scalpicin t.
    t. skin protection (TSP)
    Spectazole t.
    Staticin t.
    S-T Cort t.
    t. steroid
    Sulcosyn t.
    Sulfacet-R t.
    Sulfamylon t.
    Synacort t.
    Synalar T.
    Synalar-HP T.
    Synemol t.
    Tegrin-HC t.
    Teladar t.
    Temovate t.
    Texacort t.
    Topicycline t.
    Travase t.
    Triacet t.
    Tridesilon t.
    Triple Antibiotic t.
    Tri-Statin II t.
    T-Stat t.
    UAD t.
    U-Cort t.
    Ultra Mide t.
    Ultravate t.
    Undoguent t.
    Ureacin-20, -40 t.
    Valisone t.
    Vioform t.
    Vitec t.
    Vytone t.
    Westcort t.
    Zovirax t.

Topicort-LP
Topicycline Topical
Topigel occlusive sheeting
Topilene
Topisone
Topo I
    DNA topoisomerase I
topoisomerase
    DNA t. I (Topo I)
Toposar injection
Topsyn
Toradol injection
TORCH
    toxoplasmosis, other infections, rubella,
    cytomegalovirus infection, and herpes
    simplex
    TORCH syndrome
    TORCH viral screen
tori (*pl. of* torus)
TOR inhibitor
Tornalate
Torpedo californica
Torre syndrome
torti
    pili t.
torticollis
    dermatogenic t.
tortuous telangiectasis
tortus
    pilus t.
Torula
torula meningitis
torular meningitis
toruli tactiles

toruloidea
    Hendersonula t.
Torulopsis glabrata
torulosis
torus, pl. **tori**
    t. mandibulae
    mandibular t.
    t. palatinus
TOS
    toxic oil syndrome
Totacillin-N
total
    t. abdominal evisceration (TAE)
    t. allergy syndrome
    t. biopsy
    t. body bone mineral content
    t. body irradiation (TBI)
    t. body surface area (TBSA)
    t. contact cast
    t. counts bound (TCB)
    t. hemolytic complement
    t. lipodystrophy
    t. lung capacity (TLC)
    t. lymphoid irradiation (TLI)
    t. serum IgE
    t. serum IgE level
    t. skin electron beam (TSEB)
    t. skin score
totalis
    alopecia capitis t.
toto
    in t.
touch
    t. object maneuver
    t. prep
Toulon typhus
Touraine
    T. aphthosis
    T. centrofacial lentigo
    T. syndrome
Touraine-Solente-Golé syndrome
tourniquet
    Löfqvist t.
    t. test
Touro LA
Touton giant cell
Townes-Brock syndrome
toxemia
toxemic
toxic
    t. alopecia
    t. appearance

t. bullous epidermolysis
t. epidermal necrolysis (TEN)
t. erythema
t. nephrosis
t. oil syndrome (TOS)
t. organ damage
t. shock-like syndrome (TSLS)
t. shock syndrome (TSS)
T. Substance Control Act
t. systemic reaction
t. unit (TU)
toxica
    alopecia t.
toxicemia
toxicity
    cumulative t.
    ocular t.
    transplant-related t.
Toxicodendron
    T. dermatitis
    T. diversilobum
    T. radicans
    T. verniciferum
toxicodendron
    Rhus t.
toxicoderma
toxicodermatitis
toxicodermatosis
toxicogenic conjunctivitis
toxicopathic
toxicosis
toxicum
    erythema neonatorum t.
toxigenic
toxigenicity
toxin
    adenylate cyclase t.
    animal t.
    anthrax t.
    antitetanus t.
    Bacillus anthracis t.
    bacterial t.
    botulinus t.
    cholera t.
    Coley t.
    detoxified t.
    diagnostic diphtheria t.
    Dick test t.
    dinoflagellate t.
    diphtheria t.
    erythrogenic t.
    extracellular t.

NOTES

573

toxin *(continued)*
    fusion t.
    intracellular t.
    normal t.
    plant t.
    RNA glycosidase t.
    scarlet fever erythrogenic t.
    Schick test t.
    Shiga-like t.
    t. spectrum
    streptococcus erythrogenic t.
    tetanus t.
toxinic
toxinogenic
toxinogenicity
toxinology
toxinosis
toxipathic
toxipathy
Toxocara
    T. canis
    T. cati
toxocariasis
toxoid
    acellular pertussis vaccine combined with diphtheria and tetanus t. (DTaP)
    diphtheria and tetanus t.
    tetanus t.
toxon
toxonosis
toxophil
toxophore
toxophorous
Toxoplasma gondii
toxoplasmosis
    congenital t.
    cutaneous t.
    epidermotropic cutaneous t.
    t., other infections, rubella, cytomegalovirus infection, and herpes simplex (TORCH)
    t., other infections, rubella, cytomegalovirus infection, and herpes simplex syndrome
    t., other, rubella, cytomegalovirus, and herpes
    t., other, rubella, cytomegalovirus, and herpes viral screen
ToxR protein
toyocaensis
    Streptomyces t.
TP10
TPE
    thermoplastic elastomer
TPHA test

TPI test
TPO
    thrombopoietin
    thyroid peroxidase
TR
    thioredoxin reductase
TRAb
    TSH receptor antibody
trabecular carcinoma
trace element
trachea
    extrinsic compression of t.
    Syngamus t.
tracheal
    t. stenosis
    t. tumor
tracheitis
tracheobronchial amyloidosis
Tracheolife HME
tracheomalacia
tracheostomy
trachoma
    t. body
    t. virus
trachomatis
    Chlamydia t.
trachyonychia
tracking
    railroad t.
tracks
    tram t.
tract
    dental sinus t.
    sinus t.
traction
    t. alopecia
    t. atrophy
trade acne
traditional Chinese herbal therapy (TCHT)
tragacanth
    Gum t.
tragal
tragomaschalia
tragus, pl. tragi
    accessory t.
TRAIL
    tumor necrosis factor-related apoptosis-inducing ligand
training
    joint protection t.
trait
    autosomal recessive t.
    beta thalassemia t.
    recessive t.
    sickle cell t.

TRALI
   transfusion-related acute lung injury
tram
   t. line
   t. tracks
tramadol
tranexamic acid
Tranquility Quest
tranquilizer
transactivator
   reverse tetracycline t.
   tetracycline t.
transaldolase
transaminase
transarterial chemoembolization (TACE)
transaxillary apical bullectomy
transcapsidation
transcellular metabolism
transcervical infection
transchondral fracture
transcript
   bcr-abl chimeric t.
transcriptase
   t. inhibitor
   reverse t.
transcription
   calcium-dependent t.
   t. factor
   gene t.
   germline t.
   signal transducer and activator
      of t. (STAT)
   signal transduction and activator
      of t. (STAT)
transcutaneous
   t. electrical nerve stimulation
      (TENS)
   t. electrical neuromuscular
      stimulator (TENS)
TransCyte skin substitute
transdermal therapeutic system (TTS)
transdermic
Transderm Scōp Patch
transduce
transducer
   fluid-filled pressure t.
   force t.
transductant
transduction
   abortive t.
   complete t.

general t.
   high frequency t.
   low frequency t.
   signal t.
   specialized t.
   specific t.
Transeal transparent film
transection
transendothelial neutrophil migration
transfection
   adenoviral gene t.
   ex vivo adenoviral t.
transfer
   adenovirus-mediated gene t.
   t. factor
   t. gene
   melanin t.
   passive t.
   t. ribonucleic acid (tRNA)
   t. test
transferable T-cell suppression
transferase
   catechol-*O*-methyl t. (COMT)
transference
   passive t.
transferred immune response
transformant
transformation
   blast t.
   Box-Cox t.
   cell t.
   logit t.
   lymphocyte t.
   malignant t.
   refractory anemia with excess
      blasts in t. (RAEB-t)
   von Krogh t.
transformed lymphocyte
transforming
   t. agent
   t. gene
   t. growth factor (TGF)
   t. growth factor-alpha (TGF-alpha)
   t. growth factor-B (TGF-B)
   t. growth factor-beta (TGFB, TGF-
      beta)
   t. growth factor-induced
      immunosuppression
   t. infection
transfusion
   blood t.

NOTES

transfusion *(continued)*
    donor-specific t. (DST)
    exchange t.
    granulocyte t.
    haplotype-shared t.
    t. hepatitis
    t. nephritis
    packed red cell t.
    pretransplant donor blood t.
    t. reaction
    reciprocal t.
transfusion-associated AIDS (TA-AIDS)
transfusion-related acute lung injury (TRALI)
transgene
transgenic
    t. mice
    t. organism
transglutaminase
    tissue t. (Ttg)
transglutamination
    protein t.
transient
    t. acantholytic dermatosis (TAD)
    t. acantholytic dyskeratosis
    t. agammaglobulinemia
    t. bullous dermolysis of the
      newborn
    t. cerebral ischemia
    t. erythroporphyria of infancy
    t. hypogammaglobulinemia of
      infancy
    t. migratory infiltrate
    t. neonatal pustular melanosis
    t. neonatal systemic lupus
      erythematosus
    t. pulmonary infiltrate
transiently amplifying cell (TAC)
TransiGel impregnated gauze
transillumination of sinus
transin
transition mutation
transitory
    t. benign plaque of tongue
    t. palsy
transit time
transjugular hepatic biopsy
translation
translocation
    bacterial t.
    chromosomal t.
    unbalanced t.
transmembrane
    t. connector
    t. linker
    t. receptor

transmissible
    t. dementia
    t. enteritis
    t. gastroenteritis virus (TGE)
    t. gastroenteritis virus of swine
    t. mink encephalopathy
    t. plasmid
    t. spongiform encephalopathy (TSE)
    t. turkey enteritis virus
transmission
    airborne t.
    bedbug disease t.
    t. disequilibrium testing (TDT)
    t. electron microscopy (TEM)
    horizontal t.
    transovarian t.
    vertical t.
Transorbent hydrogel sheet
transovarian transmission
transparent facial powder
transpeptidase
transphosphorylation
transplacental infection
transplant
    allogenic t.
    allographic stem cell t. (mini-allo)
    autologous bone marrow t.
    auxiliary partial orthotopic liver t.
      (APOLT)
    bone marrow t. (BMT)
    dual kidney t.
    t. elbow
    en bloc t.
    hair t.
    hematopoietic stem cell t.
    islet cell t.
    matched unrelated donor stem
      cell t. (mini-MUD)
    PAK t.
    pancreas after kidney t. (PAK)
    reduced liver t. (RLT)
    reduced-size liver t. (RSLT)
    t. rejection classification
    related t.
    renal t.
    simultaneous pancreas-kidney t.
      (SPK)
    single-lung t. (SLT)
    SPK t.
      simultaneous pancreas-kidney
      transplant
    stem cell t. (SCT)
    syngeneic heart t.
    thoracic organ t.
Trans-Plantar Transdermal Patch
transplantation (Tx)

ABO-incompatible kidney t.
allogenic bone marrow t.
allogenic hematopoietic stem cell t.
  (allo-HSCT)
t. antigen
autologous t.
auxiliary partial heterotopic liver t.
  (APHLT)
auxiliary partial orthotopic liver t.
  (APOLT)
Bethesda Conference on Cardiac T.
bone marrow t. (BMT)
cadaver donor t.
cardiomyocyte t.
Cooperative Clinical Trials in
  Adult T. (CCTAT)
Cooperative Clinical Trials in
  Pediatric T. (CCTPT)
corneal t.
domino heart t. (DHT)
en bloc t.
European Group for Bone
  Marrow T. (EBMT)
fetal liver t.
fetal pig cell t.
fetal thymus t.
fetal ventral mesencephalic tissue t.
FISH protocol in bone marrow t.
fluorescence in situ hybridization
  protocol in bone marrow t.
heart t. (HTX)
heart-lung t. (HLT)
hematopoietic stem cell t. (HCT,
  HSCT)
heterotopic heart t. (HHT)
International Society of Heart and
  Lung T. (ISHLT)
intestinal t.
intrasplenic t. (isp-Tx)
islet t.
isolated pancreatic islet t. (IPITx)
kidney t. (KTx)
liver and intestinal t. (LITx)
liver and kidney t. (LKT)
living donor liver t. (LDLT)
living-related liver t. (LRT)
NHBD t.
nonheart-beating donor liver t.
nude bone graft t.
orthotopic heart t. (OHT)
orthotopic liver t. (OLT)
pancreas t.

pancreaticoduodenal t.
peripheral blood stem cell t.
  (PBSCT)
pigment cell t.
porcine bone marrow t. (PBMTx)
reduced-size liver t. (RSLT)
Registry of the International
  Society for Heart and Lung T.
sibling bone marrow t.
simultaneous double kidney t.
  (SDKT)
simultaneous kidney-pancreas t.
  (SKPT)
small bowel t. (SBTx)
small intestinal t. (SITx)
solid organ t. (SOT)
split-liver t. (SLT)
stem cell t.
syngeneic t.
thymic t.
vascularized bone marrow t.
  (VBMT)
xenogeneic t.
xenograft t.
xenoislet t.
transplantin
transplant-related toxicity
transport
  active t.
  basolateral t.
transpose
transposition flap
transposon
Trans-Sal
transthyretin
  t. amyloidosis
  t. Val30Met variant
transthyretin-origin amyloid deposit
transtracheal
transubstantiation
transvalensis
  Nocardia t.
transvector
transversa
  stria nasi t.
Trans-Ver-Sal Transdermal Patch
  Verukan solution
transverse
  t. furrow
  t. ligament
  t. myelitis
  t. nasal groove

NOTES

transversion mutation
Trantas dots
Tr^a antigen
Tranxene
TRAP
    tartrate-resistant acid phosphatase
trap
    Burkard spore t.
    Hirst spore t.
    Kramer-Collins Spore t.
trap-door deformity
trapped gas volume (TGV)
trapping
    air t.
TRAP-positive cell
TRAPS
    tumor necrosis factor receptor-associated
    periodic syndrome
trastuzumab
trauma
    inadvertent t.
    Parkland formula for fluid
    resuscitation for burn t.
traumatic
    t. alopecia
    t. anserine folliculosis
    t. arthritis
    t. bursitis
    t. calcinosis
    t. dermatitis
    t. fat necrosis
    t. fever
    t. herpes
    t. lesion
    t. neuroma
    t. panniculitis
    t. purpura
traumatica
    alopecia t.
    t. dermatitis
traumatically induced inflammatory
disease
traumaticum
    chloasma t.
    erythema t.
Travamine
Travase topical
Travel
    T. Aid
    T. Scrubz
    T. Tabs
Traveler
    Pulmo-Aide T.
Travelmate
Treacher Collins syndrome
treatment
    Anti-Acne Spot T.
    Ascoli t.

    AuTolo Cure Process wound t.
    Brehmer t.
    Castellani t.
    Clear Pore T.
    complementary and alternative
    medicine t.
    double drug t.
    duration of t.
    etretinate t.
    FotoFacial t.
    Gennerich t.
    Goeckerman t.
    grenz ray t.
    Histofreezer cryosurgical wart t.
    isoserum t.
    light t.
    Mother2Be skin t.
    No-Name Dandruff T.
    nonpharmacologic measure of t.
    oatmeal t.
    preventive t.
    prophylactic t.
    t. of psoriasis
    short-contact t. (SCAT)
    steroid-sparing t.
    thermescent skin t.
    triple drug t.
Trecator-SC
tree
    acacia t.
    alder t.
    American elm t.
    arbor vitae t.
    Arizona ash t.
    Arizona cypress t.
    Arizona/Fremont cottonwood t.
    ash t.
    aspen t.
    Australian pine t.
    bald cypress t.
    bayberry t.
    beech t.
    birch t.
    black locust t.
    box elder maple t.
    Brazilian rubber t.
    California peppertree t.
    Chinese elm t.
    cottonwood t.
    Douglas fir t.
    elm t.
    eucalyptus t.
    fall elm t.
    Gambel oak t.
    green ash t.
    groundsel t.
    hackberry t.
    hazelnut t.

hickory t.
Italian cypress t.
Japanese cedar t.
Japanese lacquer t.
juniper mix t.
lilac t.
live oak t.
loblolly pine t.
lodgepole pine t.
Lombardy poplar t.
malaleuca t.
maple t.
mesquite t.
Monterey cypress t.
mountain cedar t.
oak t.
olive t.
palm t.
paper mulberry t.
pecan t.
ponderosa pine t.
poplar t.
privet t.
queen palm t.
red alder t.
red cedar t.
red maple t.
red mulberry t.
redwood t.
Russian olive t.
salt cedar t.
shagbark hickory t.
slash pine t.
slippery elm t.
spruce t.
sugar maple t.
sweetgum t.
sycamore t.
walnut t.
wax myrtle t.
weeping fig t.
Western juniper t.
white ash t.
white mulberry t.
white oak t.
white pine t.
white poplar t.
willow t.
yew t.
trefoil dermatitis
Treg development
Trematoda

trematode
tremor
   epidemic t.
trench
   t. fever
   t. foot
   t. hand
   t. mouth
Trendar
Trendelenburg test
Trental
trephine
   skin t.
Treponema
   T. carateum
   T. denticola
   T. endemium
   T. pallidum
   T. pallidum hemagglutination test
   T. pallidum immobilization reaction
   T. pallidum immobilization test
   T. paraluis-cuniculi
   T. pertenue
   T. phagedenis
treponema-immobilizing antibody
treponemal
   t. antibody
   t. test
Treponema pallidum
   direct fluorescent antibody test for p. (DFA-TP)
treponemata
treponematosis
   bejel t.
   nonsyphilitic t.
   nonvenereal t.
   pinta t.
treponeme
treponemiasis
Tresilian sign
tresperimus
tretinoin
   t. cream
   mequinol and t.
triacetin
Triacet Topical
triad
   aspirin t.
   follicular occlusion t.
   Gougerot t.
   Hutchinson t.
   T. hydrocolloid

NOTES

triad *(continued)*
    T. hydrocolloid dressing
    Osler t.
    Phemister t.
    retention t.
Triaderm
trial
    GESICA t.
    Hy-C t.
    Metoprolol in Dilated
      Cardiomyopathy T.
    Outcome Measures in
      Rheumatology Clinical T.
      (OMERACT)
    Veterans' Administrative
      Cooperative T.
Triam
    T. Forte
    T. Forte Injection
Triam-A Injection
Triamcine-A
    Scheinpharm T.-A.
triamcinolone
    t. acetonide (TAA)
    t. cream (TAC)
    t. hexacetonide
    t. lotion (TAL)
    nystatin and t.
    t. ointment (TAO)
Triaminic
    T. AM Decongestant Formula
    T. Expectorant
    T. Oral Infant drops
Triamolone
Triamonide Injection
triangle
    Burow t.
triangular fibrocartilage complex (TFCC)
triangularis
    alopecia t.
Triatoma
    T. gerstaeckeri
    T. gerstaeckeri bite
    T. protracta
    T. sanguisuga
    T. sanguisuga bite
Triatominae
Triaz gel
triazolam
triazole
trichatrophia
trichatrophy
trichauxis
trichiasis
trichilemmal
    t. carcinoma
    t. cyst

trichilemmoma
    benign t.
    desmoplastic t.
Trichina
    T. spiralis
Trichinella
    T. spiralis
trichinelliasis
trichinellosis
trichiniasis
trichinosis
trichitis
trichiura
    Trichuris t.
Tri-Chlor
trichloroacetic
    t. acid (TCA)
    t. acid-tape technique
trichloroethylene
trichloromonofluoromethane
    dichlorodifluoromethane and t.
trichoadenoma
trichobezoar
trichoblastoma
trichoclasia
trichoclasis
trichocryptomania
trichocryptosis
trichocryptotillomania
Trichoderma
    T. harzianum
    T. longibrachiatum
    T. viride
trichoderma
trichodiscoma (TD)
trichodystrophy
trichoepithelioma (TE)
    acquired t.
    desmoplastic t.
    hereditary multiple t.
    multiple t.
    t. papillosum multiplex
trichofolliculoma
    sebaceous t.
trichogen
trichogenous
trichoglossia
trichogram
trichokinesis
trichokleptomania
trichokryptomania
tricholemmal differentiation
tricholemmoma
tricholith
trichologia
trichology
trichoma
trichomatose

trichomatosis
trichomatous
trichomatrioma
trichomegaly
Trichomonas vaginalis
trichomoniasis
trichomycetosis
trichomycosis
    t. axillaris
    t. axillaris nodosa
    t. axillaris nodularis
    t. chromatica
    t. favosa
    t. nigra
    t. palmellina
    t. pustulosa
    t. rubra
trichonocardiosis axillaris
trichonodosis
trichonosis
trichonosus versicolor
trichopathic
trichopathophobia
trichopathy
trichophagy
trichophobia
trichophytic
    t. dyshidrosis
    t. granuloma
trichophytica
trichophyticum
    granuloma t.
trichophyticus
    lichen t.
trichophytid
trichophytin
trichophytina
    dermatomycosis t.
Trichophyton, Trichophytum
    T. concentricum
    T. erinacei
    T. gypseum
    T. mentagrophytes
    T. purpureum
    T. rubrum
    T. schoenleinii
    T. skin test
    T. sulfureum
    T. tonsurans
    T. tonsurans fungus
    T. verrucosum
    T. violaceum

Trichophyton-induced asthma
trichophytosis
    t. barbae
    t. capitis
    t. corporis
    t. cruris
    t. unguium
Trichophytum (var. of Trichophyton)
trichopoliodystrophy
trichopoliosis
trichoptilosis
tricho-rhino-phalangeal syndrome
trichorrhea
trichorrhexis
    t. invaginata
    t. nodosa
trichorrhexomania
trichoschisia
trichoschisis
trichoscopy
trichosis
    t. carunculae
    t. sensitiva
    t. setosa
Trichosporon beigelii
trichosporonosis
trichosporosis
trichostasis spinulosa
Trichostrongylus
trichothiodystrophy syndrome
trichotillomania
trichotoxin
trichotrophy
trichrome
    Masson t.
Trichuris trichiura
Tri-Clear Expectorant
triclocarban
triclosan
Tricomine
tricone defect
Tricoplast adhesive elastic bandage
Tricosal
tricuspid valvular leaflet
tricyclic antidepressant
Triderm
Tridesilon topical
Tridione
triethylenemelamine (TEM)
trifida
    Ambrosia t.
Tri-Flow incentive spirometry

NOTES

T

trifluridine
trigeminal
  t. ganglion
  t. trophic syndrome
trigger
  t. factor
  t. finger
  Smart T.
triglyceride
trihexoside
  ceramide t. (CTH)
Tri-Immunol
triiodothyronine (T3)
Trikacide
Tri-Kort Injection
Trilafon
trilete
Trilisate
Trilog Injection
Trilone Injection
trimellitic anhydride
trimeprazine tartrate
trimer
  stable knob t.
trimethadione
trimethoprim and polymyxin b
trimethoprim-sulfamethoxazole (TMP-SMX)
trimethyl psoralen (TMP)
trimetrexate glucuronate
Trimox
Trimpex
Trinalin
Tri-Nasal Spray
trinucleotide
Triofed Syrup
trioxide
  arsenic t.
trioxsalen
Tripedia
tripelennamine
tripe palm
Tri-Phen-Chlor
Triphenyl Expectorant
triphosphatase
  adenosine t. (ATPase)
triphosphate
  adenosine t. (ATP)
  guanosine t. (GTP)
  inositol t.
  purine nucleotide adenosine t.
  uridine t.
triple
  T. Antibiotic topical
  t. drug treatment
  t. helix
  t. palm
  T. Paste

  t. response
  t. response of Lewis
  t. therapy
  T. X liquid
triple-drug therapy immunosuppression
  protocol
triple-jawed pedicellaria
triplet
  nonsense t.
Tri-P Oral Infant drops
Triposed
  T. Syrup
  T. Tablet
Triprofed
triprolidine and pseudoephedrine
TripTone Caplets
triradius
trisalicylate
  choline magnesium t.
Tris-buffered saline (TBS)
TRIS-buffered saline solution (TBS)
trisodium phosphonoformate
Trisoject Injection
trisomy
  t. 21, 22
  t. of chromosome II, dup(1)
    (q23q31)
  t. 20 syndrome
Trisoralen Oral
Tri-Statin II topical
Tristoject
Tritin
  Dr. Scholl's Maximum Strength T.
Trivagizole 3
trivalent oral poliovirus solution
TriZol reagent
tRNA
  transfer ribonucleic acid
  tRNA synthetase
TRNG
  tetracycline-resistant *Neisseria
    gonorrhoeae*
Trobicin injection
trochanteric bursitis
troche
  clotrimazole buccal t.
  Mycelex t.
trochleo-ginglymoid joint
Trolab wool alcohol test
troleandomycin
trolley-track sign
Trombicula
  T. akamushi
  T. deliensis
  T. irritans
Trombiculidae
trombidiasis
trombidiosis

tromethamine
  fosfomycin t.
  ketorolac t.
  lodoxamide t.
Tronothane ointment
Trophermyma whippleii
trophic
  t. syndrome
  t. ulcer
trophodermatoneurosis
trophoneurotic leprosy
tropica
  acrodermatitis vesiculosa t.
  elephantiasis t.
  frambesia t.
  Leishmania t.
  leishmaniasis t.
  phagedena t.
  pyosis t.
tropicae
  aphtha t.
tropical
  t. acne
  t. anhidrotic asthenia
  t. boil
  t. disease
  t. eczema
  t. eosinophilia
  t. immersion foot
  t. lichen
  t. mask
  t. measles
  t. phagedena
  t. phagedenic ulcer
  t. pyomyositis
  t. sloughing phagedena
  t. sore
  t. spastic paraparesis (TSP)
  t. swelling
  t. typhus
tropicalis
  acne t.
  Blomia t.
  Candida t.
  tinea t.
tropicalum
  pyoderma ulcerosum t.
tropic immersion foot (TIF)
tropicum
  acanthoma t.
  angiofibroma contagiosum t.
  granuloma inguinale t.

  papilloma inguinale t.
  ulcus t.
tropicus
  lichen t.
tropism
  viral t.
tropomyosin
troponin
trospectomycin sulfate
trough
  peak and t.
Trousseau
  T. spot
  T. syndrome
Tru-Area Determination measuring device
T.R.U.E.
  T. allergy patch test
  T. TEST
true
  t. progeria
  t. skin
trumpeter wart
trumpet nail
truncated
trunk dermatitis
Truphylline suppository
TruPulse
  T. CO2 laser system
Truxcillin
TruZone peak flow meter
TRX
  thioredoxin
trypan blue
trypanid
Trypanosoma
  T. brucei
  T. cruzi
trypanosome growth factor (TGF)
trypanosomiasis
  African t.
  American t.
  South American t.
trypanosomid
tryparsamide organic arsenic
trypsin, balsam Peru, and castor oil
trypsinization
tryptase
tryptophan
  t. dysmetabolism
TS
  temperature sensitive

NOTES

TSAb
  thyroid-stimulating antibody
T/Sal
    T. Neutrogena
    T. Shampoo
T/SA Shampoo
TSBP
  testis-specific binding protein
TSC
  tuberous sclerosis
  tuberous sclerosis complex
TSE
  transmissible spongiform encephalopathy
TSE-424
TSEB
  total skin electron beam
tsetse
    t. fly
    t. fly bite
TSH
  thyroid-stimulating hormone
    TSH receptor (TSH-R)
    TSH receptor antibody (TRAb)
TSH-displacing antibody
TSH-R
  thyroid-stimulating hormone receptor
  TSH receptor
TSLS
  toxic shock-like syndrome
TSP
  thrombospondin
  topical skin protection
  tropical spastic paraparesis
TSS
  toxic shock syndrome
TSTA
  tumor-specific transplantation antigen
T-Stat topical
Tsukamurella paurometabolum
tsukubaensis
    Streptomyces t.
T-suppressor cell
tsutsugamushi
    t. disease
    t. fever
    Rickettsia t.
TTBS
  Tween-TRIS-buffered saline solution
t-test
Ttg
  tissue transglutaminase
TTP
  thrombotic thrombocytopenic purpura
TTP-HUS
  thrombocytopenic purpura/hemolytic
    uremic syndrome
TTS
  transdermal therapeutic system

TU
  toxic unit
  tuberculin unit
tubba
tube
    Chaoul t.
    Eppendorf t.
    eustachian t.
    Lymphoprep T.
    t. precipitin test
    pus t.
    Shiley tracheostomy t.
    Softech endotracheal t.
    t. thoracostomy
tubercle
    anatomic t.
    anatomical t.
    butcher's t.
    dissection t.
    Lister t.
    naked t.
    necrogenic t.
    postmortem t.
    prosector's t.
    sebaceous t.
tubercula dolorosa
tubercular
    t. eruption
    t. tertiary syphilis
tuberculation
tuberculatum
    erythema t.
tuberculid
    bacillary-barren t.'s
    micronodular t.
    micropapular t.
    nodular t.
    papular t.
    papulonecrotic t.
    rosacea-like t.
tuberculin
    Koch old t.
    old t. (OT)
    purified protein derivative of t.
      (PPD)
    t. skin test
    Swedish old t.
    t. tine test
    t. titer test
    t. unit (TU)
tuberculin-type hypersensitivity
tuberculitis
tuberculization
tuberculochemotherapeutic
tuberculocidal
tuberculocide
tuberculoderma

tuberculoid
    t. leprosy
    t. rosacea
tuberculoides
    lepra t.
tuberculoprotein
tuberculosa
    dactylitis t.
tuberculosis (TB)
    adult t.
    aerogenic t.
    appendicular t.
    arthritic t.
    attenuated t.
    cestodic t.
    childhood-type t.
    chronic fibroid t.
    cutaneous t.
    t. cutis colliquativa
    t. cutis follicularis disseminata
    t. cutis indurata
    t. cutis indurativa
    t. cutis lichenoid
    t. cutis lichenoides
    t. cutis luposa
    t. cutis miliaris
    t. cutis miliaris disseminata
    t. cutis orificialis
    t. cutis papulonecrotica
    t. cutis verrucosa
    dermal t.
    disseminated t.
    extrapulmonary t.
    t. fungosa cutis
    hepatosplenic t.
    hilus t.
    t. luposa
    t. lymphadenitis
    miliary t.
    multidrug-resistant t. (MDR-TB)
    Mycobacteria other than t. (MOTT)
    Mycobacterium t. (MTB)
    open t.
    oral t.
    orificial t.
    t. orificialis
    orofacial t.
    postprimary t.
    primary inoculation t.
    reinfection t.
    rifampin-isoniazid-streptomycin-
      ethambutol-resistant t.

RISE-resistant t.
    secondary t.
    t. of serous membrane
    t. of skin
    surgical t.
    t. ulcerosa
    t. vaccine
    t. verrucosa cutis
    vertebral t.
    warty t.
tuberculostat
tuberculostatic
tuberculosus
    lupus t.
tuberculotic
tuberculous
    t. abscess
    t. arthritis
    t. chancre
    t. dactylitis
    t. nephritis
    t. phlyctenulosis
    t. pleurisy
    t. polyserositis
    t. rheumatism
    t. synovitis
    t. wart
tuberculum
    t. sebaceum
    t. syphiliticum
tuberoeruptive xanthoma
tuberosa
    urticaria t.
tuberosis
tuberositas, pl. **tuberositates**
tuberosum
    xanthoma t.
tuberous
    t. angioma
    t. sclerosis (TSC)
    t. sclerosis complex (TSC)
    t. xanthoma
Tubersol
TubiFast bandage
tubing
    Silastic t.
    Surgitube t.
    X-span t.
tubocurarine
tubular venectasia
tubule
    T t.

NOTES

tubulitis
tubulointerstitial nephritis (TIN)
tuft
>   t. of hair
>   ungual t.
tufted angioma
tuftsin
Tukey
>   T. post-hoc correction
>   T. standardized range test
tularemia
tularemic chancre
tularensis
>   *Francisella t.*
>   *Pasteurella t.*
tulip bulb dermatitis
tumbleweed weed pollen
tumbu
>   t. fly
>   t. fly myiasis
tumefaciens
>   *Agrobacterium t.*
tumefacient
tumefaction
tumentia
tumescent technique
tumid lupus erythematosus
tumidus
>   lupus erythematosus t.
tumor
>   Abrikosov t.
>   acral arteriovenous t. (AAVT)
>   adnexal t.
>   amyloid t.
>   ANGEL t.
>   t. antigen
>   Bednar t.
>   benign t.
>   Brooke t.
>   brown t.
>   t. burden index (TBI)
>   Buschke-Löwenstein t.
>   carcinoid t.
>   t. cell negative selection
>   t. cell purging
>   cutaneous t.
>   Dabska t.
>   dermal duct t.
>   desmoid t.
>   eccrine t.
>   epithelial t.
>   Ewing t.
>   filiform t.
>   t. of the follicular infundibulum (TFI)
>   genital t.
>   giant cell t.
>   glomus t.

granular cell t.
haarscheibe t.
insulin t.
Koenen t.
Landschutz t.
Leydig cell t.
t. lysis factor
Malherbe t.
malignant glomus t. (MGT)
malignant peripheral nerve sheath t.
t. marker
Merkel cell t.
mixed t.
t. necrosis factor (TNF)
t. necrosis factor-alpha (TNF-alpha)
t. necrosis factor alpha
t. necrosis factor-beta
t. necrosis factor receptor
t. necrosis factor receptor-associated periodic syndrome (TRAPS)
t. necrosis factor-related apoptosis-inducing ligand (TRAIL)
neuroendocrine t.
t., node, metastasis (TNM)
t., node, metastasis staging
osseous t.
papillary t.
peripheral nerve sheath t.
phantom t.
Pinkus t.
Pott puffy t.
precancerous t.
premalignant t.
primary neuroendocrine t.
Rous t.
sebaceous t.
Spiegler t.
Spitz t.
squamous cell lung t.
t. stage
t. suppressor gene
tomato t.
tracheal t.
turban t.
villous t.
t. virus
Wilms t.
Yaba t.
tumoral calcinosis
tumor-associated
>   t.-a. antigen
>   t.-a. transplantation antigen (TATA)
tumoriform
tumorigenic
tumorigenicity
tumor-infiltrating
>   t.-i. lymphocyte (TIL)
>   t.-i. lymphocyte cell

tumor-lysis syndrome
tumor-specific transplantation antigen
  (TSTA)
tuna fish
TUNEL method
Tunga
> *T. penetrans*
> *T. penetrans* bite

tungiasis
tunica dartos
tuning fork
tunnel of Guyon
turban tumor
turbidimetry
Turbinaire
> Decadron Phosphate T.
> Dexacort Phosphate T.

turbinate
> nasal t.

turbot
Turbuhaler
> T. inhaler
> Pulmicort T.

turgometer
turkey
> bluecomb disease of t.
> t. feather
> t. meningoencephalitis virus

Turlock virus
Turner
> T. phenotype
> T. syndrome

Turner-Kieser syndrome
turnover
> inositol phospholipid t.

Turpentine oil
turtleback nail
Tusibron-DM
Tussin
> Safe T.

Tussionex
Tussi-Organidin NR
Tuss-LA
Tusstat Syrup
Tween
Tween-TRIS-buffered saline solution
  (TTBS)
twentieth century disease
twenty-nail
> t.-n. dystrophy
> t.-n. involvement

Twice-A-Day Nasal solution

Twilite Oral
Twin Jet nebulizer
twisted
> t. chondrodysplasia
> t. hair

twitch
two-dimensional immunoelectrophoresis
two feet-one hand syndrome
Twort-d'Herelle phenomenon
Twort phenomenon
two-site immunoradiometric assay
two-stage reaction
Tx
> transplantation

TXA_2
Ty21a vaccine
tyle
Tylenol Cold Effervescent Medication
  Tablet
tyloma
Tylophora asthmatica
tylosis, pl. tyloses
> t. ciliaris
> t. lingua
> t. palmaris et plantaris

tylotic
tyloticum
> eczema t.

tympanic membrane (TM)
tympanocentesis
tympanometry
tyndallization
type
> t. 68–72
> t. A, B, C acanthosis nigricans
> t. 1, 1A, 1B diabetes
> t. II alveolar cell
> t. I, IIb antineuronal antibody
> APS t. 1, 2
> t. A synoviocyte
> axial t.
> t. B fibroblast
> blood t.
> t. I–XI, XIV collagen
> t. IV collagenase
> t. 1-24 cornification
> t. IV delayed hypersensitivity
>   reaction
> dermatosparaxis t.
> t. 1 diabetes mellitus (T1DM)
> t. 2 diabetes mellitus (T2DM)
> Duffy blood antibody t.

NOTES

T

type *(continued)*
    Ehlers-Danlos syndrome, arthrochalasia t.
    Ehlers-Danlos syndrome, hypermobility t.
    Ehlers-Danlos syndrome, kyphoscoliotic t.
    Ehlers-Danlos syndrome, vascular t.
    Ehlers-Danlos syndrome t. X
    epidermolysis bullosa, dermal t.
    epidermolysis bullosa, epidermal t.
    epidermolysis bullosa, Gravis t.
    epidermolysis bullosa, junctional t.
    epidermolysis bullosa, Mitis t.
    Fitzpatrick classification of skin t.
    t. I glycogen storage disease
    t. I–III hypersensitivity reaction
    t. III immune complex drug reaction
    t. I–IV immunologic drug reaction
    Kell blood antibody t.
    keratosis palmaris et plantaris of the Meleda t.
    Kidd blood antibody t.
    kyphoscoliotic t.
    Lewis blood antibody t.
    t. I–VII mucopolysaccharidosis
    t. I, II ocular albinism
    t. I, IA, IB, II oculocutaneous albinism
    t. I-MP, I-TS oculocutaneous albinism
    t. I, II osteoporosis
    t. II pachyonychia congenita peripheral t.
    t. II pneumocyte
    t. II procollagen gene COL2A1 skin t.
    t. strain
    t. I, II tyrosinemia
    t. V collagenase

typhi
    Rickettsia t.
    Salmonella t.

Typhim
    T. Vi
    T. Vi vaccine

typhimurium
    Salmonella t.

typhoid
    t. A&B (T.A.B.)
    t. A&B vaccine
    t. bacteriophage
    t. cholera
    t. fever
    t. osteomyelitis
    provocation t.

    t. septicemia
    t. spot

typhoid-paratyphoid A&B vaccine
typholysin
typhosepsis
typhous
typhus
    African tick t.
    t. degenerativus amstelodamensis
    endemic t.
    epidemic t.
    t. exanthematique
    exanthematous t.
    flea-borne t.
    Gubler-Robin t.
    Hildenbrand t.
    Indian tick t.
    Kenya tick t.
    louse-borne t.
    Manchurian t.
    mite t.
    mite-borne t.
    t. mitior
    Moscow t.
    murine t.
    North Asian tick t.
    North Queensland tick t.
    petechial t.
    Queensland tick t.
    recrudescent t.
    scrub t.
    shop t.
    sporadic t.
    tick t.
    Toulon t.
    tropical t.
    urban t.
    t. vaccine

typing
    bacteriophage t.
    HLA t.
    HLA-DRB and HLA-DRQ DNA t.
    LCR-based HLA t.
    skin t. I–VI

tyramine
Tyrell skin hook
Tyrocidine
Tyroglyphus
    T. longior
    T. siro

Tyrophagus putrescentiae
tyrosinase inhibitor
tyrosinase-negative oculocutaneous albinism
tyrosinase-positive oculocutaneous albinism
tyrosinase-related oculocutaneous albinism

tyrosine
    t. aminotransferase deficiency
    t. kinase
    t. kinase inhibitor
    t. metabolism
    t. phosphorylation
tyrosinemia
    neonatal t.
    type I, II t.

Tyrothricin
T-Y stent
Tyzine Nasal
Tzanck
    T. preparation
    T. smear
    T. test

NOTES

T

U3

U3 small nuclear ribonucleoprotein

U3 snRNP

U1 RNP antibody

UAD

upper airway disorder

UAD topical

UAS

undifferentiated autoimmune syndrome

ubiquitin

ubiquitin-conjugating enzyme

ubiquitinization

UBT

urea breath test

UCB

umbilical cord blood

U-cell

undefined-cell

U-cell lymphoma

UCF

urinary free cortisol

UCF study

U-Cort Topical

UCTD

undifferentiated connective tissue disease

UCTS

undifferentiated connective tissue
syndrome

Udder Butter lubricant/emollient

Uganda Cancer Institute staging system

UIFE

urine immunofixation electrophoresis

UIP

usual interstitial pneumonia

ulcer

acute decubitus u.

Aden u.

amebic u.

amputating u.

aphthous genital u.

aphthous oral u.

arterial u.

atonic u.

Bairnsdale u.

Bazin u.

Buruli u.

chiclero u.

chrome u.

chronic undermining burrowing u.

cockscomb u.

cold u.

constitutional u.

corneal u.

corrosive u.

crateriform u.

creeping u.

Curling u.

cutaneous u.

decubitus u.

diabetic foot u.

diphtheritic u.

Gaboon u.

genital aphthous u.

gravitational u.

groin u.

gummatous u.

hard u.

healed u.

herpetic u.

idiopathic giant esophageal u.

indolent u.

inflamed u.

inflammatory u.

ischemic u.

Jacob u.

Kurunegala u.

u. lesion

Lipschütz u.

lupoid u.

Malabar u.

Marjolin u.

Meleney chronic undermining u.

nasopharyngeal u.

necrotic u.

neurotrophic u.

in noma u.

oral aphthous u.

Oriental u.

Parrot u.

perambulating u.

phagedenic u.

phlegmonous u.

postencephalitic trophic u.

pressure u.

pudendal u.

recurrent u.

ring u.

rodent u.

Searl u.

serpiginous u.

sickle cell u.

skin u.

sloughing u.

snail-track u.

soft u.

stasis vascular u.

steroid u.

Sutton u.

symptomatic u.

syphilitic u.

U

ulcer *(continued)*
    tanner's u.
    trophic u.
    tropical phagedenic u.
    undermining u.
    varicose u.
    vascular u.
    venereal u.
    venous stasis u.
    Zambesi u.
ulcera
ulcerans
    Mycobacterium u.
ulcerate
ulcerated
ulcerating granuloma of pudendum
ulceration
    gastrointestinal u.
    intertrigo with u.
    intestinal u.
    mucous membrane u.
    nasal mucosal u.
    oral u.
    u. of oral mucosa
    rectal u.
ulcerative
    u. colitis
    u. dermatosis
    u. gingivitis
    u. lichen planus
    u. proctocolitis
    u. stomatitis
ulceroglandular
ulceronecrotic lesion
ulcerosa
    tuberculosis u.
ulcerous
ulcerovegetating plaque
Ulcosan Unna boot with inelastic zinc plaster bandage
ulcus
    u. ambulans
    u. ambustiforme
    u. durum
    u. hypostaticum
    u. migrans
    u. tropicum
    u. venereum
    u. vulvae acutum
ULE
    unilateral laterothoracic exanthem
ulerythema
    u. acneiforma
    u. centrifugum
    u. ophryogenes
    u. sycosiforme
ulerythematosa
    atrophoderma u.

Ulex europaeus
Ullrich-Turner syndrome
ulnar
    u. deviation
    u. nerve
ulnaris
    extensor carpi u. (ECU)
ulodermatitis
ulotrichous
ULR
ULR-LA
Ultec
    U. hydrocolloid
    U. hydrocolloid dressing
Ultra
    Grisactin U.
    U. Mide topical
    U. Tears solution
Ultracef
ultracentrifugation
Ultracortinol
UltraFine erbium laser system
ultrahigh frequency ventilation
UltraKlenz wound cleanser
Ultram
ultramicrosize griseofulvin
Ultramop
UltraPulse CO_2 laser
Ultraquin Plain
ultrasonic nebulizer
ultrasonography
    Power Doppler u.
ultrasonometer
    QUS-2 calcaneal u.
ultrasound
    Acuson 128XT u.
    A-mode u.
    B-mode u.
    Diasonic u.
    Doppler u.
    intravascular u. (IVUS)
ultrasound-guided bronchoscopy
ultrastructural
    u. analysis
    u. component
UltraThon insect repellent
Ultravate topical
ultraviolet (UV)
    u. A (UVA)
    u. A, B lamp
    u. actinotherapy
    u. B (UVB)
    u. B-range (UVB)
    u. C (UVC)
    u. light
    u. light index
    psoralen u. A (PUVA)

u. radiation
u. recall
ultravirus
Umballa sore
umbilical
u. cord
u. cord blood (UCB)
u. fungus
umbilicated
umbilication
Umbrelle sunscreen
Umbre virus
Unasyn
unbalanced translocation
uncharacteristic leprosy
Uncinaria
uncinarial dermatitis
uncinariasis
unclassified air cleaner
uncombable hair syndrome
uncomplemented
uncovertebral arthrosis
unction
unctuosa
cutis u.
undecamer
undecapeptide
undecylenic
u. acid
u. acid and derivatives
undefined-cell (U-cell)
u.-c. lymphoma
undercover cosmetic
underexcretion-type gout
undermining ulcer
Underwood disease
undifferentiated
u. autoimmune syndrome (UAS)
u. connective tissue disease (UCTD)
u. connective tissue syndrome (UCTS)
u. somatoform IA anaphylaxis
u. spondyloarthropathy
u. type fevers
Undoguent topical
undulant fever
undulin
unexpected phenotype
ungual tuft

unguent
Lasan U.
unguentum, pl. **unguenta**
unguinal
unguis
u. incarnatus
leukopathia u.
lunula u.
matrix u.
pterygium inversum u.
solum u.
stratum corneum u.
vallum u.
unguium
achromia u.
albedo u.
canities u.
defluvium u.
dystrophia u.
fragilitas u.
gryposis u.
scabrities u.
tinea u.
trichophytosis u.
unheated serum reagin (USR)
Uni-Ace
Unibase cream
Uni-Bent Cough Syrup
unicameral cyst
unicellular protozoa
unicondylar arthritis
Unicort
Uni-Decon
Uni-Dur
Uniflex polyurethane adhesive surgical dressing
unifocal Langerhans cell
unilateral
u. dermatomal superficial telangiectasia
u. hemangiomatosis
u. hemidysplasia
u. hemidysplasia cornification disorder
u. hyperhidrosis
u. laterothoracic exanthem (ULE)
u. macular degeneration
u. nevoid telangiectasia
unilateralis
nevus acneiformis u.
unilocular cyst
uninflamed

U

NOTES

Unipen
    U. injection
    U. Oral
Uniphyl
Uni-Pro
Uniserts
    Hemril-HC U.
Unisom
Unisom-C
unit
    Å u.
        Ångström unit
    alexin u.
    allercoat enzyme allergosorbent u.
      (AEU)
    allergy u. (AU)
    amboceptor u.
    Ångström u. (Å unit)
    antigen u.
    antitoxin u.
    antivenene u.
    Asepticator u.
    basic multicellular u. (BMU)
    Bell international u.
    Bethesda u. (BU)
    biologic u. (BU)
    biological allergic u. (BAU)
    biological standard u.
    Brymill CryAc cryosurgical u.
    Brymill 30 cryosurgical u.
    colony-forming u. (CFU)
    complement u.
    Cryo-Surg liquid nitrogen spray u.
    dermal microvascular u.
    diphtheria antitoxin u.
    ELISA u. (EI.U)
    environmental exposure u. (EEU)
    epidermal-melanin u.
    fetoplacental u. (FPU)
    fingertip u. (FTU)
    Flexercell Strain U.
    Florey u.
    follicular melanin u.
    Geiger electrocautery u.
    GPL u.
    hemolysin u.
    inhalation breath u.
    iontophoretic u.
    Lf u.
    musculotendinous u.
    nectary of floral u.
    noon u.
    Noon pollen u.
    ostiomeatal u. (OMU)
    Oxford u.
    u. of penicillin
    pilosebaceous u.

    plaque-forming u. (PFU)
    priming renal dialysis u.
    protein nitrogen u. (PNU)
    skin test u. (STU)
    streptomycin u.
    tetanus antitoxin u.
    toxic u. (TU)
    tuberculin u. (TU)
    Wood u.
unitarian hypothesis
United
    U. Network for Organ Sharing
      (UNOS)
    U. States Renal Data System
      (USRDS)
Unithroid
Unitrol
unius
univalent antibody
univariant
univariate regression analysis
Uni-Vent
universal
    u. acquired melanosis
    u. allergy
    u. angiomatosis
    u. donor
universale
    angiokeratoma corporis diffusum u.
    melasma u.
universalis
    albinismus u.
    alopecia u.
    calcinosis u.
    hypertrichosis u.
    protoporphyria u.
    psoriasis u.
University
    U. of Wisconsin (UVW)
    U. of Wisconsin solution (UW
      solution)
unmethylated oligodeoxynucleotide
Unna
    U. boot
    U. cell
    U. comedo extractor
    U. dermatosis
    U. disease
    U. expressor
    U. mark
    U. nevus
    U. paste
Unna-Flex leg compression dressing
Unna-Pak leg compression dressing
Unna-Thost
    U.-T. disease
    U.-T. keratoderma

keratosis palmaris et plantaris of U.-T.
U.-T. syndrome
unopsonized zymosan
UNOS
United Network for Organ Sharing
UNOS 3, 4 score
UNOS transplant listing
unusual
u. lupus erythematosus-like syndrome
u. opportunistic infection
upcurved punch
UPEP
urine protein electrophoresis
upper
u. airway disorder (UAD)
u. airway obstruction
u. dermis
U. Hands self-retaining retractor
u. respiratory tract infection (URTI)
u. respiratory tract mucosa
up-regulation
upstream
u. enzyme
u. regulatory region (URR)
urate
u. deposition
monosodium u. (MSU)
u. nephropathy
u. oxidase
urate-associated inflammation
Urbach-Oppenheim disease
Urbach-Wiethe
U.-W. disease
U.-W. syndrome
urban
u. cutaneous leishmaniasis
u. typhus
urchin
sea u.
urea
u. breath test (UBT)
Diazolidinyl u. (DiU)
u. frost
u. and hydrocortisone
imidazolidinyl u.
Ureacin
Ureacin-20, -40 topical
ureae
Actinobacillus u.

urealyticum
Ureaplasma u.
Ureaphil Injection
Ureaplasma urealyticum
urediospore, uredinospore, ureidospore
uredo
Uree
ureidospore (*var. of* urediospore)
uremia
perforating disorder of u.
uremic
u. pneumonitis
u. pruritus
Uremol
Uremol-HC
ureteric stenting
ureteroneocystostomy
Lich-Gregoire u.
urethritis
chlamydial u.
gonorrheal u.
urhidrosis
uric acid
uricase
uricemia
uricosuria
uricosuric drug
uridine
u. diphosphoglucose dehydrogenase
u. triphosphate
uridrosis
u. crystallina
urinary
u. alkalinizer
u. electrophoresis
u. free cortisol (UCF)
u. free cortisol study
u. tract infection (UTI)
urine
cellular casts in u.
u. immunofixation electrophoresis (UIFE)
mouse u.
u. myoglobin immunoassay
u. protein electrophoresis (UPEP)
u. pyridinoline collagen crosslink
urinosus
sudor u.
Urisec
Uri-Tet Oral
uritis
Urobak

U

NOTES

urolithiasis
Uroplus
    U. DS
    U. SS
uroporphyrin
urostomy dermatitis
URR
    upstream regulatory region
ursodiol
URTI
    upper respiratory tract infection
urtica
urticans
    erythema u.
    purpura u.
urticant
urticaria
    u. acuta
    acute allergic u.
    adrenergic u.
    allergic u.
    angioedema-induced u.
    aquagenic u.
    autonomic u.
    u. bullosa
    cholinergic u.
    u. chronica
    chronic familial giant u.
    chronic idiopathic u. (CIU)
    cold-induced u.
    cold reflex u.
    u. conferta
    congelation u.
    contact u.
    cyclic u.
    delayed pressure u.
    endemic u.
    u. epidemica
    exercise-induced cholinergic u.
    u. factitia
    factitious u.
    familial cold u.
    febrile u.
    u. febrilis
    generalized heat u.
    giant u.
    u. gigantea
    heat u.
    u. hemorrhagica
    heredofamilial u.
    idiopathic cold u.
    immediate contact u.
    immunological contact u. (ICU)
    immunologic contact u.
    irritant contact u.
    light u.
    u. maculosa
    u. medicamentosa

Milton u.
    u. multiformis endemica
    nonallergic contact u. (NICU)
    nonconimmunological contact u.
    (NICU)
    papular u.
    u. papulosa
    u. perstans
    u. photogenica
    physical u.
    u. pigmentosa
    u. pigmentosum
    pressure u.
    pressure-induced u.
    recall u. (RU)
    recurrent u.
    solar u.
    solaris u.
    u. subcutanea
    u. tuberosa
    u. vesiculosa
    vibratory u.
urticarial
    u. dermatographia
    u. plaque
    u. vasculitis
    u. xanthoma
urticariogenic
urticarioides
    acarodermatitis u.
urticata
    acne u.
urticate
urtication
urticatus
    lichen u.
urushiol
use test
USR
    unheated serum reagin
USRDS
    United States Renal Data System
USSC stapler
ustilaginism
Ustilago
ustus
    Aspergillus u.
usual interstitial pneumonia (UIP)
uta
uterine leiomyoma
uterus, pl. **uteri**
    ichthyosis uteri
UTI
    urinary tract infection
Uticort
utility scissors
utilization

UV
 ultraviolet
  UV solution
UVA
 long-wavelength ultraviolet light
 ultraviolet A
  UVA lamp
  photochemotherapy with oral
   methoxypsoralen therapy followed
   by UVA (PUVA)
Uvadex
UVB
 midrange-wavelength ultraviolet light
 ultraviolet B
 ultraviolet B-range
  UVB lamp
  narrowband UVB (NBUVB)
  UVB phototherapy

UVC
 ultraviolet C
uveitis
  anterior u.
  idiopathic posterior u.
  lens-induced u.
  phacoanaphylactic u.
uveomeningoencephalitis
uviofast
uviol lamp
uvioresistant
uviosensitive
UVW
 University of Wisconsin
UW solution

NOTES

U

V
    V antigen
    Big V
    V gene
V-2 carcinoma
Va
    coagulation factor Va
vaccae
    Mycobacterium v.
vaccina
vaccinal areola
vaccinate
vaccination
    cancer v.
    DNA v.
vaccinator
vaccinatum
    eczema v.
vaccine
    ActHIB v.
    adjuvant v.
    V. Adverse Events Reporting
      System (VAERS)
    AIDS v.
    allergy v.
    antiidiotype v.
    aqueous v.
    attenuated live mumps virus v.
    autogenous v.
    Avicine v.
    bacille Calmette-Guérin v.
    bacillus Calmette-Guérin v.
    bacterial v.
    BCG v.
    Biken-CAM v.
    brucella strain 19 v.
    Calmette-Guérin v.
    chickenpox v.
    cholera v.
    crystal violet v.
    diphtheria, tetanus toxoid, and
      acellular pertussis v.
    diphtheria, tetanus toxoid, and
      whole-cell pertussis v.
    diphtheria, tetanus toxoid, and
      whole-cell pertussis vaccine and
      Haemophilus b conjugate v.
    diphtheria toxoid, tetanus toxoid,
      and pertussis v. (DTP)
    DNA v.
    duck embryo origin v. (DEV)
    Edmonston-Zagreb v.
    Flury strain v.
    foot-and-mouth disease virus v.
    gene-based v.

    Haffkine v.
    Havrix v.
    HbOC v.
    HbOC/DTP v.
    heat-phenol inactivated v.
    hepatitis A v.
    hepatitis B v.
    heterogenous v.
    HGP-30W v.
    Hib-TT v.
    high-egg-passage v.
    hog cholera v.
    human diploid cell v. (HDCV)
    human diploid cell rabies v.
      (HDCV)
    Imovax Rabies intradermal v.
    Imovax Rabies intramuscular v.
    ImuLyme v.
    inactivated poliovirus v. (IPV)
    Infanrix v.
    influenza virus v.
    IR502 psoriasis v.
    Japanese encephalitis virus v. (JE-
      VAX)
    killed-virus v.
    Lipomel melanoma v.
    lipopolysaccharide v.
    live oral polio v.
    live oral poliovirus v.
    low-egg-passage v.
    low virulence v.
    v. lymph
    measles, mumps, and rubella v.
      (MMR)
    measles virus v.
    Melacine v.
    meningococcal v.
    MMR v.
    multivalent v.
    mumps virus v.
    oil v.
    Oka v.
    oral polio v. (OPV)
    Pasteur v.
    pertussis v.
    plague v.
    PncCRM v.
    pneumococcal polysaccharide v.
    pneumococcal polysaccharide/protein
      conjugate v.
    poliomyelitis v.
    poliovirus v.
    polyvalent v.
    rabies virus v.
    rheumatoid arthritis v.

V

vaccine *(continued)*
    Rocky Mountain spotted fever v.
    Rotamune v.
    RotaShield v.
    Sabin v.
    Salk v.
    Semple v.
    smallpox v.
    split-virus v.
    Staphylococcus aureus v.
    stock v.
    subunit v.
    T.A.B. v.
    tetanus v.
    v. therapy
    Theratope-STn v.
    tuberculosis v.
    Ty21a v.
    Typhim Vi v.
    typhoid A&B v.
    typhoid-paratyphoid A&B v.
    typhus v.
    varicella virus v.
    variola v.
    viral v.
    v. virus
    vital v.
    whooping-cough v.
    yellow fever v. (YF-VAX)
vaccinia
    disseminated v.
    v. gangrenosa
    generalized v.
    v. immune globulin
    v. infection
    v. necrosum
    Orthopoxvirus v.
    progressive v.
    roseola v.
    variola v.
    v. virus
vaccinial
vacciniform
    estival v.
vacciniforme
    hydroa v.
vaccinist
vaccinization
vaccinogen
vaccinogenous
vaccinoid reaction
vaccinostyle
vaccinum
Vacu-Aide portable suction device
vacuolar
    v. change
    v. myelopathy
    v. myopathy

vacuolated
vacuolating virus
vacuole
vacuolization
    basket-weave v.
vacutome
vacuum
    v. phenomenon
    Rainbow v.
    v. tube apparatus
    v. tube cutting current
VAERS
    Vaccine Adverse Events Reporting System
vagabond's disease
Vaginal
    Cleocin V.
    Dalacin V.
vaginalis
    Trichomonas v.
Vaginex
vaginitis
    Gardnerella v.
    granular v.
vaginosis
vagrant's disease
vagus nerve
valacyclovir HCl
valdecoxib
valency
valerate
    betamethasone v.
    hydrocortisone v.
valgum
    genu v.
valgus
    hallux v.
Valisone Topical
Valium
    V. injection
    V. Oral
vallum unguis
valproic acid and derivatives
Valrelease Oral
Valsalva maneuver
Valtrex
value
    negative predictive v. (NPV)
    positive predictive v. (PPV)
    threshold limit v. (TLV)
valve
    Passy-Muir tracheostomy speaking v.
valvulae conniventes
valvular disease
Vamate
Van
    V. Buchem disease

V. der Bend chamber
V. Lohuizen syndrome
van
v. der Heijde modification of Sharp method
v. der Waals force
vanA
v., vanH. vanS gene
VanA phenotype
Vancenase
V. AQ
V. AQ Inhaler
V. Nasal Inhaler
V. Pockethaler
Vanceril
V. Double Strength
V. Oral Inhaler
Vancocin
V. injection
V. Oral
Vancoled injection
vancomycin
v. hydrochloride
kanamycin and v. (KV)
vancomycin-resistant
v.-r. enterococci (VRE)
v.-r. *Enterococcus* (VRE)
v.-r. *Enterococcus faecium* (VREF)
v.-r. *Enterococcus faecium* bacteremia
Vanex-LA
Vanicream
vanilla
vanilla-fudge cyst
vanillism
Vaniqa cream
Vanoxide
Vanoxide-HC
Vansil
Vantin
vapocoolant spray
Vaponefrin
Vaporisateur Nasal Decongestionnant
VAPS
volume-assured pressure support
Varady phlebectomy hook
variabilis
Dermacentor v.
erythrokeratodermia figurata v.

variable
v. numbers of tandem repeats (VNTR)
v. region
variance
analysis of v. (ANOVA)
multivariate analysis of v. (MANOVA)
variance-covariance matrix
variant
v. amyloidogenic protein
v. asthma
dystrophic epidermolysis bullosa, albopapuloid v.
generalized morphea v.
junctional v.
linear scleroderma v.
Miller-Fisher v.
morphea v.
v. neurofibromatosis
simplex v.
transthyretin Val30Met v.
variation
antigenic v.
coefficient of v. (CV)
varicella
congenital v.
v. disease
v. encephalitis
v. gangrenosa
v. inoculata pustulosa
v. virus vaccine
v. virus vaccine live
varicellation
varicella-zoster (VZ)
v.-z. immune globulin
v.-z. immunoglobulin (VZIG)
v.-z. infection
v.-z. virus (VZV)
v.-z. virus retinitis
varicelliform
v. lesion
varicelloid
varicellosus
herpes zoster v.
varices (*pl. of* varix)
varicography
varicose
v. eczema
v. ulcer
varicosis

V

NOTES

varicosity
> venous v.

varicosum
> lymphangioma capillare v.

variegata
> parakeratosis v.
> parapsoriasis v.
> porphyria v.

variegated

variegate porphyria (VP)

variegatum
> *Hyalomma* v.

Vari/Moist wound dressing

variola
> v. benigna
> v. crystallina
> v. hemorrhagica
> v. inserta
> v. major
> v. maligna
> v. miliaris
> v. minor
> v. mitigata
> v. pemphigosa
> v. siliquosa
> v. sine eruptione
> v. vaccine
> v. vaccinia
> v. vera
> v. verrucosa
> v. virus

variolar

variolate

variolation

variolic

varioliformis
> acne v.
> folliculitis v.
> molluscum v.
> parapsoriasis acuta et v.

varioliform syphilid

variolization

varioloid

variolosa
> impetigo v.
> osteomyelitis v.
> purpura v.

variolous

variolovaccine

variotii
> *Paecilomyces* v.

Varivax

varix, pl. **varices**
> lymph v.
> v. lymphaticus
> venous v.

varus
> hallux v.
> v. intertrochanteric
> v. malalignment

VAS
> visual analog scale
> VAS 972

vasa nervorum

vascular
> v. arcade
> v. cell adhesion molecule (VCAM)
> v. cell adhesion molecule-1 (VCAM-1)
> v. dermatosis
> v. disorder
> v. dysfunction
> v. endothelial growth factor (VEGF)
> v. endothelial growth factor-2 (VEGF2)
> endothelium v.
> v. FLPD
> v. malformation birthmark
> v. nevus
> v. permeability
> v. permeability factor/vascular endothelial cell growth factor (VPF/VEGF)
> v. reaction
> v. type Ehlers-Danlos syndrome
> v. ulcer

vasculare
> poikiloderma atrophicans v.

vascularis
> nevus v.

vascularized
> v. bone marrow transplantation (VBMT)
> v. xenograft

vasculature

Vasculight laser

vasculitic lesion

vasculitis, pl. **vasculitides**
> allergic v.
> ANCA-associated v. (AAV)
> ANCA-positive v. (APV)
> Churg-Strauss v.
> coronary v.
> cutaneous leukocytoclastic v.
> cutaneous necrotizing v.
> granulomatous v.
> Henoch-Schönlein v.
> hypersensitivity v.
> hypocomplementemic urticarial v.
> immune complex v.
> large vessel v.
> leukocytoclastic v. (LCV)
> livedo v.
> livedoid v.
> lymphocytic v.
> mesenteric v.
> necrotizing v.

nodular granulomatous v.
primary systemic v. (PSV)
rheumatoid rheumatic v.
segmental hyalinizing v.
small vessel v.
systemic necrotizing v. (SNV)
urticarial v.
vasculopathy
basilar v.
cardiac allograft v. (CAV)
Churg-Strauss v.
pulmonary occlusive v.
vasculosus
nevus v.
Vaseline
V. Intensive Care moisturizer
V. Lip Therapy
V. petroleum jelly
Vaselinoderma
vasoactive
v. intestinal peptide (VIP)
v. mediator
Vasocidin Ophthalmic
Vasocon
vasoconstriction
hypoxic v.
vasoconstrictor
topical ophthalmic v.
Vasodilan
vasodilatation
vasodilation
Vasofrinic
vasomotor
v. reaction
v. rhinitis (VMR)
vasoocclusive
v. disease
vasopressor
vasospasm
cold-induced v.
Vasosulf Ophthalmic
vasovagal reaction
Vater-Pacini corpuscle
VATS
video-assisted thoracic surgery
Vaughn-Jackson
V.-J. lesion
V.-J. sign
Vav/Rac pathway
VaxGen
VaxSyn
Vbeam pulse dye laser system

VBMT
vascularized bone marrow transplantation
VC
vital capacity
VC25
Gravicon V.
VCAM
vascular cell adhesion molecule
VCAM-1
vascular cell adhesion molecule-1
V-Cillin K Oral
V-Dec-M
V-D-J
V-D-J gene
V-D-J gene arrangement
VDRL
Venereal Disease Research Laboratories
VDRL test
VDS
venereal disease-syphilis
VDT
visual display terminal
vection
vector
attenuated poxvirus v.
biological v.
gene-based v.
mechanical v.
pBluescript v.
v. of plague
recombinant v.
retroviral v.
viral v.
vector-borne disease
vectorial
vector-transfected cell clone
Vectrin
vecuronium
VEE
Venezuelan equine encephalomyelitis
VEE virus
Veetids Oral
vegetable gum
vegetans
benign pemphigus v.
dermatitis v.
herpes v.
hyperkeratosis follicularis v.
keratosis v.
pemphigus v.
pyoderma v.
pyostomatitis v.

V

NOTES

vegetating
    v. bromidism
    v. halogenosis
vegetative bacteriophage
VEGF
    vascular endothelial growth factor
VEGF2
    vascular endothelial growth factor-2
Veiel paste
veiled cell
vein
    broken v.
Veingard dressing
Vel antigen
Velban
Velband orthopedic padding wool
Velbe
Velcro closure
"Velcro" crackle
Veldona
veldt sore
Velella velella **dermatitis**
vellus
    v. hair
    v. olivae
velocardiofacial syndrome
velocimetry
    laser Doppler v.
velocity
    nerve conduction v.
velogenic
Velosef
Veltane Tablet
Velvelan
velvet grass
venae cavae
Ven antigen
venectasia
    tubular v.
venenata
    acne v.
    cheilitis mycotic v.
    dermatitis v.
    Rhus v.
venenatum
    erythema v.
venerea
    lues v.
venereal
    v. bubo
    v. disease
    V. Disease Research Laboratories
    (VDRL)
    v. disease-syphilis (VDS)
    v. sore
    v. ulcer
    v. wart
venereal-associated arthritis

venereum
    granuloma v.
    lymphogranuloma v. (LGV, LVG)
    lymphopathia v.
    papilloma v.
    ulcus v.
veneris
    corona v.
Venezuelan
    V. equine encephalomyelitis (VEE)
    V. equine encephalomyelitis virus
venezuelensis
    Strongyloides v.
venoarterial shunting
venocclusion
Venodyne compression stocking
Venoglobulin-I, -S
venom
    bee v.
    v. extract
    flea v.
    v. hemolysis
    Hymenoptera v.
    v. immunotherapy (VIT)
    snake v.
    spider v.
    v. testing
venom-bathed nematocyst
venom-bearing spine
venomous snake
venoocclusive disease (VOD disease)
venoplasty
venoscope
venosus
    nevus v.
venous
    v. gangrene
    v. lake
    v. malformation
    v. nevus
    v. star
    v. stasis ulcer
    v. varicosity
    v. varix
Ventex composite dressing
ventilated alveolus
ventilation
    airway pressure release v. (APRV)
    alveolar v.
    high-frequency jet v.
    high-frequency positive pressure v.
    intermittent mandatory v.
    inverse ratio v. (IRV)
    maximal v. (MV)
    maximal voluntary v. (MVV)
    mechanical v. (MV)
    minute v.
    pressure-controlled inverse ratio v.

pressure-regulated volume control v.
pressure support v. (PSV)
proportional assist v.
synchronized intermittent mechanical v.
synchronous intermittent mandatory v.
ultrahigh frequency v.
volume-cycled decelerating-flow v.

ventilation/perfusion (V/Q)
v./p. lung scan (V/Q lung scan)
v./p. ratio

ventilator
High Frequency Oscillatory v.
mechanical v.
volume-limited v.

ventilator-associated pneumonia
ventilatory failure
Ventolin
V. nebules
V. Rotacaps

VenTrak respiratory mechanics monitor
ventral
ventricosus
dermatitis pediculoides v.
Pediculoides v.
Pyemotes v.

ventricular pseudoaneurysm (PVA)
ventriculography
radionuclide v.

ventriculoperitoneal shunt (VP)
Venture demand oxygen delivery device
venular lesion
venule
dilated v.
high endothelial v. (HEV)

venulitis
cutaneous necrotizing v.

Venus
collar of V.
crown of V.
necklace of V.

VePesid
V. injection
V. Oral

vera
cutis v.
polycythemia v.
variola v.

verdoperoxidase
verge
nasal v.

vergeture
Vergogel Gel
Vergon
Verhoeff-van Gieson stain
Veriderm
Medrol V.

vermicular
vermicularis
atrophoderma v.
Enterobius v.
Oxyuris v.

vermiculate atrophoderma
vermiculation
vermiculatum
atrophoderma v.

vermiculous
vermifugal
vermifuges
vermilion border
verminous abscess
Vermizine
Vermox
vernal
v. conjunctivitis
v. encephalitis
v. grass
v. keratoconjunctivitis
sweet v.

Verner syndrome
Verneuil
hidradenitis axillaris of V.
V. neuroma

verniciferum
Toxicodendron v.

vernix
Rhus v.

Vero cell
veronii
Aeromonas v.

Verrex-C&M
verruca, pl. verrucae
v. acuminata
v. digitata
v. filiformis
v. glabra
v. mol2usciformis
v. necrogenica
v. palmaris et plantaris
v. peruana
v. peruviana

V

*verrucae
vulgares
) plural
vulgares*

verruca *(continued)*
   Phialophora v.
   v. plana
   v. plana juvenilis
   v. plana senilis
   v. planta
   seborrheic v.
   v. simplex
   v. vulgaris
Verruca-Freeze
verruciformis
   acrokeratosis v.
   dermatodysplasia v.
   epidermodysplasia v.
verruciforms
verruciform xanthoma
verrucosa
   Betula v.
   v. cutis
   dermatitis v.
   elephantiasis nostra v.
   pachyderma v.
   Phialophora v.
   telangiectasia v.
   tuberculosis cutis v.
   variola v.
verrucose
   v. dermatitis
verrucosis
   lymphostatic v.
verrucosum
   eczema v.
   erysipelas v.
   molluscum v.
   pyoderma v.
   Trichophyton v.
verrucosus
   lichen planus v.
   lichen ruber v.
   lupus v.
   nevus v.
verrucous
   v. angiokeratoma
   v. carcinoma
   v. hemangioma
   v. hypertrophicum
   v. nevus
   v. scrofuloderma
   v. xanthoma
verruga peruana
Versacaps
VersaLight laser
VersaPulse laser
Versed
Versel
versican CS/DS
Versiclear

versicolor
   Aspergillus v.
   pityriasis v.
   tinea v.
   trichonosus v.
vertebra, pl. **vertebrae**
   codfish vertebrae
vertebral tuberculosis
vertex
vertical
   v. growth phase
   v. mattress stitch
   v. section
   v. transmission
Verticillium alboatrum
Verukan solution
very
   v. late activation antigen (VLA-1 antigen)
   v. late antigen-4 (VLA-4)
very-low-density
   v.-l.-d. lipoprotein (VLDL)
   v.-l.-d. lipoprotein cholesterol
vesica, pl. **vesicae**
   pachyderma v.
vesicant
vesicate
vesication
vesicatoria
   Lytta v.
vesicatory
vesicle
   spongiotic v.
vesicobullous
   v. lesion
vesicopustular
   v. eruption
vesicopustule
vesicular
   v. dermatitis
   v. eruption
   v. exanthem
   v. exanthema
   v. exanthema of swine virus
   v. stomatitis
   v. stomatitis virus
   v. viral infection
vesiculate
vesiculated
vesiculation
   creeping v.
   intraepidermal v.
   subepidermal v.
vesiculiform
vesiculobullous disease
vesiculopapular
vesiculopustular lesion

vesiculosa
 miliaria v.
 urticaria v.
vesiculose
vesiculosum
 eczema v.
 erysipelas v.
 hydroa v.
vesiculotomy
vesiculous
Vesiculovirus
vespid
 v. antigen
 Hymenopterous v.
Vespula
 V. crabro
 V. sting
vessel-based lobular panniculitis
vessel blockage
vest
 halo v.
vestibular
 v. adenitis
 v. cyst
 v. papilla
vestibulum nasi
vestimenti
 pediculosis v.
vestimentorum
 pediculosis corporis vel v.
Veterans' Administrative Cooperative Trial
veto effect
Vexol Ophthalmic suspension
V-Gan injection
VH
 viral hepatitis
 VH gene
VHF
 viral hemorrhagic fever
VHL
 von Hippel-Lindau gene
Vi
 Vi antibody
 Vi antigen
 Typhim Vi
Viasorb composite dressing
Viaspan
vibesate
vibex, pl. **vibices**

Vibramycin
 V. injection
 V. Oral
Vibra-Tabs
vibration
 chest percussion and v.
vibration-induced white finger (VWF)
vibratory
 v. angioedema
 v. urticaria
Vibrio
 V. cholerae
 V. vulnificus
vibrio
 Nasik v.
vibriocidal
Vibrios vulnificus
vicious cicatrix
Vicks
 V. DayQuil Allergy Relief 4 Hour Tablet
 V. DayQuil Sinus Pressure & Congestion Relief
 V. 44D Cough & Head Congestion
 V. 44 Non-Drowsy Cold & Cough Liqui-Caps
 V. Sinex
 V. Sinex Long-Acting Nasal solution
Vicryl suture
VIDA
 vitiligo disease activity
Vidal disease
vidarabine
video
 Sony VHS HQ Digital Picture v.
video-assisted thoracic surgery (VATS)
videomicroscopic imaging
Videx Oral
Vierra sign
view
 coronal v.
 Waters v.
Vif
vigabatrin
Vigilon
 V. dressing
 V. hydrogel sheet
vigorous hydration
VIIIa
 factor V.

V

NOTES

villi (*pl. of* villus)
villoma
villonodular synovitis
villous
 v. atrophy
 v. fold
 v. frond
 v. tumor
villus, pl. **villi**
 blunted v.
vimentin
VIMRxyn light-activated therapy
vinblastine sulfate
Vinca **alkaloid**
Vincasar PFS
Vincent
 V. angina
 V. disease
 V. infection
 V. white mycetoma
vincristine
vine
 Thunder God v.
vinegar solution
vinosus
 nevus v.
vinyl
 v. chloride
 v. chloride disease
 v. chloride exposure
vinyl-alternating air mattress
Vioform topical
violaceous
 v. plaque
 v. shawl pattern rash
 v. V neck pattern rash
violaceum
 Trichophyton v.
violet
 crystal v.
 gentian v.
 hexamethyl v.
 Hofmann v.
 Lauth v.
violet-blue erythema
violin-back
 v.-b. spider
 v.-b. spider bite
violin deformity
Vioxx
VIP
 vasoactive intestinal peptide
Vira-A Ophthalmic
Viracept
viral
 v. arthritis
 v. capsid antigen
 v. conjunctivitis

 v. disease
 v. dysenteriae
 v. encephalomyelitis
 v. envelope
 v. exanthema
 v. gastroenteritis
 v. genome
 v. hemagglutination
 v. hemorrhagic fever (VHF)
 v. hemorrhagic fever virus
 v. hepatitis (VH)
 v. hepatitis type A–E
 v. immunization
 v. neurolabyrinthitis
 v. neutralization
 v. pneumonia
 v. probe
 v. protein gag
 v. protein tax
 v. respiratory infection
 v. sandfly fever
 v. strand
 v. tropism
 v. vaccine
 v. vector
 v. wart
Viramune
Virazole Aerosol
virchowian leprosy
viremia
Virend
virginium
 chloasma periorale v.
viricidal
viricide
viridans
 v. hemolysis
 Streptococcus v.
viride
 Trichoderma v.
Viridis pulsed laser
virilization
 frank v.
virion
Virivac
viroceptor
viroid
virokine
virologist
virology
viropexis
Viroptic Ophthalmic
virosis, pl. **viroses**
virostatic effect
virucidal
virucide
virucopria
virulence

virulent bacteriophage
viruliferous
viruria
    BK v.
virus
    2060 v.
    Abelson murine leukemia v.
    acquired immunodeficiency
      syndrome-related v. (ARV)
    adeno-associated v. (AAV)
    adenoidal-pharyngeal-conjunctival v.
    adenosatellite v.
    African horse sickness v.
    African swine fever v. (ASFV)
    African tick v.
    v. A hepatitis
    AIDS-related v. (ARV)
    Akabane v.
    Aleutian mink disease v.
    Amapari v.
    amphotropic v.
    Andes v.
    animal v.
    anti-Epstein-Barr v. (anti-EBV)
    antihepatitis A v.
    A-P-C v.
    Arenaviridae v.
    Argentine hemorrhagic fever v.
    arthropod-borne v.
    Astroviridae v.
    attenuated v.
    attenuate vaccinia v.
    Aujeszky disease v.
    Australian X disease v.
    avian encephalomyelitis v.
    avian erythroblastosis v.
    avian infectious laryngotracheitis v.
    avian influenza v.
    avian leukosis-sarcoma v.
    avian lymphomatosis v.
    avian myeloblastosis v.
    avian neurolymphomatosis v.
    avian pneumoencephalitis v.
    avian sarcoma v.
    avian viral arthritis v.
    B v.
    B19 v.
    bacterial v.
    Barmah Forest v.
    Bittner v.
    BK v.
    Black Lagoon v.

    v. blockade
    bluecomb v.
    bluetongue v.
    Borna disease v.
    Bornholm disease v.
    bovine leukemia v. (BLV)
    bovine leukosis v.
    bovine papular stomatitis v.
    bovine virus diarrhea v.
    Bunyamwera v.
    Bwamba v.
    CA v.
    Caliciviridae v.
    California v.
    canarypox v.
    canine distemper v.
    Capim v.
    Caraparu v.
    cat distemper v.
    cattle plague v.
    Catu v.
    CELO v.
    Central European tick-borne
      encephalitis v.
    C group v.
    Chagres v.
    chicken embryo lethal orphan v.
    chickenpox v.
    chikungunya v.
    Coe v.
    cold v.
    Colorado tick fever v. (CTF virus)
    Columbia S. K. v.
    common cold v.
    contagious pustular stomatitis v.
    Coronaviridae v.
    cowpox v.
    Coxsackie B v.
    Crimean-Congo hemorrhagic
      fever v.
    croup-associated v.
    CTF
      Colorado tick fever virus
    cytopathogenic v.
    Dakar bat v.
    defective v.
    delta v.
    dengue v.
    distemper v.
    DNA v.
    dog distemper v.
    duck hepatitis v.

V

NOTES

virus *(continued)*
    duck influenza v.
    duck plague v.
    Duvenhaga v.
    eastern equine encephalomyelitis v.
    EB v.
    Ebola v.
    ECBO v.
    ECHO v.
    ECMO v.
    ecotropic v.
    ECSO v.
    ectromelia v.
    EEE v.
    EMC v.
    emerging v.
    encephalitis v.
    v. encephalomyelitis
    encephalomyocarditis v.
    enteric cytopathogenic bovine
      orphan v.
    enteric cytopathogenic human
      orphan v.
    enteric cytopathogenic monkey
      orphan v.
    enteric cytopathogenic swine
      orphan v.
    enzootic encephalomyelitis v.
    ephemeral fever v.
    epidemic gastroenteritis v.
    epidemic keratoconjunctivitis v.
    epidemic myalgia v.
    epidemic parotitis v.
    epidemic pleurodynia v.
    Epstein-Barr v. (EBV)
    equine abortion v.
    equine arteritis v.
    equine coital exanthema v.
    equine infectious anemia v.
    equine influenza v.
    equine rhinopneumonitis v.
    FA v.
    feline leukemia v. (FeLV)
    feline panleukopenia v. (FPV)
    feline rhinotracheitis v.
    fibrous bacterial v.
    filamentous bacterial v.
    Filoviridae v.
    filtrable v.
    fixed v.
    Flury strain rabies v.
    FMD v.
    foamy v.
    foot-and-mouth disease v.
    fowl erythroblastosis v.
    fowl lymphomatosis v.
    fowl myeloblastosis v.
    fowl neurolymphomatosis v.

    fowl plague v.
    fowlpox v.
    fox encephalitis v.
    Friend leukemia v.
    GAL v.
    gallus adeno-like v.
    gastroenteritis v. type A, B
    genital herpes simplex v.
    German measles v.
    Germiston v.
    goatpox v.
    Graffi v.
    green monkey v.
    Gross leukemia v.
    Guama v.
    Guaroa v.
    HA1, HA2 v.
    hand-foot-and-mouth disease v.
    Hantaan v.
    hard pad v.
    Harvey murine sarcoma v.
    helper v.
    hemadsorption v. type 1, 2
    Hendra v.
    hepatitis A v. (HAV)
    hepatitis B v. (HBV)
    hepatitis C v. (HCV)
    hepatitis D v. (HDV)
    hepatitis E v. (HEV)
    hepatitis G v. (HGV)
    herpes simplex v. (HSV)
    herpes simplex v. type I, II
    herpes zoster v.
    hog cholera v.
    horsepox v.
    human immunodeficiency v. (HIV)
    human T-cell leukemia v. (HTLV)
    human T-cell leukemia v. I
      (HTLV I)
    human T-cell leukemia v. III
      (HTLV III)
    human T-cell
      leukemia/lymphoma v. (HTLV)
    human T-cell lymphotrophic v.
      (HTLV)
    human T-cell lymphotrophic v.
      type I (HTLV-I)
    human T-cell lymphotrophic v.
      type II (HTLV-II)
    human T-cell lymphotrophic v.
      type III (HTLV-III)
    Ibaraki v.
    IBR v.
    v. III of rabbit
    Ilhéus v.
    inclusion conjunctivitis v.
    infantile gastroenteritis v.
    infectious bovine rhinotracheitis v.

infectious bronchitis v. (IBV)
infectious ectromelia v.
infectious hepatitis v.
infectious papilloma v.
infectious porcine
  encephalomyelitis v.
influenza v.
insect v.
iridescent v.
Jamestown Canyon v. (JCV)
Japanese B encephalitis v.
JC v.
JH v.
Junin v.
K v.
Kelev strain rabies v.
v. keratoconjunctivitis
Kilham rat v.
Kisenyi sheep disease v.
Koongol v.
Korean hemorrhagic fever v.
Kotonkan v.
Kyasanur Forest disease v.
labial herpes simplex v.
La Crosse v.
lactate dehydrogenase v.
Lassa v.
latent rat v.
LCM v.
    lymphocytic choriomeningitis virus
Lipovnik v.
louping ill v.
Lucké v.
Lunyo v.
lymphadenopathy-associated v.
  (LAV)
lymphocytic choriomeningitis v.
  (LCM virus)
lymphogranuloma venereum v.
lytic Epstein-Barr v.
Machupo v.
maedi v.
malignant catarrhal fever v.
Maloney leukemia v.
Marburg v.
Marek disease v.
marmoset v.
masked v.
Mason-Pfizer v.
Mayaro v.
measles v.
medi v.

Mengo v.
milkers' nodule v.
mink enteritis v.
MM v.
Mokola v.
molluscum contagiosum v. (MCV)
Moloney v.
Moloney murine leukemia v.
monkey B v.
monkeypox v.
mouse encephalomyelitis v.
mouse hepatitis v.
mouse leukemia v.
mouse mammary tumor v.
mouse parotid tumor v.
mouse poliomyelitis v.
mousepox v.
mouse thymic v.
mucosal disease v.
Muerto Canyon v.
mumps v.
murine sarcoma v.
Murray Valley encephalitis v.
Murutucu v.
MVE v.
myxomatosis v.
Nairobi sheep disease v.
naked v.
ND v.
Nebraska calf scours v.
Neethling v.
negative strand v.
Negishi v.
neonatal calf diarrhea v.
neonatal herpes simplex v.
neurotrophic v.
neurotropic v.
v. neutralization test
Newcastle disease v.
non-A non-B hepatitis v.
nonoccluded v.
Norwalk v.
occluded v.
Omsk hemorrhagic fever v.
oncogenic v.
o'nyong-nyong v.
orf v.
Oriboca v.
ornithosis v.
orphan v.
Orthomyxoviridae v.
Oscar v.

V

NOTES

virus *(continued)*
    Pacheco parrot disease v.
    pantropic v.
    papilloma v.
    pappataci fever v.
    parainfluenza v.
    Paramyxoviridae v.
    paravaccinia v.
    parrot v.
    Patois v.
    pharyngoconjunctival fever v.
    Phlebotomus fever v.
    Picornaviridae v.
    Pirital v.
    plant v.
    v. pneumonia of pig
    poliomyelitis v.
    polymerase chain reaction-based
      detection of hepatitis G v.
    porcine hemagglutinating
      encephalomyelitis v.
    Powassan v.
    primary genital herpes simplex v.
    progressive pneumonia v.
    pseudocowpox v.
    pseudolymphocytic
      choriomeningitis v.
    pseudorabies v.
    psittacosis v.
    Puumala v.
    PVM v.
    quail bronchitis v.
    Quaranfil v.
    rabbit fibroma v.
    rabbit myxoma v.
    rabbitpox v.
    rabies v.
    Rauscher leukemia v.
    recurrent genital herpes simplex v.
    recurrent intraoral herpes
      simplex v.
    recurrent labial herpes simplex v.
    REO v.
    respiratory enteric orphan v.
    respiratory syncytial v. (RSV)
    Rida v.
    Rift Valley fever v.
    rinderpest v.
    RNA tumor v.
    Ross River v.
    Rous-associated v. (RAV)
    Rous sarcoma v. (RSV)
    Rous sarcoma v. immune globulin
      intravenous (RSV-IGIV)
    Rs v.
    Rubarth disease v.
    rubella vaccine v.
    rubeola v.

    Russian autumn encephalitis v.
    Russian spring-summer
      encephalitis v.
    Salisbury common cold v.
    salivary gland v.
    sandfly fever v.
    San Miguel sea lion v.
    Semliki Forest v.
    Sendai v.
    serum hepatitis v.
    v. shedding
    sheep-pox v.
    shipping fever v.
    Shope fibroma v.
    Shope papilloma v.
    Simbu v.
    simian v. (SV)
    simian vacuolating v. No. 40
      (SV40)
    Sindbis v.
    slow v.
    smallpox v.
    snowshoe hare v.
    soremouth v.
    Spondweni v.
    Stealth v.
    St. Louis encephalitis v.
    street v.
    swamp fever v.
    swine encephalitis v.
    swine fever v.
    swine influenza v.
    swinepox v.
    Swiss mouse leukemia v.
    syncytial v.
    Tacaribe complex of v.
    Tahyna v.
    temperate v.
    Teschen disease v.
    Tete v.
    TGE v.
    Theiler mouse encephalomyelitis v.
    Theiler original strain of mouse
      encephalomyelitis v. (TO)
    tickborne encephalitis v.
    TO v.
    Togaviridae v.
    trachoma v.
    transmissible gastroenteritis v.
      (TGE)
    transmissible turkey enteritis v.
    tumor v.
    turkey meningoencephalitis v.
    Turlock v.
    Umbre v.
    vaccine v.
    vaccinia v.
    vacuolating v.

varicella-zoster v. (VZV)
variola v.
VEE v.
Venezuelan equine
  encephalomyelitis v.
vesicular exanthema of swine v.
vesicular stomatitis v.
viral hemorrhagic fever v.
visceral disease v.
visna v.
VS v.
WEE v.
Wesselsbron disease v.
western equine encephalitis v.
western equine encephalomyelitis v.
West Nile encephalitis v.
v. X disease
xenotropic v.
Yaba monkey v.
yellow fever v.
Zika v.
virus-1
  human immunodeficiency v. (HIV-
    1)
virus-2
  human immunodeficiency v. (HIV-
    2)
virus-inactivating agent
virus-induced
  v.-i. asthma
  v.-i. wheezing
virus-infected cell
virusoid
virus-transformed cell
visage
  Hippocratic v.
viscera
visceral
  v. disease virus
  v. larva migrans
  v. leishmaniasis (VL)
  v. lymphomatosis
  v. schistosomiasis
  v. sporotrichosis
  v. syphilis
viscerocutaneous loxoscelism
viscerotropic leishmaniasis (VTL)
viscosity
Visine
  V. L.R. Ophthalmic
  V. Workplace
Visiport

visna virus
Vistacrom
Vistaquel
Vistaril
  V. Injection
  V. Oral
Vistazine Injection
Vistide
visual
  v. analog scale (VAS)
  v. analog scale (VAS)
  v. display terminal (VDT)
VIT
  venom immunotherapy
VitaCuff
Vitadye makeup by Elder
Vita-E
vitae
  arbor v.
vital
  v. capacity (VC)
  v. vaccine
vitamin
  v. A
  v. A deficiency
  antioxidant v.
  v. A and vitamin D
  v. B$_6$
  v. B deficiency
  v. B$_1$ deficiency
  v. B$_5$ deficiency
  v. B$_6$ deficiency
  v. B$_{12}$ deficiency
  v. B therapy
  v. C
  v. C deficiency
  v. C test
  v. D deficiency
  v. D synthesis
  v. E
  v. E deficiency
  v. K deficiency
  v. K therapy
  microbial v.
vitamin-related obesity
Vita-Plus E Softgels
viteae
  Acanthocheilonema v.
Vitec topical
Vite E Creme
vitiligines
vitiliginous

NOTES

vitiligo
    acral v.
    acrofacial v.
    v. antibody
    v. capitis
    Cazenave v.
    Celsus v.
    v. disease activity (VIDA)
    v. disease activity score
    facial v.
    generalized v.
    localized v.
    occupational v.
    perinevic v.
    perinevoid v.
    segmental v.
vitiligoidea
vitlata
    Epicauta v.
Vitrasert intraocular device
Vitrax
    AMO V.
vitreitis
vitreous body
vitro
    in v.
vitronectin
vittatus
    Centruroides v.
Viva-Drops solution
vivax
    Plasmodium v.
Vivelle
viviparus
    Dictyocaulus v.
vivo
    in v.
Vivonex formula
Vivotif Berna Oral
VK
    Apo-Pen V.
VKH
    Vogt-Koyanagi-Harada
VKHS
    Vogt-Koyanagi-Harada syndrome
VL
    visceral leishmaniasis
VLA-4
    very late antigen-4
VLA-1 antigen
VLDL
    very-low-density lipoprotein
Vlemasque
Vleminckx solution
VM-301
Vmax
VMR
    vasomotor rhinitis

VNTR
    variable numbers of tandem repeats
VO$_2$
    oxygen consumption per minute
        VO$_2$ max
vocational intervention
voces (*pl. of* vox)
VOD disease
Voerner disease
Vofenal
Vogt-Koyanagi-Harada (VKH)
    V.-K.-H. syndrome (VKHS)
Vogt-Koyanagi syndrome
Vohwinkel
    mutilating keratoderma of V.
    V. syndrome
Voigt line
volar
    v. psoriasis
    v. skin
volatile odor
volcanic border
vole bacillus
Volkmann cheilitis
Vollmer test
Volmax
voltage-gated potassium channel
voltametry
    adsorptive v.
Voltaren
    V. Oral
    V. Rapide
Voltaren-XR Oral
volume
    erosion v.
    expiratory residual v. (ERV)
    forced expiratory v. (FEV)
    high lung v.
    intrathoracic blood v. (ITBV)
    pulmonary blood v. (PBV)
    residual v.
    stroke v. (SV)
    v. test
    v. thickness index (VTI)
    tidal v.
    trapped gas v. (TGV)
volume-assured pressure support (VAPS)
volume-cycled decelerating-flow ventilation
volume-limited ventilator
volumetric
    v. magnetization transfer imaging
    v. method
    v. technique
volutrauma
volvae
volvulosis

volvulus
> *Onchocerca v.*

vomiting
> epidemic v.
> explosive v.

von
> v. Behring law
> v. Economo disease
> v. Economo encephalitis
> v. Gierke glycogen storage disease
> v. Hippel-Landau syndrome
> v. Hippel-Lindau gene (VHL)
> v. Krogh transformation
> v. Recklinghausen disease
> v. Willebrand disease (vWD)
> v. Willebrand factor (vWF)
> v. Zumbusch disease
> v. Zumbusch pustular psoriasis

Vontrol
vorax
> lupus v.

Vornado
> V. Air Quality System

Vorner variant of Unna-Thost keratoderma
vortices pilorum
VoSol HC Otic
vox, pl. **voces**
> v. cholerica

VP
> variegate porphyria
> ventriculoperitoneal shunt

VPF/VEGF
> vascular permeability factor/vascular
> endothelial cell growth factor

V-plasty to Y-plasty
Vpr
Vpu
V/Q
> ventilation/perfusion
> V/Q lung scan

VRE
> vancomycin-resistant enterococci
> vancomycin-resistant *Enterococcus*

VREF
> vancomycin-resistant *Enterococcus*
> *faecium*
> VREF bacteremia

VS virus
VTI
> volume thickness index

VTL
> viscerotropic leishmaniasis

V-type microtiter plate
vulgaris
> acne v.
> apple jelly papule of lupus v.
> *Artemis v.*
> *Faba v.*
> ichthyosis v.
> impetigo v.
> lupus v.
> pemphigus v. (PV)
> *Proteus v.*
> sycosis v.
> *Thermoactinomyces v.*
> verruca v.
> xerosis v.

vulnificus
> *Vibrio v.*
> *Vibrios v.*

vulva, pl. **vulvae**
> kraurosis v.
> leukoplakia v.
> pruritus v.

vulvar
> v. dermatosis
> v. intraepithelial neoplasia
> v. itch
> v. lesion
> v. nevus
> v. vestibulitis syndrome
> v. wart

vulvitis
> chronic atrophic v.
> follicular v.
> leukoplakic v.
> plasma cell v.

vulvodynia
vulvovaginal candidiasis (VVC)
vulvovaginitis
> herpetic v.

Vumon injection
VVC
> vulvovaginal candidiasis

Vw antigen
vWD
> von Willebrand disease

VWF
> vibration-induced white finger

vWF
> von Willebrand factor

VX-497

V

NOTES

VX-740
VX-745
Vytone topical
VZ
    varicella-zoster

VZIG
    varicella-zoster immunoglobulin
VZV
    varicella-zoster virus
      VZV retinitis

W
>Benzac W
>Compound W

W-135
>meningococcal polysaccharide
>vaccine, groups A, C, Y, W.

Waardenburg-Shah syndrome
Waardenburg syndrome
Wagner-Meissner tactile corpuscle
Wagner potion
Waldenström
>hypergammaglobulinemia of W.
>W. macroglobulinemia (WM)
>W. purpura
>W. syndrome

Walker-Murdoch sign
walking
>chromosome w.

wall
>nail w.
>w. pellitory
>shaggy thick w.

Wallgren aseptic meningitis
walnut
>black w.
>shaking of w.'s
>w. tree

walnut-juice stain
Walsh pressure ring
Walter
>W. Reed classification
>W. splinter forceps

Walton
>W. expressor
>W. extractor

wandering
>w. erysipelas
>w. rash

waning
>waxing and w.

warble
Wardrop disease
warehouseman's itch
warfare
>biological w. (BW)
>Skin Exposure Reduction Paste
>Against Chemical W.

warfarin sodium
warm
>w. agglutinin
>w. autoantibody
>w. spot
>w. water immersion foot (WWIF)

warm-cold hemolysin
warm-reactive antibody

wart
>acuminate w.
>anatomic w.
>anatomical w.
>asbestos w.
>black seeds in w.
>cattle w.
>common w.
>digitate w.
>doughnut w.
>fig w.
>filiform w.
>flat w.
>fugitive w.
>genital w.
>infectious w.
>moist w.
>mosaic w.
>myrmecia w.
>nail w.
>necrogenic w.
>palmar w.
>paronychial w.
>periungual w.
>Peruvian w.
>pitch w.
>plane w.
>plantar w.
>pointed w.
>postmortem w.
>prosector's w.
>recalcitrant w.
>W. Remover
>ridged w.
>seborrheic w.
>seed w.
>senile w.
>soft w.
>soot w.
>subungual w.
>telangiectatic w.
>trumpeter w.
>tuberculous w.
>venereal w.
>viral w.
>vulvar w.
>water w.

Wart-Away
Wartenberg symptom
Warthin-Finkeldey cell
Warthin-Starry stain
Warthin-Starry-staining bacillus
wart-like excrescence
wartpox

W

warty
    w. dyskeratoma
    w. horn
    w. keratotic plaque
    w. tuberculosis
WAS
    Wiskott-Aldrich syndrome
Wash
    Benzac AC W.
    Benzac W W.
    Desquam-X W.
    Dryox W.
    Fostex 10% W.
    Oil-Free Acne W.
    Oxy 10 W.
    SAStid Plain Therapeutic Shampoo
     and Acne W.
    Theroxide W.
washed maternal platelet
washerman's mark
washerwoman's itch
WASP
    Wiskott-Aldrich syndrome protein
wasp
    paper w.
    w. sting
Wassermann
    W. antibody
    W. fast test
    W. reaction (W.r.)
Wassilieff disease
wasting
    w. disease
    w. syndrome
Watch
    Oxy Night W.
water
    W. Babies
    w. blister
    w. canker
    extravascular lung w. (EVLW)
    w. itch
    w. moccasin snake
    w. sore
    w. wart
water-based
    w.-b. facial foundation
    w.-b. mascara
water-buffalo leprosy
water-free facial foundation
Waterhouse-Friderichsen syndrome
water-impermeable, nonsilicone-based
  occlusive dressing
water-in-oil ointment
watermelon stomach
waterpox
water-repellent ointment
water-soluble ointment

Waters view
water-washable cream
waveform
    high-energy, pulse-doublet w.
wave splash
wax
    w. epilation
    w. myrtle
    w. myrtle tree
waxing and waning
waxy
    w. finger
    w. skin
4-Way Long Acting Nasal Solution
Ways of Coping Scale
WBC
    white blood cell
    WBC count
WBI
    whole body irradiation
WCD
    Weber-Christian disease
WCS-90
    Clorpactin W.
WDE
    wound dressing emulsion
    Biafine WDE
weakness
    generalized w.
    motor neuron w.
    muscle w.
weal *wheal*
weanling diarrhea
Webb antigen
webbed pattern
Weber-Christian disease (WCD)
Weber-Cockayne
    W.-C. disease
    W.-C. syndrome
Weber test
web formation
Webril
Webster needle holder
wedge renal biopsy
WEE
    western equine encephalomyelitis
    WEE virus
weed
    careless w.
    poverty w.
weeping
    w. dermatitis
    w. eczema
    w. fig
    w. fig tree
    w. lesion
    w. willow

Wegener
  W. granulomatosis (WG)
  W. granulomatosus syndrome
Weibull regression model
Weichselbaum lacunar resorption
weight
  high molecular w. (HMW)
  w. loss
Weil disease
Weil-Felix
  W.-F. reaction
  W.-F. test
Weill-Marchesani syndrome
Weinberg reaction
Weissenbach syndrome
Weissenbach-Zweymuller syndrome
weld
  spot w.
Well
  W. disease
  W. syndrome
Wellcovorin
  W. injection
  W. Oral
well-demarcated skin reaction
Wells
  W. Johnson pump
  W. syndrome
welt
  indurated w.
wen
Werlhof
  W. disease
  W. purpura
werneckii
  Cladosporium w.
  Exophiala w.
Werner syndrome
Wernicke-Korsakoff syndrome
Werther
  W. disease
  W. nevus
Wesselsbron
  W. disease
  W. disease virus
  W. fever
Wessely ring
West
  W. African fever
  W. Indian smallpox
  W. Nile encephalitis virus
  W. Nile fever

Westcort Topical
Westergren sedimentation rate
westermani
  Paragonimus w.
western
  w. black-legged tick
  W. blot
  W. blot electrotransfer test
  W. blot infection
  W. blot vaccine profile
  w. equine encephalitis virus
  w. equine encephalomyelitis (WEE)
  w. equine encephalomyelitis virus
  W. juniper
  W. juniper tree
  W. Ontario and McMaster
    Universities Osteoarthritis Index
    (WOMAC)
  W. Ontario and McMaster
    Universities Osteoarthritis Index
    Physical Functioning subscale and
    chair-stand performance
    (WOMAC-PF)
  w. poison oak
  W. ragweed
  W. ragweed weed pollen
  W. red cedar
  w. water hemp
Westrim LA
wet
  w. cutaneous leishmaniasis
  w. dressing
  w. flush
  w. gangrene
  w. pellagra
  w. smear
  w. tetter
WG
  Wegener granulomatosis
whale finger
Whatman 3MM
wheal
  w. and erythema radiation
  erythematous w.
  w. and flare
  skin w.
wheal-and-erythema reaction
wheal-and-flare reaction
whealing
wheat
  w. flour

NOTES

W

wheat *(continued)*
    w. grain dust mite
    whole w.
wheeze
    monophonic w.
wheezing
    intractable w.
    nocturnal w.
    virus-induced w.
wheezy bronchitis
Whiff test
whiplash injury
Whipple
    W. bacillus
    W. disease
whippleii
    Trophermyma w.
whistling face syndrome
white
    w. ash
    w. ash tree
    w. blood cell (WBC)
    w. blood cell count
    w. burrobrush
    w. dermatographia
    w. dermographism
    w. finger
    w. frontal forelock
    w. gangrene
    w. graft
    w. lesion
    w. line
    w. line response
    w. melanin
    w. mulberry
    w. mulberry tree
    w. oak
    w. oak tree
    w. petrolatum
    w. piedra
    w. pine
    w. pine tree
    w. poplar tree
    w. scar
    w. sponge nevus
    w. spot disease
    w. spots of the nail plate
    w. spots of skin
    w. strawberry tongue
white-faced hornet
whitegraft reaction
whitehead
whitepox
Whitewater Arroyo
Whitfield ointment
whitlow
    herpes w.

    herpetic w.
    melanotic w.
Whitmore
    W. disease
    W. fever
    W. melioidosis
WHO
    World Health Organization
    WHO Class IV
    WHO criteria
WHO/ILAR
    World Health Organization/International
    League of Associations for
    Rheumatology
whole
    w. blood
    w. body irradiation (WBI)
    w. ragweed extract (WRE)
    w. wheat
whole-body
    w.-b. antibody technique (IMX)
    w.-b. extract
whooping cough
whooping-cough vaccine
whorl
    digital w.
whorled
Whytt disease
wickerhamii
    Prototheca w.
Wickham stria
Widal
    W. reaction
    W. serum test
    W. syndrome
wide
    w. excision
    w. spectrum
widow's peak
Wigraine
Wilcoxon rank sum test
wild
    w. oat grass pollen
    w. rye
    w. rye grass
    w. tobacco
wildfire rash
Willan
    W. disease
    W. lepra
Willebrand factor
willow
    w. tree
    w. tree pollen
    weeping w.
Wilms tumor

Wilson
>W. disease
>W. lichen

Wilson-Brocq erythroderma

Wimberger sign

Win
>wound-induced

windborne pollen

windburn

Windmill-Vane-Hand syndrome

window
>core w.
>nasoantral w.
>Rebuck skin w.

wine-induced asthma

Winer
>dilated pore of W.
>pore of W.

wingscale

Winkler disease

Winks

Winn test

Winpred

WinRho
>W. SD
>W. SD antibody

Winstrol

winter
>w. dysentery of cattle
>w. eczema
>w. itch
>w. protoporphyria
>w. pruritus
>w. vomiting disease

Winterbottom sign

Wipes
>Sport W.

wire-loop
>w.-l. lesion
>w.-l. shaped telangiectasia

Wisconsin
>University of W. (UVW)

Wiskott-Aldrich
>W.-A. syndrome (WAS)
>W.-A. syndrome protein (WASP)

Wissler-Fanconi syndrome

Wissler syndrome

Wistar rats

witch hazel

witkop

Witkop-Von Sallman disease

WM
>Waldenström macroglobulinemia

Wohlfahrtia

wolf-biter habit

WOMAC
>Western Ontario and McMaster
>Universities Osteoarthritis Index
>WOMAC pain score
>WOMAC Physical Function
>subscale
>WOMAC stiffness scale

WOMAC-PF
>Western Ontario and McMaster
>Universities Osteoarthritis Index
>Physical Functioning subscale and
>chair-stand performance

women
>teratogenic effect on pregnant w.

wood
>W. glass
>W. lamp
>W. light
>W. light examination
>pao ferro w.
>w. tar
>w. tick
>W. unit

woodcutter's encephalitis

wood-pulp worker's disease

wool
>sheep w.
>Sofban orthopedic padding w.
>Velband orthopedic padding w.
>w. wax alcohol

woolly hair

woolly-hair nevus

Wor Ditchling agent

Woringer-Kolopp disease

Workplace
>Visine W.

Work-Station Sun-Sparcs 20

World
>W. Health Organization (WHO)
>W. Health Organization
>classification of lupus nephritis (I,
>IIA, IIB, III, IV, V)
>W. Health Organization criteria
>W. Health Organization/International
>League of Associations for
>Rheumatology (WHO/ILAR)

worm
>biting reef w.

W

NOTES

worm *(continued)*
    blood w.
    Guinea w.
    medina w.
worm-like
wormwood
Woronoff ring
wortmannin
wound
    abraded w.
    w. botulism
    w. contraction
    w. dressing emulsion (WDE)
    w. fever
    fish-mouth w.
    w. grading 1-6
    w. healing
    w. myiasis
    puncture w.
    W. Span Bridge II dressing
    W. Stick measuring system
wound-induced (Win)
Woun'Dres
    W. collagen
    W. hydrogel dressing
W-plasty
W.r.
    Wassermann reaction
Wr^a
    Wright antigen
    Wr^a antigen
wrap
    Coban w.
    Coflex flexible w.
    Comprilan w.
    elastic w.
WRE
    whole ragweed extract
wreath
    Hippocratic w.
wrestler herpes
Wright
    W. antigen (Wr^a)
    W. nebulizer
    W. stain
wrinkle
wrinkling
    cigarette-paper w.
writing
    skin w.
wt gene
wucher atrophy
Wuchereria bancrofti
wuchereriasis
Wu-Kabat plot
WWIF
    warm water immersion foot
Wyamycin S
Wyburn-Mason syndrome
Wycillin injection
Wydase
Wyeth bifurcated needle
Wymox

X

X chromosome
X factor
Histalet X
histiocytosis X
XAb
Xanar 20 Ambulase CO$_2$ laser
Xanax
xanchromatic
xanthelasma
generalized x.
x. palpebrarum
xanthelasmoidea
xanthelasmoideum
lymphangioma x.
xanthine
x. crystal
x. inhibition
x. stone excretion
xanthinuria
xanthism
xanthochroia
xanthochromatic
xanthochromia striata palmaris
xanthochromic
xanthochrous
xanthoderma
xanthoerythrodermia perstans
xanthogranuloma (XG)
juvenile x. (JXG)
necrobiotic x.
xanthoma, pl. xanthomata
x. diabeticorum
diffuse plane x.
x. dissemination
x. disseminatum (XD)
eruptive x.
fibrous x.
generalized plane x.
hypercholesteremic x.
hyperlipemic x.
juvenile x.
x. multiplex striatum palmare
nodular x.
normocholesteremic x.
palmar x.
palpebrarum x.
x. palpebrarum
papular x.
planar x.
plane x.
x. planum
x. striata palmaris
x. tendinosum
tendinous x.

tendon x.
tuberoeruptive x.
x. tuberosum
x. tuberosum multiplex
tuberous x.
urticarial x.
verruciform x.
verrucous x.
xanthomatosis
cerebrotendinous x.
generalized plane x.
normolipemic x.
normolipoproteinemic x.
xanthomatous biliary cirrhosis
Xanthomonas maltophilia
xanthopathy
xanthopsydracia
xanthosis diabeticorum
Xcellerate T-cell product
XD
xanthoma disseminatum
Xe
xenon
XeCl excimer laser
X-encoded immune system gene
XenoDerm graft
xenogeneic
x. cellular immune response
x. graft
x. transplantation
xenogenic
xenogenous
xenograft
discordant cellular x.
discordant organ x.
free-tissue x.
organ x.
x. rejection
x. transplantation
vascularized x.
xenoislet transplantation
xenon (Xe)
x. arc lamp
xenoparasite
xenopi
Mycobacterium x.
Xenopsylla
X. cheopis
X. cheopis bite
xenoreactive natural antibody (XNA)
xenorecognition
T-cell x.
xenosis
xenotransplant

X

xenotransplantation
  cellular x.
  pig-to-primate model of x.
xenotropic virus
xenozoonoses
Xerac AC
xerasia
xerochilia
xeroderma, xerodermia
  Kaposi x.
  x. pigmentosum
Xeroform
Xero-Lube
xeronosus
xerophthalmia
xerosis vulgaris
xerostomia
xerotes
xerotica
xerotic eczema
xerotripsis
XG
  xanthogranuloma
Xg antigen
X-inactivation
xinafoate
  salmeterol x.
XL
  Biaxin XL
X-linked
  X.-l. agammaglobulinemia
  X.-l. Ehlers-Danlos syndrome
  X.-l. hypogammaglobulinemia
  X.-l. ichthyosis
  X.-l. immunodeficiency with hyper IgM
  X.-l. lymphoproliferative disease (XLP)
  X.-l. lymphoproliferative syndrome
  X.-l. mucopolysaccharidosis
  X.-l. ocular albinism (XOAN)
  X.-l. recessive inheritance
  X.-l. severe combined immunodeficiency (XSCID)
XLP
  X-linked lymphoproliferative disease
XMMEN-OE5 monoclonal antibody
XNA
  xenoreactive natural antibody
XOAN
  X-linked ocular albinism
Xolair
Xopenex
Xosten
x-radiation
x-ray
  x.-r. alopecia
  x.-r. crystallographic data
  x.-r. dermatitis
  x.-r. finding
XSCID
  X-linked severe combined immunodeficiency
X-Seb T
X-span tubing
x-square test
XT
  Contuss XT
XXMEN-OE5
  X.-O. antiendotoxin
XXYY genotype
xylene
Xylocaine
  X. with epinephrine
xylol prep
xylometazoline
xylose
xylosoxidans
  Achromobacter x.
  Alcaligenes x.
XYY syndrome

Y
histiocytosis Y
Y12 monoclonal antibody
Yaba
Y. monkey virus
Y. tumor
YAC
yeast artificial chromosome
YAG
yttrium-aluminum-garnet
YAG laser
YagLazr system
Yangtze edema
Yates corrected chi square test
yaw
bosch y.
bush y.
crab y.
early y.
foot y.
forest y.
guinea corn y.
late y.
mother y.
osseous y.
ringworm y.
tertiary y.
yeast
y. artificial chromosome (YAC)
y. form
y. infection
lipophilic y.
y. meningitis
Yeast-Gard Medicated Douche
yellow
y. disease
y. dock
y. fever
y. fever vaccine (YF-VAX)

y. fever virus
y. hornet
y. jacket
y. jacket sting
y. lesion
y. mustard
y. mutant albinism
y. nail
y. nail syndrome
y. oculocutaneous albinism
y. papule
y. skin
Yergason supination sign
Yersinia
Y. antigen
Y. arthritis
Y. *enterocolitica*
Y. *pestis*
Y. *pestis* bite
Y. *pseudotuberculosis*
Y. pseudotuberculosis agglutinin
yew tree
YF-VAX
yellow fever vaccine
ying-yang fashion
YKL-40 antigen
ylang-ylang oil
Yodoxin
young
maturity-onset diabetes of the y. (MODY)
Y. syndrome
Y-plasty
V-plasty to Y.-p.
Yt^a antigen
Yttrium-90
yttrium-aluminum-garnet (YAG)
y.-a.-g. laser
yucca

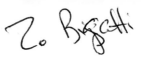

Zaditen
Zaditor
zafirlukast
Zagam
Zahorsky disease
Zaire subtype
zalcitabine (ddC)
Zambesi ulcer
Zambusch (*See* Zumbusch)
    generalized pustular psoriasis of Z.
Zanfel cream
Zantac
    Z. injection
    Z. Oral
ZAP-70 deficiency
Zartan
ZDV
   zidovudine
Zeasorb-AF Powder
zebra body
zebra-like hyperpigmentation
ZEEP
   zero end-expiratory pressure
Zefazone
Zeis gland
Zenapax
Zen macrobiotic diet
Zephiran mouthwash
Zephrex LA
Zerit (d4T)
zero end-expiratory pressure (ZEEP)
zeta
    z. potential
    z. sedimentation rate
Zetar
Zetone cream
Zetran injection
Ziagen
zidovudine (ZDV)
    z. and lamivudine
Ziehl-Neelsen
    Z.-N. smear
    Z.-N. stain
zigzag approximation
Zika
    Z. fever
    Z. virus
zileuton
Zimmerman-Laband syndrome
Zimmerman-Walton expressor
Zimmer Pulsavac wound debridement
  system
Zinacef injection
Zinaderm

Tzanck smear

zinc
    z. chloride paste
    z. deficiency
    DHS z.
    z. finger protein
    z. gluconate lozenge
    z. oxide
    z. oxide, cod liver oil, and talc
    z. oxide microfine
    z. pox
    z. protoporphyrin (ZPP)
    z. protoporphyrin:heme ratio
    pyrithione z.
    z. pyrithione
    z. sulfate
Zincoderm
Zincofax
Zincon Shampoo
Zindaclin
Zino
    Scholl Z.
Zinsser-Cole-Engman syndrome
Zinsser-Engman-Cole syndrome
ZIP
   zoster immune plasma
Zipzoc
    Z. stocking
    Z. Stocking leg compression
     dressing
zirconium granuloma
zit
Zithromax
ZLN
   zosteriform lentiginous nevus
Zn-dependent endopeptidase
ZNP bar
zoacanthosis
Zolicef
Zoloft
zona, pl. zonae
    z. corona
    z. dermatica
    z. epithelioserosa
    z. facialis
    z. fasciculata
    z. glomerulosa
    z. ignea
    z. ophthalmica
    z. reticularis
    z. serpiginosa
Zonalon Topical cream
zonal type reaction
zonary
zone
    barrier z.

Z

zone (*continued*)
>   basement membrane z. (BMZ)
>   equivalence z.
>   floristic z.
>   Head z.
>   z. of hyperalgesia
>   z. of hyperemia
>   hyperesthetic z.
>   keratogenous z.
>   perinuclear z.
>   T z.

zonesthesia
zoniform nevus
zonula occludens
zoograft
Zoon
>   balanitis of Z.
>   Z. disease
>   Z. erythroplasia

zoonosis
zoonotic
>   z. cutaneous leishmaniasis
>   z. erysipelas
>   z. infection
>   z. potential

zoophilic fungus
zootoxin
ZORprin
zoster
>   acute herpes z.
>   dermatomal z.
>   disseminated herpes z.
>   z. encephalomyelitis
>   herpes z. (HZ)
>   z. immune globulin
>   z. immune plasma (ZIP)
>   ophthalmic z.
>   z. sine herpetic

zosteriform
>   z. distribution of lesion

>   z. lentiginous nevus (ZLN)
>   z. lichen planus
>   z. pattern

zosteroid
Zostrix
Zostrix-HP
Zosyn
Zovirax
>   Z. injection
>   Z. Oral
>   Z. topical

Zoysia
ZP 11
Z-plasty
>   O-plasty to Z.-p.
>   Z.-p. procedure

ZPP
>   zinc protoporphyrin

z score
Zumbusch
>   Z. disease
>   generalized pustular psoriasis of
>   von Z.

Zyderm
>   Z. collagen implant
>   Z. II collagen

Zygomycetes
zygomycosis
zygospore
Zyloprim
zymography
>   gelatin z.

zymosan
>   unopsonized z.

zymotic papilloma
Zyplast
>   Z. collagen
>   Z. collagen implant

Zyrtec

Tzanck smear

Anatomical Illustrations

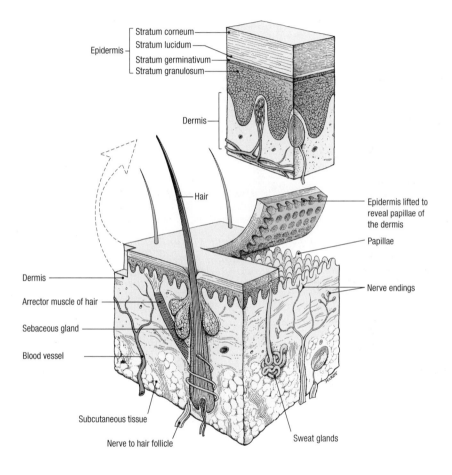

Figure 1. Skin components and layers.

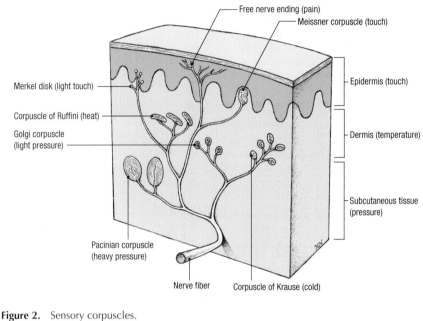

Figure 2. Sensory corpuscles.

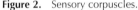

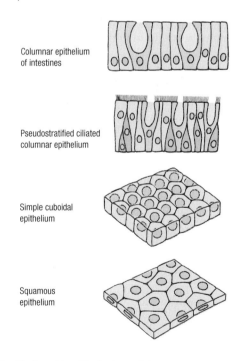

Figure 3. Types of epithelium (simplified schematic).

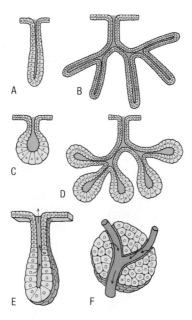

Figure 4. Types of glands: tubular (A), compound tubular (B), acinous (C), compound acinous (D), exocrine (E), endocrine (F).

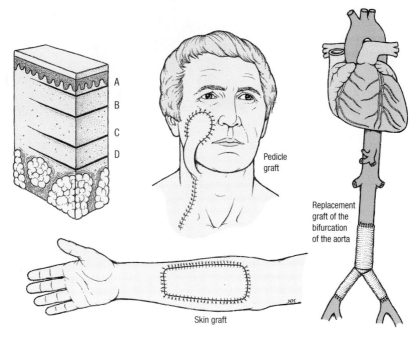

Figure 5. Graft types: split-thickness grafts (A, B, C), full-thickness graft (D).

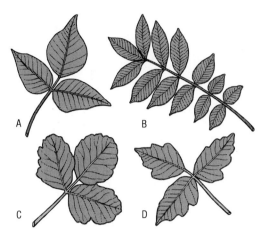

Figure 6.   *Toxicodendron:* poison ivy (A), poison sumac (B), Western poison oak (C), Eastern poison oak (D).

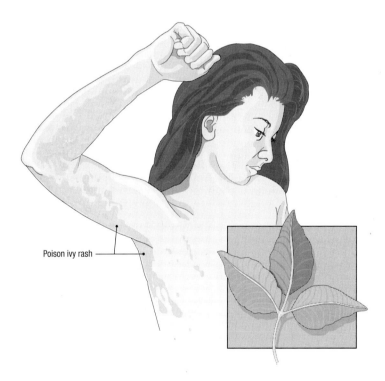

Poison ivy rash

Figure 7.   Young girl with arm lifted to show typical poison ivy rash with weepy blisters on underside of arm and wrist; inset shows poison ivy leaflet of three.

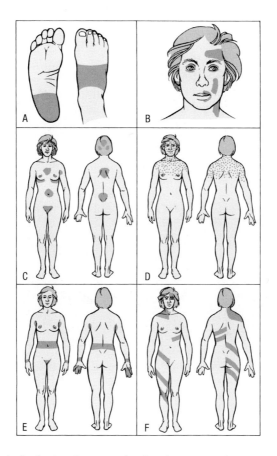

Figure 8. Anatomic distribution of common skin disorders: contact dermatitis from shoes (A), contact dermatitis from cosmetics, perfumes and earrings (B), seborrheic dermatitis (C), acne (D), scabies (E), herpes zoster (shingles) (F). This image, created by Mikki Senkarik, for Smeltzer SC & Bare GB, *Brunner & Suddarth's Textbook of Medical Surgical-Nursing, 8th Edition,* Philadelphia, J. B. Lippincott Company, 1996, fig. 53.5, appears here with permission and courtesy of Lippincott Williams & Wilkins.

Appendix 1

Primary lesions

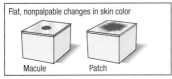

Flat, nonpalpable changes in skin color

Macule   Patch

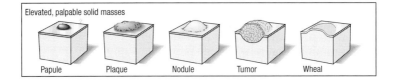

Elevated, palpable solid masses

Papule   Plaque   Nodule   Tumor   Wheal

Elevation formed by fluid in a cavity

Vesicle   Bulla   Pustule

Secondary lesions

Loss of skin surface

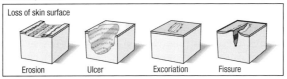

Erosion   Ulcer   Excoriation   Fissure

Material on skin surface

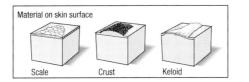

Scale   Crust   Keloid

Vascular lesions

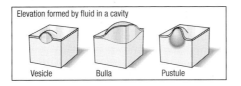

Cherry angioma   Telangiectasia   Petechia   Ecchymosis

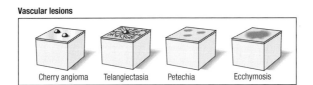

Figure 9. Lesions. Types of primary, secondary and vascular lesions. This image, from Willis MC, *Medical Terminology: The Language of Health Care,* Baltimore, Williams & Wilkins, 1996, fig. 53.5, appears here with permission and courtesy of Lippincott Williams & Wilkins.

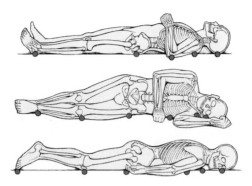

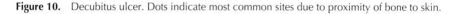

Figure 10. Decubitus ulcer. Dots indicate most common sites due to proximity of bone to skin.

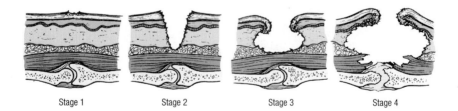

Stage 1   Stage 2   Stage 3   Stage 4

Figure 11. Cross-section of skin showing 4 stages of pressure sore and ulcer classification. Stage 1: inflammation, redness of epidermis. Stage 2: loss of epidermis, damage to dermis. Stage 3: involvement of subcutaneous tissue. Stage 4: damage to tendon, muscle and bone.

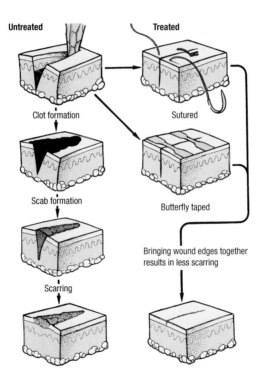

Figure 12. Wound healing.

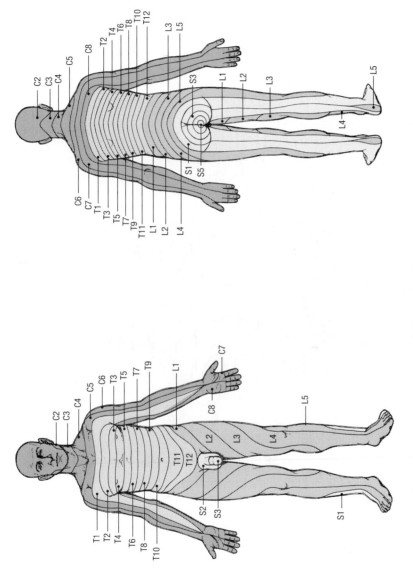

Figure 13. Dermatomes. Areas of skin supplied by cutaneous branches of spinal nerves.

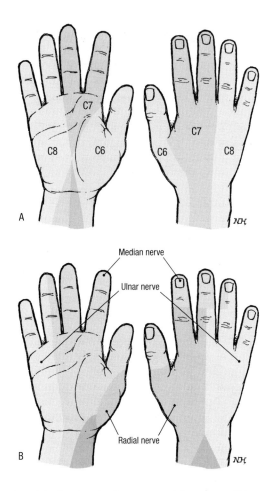

Figure 14. Innervation of the hand and wrist: segmental dermatomes (A), cutaneous nerve distribution (B).

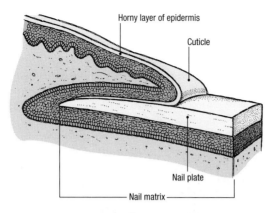

Figure 15. Structure of the nail (unguis).

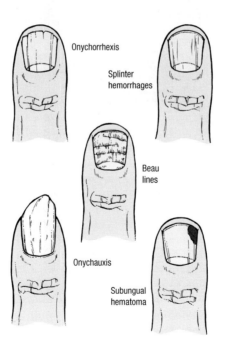

Figure 16. Nail abnormalities. This image, created by Larry Ward, for Fuller J & Schaller-Ayers J, *A Nursing Approach, 2nd Edition,* Philadelphia, J. B. Lippincott Company, 1994, p. 143, appears here with permission and courtesy of Lippincott Williams & Wilkins.

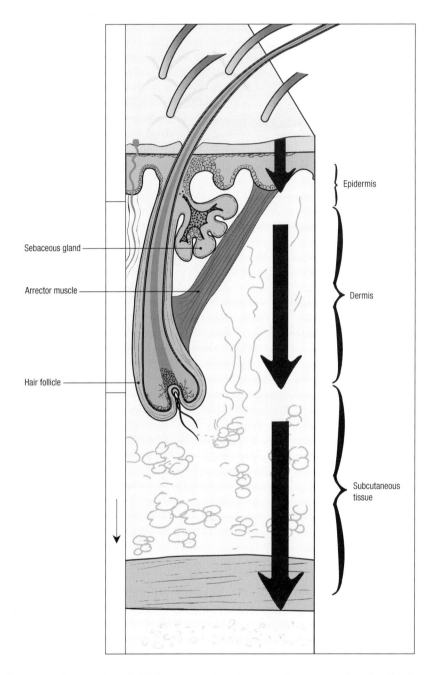

Figure 17. Cross-section of skin layers, muscle and bone, with corresponding classification of burn depths.

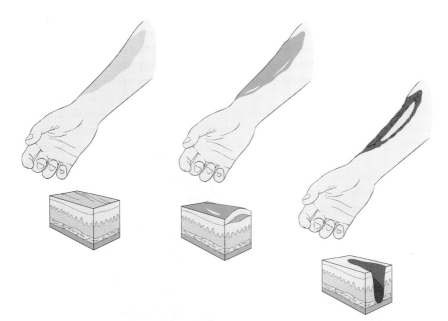

Figure 18. Three types of burns shown on arm and in cross-section of skin. Superficial burn (left). Partial-thickness burn (center). Full-thickness burn (right).

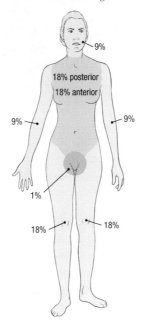

Figure 19. Adult female illustrating the rule of nines used when assessing burn damage to various body parts.

Appendix 1

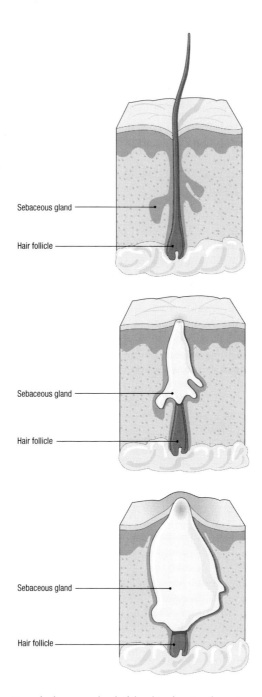

Figure 20. Cross-section of sebaceous gland of the skin showing three stages in the development of acne.

Antibiotic groups

Aminoglycosides
(e.g., streptomycin, gentamicin, sisomicin, tobramycin, amicacin)

Ansamycins
(e.g., rifamycin)

Antimycotics
Polyenes
(e.g., nystatin, pimaricin, amphotericin B, pecilocin)
Benzofuran derivatives
(Griseofulvin)

β–lactam antibiotics
Penicillins
(Penicillin G and its derivatives, oral penicillins, penicillinase-fixed penicillins, broad-
-spectrum penicillins, penicillins active against *Proteus* and *Pseudomonas*)
Cephalosporins
(e.g., cephalothin, cephaloridine, cephalexin, cefazolin, cefotaxime)

Chloramphenicol group
(Chloramphenicol, thiamphenicol, azidamphenicol)

Imidazole
Fluconazole, itraconazole

Linosamides
(Lincomycin, clindamycin)

Macrolides
(e.g., azithromycin, erythromycin, oleandomycin, spiramycin, clarithromycin)

Peptides, peptolides, polypeptides
(e.g., polymyxin B and E, bacitracin, tyrothricin, capreomycin, vancomycin)

Quinolones
(Nalidixic acid, ofloxacin, ciprofloxacin, norfloxin)

Tetracyclines
(e.g., tetracycline, oxytetracycline, minocycline, doxycycline)

Other antibiotics
(Phosphomycin, fusidic acid)

Figure 21. Antibiotic groups. This table, created by Susan Caldwell for *Stedman's Medical Dictionary, 27th Edition,* Baltimore, Lippincott Williams & Wilkins, 2000, p. 96, appears here with permission and courtesy of Lippincott Williams & Wilkins.

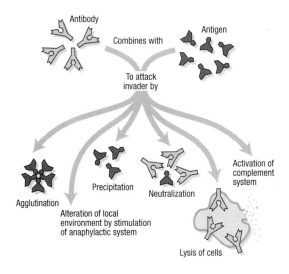

Figure 22. Humoral immunity. This image, created by Mary Anna Barratt for *Stedman's Medical Dictionary, 27th Edition,* Baltimore, Lippincott Williams & Wilkins, 2000, p. 879, appears here with permission and courtesy of Lippincott Williams & Wilkins.

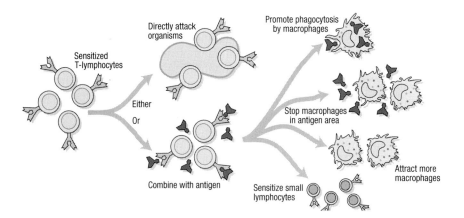

Figure 23. Cell-mediated immunity. This image, created by Mary Anna Barratt for *Stedman's Medical Dictionary, 27th Edition,* Baltimore, Lippincott Williams & Wilkins, 2000, p. 878, appears here with permission and courtesy of Lippincott Williams & Wilkins.

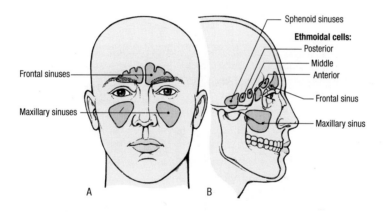

Figure 24. Paranasal sinuses: anterior (A) and lateral (B) views of the head.

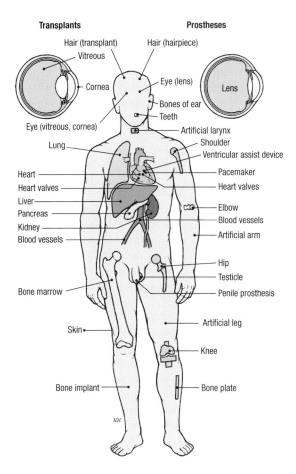

Figure 25. Transplants and prostheses.

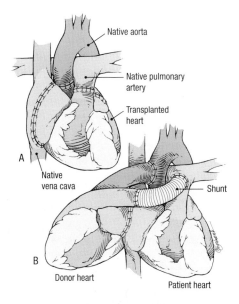

Figure 26. Heart transplantation: orthotopic method (A), heterotopic method (B). This image, created by Mikki Senkarik, for Smeltzer SC & Bare BG, *Brunner & Suddarth's Textbook of Medical Surgical-Nursing, 8th Edition,* Philadelphia, J. B. Lippincott Company, 1996, fig. 30.3, appears here with permission and courtesy of Lippincott Williams & Wilkins.

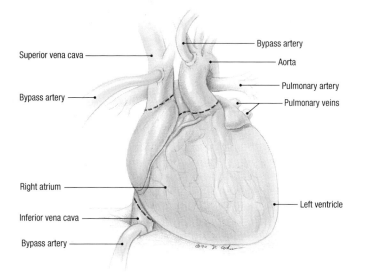

Figure 27. Anterior view of recipient heart prior to removal. Resection lines are shown dashed.

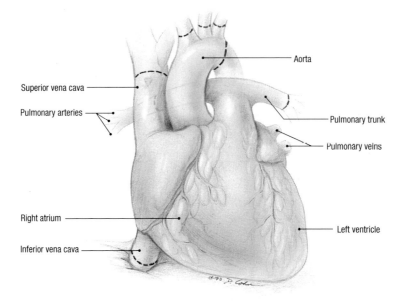

Figure 28. Anterior view of donor heart prior to transplantation showing dissection lines.

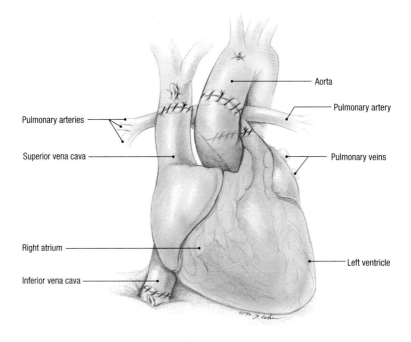

Figure 29. Anterior view of transplanted heart showing sutured areas.

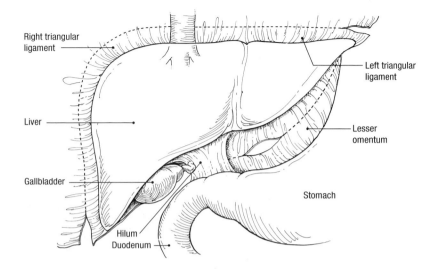

Figure 30. Mobilizing the liver. The lesser omentum and left triangular ligament are divided. The right triangular ligament and peritoneal reflections on the bare area are divided. The mobilization of the right lobe of the liver may be reserved until venovenous bypass has been initiated, and the liver has been devascularized. Figures 30–34, from Kaplowitz N, *Liver & Biliary Disease, 2nd Edition,* Baltimore, Lippincott Williams & Wilkins, 1996, figs. 37.1–5, appear here with permission and courtesy of Lippincott Williams & Wilkins.

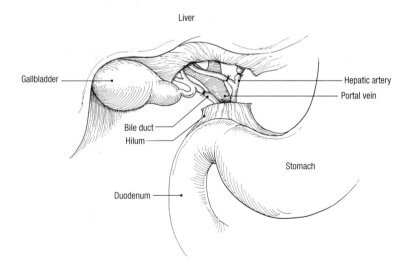

Figure 31. Dissection of the hilum. The peritoneum and adventitial structures are divided. Nerve, lymphatics, and particularly large venous collaterals are dissected. The hepatic artery is ligated and divided, and the bile duct is divided.

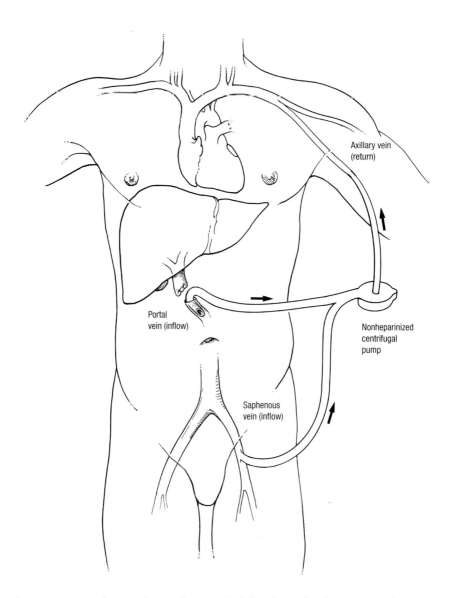

Figure 32. Venous bypass. The portal vein is divided and cannulated, and a second cannula is placed into the inferior vena cava. The blood is pumped in a nonheparinized system and returned to the patient via cannula in the axillary vein.

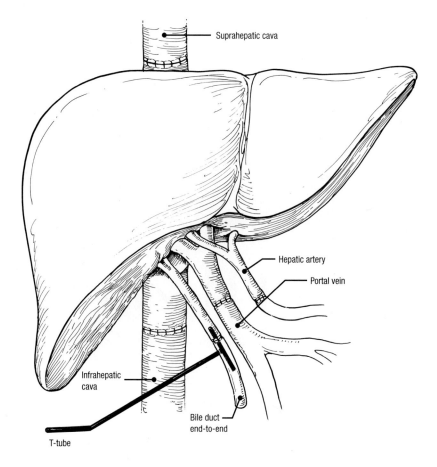

Figure 33. Completed transplant of the liver. Vascular anastomoses include the suprahepatic vena cava, the infrahepatic vena cava, the portal vein, and the hepatic artery. A choledochocholedochostomy biliary reconstruction is depicted.

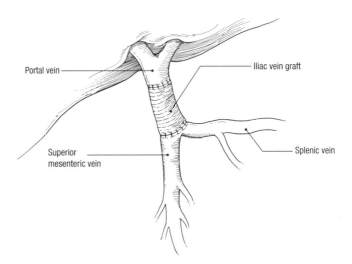

Figure 34.   Iliac vein graft to the portal vein confluence.

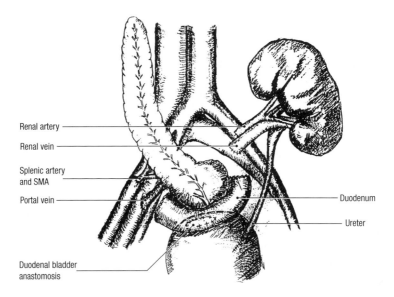

Figure 35.   Simultaneous pancreas-kidney transplant with bladder drainage. This image, from Howard, Idezuki & Prinz, *Surgical Diseases of the Pancreas, 3rd Edition,* Baltimore, Lippincott Williams & Wilkins, 1997, fig. 86.3, appears here with permission and courtesy of Lippincott Williams & Wilkins.

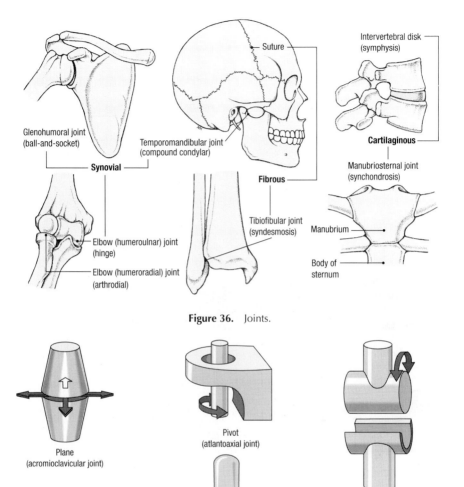

Figure 36. Joints.

Plane
(acromioclavicular joint)

Pivot
(atlantoaxial joint)

Hinge
(elbow joint)

Condyloid
(metacarpophalangeal joint)

Ball and socket
(hip joint)

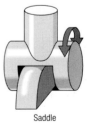

Saddle
(carpometacarpal joint)

Figure 37. Illustration of different types of movements of joints as demonstrated by mechanical models.

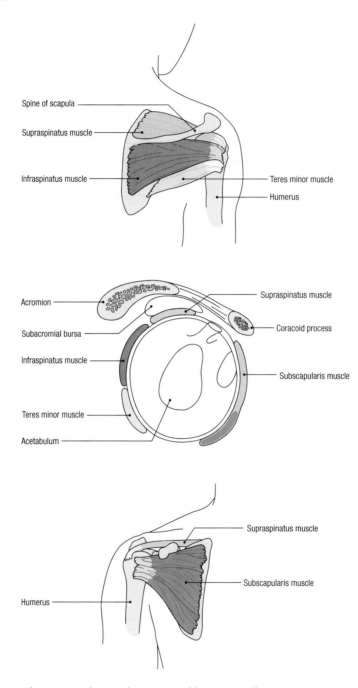

Figure 38. Three images showing the anatomy of the rotator cuff area. Posterior view (top), lateral view (middle) and anterior view (bottom).

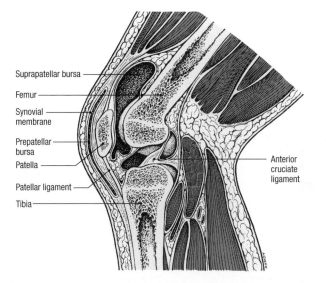

Figure 39. Knee joint. Sagittal section showing prepatellar and suprapatellar bursae.

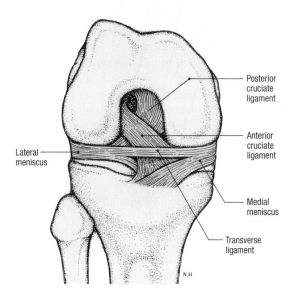

Figure 40. Cruciate ligaments of the knee.

Appendix 1

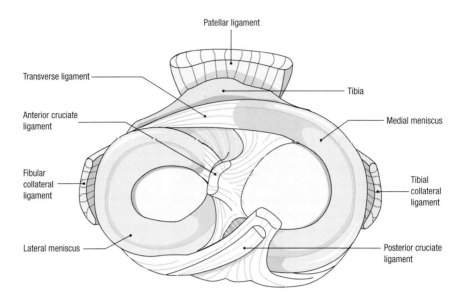

Figure 41. Knee joint viewed from above showing the crescent-shaped menisci that serve as cushions between the bones of the joint.

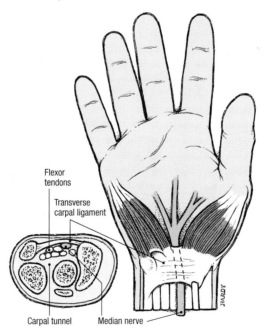

Figure 42. The carpal tunnel contains the median nerve and the flexor tendons of the fingers and thumb.

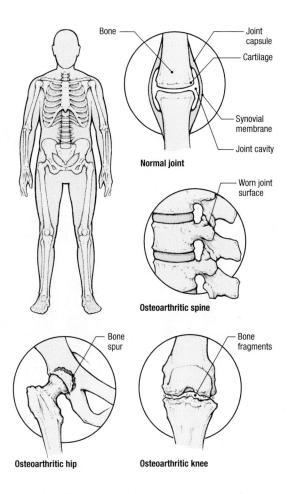

Figure 43. Osteoarthritis. Problems associated with osteoarthritis and some sites where they commonly occur. This image, created by Duckwall Productions, for *Stedman's Medical Dictionary, 27th Edition,* Baltimore, Lippincott Williams & Wilkins, 2000, p. 1282, appears here with permission and courtesy of Lippincott Williams & Wilkins.

Appendix 1

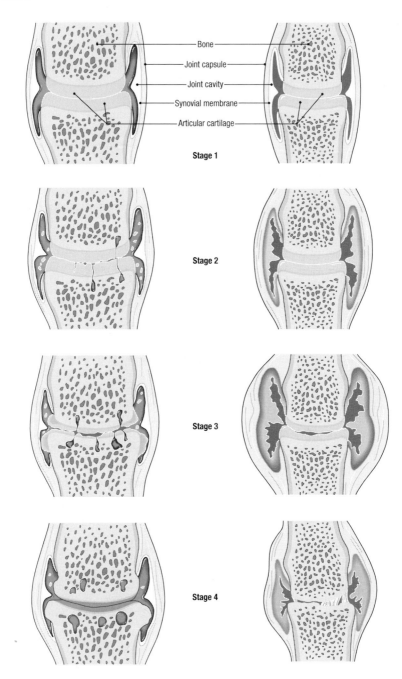

Figure 44. Cross-sections of synovial joints showing the progression of osteoarthritis (left) and rheumatoid arthritis (right) in four stages.

Appendix 2
Normal Lab Values

Test	Conventional Units	SI Units
*Alanine Aminotransferase (ALT, SGPT), serum		
Male	13–40 U/L (37°C)	0.22–0.68 μkat/L (37° C)
Female	10–28 U/L (37°C)	0.17–0.48 μkat/L (37° C)
*Aldolase, serum	1.0–7.5 U/L (30° C)	0.02–0.13 μkat/L (30° C)
Ammonia		
Plasma (Hep)	9–33 μmol/L	9–33 μmol/L
*Aspartate aminotransferase (AST, SGOT), serum	10–59 U/L (37°C)	0.17–1.00 −2 to +3 kat/L (37°C)
*Bilirubin		
Serum		
Adult		
Conjugated	0.0–0.3 mg/dL	0–5 μmol/L
Unconjugated	0.1–1.1 mg/dL	1.7–19 μmol/L
Delta	0–0.2 mg/dL	0–3 μmol/L
Total	0.2–1.3 mg/L	3–22 μmol/L
Neonate		
Conjugated	0–0.6 mg/dL	0–10 μmol/L
Unconjugated	0.6–10.5 mg/dL	10–180 μmol/L
Total	1.5–12 mg/dL	1.7–180 μmol/L
Urine, qualitative	Negative	Negative
Ceruloplasmin, serum	20–60 mg/dL	0.2–6.0 g/L
Coagulation tests		
Antithrombin III (synthetic substrate)	80–120% of normal	0.8–1.2 of normal
Bleeding time (Duke)	0–6 min	0–6 min
Bleeding time (Ivy)	1–6 min	1–6 min
Bleeding time (template)	2.3–9.5 min	2.3–9.5 min
Clot retraction, qualitative	50–100% in 2 h	0.5–1.0/2 h
Coagulation time (Lee-White)	5–15 min (glass tubes) 19–60 min (siliconized tubes)	5–15 min (glass tubes) 19–60 min (siliconized tubes)
Cold hemolysin test (Donath-Landsteiner)	No hemolysis	No hemolysis
Complement components		
Total hemolytic complement activity, plasma (EDTA)	75–160 U/mL	75–160 kU/L
Total complement decay rate (functional), plasma (EDTA)	10–20% Deficiency >50%	Fraction decay rate: 0.10–0.20 >0.50
C1q, serum	14.9–22.1 mg/dL	149–221 mg/L
C1r, serum	2.5–10.0 mg/dL	25–100 mg/L

continued

Test	Conventional Units	SI Units
C1s(C1 esterase), serum	5.0–10.0 mg/dL	50–100 mg/L
C2, serum	1.6–3.6 mg/dL	16–36 mg/L
C3, serum	90–180 mg/dL	0.9–1.8 g/L
C4, serum	10–40 mg/dL	0.1–0.4 g/L
C5, serum	5.5–11.3 mg/dL	55–113 mg/L
C6, serum	17.9–23.9 mg/dL	179–239 mg/L
C7, serum	2.7–7.4 mg/dL	27–74 mg/L
C8, serum	4.9–10.6 mg/dL	49–106 mg/L
C9, serum	3.3–9.5 mg/dL	33–95 mg/L
Coombs test		
Direct	Negative	Negative
Indirect	Negative	Negative
Copper		
Serum		
Male	70–140 μg/dL	11–22 μmol/L
Female	80–155 μg/dL	13–24 μmol/L
Urine	3–35 μg/24 h	0.05–0.55 μmol/24 h
Corpuscular values of erythrocytes (values are for adults; in children values vary with age)		
Mean corpuscular hemoglobin (MCH)	27–31 pg	0.42–0.48 fmol
Mean corpuscular hemoglobin concentration (MCHC)	33–37 g/dL	330–370 g/L
Mean corpuscular volume (MCV)	Male 80–94 μ^3	80–94 fL
	Female 81–99 μ^3	81–99 fL
[†]*Creatine kinase (CK), serum		
Male	15–105 U/L (30°C)	0.26–1.79 μkat/L (30°C)
Female	10–80 U/L (30°C)	0.17–1.36 μkat/L (30°C)
Note: Strenuous exercise or intramuscular injections may cause transient elevation of CK.		
*Creatine kinase MB isoenzyme, serum	0–7 ng/mL	0–7 μg/L
*Creatinine		
Serum or plasma, adult		
Male	0.7–1.3 mg/dL	62–115 μmol/L
Female	0.6–1.1 mg/dL	53–97 μmol/L
Urine		
Male	14–26 mg/kg body weight/24 h	124–230 μmol/kg body weight/24 h
Female	11–20 mg/kg body weight/24 h	97–177 μmol/kg body weight/24 h
*Creatinine clearance, serum or plasma and urine		
Male	94–140 mL/min/1.73 m²	0.91–1.35 mL/s/m²
Female	72–110 mL/min/1.73 m²	0.69–1.06 mL/s/m²
Cryoglobulins, serum	0	0

continued

Test	Conventional Units	SI Units
C-Reactive protein, serum	<0.5 mg/dL	<5 mg/L
‡*Cyclosporine, whole blood		
Therapeutic, trough	100–200 ng/mL	83–166 nmol/L
Fibrin degradation products	<10 μg/mL	<10 mg/L
γ-Glutamyltransferase (GGT), serum		
Male	2–30 U/L (37°C)	0.03–0.51 μkat/L (37°C)
Female	1–24 U/L (37°C)	0.02–0.41 μkat/L (37°C)
Haptoglobin, serum	30–200 mg/dL	0.3–2.0 g/L
Immunoglobulins, serum		
IgG	700–1600 mg/dl	7–16 g/L
IgA	70–400 mg/dl	0.7–4.0 g/L
IgM	40–230 mg/dl	0.4–2.3 g/L
IgD	0–8 mg/dl	0–80 mg/L
IgE	3–423 mg/dl	3–423 kIU/L
Immunoglobulin G (IgG), CSF	0.5–6.1 mg/dL	0.5–6.1 g/L
Insulin, plasma (fasting)	2–25 μU/mL	13–174 pmol/L
*Iron, serum		
Male	65–175 μg/dL	11.6–31.3 μmol/L
Female	50–170 μg/dL	9.0–30.4 μmol/L
Iron binding capacity, serum total (TIBC)	250–425 μg/dL	44.8–71.6 μmol/L
Iron saturation, serum		
Male	20–50%	0.2–0.5
Female	15–50%	0.15–0.5
L-Lactate		
Plasma (NaF)		
Venous	4.5–19.8 mg/dL	0.5–2.2 mmol/L
Arterial	4.5–14.4 mg/dL	0.5–1.6 mmol/L
Whole blood (Hep), at bed rest		
Venous	8.1–15.3 mg/dL	0.9–1.7 mmol/L
Arterial	<11.3 mg/dL	<1.3 mmol/L
Urine, 24 h	496–1982 mg/d	5.5–22 mmol/d
CSF	10–22 mg/dL	1.1–2.4 mmol/L
*Lactate dehydrogenase (LDH) Total (L→P), 37°C, serum		
Newborn	290–775 U/L	4.9–13.2 μkat/L
Neonate	545–2000 U/L	9.3–34 μkat/L
Infant	180–430 U/L	3.1–7.3 μkat/L
Child	110–295 U/L	1.9–5 μkat/L
Adult	100–190 U/L	1.7–3.2 μkat/L
>60 y	110–210 U/L	1.9–3.6 μkat/L
*Isoenzymes, serum by agarose gel electrophoresis		
Fraction 1	14–26% of total	0.14–0.26 fraction of total
Fraction 2	29–39% of total	0.29–0.39 fraction of total

continued

Test	Conventional Units	SI Units
Fraction 3	20–26% of total	0.20–0.26 fraction of total
Fraction 4	8–16% of total	0.08–0.16 fraction of total
Fraction 5	6–16% of total	0.06–0.16 fraction of total
*Lactate dehydrogenase, CSF	10% of serum value	0.10 fraction of serum value
Magnesium		
Serum	1.3–2.1 mEq/L	0.65–1.07 mmol/L
	1.6–2.6 mg/dL	16 26 mg/L
Urine	6.0–10.0 mEq/24 h	3.0–5.0 mmol/24 h
Methotrexate, serum or plasma (Hep or EDTA)		
Therapeutic	Variable	Variable
Toxic		
1–2 wk after low dose therapy	≥0.02 mmol/L	≥0.02 mmol/L
post-IV infusion 24 h	≥5 μmol/L	≥5 μmol/L
48 h	≥0.5 μmol/L	≥0.5 μmol/L
72 h	≥0.05 μmol/L	≥0.05 μmol/L
Partial thromboplastin time activated (APTT)	<35 sec	<35 sec
Phenosulfonphthalein excretion (PSP), urine	28–51% in 15 min	0.28–0.51 in 15 min
	13–24% in 30 min	0.13–0.24 in 30 min
	9–17% in 60 min	0.09–0.17 in 60 min
	3–10% in 2 h	0.03–0.10 in 2 h
	(After injection of 1 mL PSP intravenously)	(After injection of 1 mL PSP intravenously)
*Phosphatase, alkaline, total, serum	38–126 U/L (37°C)	0.65–2.14 μkat/L
*Protein, serum		
Total	6.4–8.3 g/dL	64–83 g/L
Albumin	3.9–5.1 g/dL	39–51 g/L
Globulin		
α_1	0.2–0.4 g/dL	2–4 g/L
α_2	0.4–0.8 g/dL	4–8 g/L
β	0.5–1.0 g/dL	5–10 g/L
γ	0.6–1.3 g/dL	6–13 g/L
Urine		
Qualitative	Negative	Negative
Quantitative	50–80 mg/24 h (at rest)	50–80 mg/24 h (at rest)
CSF, total	8–32 mg/dL	80–320 mg/dL
*Prothrombin time (PT)	12–14 sec	12–14 sec
Sedimentation rate		
Wintrobe		
Male	0–10 mm in 1 h	0–10 mm/h
Female	0–20 mm in 1 h	0–20 mm/h

continued

Test	Conventional Units	SI Units
Westergren		
Male (<50 yr)	0–15 mm in 1 h	0–15 mm/h
Female (<50 yr)	0–20 mm in 1 h	0–20 mm/h
Theophylline, serum or plasma		
(Hep or EDTA)		
Therapeutic		
Bronchodilator	8–20 μg/mL	44–111 μmol/L
Prem. apnea	6–13 mg/mL	33–72 μmol/L
Toxic	>20 μg/mL	>110 μmol/L
Transferrin, serum		
Newborn	130–275 mg/dL	1.30–2.75 g/L
Adult	212–360 mg/dL	2.12–3.60 g/L
>60 yr	190–375 mg/dL	1.9–3.75 g/L
Urea nitrogen, serum	6–20 mg/dL	2.1–7.1 mmol Urea/L
Urea nitrogen/creatinine ratio, serum	12:1 to 20:1	48–80 urea/creatinine mole ratio
*Uric acid		
Serum, enzymatic		
Male	4.5–8.0 mg/dL	0.27–0.47 mmol/L
Female	2.5–6.2 mg/dL	0.15–0.37 mmol/L
Child	2.0–5.5 mg/dL	0.12–0.32 mmol/L
Urine	250–750 mg/24 h (with normal diet)	1.48–4.43 mmol/24 h (with normal diet)

*Test values are method dependent.

†Test values are race dependent.

‡Actual therapeutic range should be adjusted for individual patient.

§"Fatty acids" include a mixture of different aliphatic acids of varying molecular weight; a mean molecular weight of 284 daltons has been assumed.

Common Allergens

Dander (epithelia)
cat
cattle
chicken feather
cockatiel feather
cow
deer
dog
duck feather
ferret
French poodle
gerbil
goat
goose feather
guinea pig
hamster
horse
mixed feathers
mohair
monkey
moth
mouse
rabbit
rat
sheep
silk
swine
turkey feather

Environmental
acacia
Acarus
aerosol sprays
automobile exhaust
barn dust
Bermuda smut
cat
cigarette smoke
cotton linters
cottonseed

Dermatophagoides
dog
elevator grain dust mite
flaxseed
grain dust
house dust
house dust mite F
   (Dermatophagoides farinae)
house dust mite P
   (Dermatophagoides pteronyssinus)
jute
kapok
karaya
mite
newsprint
nylon
orris root
parakeet feather
parrot feather
pigeon feather
perfume
pyrethrum
silk
soybean grain dust mite
tobacco
tragacanth
Tyrophagus
wheat grain dust mite
wool

Foods
almond
apple
apricot
arrowroot
artichoke
asparagus
banana
barley
bass

beef
beet
blackberry
black mulberry
black pepper
Brazil nut
broccoli
Brussel sprouts
buckwheat
cabbage
cantaloupe
carrot
cashew
cauliflower
celery
cheese
cherry
chicken
chive
chocolate
cinnamon
clam
cocoa
coconut
codfish
coffee
corn
cornmeal
cottonseed
cow milk
crab
cucumber
currant
date
duck
eggplant
egg white
egg yolk
garlic
gelatin
ginger
goat milk
gooseberry

grape
grapefruit
green bean
green pepper
hazelnut
kale
Karaya gum
kidney bean
lamb
leek
lemon
lettuce
lentil
licorice
lima bean
lobster
malt
monosodium glutamate
mustard
navy bean
oat
onion
orange
parsley
parsnip
pea
peach
peanut
pear
perch
pineapple
pistachio
plum
pork
potato
prune
pumpkin
radish
raisin
rhubarb
rice
rye meal
salmon

sardine
sesame seed
shrimp
sole
soybean meal
spinach
squash
strawberry
string bean
sweet potato
Swiss chard
Swiss cheese
tea
tomato
tuna fish
turkey
turnip
vanilla
walnut
watermelon
whole wheat
yeast

Grasses

alfalfa
annual bluegrass
Bahia
Bermuda
bromegrass
Canada bluegrass
canary
common reed
crab grass
cultivated barley smut
cultivated corn smut
cultivated oat smut
cultivated rye smut
cultivated wheat smut
Cynodon dactylon
Dactylis glomerata
grama
Johnson

June
Kentucky bluegrass
meadow fescue
meadow foxtail
oat
orchard
perennial rye
Phleum pratense
Poa pratensis
redtop A
reed canary
rye
salt
sorghum grass
sweet vernal
timothy
velvet
wild rye
Zoysia

Insects

American cockroach
bee venom
black ant
black fly
blood worm
bumblebee
cockroach
cricket
deer fly
fire ant
flea
German cockroach
honeybee
horsefly
housefly
Hymenopterous vespid
louse
mayfly
mosquito
moth
nimitti midge

paper wasp
red ant
sweat bee
wasp
white-faced hornet
yellow hornet
yellow jacket

Molds and Fungi

Alternaria
Aspergillus
Aureobasidium
Botryomyces
Candida
Cephalosporium
Chaetomium
Chrysosporium
Cladosporium
Curvularia
Dematiaceae mix
Drechslera
Epicoccum
Epidermophyton
Fusarium
Gliocladium
Helminthosporium
Hormodendrum
Micropolyspora
Microsporum
Monilia
Mucor
Neurospora
Nigrospora
Paecilomyces
Penicillium
Phoma
Phycomycetes
Phytophthora infestans
Pullularia
Rhizopus
Rhodotorula
Saccharomyces

Spondylocladium
Sporobolomyces
Sporotrichum
Stemphylium
Torulopsis
Trichoderma
Trichophyton
Verticillium
Zygomycetes

Preservatives

formaldehyde
quaternium-15
hydantoin/EDTA
Kathon-CG

Occupational

amprolium hydrochloride
anthroquinone
azoquinone
benzene
carbamate
chicken feathers
chromate
diisocyanate
Effersyl
epoxy resin
ethylenediamine
formaldehyde
gelatin
green coffee bean
hexahydrophthalic anhydride
himic anhydride
Ispaghula (laxative)
latex
mercaptobenzothiazole
Metamucil
MSP (mouse serum protein)
MUP (mouse urine protein)
nickel salts
persulfate salts
phthalic anhydride
pigeon droppings

piperazine hydrochloride
platinum salts
polydivinyl
polyvinyl difluoride
PSP (pigeon serum protein)
RSP (rat serum protein)
RUP (rat urine protein)
Sof-Cil
Syllamalt
tetrachlorophthalic anhydride
thiuram
toluene
trichloroethylene
triethylene tetramine
tryptophan
vinyl chloride
xylene

Trees and Shrubs
acacia
alder
Alnus glutinosa
arbor vitae
American elm
Arizona ash
Arizona cypress
Arizona/Fremont cottonwood
aspen
Australian pine
bald cypress
bayberry
beech
Betula verrucosa
birch
black locust
black walnut
box elder maple
Brazilian rubber
California peppertree
Carpinus betulus
Chinese elm
Corylus avellana
cottonwood

Cryptomeria japonica
Cupressaceae
cypress
elm
eucalyptus
Douglas fir
fall elm
Gambel oak
green ash
groundsel
hackberry
hazelnut
hickory
Italian cypress
Japanese cedar
jasmine
juniper mix
lilac
Liquidambar
live oak
loblolly pine
lodgepole pine
Lombardy poplar
Melaleuca
maple
marsh elder
mesquite
Monterey cypress
mountain cedar
mulberry
oak
Olea europa
olive
orange blossom
Oregon ash
palm
paper mulberry
pecan
pepper
poison oak
poison sumac
ponderosa pine
poplar

privet
queen palm
red alder
red birch
red cedar
red maple
red mulberry
redwood
river birch
rough marsh elder
Russian olive
Russian thistle
saltbush
salt cedar
saltwort
shagbark hickory
slash pine
slippery elm
spruce
sugar maple
sweetgum
sycamore
walnut
wax myrtle
weeping fig
weeping willow
Western juniper
Western red cedar
white ash
white mulberry
white oak
white pine
white poplar
willow

Weeds

Ambrosia trifida
Ambrosia artemisiifolia
bitter dock
burrobrush
burweed
careless
canyon ragweed

castor bean
Chenopodium
coast sage
cocklebur
dandelion
desert ragweed
dog fennel
elder
English plantain
false ragweed
firebush
fireweed
giant ragweed
goldenrod
greasewood
green amaranth
hops
iodine bush
kochia
lamb's quarter
mugwort
mustard
nettle
oxeye daisy
pigweed
poverty weed
rabbit bush
ragweed
ragwort
redroot pigweed
rough marsh elder
Russian thistle
sagebrush
Salsola pestifer
scale
Seneca snakeroot
sheep sorrel
short ragweed
slender ragweed
smotherweed
spiney pigweed
sugar beet
tall dock

tumbleweed
Ustilago
Western ragweed
western water hemp
white burrobrush

wild tobacco
wormwood
yellow dock
yellow mustard

Appendix 4
Sample Reports

ARTHROSCOPIC PARTIAL MEDIAL MENISCECTOMY AND CHONDROPLASTY

TITLE OF OPERATION 1. Arthroscopy.
2. Arthroscopic partial medial meniscectomy.
3. Arthroscopic chondroplasty, degenerative medial femoral condyle.

PREOPERATIVE DIAGNOSIS: Torn medial meniscus, left knee.

POSTOPERATIVE DIAGNOSIS: Torn medial meniscus and degenerative arthritis, left knee.

PROCEDURE IN DETAIL: The patient was taken to the operating room, and after adequate anesthesia was attained, the left lower extremity was prepped with Betadine gel and draped in a sterile fashion. The knee was inflated with Ringer lactate, and the arthroscope was introduced in the anterolateral portal. The patellofemoral joint was identified. There was mild degenerative change in the posterior aspect of the patella. The medial joint was then visualized. There was prominent degenerative change noted on much of the medial femoral condyle, including the majority of the weightbearing surface of the femoral condyle. There was also noted to be a complex tear of the posterior horn of the medial meniscus.

An anteromedial portal was made. The shaver with the incisor blade was introduced and used to debride the undersurface and posterior horn of the medial meniscus, removing the complex tear. A nice, smooth superior and peripheral rim of the meniscus remained after debridement of the undersurface of the meniscus. It was transitioned back to the more normal midportion of the meniscus. The Dyonics shaver with the turbo-whisker blade was then introduced and used to smooth the inner aspect of the meniscus. Following this, nonaggressive shaving was performed on the femoral condyle with the turbo-whisker blade. This was used to shave any irregularities of the articular cartilage of the femoral condyle. There were grade 2 and 3 changes, which were shaved.

The rest of the joint was visualized, and the anterior cruciate appeared intact. The lateral joint was visualized. The lateral meniscus appeared intact throughout its entirety without any signs of a tear. It was probed with a probe, without signs of a tear. The rest of the joint appeared in general good condition.

The knee was copiously irrigated. The cannula and arthroscope were removed. Marcaine was injected, and the puncture holes were sutured with 4–0 nylon. A dry, sterile bulky dressing was applied.

The patient tolerated the procedure well and was sent to the recovery room in good condition.

EROSIVE POLYARTICULAR RHEUMATOID ARTHRITIS FOLLOWUP NOTE

HISTORY OF PRESENT ILLNESS: The patient returned to the Rheumatology Clinic today for a routine followup visit. The patient has erosive polyarticular rheumatoid arthritis but now appears under excellent control. His current antiarthritics consist of methotrexate 10 mg once weekly, Plaquenil 400 mg daily, and prednisone 10 mg daily. He is not using a nonsteroidal antiinflammatory drug because of concerns about the Coumadin he is taking for a cardiac arrhythmia. All his medications are well tolerated, taken without side effect or toxicity, and all methotrexate-related blood monitoring is normal.

The patient appears to have had very good relief of joint pain and early morning stiffness, and only has residual problems in two areas, his left knee and right shoulder. He notes pain in the shoulder when he rolls over onto it at night and then a little pain through the day that is not as much of a problem. He also notes significant left knee pain, much exacerbated by walking. I understand that the patient has longstanding degenerative arthritis involving the left knee, and this probably accounts for his knee pain to a much greater extent than does any coincidental rheumatoid arthritis in that joint.

PERTINENT PHYSICAL FINDINGS: On musculoskeletal examination, the small joints of the hands, the wrists, the elbows, the cervical spine, the lumbosacral spine, the hips, the ankles, and the feet were unremarkable. There was inability to abduct the right shoulder beyond 45 degrees, and in addition, both internal and external rotation was uncomfortable and much limited. The left shoulder was normal. On examination of the knees, the left was swollen. There did appear to be free synovial fluid within the joint; however, there was no joint margin tenderness. The knee moved fully and freely, and was stable, although there was significant coarse and fine crepitus through the full range of movement. The right knee was unaffected.

ASSESSMENT/PLAN: After discussion with the patient, and after appropriate local antisepsis and anesthesia, I injected 80 mg of Kenalog into the left knee; I was unable to withdraw any synovial fluid preceding this injection. I hope this has the desired effect in settling down his knee pain. If not, it is possible that he may be a candidate for an arthroscopy and arthroscopic surgery, but that would be preceded by some more focused investigations of his knee anatomy. An MRI scan would probably be the most productive approach. Again, while it is possible he has some significant rheumatoid arthritis activity in the knee, I think it is much more likely that the knee pain is as a result of longstanding degenerative arthritis.

On this occasion, I did not offer to inject the patient's right shoulder, but would certainly be prepared to do this at some time in the future, and I invited him to contact me by telephone if he wished this to be performed. I asked the patient to return for the next visit in four months' time, or to contact me earlier by telephone if he has any intercurrent concerns.

EXCISION OF BASAL CELL CARCINOMA OF THE NOSE

TITLE OF OPERATION
1. Excision of lesion, right side of bony nasal pyramid.
2. Frozen section to pathology consultation showing basal cell carcinoma with clear margins.
3. V-Y closure.

PROCEDURE IN DETAIL: With the patient in the supine position and after satisfactory induction of general LMA anesthesia, the patient was prepped with Betadine scrub and draped with sterile towels and drapes. The line of proposed circular excision of the lesion of the right dorsum of the bony nasal pyramid of the nose was outlined with a marking pen. It was infiltrated with local anesthetic solution, and the lesion was excised as outlined. The 12 o'clock border was marked with a marking pen and was submitted for frozen section pathology consultation, showing basal cell carcinoma with margins clear. V-Y flaps were outlined approximately 1.2 cm wide by about 2.5 cm long, one on the left side and one on the right side of the nose. These areas were infiltrated with local anesthetic solution. The flaps were elevated as outlined. Several small bleeders were controlled with electrocautery. The flaps were rotated into the defect, and the wound edges were approximated with interrupted 5–0 black nylon sutures. The patient was dressed with Steri-Strips. He tolerated the procedure very well. Total estimated blood loss was about 5 cc. He was taken to the recovery room in satisfactory condition.

EYELID FULL-THICKNESS RESECTION AND RECONSTRUCTION

TITLE OF OPERATION: Left lower eyelid full-thickness resection and reconstruction.

PREOPERATIVE DIAGNOSIS: Left lower eyelid mass, rule out tumor.

POSTOPERATIVE DIAGNOSIS: Left lower eyelid mass, rule out tumor.

INDICATION FOR OPERATION: The patient has had a left lower lid lesion off and on for one year that has not gone away. Examination revealed an elevated vascular lesion of the left lower lid. There was possible thickening of the tarsus associated with this. It was felt that this could conceivably be a sebaceous carcinoma or some other type of eyelid cancer, and therefore a full-thickness lid resection was appropriate to absolutely exclude sebaceous carcinoma. Other possibilities included a benign chronic inflammatory condition refractory to treatment.

PROCEDURE IN DETAIL: Topical tetracaine was applied to each eye. The face was prepped and draped in the usual manner. A protective contact lens was placed in the left eye. Lidocaine 1% with epinephrine was injected in the central left upper lid, and a 5–0 Mersiline was placed through the skin, orbicularis, and superficial tarsus to retract the upper lid out of the way. A small pentagon was constructed, surrounding the left lower lid lesion. This measured 4 mm in horizontal dimension. Lidocaine 1% with epinephrine was injected, a 15 blade incised the skin, and Westcott scissors removed the pentagon. Cautery was used for hemostasis. The specimen was sent for permanent pathological examination. The lid margin was reconstructed with two 6–0 silk sutures; the tarsus was reconstructed with a 6–0 Vicryl suture. The skin was closed with additional 6–0 silk, and 6–0 silk sutures were tied in order to keep them out of the eye. Polysporin ointment was applied, and ice was applied. The patient tolerated the procedure well and left the operating room in good condition.

LIVER TRANSPLANT AND BROVIAC CATHETER PLACEMENT

TITLE OF OPERATION 1. Liver transplant
2. Broviac catheter placement.

PREOPERATIVE DIAGNOSIS: Biliary atresia.

POSTOPERATIVE DIAGNOSIS: Biliary atresia.

INDICATION FOR OPERATION: This child has biliary atresia. She was evaluated by our multidisciplinary transplant committee, and a liver transplant was recommended. The parents gave informed written consent to proceed.

PROCEDURE IN DETAIL: The patient was brought to the operating room, and general anesthesia was induced. A urinary catheter was subsequently placed in the bladder, and anesthesiology placed monitoring devices and infusion lines. The abdomen, neck, and chest were prepped with Betadine and draped in sterile styles. An incision over the right neck was made and carried down until the external jugular vein was identified. It was divided proximally, and then a 7-French double-lumen Broviac catheter was placed in the subcutaneous tunnel exiting in the anterior chest and guided down through the external jugular vein and into the central venous system. Fluoroscopy revealed the catheter to be in satisfactory position. The wound was closed with two layers of absorbable suture after securing the catheter to the vein with a silk suture. The catheter was affixed to the skin at the exit site with nylon suture.

The bilateral subcostal incision was made at the site of the portoenterostomy. When the peritoneal cavity was entered, it was apparent there was a dense amount of adhesions throughout the abdomen. These were painstakingly dissected free, exposing the liver. During the course of the dissection, a colotomy occurred at the splenic flexure on the transverse colon. This was closed with a single layer of silk suture. Attention was turned to the portal, which was skeletonized. The previous Roux-en-Y limb was identified and dissected free. It was divided as close as possible to the liver. The hepatic artery was identified, and we divided the right and left hepatic arteries individually. There were numerous large lymph nodes present, which were carefully dissected free and resected. The lymphatics were ligated with silk sutures. The portal limb was identified and was noted to be extremely diminutive. This had been expected based on the MRA. It was carefully dissected free up to the bifurcation and divided. It was noted that there was very little flow in the portal vein.

The attachments of the liver to retroperitoneum were then divided medially and laterally. It was apparent that the caudate lobe encircled the vena cava, and it was not possible to remove the liver with the cava in situ. Therefore, clamps were placed on the cava above and below the liver, and the liver was resected. It was apparent that the portal vein would not be satisfactory for portal inflow, but the inferior vena cava appeared satisfactory in position and size. Therefore, the decision was made to use the vena cava as portal inflow.

The new liver was then sutured into place using a 5–0 Prolene running suture for the suprahepatic anastomosis and a 7–0 Prolene suture for the hepatic artery anastomosis, which was from an aortic patch of the donor to a branch going to the right and left hepatic arteries on the recipient. The portal vein of the donor was then anastomosed to the inferior vena cava of the recipient using running 6–0 sutures. The clamps were released, and the liver flushed nicely. Prior to releasing the clamps, the infrahepatic cava of the donor was oversewn with 4–0 Prolene suture. The liver achieved satisfactory color and texture and began to make bile. There was a strong pulse palpable in the hepatic artery, and the portal vein anastomosis appeared satisfactory. The previous Roux-en-Y limb was then used to fashion a hepaticojejunostomy using interrupted 5–0 PDS sutures. This was fashioned over a 5-French biliary stent that had been placed on the back table through the donor cystic duct and guided up the gallbladder fossa, where the peritoneum had been oversewn. Some silk sutures were used to suture the Roux-en-Y limb up to the porta and some connective tissue to relieve any tension that might occur at a later time. There was no tension on the anastomosis at this time. It was checked by infusion of the biliary catheter with saline, and there was no evidence of a leakage. The catheter was then brought out the right flank and secured with nylon suture to the skin.

The abdomen was irrigated with warm saline and, after a final check for hemostasis, was closed with running 2–0 Prolene suture in the fascia and running subcuticular stitch in the skin. The patient tolerated the procedure well.

OPEN DONOR NEPHRECTOMY

TITLE OF OPERATION: Open left donor nephrectomy.

PREOPERATIVE DIAGNOSIS: The patient is acting as a living, related kidney donor to her brother.

POSTOPERATIVE DIAGNOSIS: The patient is acting as a living, related kidney donor to her brother.

INDICATION FOR OPERATION: The patient has volunteered to be a living, related kidney donor to her brother, who suffers from end-stage renal disease. The patient was referred for evaluation as a prospective live kidney donor, and she was deemed to be a suitable candidate.

PROCEDURE IN DETAIL: After informed consent was obtained from the patient, she was brought to the operating room and placed supine on the operative table. After successful induction of general endotracheal anesthesia, a Foley catheter as well as an IV line were placed. An orogastric tube was also placed. The patient was then placed in the left lateral decubitus position, at which time her entire left side was placed perpendicular to the operating table. A kidney rest was then applied to an area superior to the iliac crest to make the skin by the left-sided kidney tense. Her left shoulder was also placed over on top of her, and so she was essentially perpendicular to the operating table. After we were content with how she was placed on the operating table, we next prepped in the usual sterile fashion for a donor nephrectomy. We identified the twelfth rib, and approximately one fingerbreadth below the twelfth rib an incision was made for an approximate length of about 18 cm. The incision ended close to the lateral border of the rectus muscle. Electrocautery was then used to cut the skin and the subcutaneous fat. The latissimus dorsi, as well as the three layers of the abdominal wall, was then excised in its entirety. This was done with cautery. Once this was done, we were able to gently palpate the kidney, which was superior and lateral, and using careful blunt as well as cautery dissection, we were able to find the peritoneum. We were able to reflect this medially while keeping the kidney in the retroperitoneal space.

Once this was done, a Bookwalter retractor was placed into the operative field for retraction both cephalad and caudad, and laterally and medially. Using careful dissection, we were able to open up Gerota fascia, the plane on top of the kidney. This was extended with electrocautery superiorly, and we were able to use the cautery to excise all of the attachments this had in adventitia to the superior pole of the kidney.

We next identified the adrenal gland, which was noted in its entirety. We found the adrenal vein. This was divided between silk sutures. We were able to essentially circumferentially dissect out the entire kidney, first at the superior pole, then extending medially and inferiorly, and then finally the inferior pole. We next found a large ovarian vein, and this was divided between silk ties. In addition, a posterior-lying lumbar vein was identified and also divided between silk sutures. We reflected the kidney, observing its inferior side, and we found the ureter. We dissected this on top of the psoas, and we left a large amount of adventitious tissue around the entire circumference of the ureter.

Once the veins were identified, we were able to manipulate the kidney and find both renal arteries. The superior pole, which was the main renal artery, had a diameter of approximately 4 to 5 mm. We dissected this with some difficulty to its entrance into the aorta. The lower pole artery, which was approximately 3 mm, was also found and dissected along its entire length to the aorta. The dissection was a little bit difficult based upon the size of the kidney, which was large, and the fact that the patient was relatively big herself and the kidney lay relatively deep. We then carefully inspected the hilum of the kidney, and it was noted to be intact.

Once this major dissection was completed, we placed a right-angle clamp quite distally on the ureter. We did not trace it on top of the iliac, and we divided it and we tied off the distal end with a 3–0 silk tie. A very minimal amount of urine was noted to emanate from the ureter. Once this was done, we had vessel loops placed around all the major vessels. We clamped off the inferior artery with a right-angle clamp right on top of the aorta; the vessel was cut. We placed a right-angle clamp on top of the main artery, which was the more superior one; this was cut. Finally, we placed a Satinsky clamp on the renal vein, and we cut on top of this. Once this was done, the kidney was removed.

On the back table, both renal arteries, the major one and the lower pole one, were irrigated with approximately 200 to 300 cc of Urecholine. We placed 200 cc through the main renal artery and approximately 100 cc through the inferior artery. The kidney was noted to blanch well, and there was good emanation of the effluent through the renal vein. The kidney was then packaged in three sterile bags and taken to the operating room for implantation.

We next turned our attention back to the donor. We tied off both renal arteries with double suture of 2–0 silk. Our attention was then directed towards the cut renal vein. The renal vein orifice was oversewn using a 5–0 Prolene suture, which was sutured in a double-row fashion. When we removed the Satinsky, there was excellent hemostasis.

The operative field was then flooded with antibiotic saline, and hemostasis was really quite excellent. We next turned our attention to closing the wound. The wound was closed in two running layers of 1–0 Novofil. The transversalis muscle was closed first with a buried stitch of running Novofil, and once this was closed the external and internal oblique muscles were closed in a single layer of running Novofil. The fascia was noted to coapt together very well. Prior to closing the fascia, we brought down the kidney rest and repositioned the table. Finally, the skin was closed using a subcuticular stitch of 4–0 Monocryl. The skin was noted to coapt together very well. Once this was done, the skin was washed off of all preparatory Betadine, and Steri-Strips were placed on top of the wound. Finally, sterile gauze was placed on top of this.

OSTEOARTHRITIS CONSULTATION NOTE

HISTORY OF PRESENT ILLNESS: The patient has a history of chronic pain in the lumbosacral spine, which has progressively gotten worse over the past two years. She was scheduled to have an MRI but never completed it because of claustrophobia. She also has pain in the hands and both shoulders, with significant morning stiffness. She has difficulty getting up from a sitting position. She reports pain in the knee with swelling of the left knee. She has moderate swelling of both ankles, which may be related more to her history of hypertension. She has just recently had an angiogram and is currently on Coumadin.

PERTINENT PHYSICAL FINDINGS: Hands have no evidence of synovitis. There are Heberden and Bouchard nodes, with changes of osteoarthritis. Wrist movement is normally maintained. There is tenderness of both shoulders with decreased range of mobility. There is also gluteal tenderness. Hip movement is decreased. There is bilateral crepitus of the knees with decreased range of mobility. The ankles have no swelling. The feet are normal.

ASSESSMENT: Osteoarthritis of the knees.

PLAN: We will start Vioxx at 12.5 mg q.d., and if no response, can be increased to 12.5 mg b.i.d. We will check for inflammation with a sedimentation rate, C-reactive proteins, rheumatoid factor, ANA and uric acid levels. Physical therapy was recommended. Local injections are an option to consider in the future.

PSORIATIC ARTHRITIS FOLLOWUP NOTE

HISTORY OF PRESENT ILLNESS: I saw the patient for the first time in over 6 months. He has gotten along reasonably well with Celebrex taken to subdue arthritic pains. His psoriasis has been variably active, helped along some by topical agents you have recently prescribed and found to be useful from personal experience. He describes a gouty attack occurring in his right foot a few weeks back. He called here and was heard by the "rheumatologist on call," who tried a Medrol Dosepak to good effect.

Lately, his knees have been sore, particularly the right, which feels stiff as well.

He recently went to you for a head-to-toe physical evaluation and brought with him papers from that visit. Laboratory work included slightly raised total cholesterol of 228 with an HDL of 38, along with a uric acid of 11.4.

He recalls receiving allopurinol before and having a "reaction," but upon closer questioning, this turned out to have been exacerbation of an existing gout attack by prescribed full-strength allopurinol. This is not unexpected and does not indicate any particular "sensitivity" to the drug.

PERTINENT PHYSICAL FINDINGS: The patient has scattered fading of plaques of psoriasis about his hands, elbows, and legs. There is restriction of motion about his hand joints. There is tenderness at the base of the thumb on the right, the hand he says he has been working with quite extensively lately. The elbows are okay except for the psoriatic changes. His right knee has a tense effusion with ulcers about the popliteal fossa. The left knee is normal by comparison. The toes are okay today.

I tapped his right knee, obtaining about 45 cc of type 2 fluid. In this, I instilled triamcinolone 40 mg and some associated lidocaine to make up 10 cc.

ASSESSMENT/PLAN: He wonders about having a different medication than Celebrex. I have provided him with some samples of Vioxx. He can take 25 mg to 50 mg a day. I also started him on a low dose of allopurinol at 50 mg a day to be increased every two weeks until he is on a full dose of 300 mg a day.

I think he is generally coping well with his psoriatic arthritis. I think the gout is probably contributing from time to time preemptively to his migratory arthralgias. He has been hyperuricemic for a while, but I think it is now time to begin to bring it down. I will see him back in three to four months or earlier, if needed.

RHEUMATOID ARTHRITIS CONSULTATION NOTE

HISTORY OF PRESENT ILLNESS: For several years, the patient had pain in the small joints of the hands that was localized to one or two fingers only and was of short duration without any evidence of inflammation. These episodes were infrequent. In November 1998, however, the patient had for the first time a very well organized onset of joint pain and inflammation located in the PIP joints, wrists, and MCP joints. The pain was associated with morning stiffness of up to two hours. Regarding major joints, she has had only mild pain in the left shoulder. At some point in her disease, the patient apparently had involvement of tendons with pain in the arms and both hands. When the inflammation has been at the highest point, the patient was unable to make a fist, and it was difficult for her to perform activities of daily life and take care of herself. However, the patient could massage herself, give herself baths with warm water, and remain active and working. On two occasions, the patient received steroids in systemic form with very significant improvement of her symptoms. Since September 1998, the patient has been taking hydroxychloroquine 400 mg a day; however, her synovitis has persisted. Currently, the patient has morning stiffness of about one hour as well as pain and inflammation in the MCP and PIP joints.

The patient denies fever, hair loss, mouth ulcers, adenopathy, shortness of breath, chest pain, abdominal pain, or skin rashes. Before her illness, the patient used to exercise regularly, riding a bike.

PERTINENT PHYSICAL FINDINGS: Musculoskeletal examination shows normal range of motion in all joints with evident synovitis localized to the second, third, and fourth PIP joints and over the styloid apophysis in the right hand. There is a subluxation of both first CMC joints bilaterally and significant tenderness to palpation in the right MCP joints. The left shoulder is minimally tender on mobilization.

PERTINENT LABORATORY FINDINGS: CBC with WBC 15.3, hemoglobin 12.3 and platelets 362,000. LFTs normal. TSH 0.33. Rheumatoid factor negative and ANA negative. X-rays of the hands in June 1999 show only a very mild osteopenia in the carpus; feet from April 1999 are normal. There are no erosions at any level.

ASSESSMENT/PLAN: We agree with your impression that this patient has a seronegative rheumatoid arthritis. Despite the use of hydroxychloroquine for five months, the patient is still showing signs of active inflammation. We think that the patient may benefit with the addition of a second drug, and we are recommending the initiation of methotrexate. The benefits and risks of this medication were explained to the patient, who accepted the treatment. On the other hand, given the acute inflammation, we are also recommending the initiation of prednisone 5 mg a day. We expect that after probably one or two months the patient may be able to discontinue prednisone. Regarding her treatment, there is duplication on cyclooxygenase-2 inhibitors, and we suggested to the patient to continue with only one of them. The patient will discontinue Vioxx. The patient will obtain an appointment with her ophthalmologist to initiate her regular checking for hydroxychloroquine. Finally, given the fact that the patient has early disease and is in to see us regarding treatment and is a very active person, we think that she may have a good prognosis. We are scheduling an appointment in two months.

RHEUMATOID ARTHRITIS FOLLOWUP NOTE

HISTORY OF PRESENT ILLNESS: The patient is a 38-year-old woman who has an illness of about three to four years, characterized by myalgias, arthralgias, and arthritis located in the MCP joints, PIP joints, wrists, and ankles. In addition, the patient has had intermittent Raynaud, mild hair loss, and a transient rash located on the face and the neck. Other problems are sleep abnormalities and problems with equilibrium that are under evaluation by neurology. In our initial evaluation, we considered that the patient may have an undifferentiated connective tissue disease, and the possibilities were rheumatoid arthritis, lupus, or scleroderma. A trial of prednisone 15 mg was initiated. Two days after the patient started taking prednisone, she felt an impressive improvement that she describes as a miracle. The chronic sensation of fatigue was almost eliminated, and the myalgias are very mild, as well as the arthritis. The patient has not had episodes of arthritis since. The patient has been unusually active at work with energy and is able to do gardening. There is no significant change in morning stiffness, and this is still about 30 minutes in duration.

PERTINENT PHYSICAL FINDINGS: The general examination is benign. There is no hair loss. There is very mild erythema on the neck with fine telangiectasis that was mentioned before. There are no other skin lesions, and there are no mucosal lesions either. Musculoskeletal examination shows a motor power of 5/5 in all four extremities, range of motion is normal in all joints, and there is no evidence of synovitis at any level.

PERTINENT LABORATORY FINDINGS: CBC showed a WBC of 10,000, hemoglobin 12.9, and hematocrit 37.3. Sodium was 139, potassium 3.3, chloride 104, CO2 24, BUN 21, creatinine 0.9, and glucose 87. Liver function tests are normal. Sedimentation rate is 28, and CRP is 0.9; both of them are only slightly elevated. Normal C3 at 143, normal C4 at 25. CK 70 and aldolase 3, both normal, and immunoelectrophoresis is normal. All of her antibodies are negative, including rheumatoid arthritis. These antibodies are Scl-70, SM, RNP, RO, LA, GF-1, Eastern, VNA, ANCA, and antiphospholipid IgG and IgM.

X-rays of hands show only mild osteopenia around the MCP and PIP joints. There are no erosions.

ASSESSMENT/PLAN: The patient is a 38-year-old woman with an undifferentiated inflammatory polyarthritis. Considering the family history of a father and a brother with rheumatoid arthritis, it is possible that the patient is at the stage of an early rheumatoid arthritis, which is seronegative. Given the presence of Raynaud and fine telangiectasis, we have to keep in mind the possibility of this illness evolving to scleroderma. We do not have serologic evidence of lupus, and there is no biochemical evidence of myositis. Our plan at the moment will be to initiate high-dose chloroquine at 400 mg q.d., evaluation by an ophthalmologist, and a slow reduction of prednisone to 10 mg in one month and then 1 mg per week. We are scheduling an appointment in two months and requesting a CBC and sedimentation rate for the next visit.

TOTAL HIP ARTHROPLASTY WITH SALZER APR II PROSTHESIS

TITLE OF OPERATION: Left total hip arthroplasty with Salzer APR II prosthesis.

PREOPERATIVE DIAGNOSIS: Osteoarthritis, left hip.

POSTOPERATIVE DIAGNOSIS: Osteoarthritis, left hip.

PROCEDURE IN DETAIL: Under epidural anesthesia supplemented by general anesthesia, the patient was placed in the left lateral decubitus position. The left hip was prepped and draped in the usual fashion. A 10-inch incision was made, centering over the greater trochanter. The incision was deepened, and small bleeders were cauterized. The short external rotator was divided close to bone, together with the posterior capsule. The hip was dislocated posteriorly. Severe osteoarthritis was noted.

The femoral neck was cut at the appropriate level and angle. The acetabulum was exposed. Osteophytes were excised. The floor was cleared of soft tissue. The acetabulum was reamed progressively to 53 mm in diameter. This was under-reamed by 2 mm. A trial with a 54-mm trial acetabular component was done. Fit and alignment were excellent. The trial component was removed. The 55-mm porous-coated acetabular component was press-fit into place. Excellent alignment and fixation were noted. The liner was inserted with the overhang posteriorly and inferiorly. The femoral canal was then prepared by reaming and broaching to 13.5-mm stem size. A trial was made with the neutral neck 32-mm head component. The hip was reduced, and a stable range of movement was noted. An AP view taken showed good position and length.

The hip was re-dislocated, and the trial femoral component was removed. The femoral canal was prepared for cementing by brushing and washing. The canal was plugged with the Universal cement restrictor plug. The canal was lavaged with pulsatile lavage and dried thoroughly. Two bags of cement were mixed in the vacuum mixer, and using the cement syringe, a 13.5-mm nonporous stem with a 14-mm centralizer was cemented in place. On setting of the cement, excellent alignment and fixation were noted. The 4-mm neck, 32-mm head component was tapped onto the femoral stem, and the hip was reduced. A stable range of movement was noted. Hemostasis was checked. The hip was drained with one Hemovac drain.

Closure was done using #1 Vicryl to reattach the short external rotators and the posterior capsule. The fascial layer was closed with #1 Vicryl, the subcutaneous layer with 2–0 and 3–0 Vicryl, and the skin with staples. The incision was dressed with Xeroform gauze, 4 x 4 gauze, and a Cover-Roll dressing.

The patient tolerated the procedure well and left for the recovery room in stable condition.

TOTAL KNEE ARTHROPLASTY AND SYNOVECTOMY

TITLE OF OPERATION: 1. Right total knee arthroplasty with Salzer Natural Knee II prosthesis.
2. Synovectomy, medial release, right knee.

PREOPERATIVE DIAGNOSIS: Severe osteoarthritis, right knee.

POSTOPERATIVE DIAGNOSIS: Severe osteoarthritis, right knee.

PROCEDURE IN DETAIL: Under spinal anesthesia, the patient was placed in the supine position. The right leg was prepped and draped in the usual fashion. The leg was draped with Esmarch, and a tourniquet on the right upper thigh was inflated to 350 mmHg pressure. A 10-inch midline incision was made, centering over the patella. The incision was deepened, and a trivector-sparing incision was made to enter the joint. Osteoarthritis was noted.

A synovectomy was done. Remnants of the menisci and anterior cruciate ligament were excised. Osteophytes were removed. Using the Intermedics instrument, a hole was made in the intercondylar notch of the femur, followed by insertion of the intramedullary rod. The distal femoral alignment guide was aligned, and the cutting block fixed with two pins. The distal femoral cut was made. The femur was sized, and #2-size anchoring holes were made. The #2 femoral cutting block was inserted, and the anterior and posterior femoral cuts were made. The beveled cutting block was inserted, and the beveled cuts were made. The area was irrigated, and the femoral canal packed with Gelfoam and bone graft.

The proximal tibia was then exposed. The alignment guide was aligned, and the cutting block fixed with two pins. The proximal alignment was checked, and the proximal tibial cut was made. The posterior cruciate ligament was taken with the cut. The

A55

tibia took a #2 size. Anchoring holes were made. A trial tibial and trial femoral component with alignment with a 9-mm insert were done. Medial release was done distally for soft tissue balance. Good extension was noted with flexion to 120 degrees with good stability.

The patella was prepared by excising the appropriate thickness of the articular surface. The patella took #1-size anchoring holes, which were made. A trial with the #1, 7-mm trial patellar component was done. Fit was excellent, and patellar tracking was excellent. The trial components were removed. Exposed bones were irrigated and lavaged with pulsatile lavage and dried thoroughly.

Two bags of cement were mixed in the vacuum mixer, and the #2 tibial base was cemented in place followed by insertion of the 9-mm outer congruent insert. A #2 femoral component was cemented as well, and the knee carried to full extension. The 7-mm polyethylene patellar component was cemented as well. On setting of the cement, excellent alignment and fixation were noted. The range of movement was stable from 0 to 120 degrees.

The tourniquet was released. Small bleeders were cauterized. No excessive bleeding was noted at the time of closure. The knee was drained with two Hemovac drains. Closure was done using #1 Vicryl for the fascia and capsular layer, and #2 and #3 Vicryl subcutaneously with staples for the skin. The incision was dressed with Xeroform gauze, followed by 4 x 4's, followed by a soft roll and Ace bandages.

The patient had approximately 800 cc of estimated and anticipated blood loss. She was transfused two units of autologous packed cells. She tolerated the procedure well and was sent to the recovery room in stable condition.

Appendix 5

Common Terms by Procedure

Arthroscopic Partial Medial Meniscectomy and Chondroplasty

anterolateral portal
anteromedial portal
arthroscopy
chondroplasty
Dyonics shaver
incisor blade
medial femoral condyle
medial meniscus
meniscectomy
patellofemoral joint
shaver
turbo-whisker blade

Erosive Polyarticular Rheumatoid Arthritis Followup

coarse crepitus
degenerative arthritis
erosive polyarticular rheumatoid arthritis
fine crepitus
Kenalog
methotrexate
Plaquenil
synovial fluid

Excision of Basal Cell Carcinoma of the Nose

basal cell carcinoma
Betadine scrub
bony nasal pyramid
circular excision
dorsum
electrocautery
frozen section
Steri-Strips
V-Y closure

Eyelid Full-Thickness Resection and Reconstruction

full-thickness resection
hemostasis
lidocaine 1% with epinephrine
Mersiline suture
orbicularis
pentagon
permanent pathological examination
Polysporin ointment
protective contact lens
sebaceous carcinoma
tarsus
topical tetracaine
Westcott scissors

Liver Transplant and Broviac Catheter Placement

biliary atresia
biliary stent
caudate lobe
central venous system
donor cystic duct
double-lumen Broviac catheter
external jugular vein
fluoroscopy
hepatic artery anastomosis
hepaticojejunostomy
inferior vena cava
infrahepatic cava
portal inflow
portal limb
portal vein
portoenterostomy
Roux-en-Y limb
subcutaneous tunnel
suprahepatic anastomosis

Open Donor Nephrectomy

adventitious tissue

antibiotic saline
blunt dissection
Bookwalter retractor
cautery dissection
double-row suturing
electrocautery
end-stage renal disease
external oblique muscle
Foley catheter
Gerota fascia
hemostasis
hilum
iliac crest
inferior pole
internal oblique muscle
kidney rest
lateral decubitus position
latissimus dorsi
Novofil
open donor nephrectomy
orogastric tube
psoas
related kidney donor
renal vein orifice
retroperitoneal space
Satinsky clamp
Steri-Strips
subcutaneous fat
superior pole
transversalis muscle
Urecholine

Osteoarthritis Consultation

ANA test
Bouchard nodes
C-reactive protein
crepitus
Heberden nodes
inflammation
osteoarthritis
rheumatoid factor
sedimentation rate
synovitis

uric acid level
Vioxx

Psoriatic Arthritis Followup

allopurinol
Celebrex
gouty attack
hyperuricemic
migratory arthralgia
plaques of psoriasis
psoriasis
psoriatic arthritis
psoriatic change
tense effusion
triamcinolone
uric acid level
Vioxx

Rheumatoid Arthritis Consultation

ANA test
CMC joint
cyclo-oxygenase-2 inhibitor
erosions
hydroxychloroquine
inflammation
joint pain
MCP joint
methotrexate
osteopenia
PIP joint
prednisone
rheumatoid factor
seronegative rheumatoid arthritis
styloid apophysis
subluxation
synovitis

Rheumatoid Arthritis Followup

ANCA antibody
antiphospholipid IgG antibody
arthralgia
arthritis

chloroquine
C-reactive protein
C3
C4
Eastern antibody
erosion
fine telangiectasis
GF-1 antibody
IgM antibody
immunoelectrophoresis
LA antibody
lupus
MCP joint
myalgia
myositis
osteopenia
PIP joint
prednisone
Raynaud phenomenon
rheumatoid arthritis
RNP antibody
RO antibody
Scl-70 antibody
scleroderma
sedimentation rate
SM antibody
synovitis
transient rash
undifferentiated connective tissue
    disease
undifferentiated inflammatory
    polyarthritis
VNA antibody

Total Hip Arthroplasty with Salzer APR II Prosthesis

acetabulum
broaching
cement syringe
centralizer
Cover-Roll dressing
epidural anesthesia
femoral canal

femoral neck
femoral stem
general anesthesia
greater trochanter
head component
Hemovac drain
liner
nonporous stem
osteoarthritis
osteophyte
overhang
porous-coated acetabular component
posterior capsule
press-fit
pulsatile lavage
reaming
re-dislocated
Salzer APR II prosthesis
short external rotator
total hip arthroplasty
trial component
universal cement restrictor plug
vacuum mixer
Xeroform gauze

Total Knee Arthroplasty and Synovectomy

anchoring hole
anterior cruciate ligament
articular surface
beveled cutting block
bone graft
distal femoral alignment guide
Esmarch
femoral cutting block
Gelfoam
Hemovac drains
intercondylar notch
Intermedics instrument
intramedullary rod
medial release
meniscus
osteoarthritis

osteophyte
outer congruent insert
patellar tracking
polyethylene patellar component
posterior cruciate ligament
pulsatile lavage
Salzer Natural Knee II prosthesis
spinal anesthesia
synovectomy

tibial base
total knee arthroplasty
tourniquet
trial femoral component
trial patellar component
trial tibial component
trivector-sparing incision
vacuum mixer
Xeroform gauze

Drugs by Indication

ACNE
Acne Products
  Acetoxyl (Can)
  Acnomel BP 5 (Can)
  adapalene
  Advanced Formula Oxy® Sensitive
    Gel [OTC]
  Akne-Mycin® Topical
  Ambi 10® [OTC]
  A/T/S® Topical
  Ben-Aqua® [OTC]
  Benoxyl®
  Benzac AC® Gel
  Benzac AC® Wash
  Benzac W® Gel
  Benzac W® Wash
  5-Benzagel®
  10-Benzagel®
  Benzagel (Can)
  Benzamycin®
  Benzashave® Cream
  benzoyl peroxide
  benzoyl peroxide and hydrocortisone
  BlemErase® Lotion [OTC]
  Brevoxyl® Gel
  Clearasil® B.P. Plus (Can)
  Clear By Design® Gel [OTC]
  Clearsil® Maximum Strength [OTC]
  Cleocin HCl® Oral
  Cleocin Pediatric® Oral
  Cleocin Phosphate® Injection
  Cleocin T® Topical
  Cleocin® Vaginal
  Clinda-Derm® Topical
  clindamycin
  Dalacin® C (Can)
  Dalacin T (Can)
  Dalacin Vaginal (Can)
  Del Aqua-5® Gel
  Del Aqua-10® Gel

Del-Mycin® Topical
Dermacne (Can)
Dermoxyl (Can)
Desquam-E™ Gel
Desquam-X® Gel
Desquam-X® Wash
Differin®
Dryox® Gel [OTC]
Dryox® Wash [OTC]
Emgel™ Topical
Eryderm® Topical
Erygel® Topical
Erymax® Topical
erythromycin and benzoyl peroxide
erythromycin (ophthalmic/topical)
E-Solve-2® Topical
ETS-2%® Topical
Exact® Cream [OTC]
Fostex® 10% BPO Gel [OTC]
Fostex® 10% Wash [OTC]
Fostex® Bar [OTC]
H₂ Oxyl (Can)
Ilotycin® Ophthalmic
Loroxide® [OTC]
Neutrogena® Acne Mask [OTC]
Neutrogena® On-The-Spot Acne
  Lotion (Can)
Oxy-5® Advanced Formula for
  Sensitive Skin [OTC]
Oxy 5 (Can)
Oxy-5® Tinted [OTC]
Oxy-10® Advanced Formula for
  Sensitive Skin [OTC]
Oxy 10® Wash [OTC]
Oxyderm (Can)
PanOxyl®-AQ
PanOxyl® Bar [OTC]
Perfectoderm® Gel [OTC]
Peroxin A5®
Peroxin A10®

Persa-Gel®
Solugel (Can)
Staticin® Topical
Theroxide® Wash [OTC]
T-Stat® Topical
Vanoxide® [OTC]
Vanoxide-HC®
Antibiotic, Topical
  Apo®-Metronidazole (Can)
  Flagyl® Oral
  Meclan® Topical
  meclocycline
  Metrocream (Can)
  MetroGel® Topical
  MetroGel®-Vaginal
  Metro I.V.® Injection
  metronidazole
  Neo-Metric (Can)
  NidaGel (Can)
  Noritate (Can)
  Novo-Nidazol (Can)
  Protostat® Oral
  Trikacide (Can)
Antiseborrheic Agent, Topical
  Anti-Acne Formula for Men (Can)
  Aveeno® Cleansing Bar [OTC]
  Fostex® [OTC]
  Meted (Can)
  Night Cast R (Can)
  Novacet® Topical
  Pernox® [OTC]
  SAStid® Plain Therapeutic Shampoo
    and Acne Wash [OTC]
  Sebulex (Can)
  Sulfacet-R® Topical
  sulfur and salicylic acid
  sulfur and sulfacetamide
  Sulsal (Can)
Keratolytic Agent
  Acnex (Can)
  Acnomel Acne Mask (Can)
  Anti-Acne Control Formula (Can)
  Anti-Acne Spot Treatment (Can)

Blemish Control (Can)
Callus Salve (Can)
Clean & Clear Deep Cleaning
  Astringent (Can)
Clean & Clear Invisible Clearasil
  Clearstick (Can)
Clearasil® Pads (Can)
Clear Away® Disc [OTC]
Clear Pore Treatment (Can)
Compound W (Can)
Compound W Plus (Can)
Duoforte (Can)
Fostex® Medicated Cleansing (Can)
Freezone® Solution [OTC]
Gordofilm® Liquid
Ionil (Can)
Keralyt (Can)
Mediplast® Plaster [OTC]
Mosco (Can)
Mudd Acne (Can)
Neutrogena® Healthy Scalp Anti-
  Dandruff (Can)
Nova Perfecting Lotion (Can)
Occlusal (Can)
Occlusal®-HP Liquid
Off-Ezy® (Can)
Oil-Free Acne Wash (Can)
Oxy Control (Can)
Oxy Deep Pore (Can)
Oxy Medicated Pads (Can)
Oxy Night Watch (Can)
Oxy Power Pads (Can)
Panscol® Lotion [OTC]
Panscol® Ointment [OTC]
PediaPatch Transdermal Patch [OTC]
Propa PH (Can)
P&S® Shampoo [OTC]
Salac (Can)
Salacid® Ointment
Sal-Acid® Plaster
salicylic acid
Salseb (Can)
Scholl 2-Drop Corn Remedy (Can)

Scholl Corn, Callus Plaster
  Preparation (Can)
Scholl Corn Salve (Can)
Scholl Wart Remover (Can)
Scholl Zino (Can)
Sebcur (Can)
Soluver (Can)
tazarotene
Tazorac®
Ten-O-Six (Can)
Trans-Plantar® Transdermal Patch
  [OTC]
Trans-Ver-Sal® Transdermal Patch
  [OTC]
Vergogel® Gel [OTC]
Verukan® Solution
Wart Remover (Can)
X-Seb® (Can)
Retinoic Acid Derivative
  Accutane®
  Avita®
  isotretinoin
  Isotrex® (Can)
  Renova®
  Retin-A™ Micro Topical
  Retin-A™ Topical
  Retisol-A® (Can)
  Stieva-A® (Can)
  Stieva-A® Forte (Can)
  tretinoin (topical)
Tetracycline Derivative
  Achromycin® Ophthalmic
  Achromycin® Topical
  Achromycin V (Can)
  Apo®-Minocycline (Can)
  Apo®-Tetra (Can)
  Declomycin®
  demeclocycline
  Dynacin® Oral
  Minocin®
  Minocin® IV Injection
  minocycline
  Nor-tet® Oral

Novo-Tetra (Can)
Nu-Tetra (Can)
Panmycin® Oral
Robitet® Oral
Sumycin® Oral
Syn-Minocycline (Can)
Tetracap® Oral
tetracycline
Tetracyn (Can)
Topicycline® Topical
Vectrin®
Topical Skin Product
  azelaic acid
  Azelex®

ACQUIRED IMMUNODEFICIENCY SYNDROME (AIDS)

Antiviral Agent
  abacavir
  adefovir
  Agenerase™
  amprenavir
  Apo®-Zidovudine (Can)
  Combivir™
  Crixivan®
  delavirdine
  didanosine
  efavirenz
  Epivir®
  Epivir®-HBV™
  Fortovase®
  Heptovir® (Can)
  Hivid®
  indinavir
  Invirase®
  Kaletra™
  lamivudine
  lopinavir and ritonavir
  nelfinavir
  nevirapine
  Norvir®
  Novo-AZT (Can)

Preveon®
Rescriptor®
Retrovir®
ritonavir
saquinavir
stavudine
Sustiva™
3TC® (Can)
Videx®
Viracept®
Viramune®
zalcitabine
Zerit®
zidovudine
zidovudine and lamivudine
Ziagen™

ALLERGIC DISORDERS

Adrenal Corticosteroid
  Acthar®
  Actharn (Can)
  Adlone® Injection
  Aeroseb-Dex®
  Ak-Tate (Can)
  Amcort® Injection
  A-methaPred® Injection
  Apo®-Prednisone (Can)
  Aristocort® Forte Injection
  Aristocort® Intralesional Injection
  Aristocort® Oral
  Aristospan® Intra-articular Injection
  Aristospan® Intralesional Injection
  Atolone® Oral
  Balpred (Can)
  betamethasone (systemic)
  Celestone® Oral
  Celestone® Phosphate Injection
  Celestone® Soluspan®
  Cel-U-Jec® Injection
  Cortef®
  corticotropin
  cortisone acetate
  Cortone® Acetate

Decadron® Injection
Decadron®-LA
Decadron® Oral
Decadron® Phosphate
Decaject®
Decaject-LA®
Delta-Cortef® Oral
Deltasone®
depMedalone® Injection
Depoject® Injection
Depo-Medrol® Injection
Depopred® Injection
dexamethasone (systemic)
dexamethasone (topical)
Dexasone®
Dexasone® L.A.
Dexone®
Dexone® LA
Diopred (Can)
D-Med® Injection
Duralone® Injection
Haldrone®
Hexadrol®
H.P. Acthar® Gel
hydrocortisone (systemic)
Hydrocortone® Acetate
Inflamase (Can)
Jaa-Prednisone® (Can)
Kenacort® Oral
Kenaject® Injection
Kenalog® Injection
Key-Pred® Injection
Key-Pred-SP® Injection
Liquid Pred®
Medralone® Injection
Medrol® Oral
Medrol Veriderm (Can)
methylprednisolone
Meticorten®
M-Prednisol® Injection
Novo-Prednisolone (Can)
Orasone®
paramethasone acetate

Pediapred® Oral
  PMS-Dexamethasone (Can)
Prednicen-M®
prednisolone (systemic)
Prednisol® TBA Injection
prednisone
Prelone® Oral
RO-Predphate (Can)
Scheinpharm Triamcine-A (Can)
Solu-Cortef®
Solu-Medrol® Injection
Solurex L.A.®
Stemex®
Tac™-3 Injection
Tac™-40 Injection
Triam-A® Injection
triamcinolone (systemic)
Triam Forte® Injection
Triamonide® Injection
Tri-Kort® Injection
Trilog® Injection
Trilone® Injection
Trisoject® Injection
Ultracortenol (Can)
Winpred (Can)
Adrenergic Agonist Agent
Adrenalin® Chloride
AsthmaHaler® Mist [OTC]
AsthmaNefrin® [OTC]
Bronitin® Mist [OTC]
Bronkaid® Mist [OTC]
Dysne-Inhal (Can)
Epi EZ (Can)
Epifrin®
epinephrine
EpiPen®
EpiPen® Jr
Glaucon®
Medihaler-Epi (Can)
microNefrin® [OTC]
Primatene® Mist [OTC]
Sus-Phrine®
Vaponefrin® [OTC]

Antihistamine
Allegra®
Aller-Aide (Can)
Aller-Chlor® Oral [OTC]
Allerdryl® (Can)
Allergy Elixir (Can)
Allergy Relief (Can)
Allergy Tablets (Can)
AllerMax® Oral [OTC]
Allernix® (Can)
AL-Rr® Oral [OTC]
Antihist-1® [OTC]
Apo®-Cetirizine (Can)
azatadine
Banophen® Oral [OTC]
Belix® Oral [OTC]
Benadryl® Injection
Benadryl® Oral [OTC]
Benadryl® Topical
Ben-Allergin-50® Injection
Benylin® Cough Syrup [OTC]
Bydramine® Cough Syrup [OTC]
Calmex (Can)
Calm-X® Oral [OTC]
cetirizine
Children's Motion Sickness Liquid
  (Can)
Chlo-Amine® Oral [OTC]
Chlorate® Oral [OTC]
chlorpheniramine
Chlor-Pro® Injection
Chlor-Trimeton® Injection
Chlor-Trimeton® Oral [OTC]
Chlor-Tripolon (Can)
Claritin®
Claritin® RediTab®
Clear Caladryl Spray (Can)
clemastine
Compoz® Gel Caps [OTC]
Compoz® Nighttime Sleep Aid
  [OTC]
Contac Allergy Formula (Can)
cyproheptadine

Dexchlor®
dexchlorpheniramine
Dihyrex® Injection
dimenhydrinate
Dimetabs® Oral
Dinate® Injection
Diphenacen-50® Injection [OTC]
Diphen® Cough [OTC]
Diphenhist [OTC]
diphenhydramine
Dormarex® 2 Oral [OTC]
Dormex (Can)
Dormin® Oral [OTC]
Dormiphen (Can)
Dramamine® Oral [OTC]
Dramilin® Injection
Dymenate® Injection
fexofenadine
Genahist® Oral
Gen-Cyproterone (Can)
Gravol (Can)
Histalon (Can)
Hydramyn® Syrup [OTC]
Hydrate® Injection
Hyrexin-50® Injection
Insomnal (Can)
Klorominr® Oral [OTC]
loratadine
Marmine® Injection
Marmine® Oral [OTC]
Maximum Strength Nytol® [OTC]
Miles Nervine® Caplets [OTC]
Nauseatol (Can)
Nausex (Can)
Nolahist® [OTC]
Nordryl® Injection
Nordryl® Oral
Novo-Dimenate (Can)
Novo-Pheniram (Can)
Nytol® Oral [OTC]
Optimine®
Periactin®

Phendry® Oral [OTC]
phenindamine
PMS-Cyproheptadine (Can)
Poladex®
Polaramine®
Pyribenzamine (Can)
Reactine (Can)
Siladryl® Oral [OTC]
Silphen® Cough [OTC]
Sleep Aid (Can)
Sleep-eze 3® Oral [OTC]
Sleep-Eze D (Can)
Sleepinal® [OTC]
Sleepwell 2-nite® [OTC]
Sominex® Oral [OTC]
Tavist®
Tavist®-1 [OTC]
Tega-Vert® Oral
Telachlor® Oral
Teldrin® Oral [OTC]
terfenadine
Travamine (Can)
Travel Aid (Can)
Travelmate (Can)
Travel Tabs (Can)
tripelennamine
TripTone® Caplets® [OTC]
Tusstat® Syrup
Twilite® Oral [OTC]
Uni-Bent® Cough Syrup
Unisom (Can)
Unisom-C (Can)
Vaginex (Can)
Winks® [OTC]
Zyrtec®
Antihistamine/Decongestant
  Combination
  Biohist-LA®
  carbinoxamine and pseudoephedrine
  Carbiset® Tablet
  Carbiset-TR® Tablet
  Carbodec® Syrup

Carbodec® Tablet
Carbodec® TR Tablet
Cardec-S® Syrup
Rondec® Drops
Rondec® Filmtab®
Rondec® Syrup
Rondec-TR®
Phenothiazine Derivative
Histantil (Can)
Phenazine® Injection
Phenergan® Injection
Phenergan® Oral
Phenergan® Rectal
promethazine
Prorex® Injection

ALLERGIC DISORDERS (NASAL)
Corticosteroid, Topical
Nasacort®
Nasacort® AQ
triamcinolone (inhalation, nasal)
Mast Cell Stabilizer
cromolyn sodium
Nalcrom (Can)
Nasalcrom® [OTC]

ALLERGIC DISORDERS (OPHTHALMIC)
Adrenal Corticosteroid
HMS Liquifilm®
medrysone

ALLERGIC RHINITIS
Antihistamine
Astelin® Nasal Spray
azelastine

ALOPECIA
Antiandrogen
finasteride
Proscar®
Progestin

hydroxyprogesterone caproate
Hylutin®
Hyprogest® 250
Topical Skin Product
Apo®-Gain (Can)
Loniten® Oral
minoxidil
Minoxigaine® (Can)
Rogaine® Topical

ANAPHYLACTIC SHOCK
Adrenergic Agonist Agent
Adrenalin® Chloride
AsthmaHaler® Mist [OTC]
AsthmaNefrin® [OTC]
Bronitin® Mist [OTC]
Bronkaid® Mist [OTC]
Dysne-Inhal (Can)
Epi EZ (Can)
Epifrin®
epinephrine
EpiPen®
EpiPen® Jr
Glaucon®
Medihaler-Epi (Can)
microNefrin® [OTC]
Primatene® Mist [OTC]
Sus-Phrine®
Vaponefrin® [OTC]

ANAPHYLACTIC SHOCK (PROPHYLAXIS)
Plasma Volume Expander
dextran 1
Promit®

ANGIOEDEMA (HEREDITARY)
Anabolic Steroid
stanozolol
Winstrol®
Androgen
Cyclomen® (Can)

danazol
Danocrine®

ANTHRAX
Vaccine
  anthrax vaccine, adsorbed
  Biothrax®

ARTHRITIS (SEE ALSO RHEUMATIC DISORDERS)
Aminoquinoline (Antimalarial)
  Aralen® Phosphate
  chloroquine phosphate
  hydroxychloroquine
  Plaquenil®
Analgesic, Topical
  Axsain (Can)
  capsaicin
  Capsin® [OTC]
  Capzasin-P® [OTC]
  Dolorac™ [OTC]
  No Pain-HP® [OTC]
  R-Gel® [OTC]
  Zostrix® [OTC]
  Zostrix®-HP [OTC]
Anti-inflammatory Agent
  Arava™
  leflunomide
Antineoplastic Agent
  cyclophosphamide
  Cytoxan®
  Folex® PFS™
  methotrexate
  Neosar®
  Procytox® (Can)
  Rheumatrex®
Antirheumatic, Disease Modifying
  Enbrel®
  etanercept
Chelating Agent
  Cuprimine®
  Depen®
  penicillamine

Gold Compound
  auranofin
  Aurolate®
  aurothioglucose
  gold sodium thiomalate
  Myochrysine (Can)
  Ridaura®
  Solganal®
Immunosuppressant Agent
  azathioprine
  cyclosporine
  Imuran®
  Neoral®
  Sandimmune®
  SangCya™
Nonsteroidal Anti-inflammatory Drug (NSAID)
  Aches-N-Pain® [OTC]
  Actiprofen® (Can)
  Actron® [OTC]
  Advil® [OTC]
  Aleve® [OTC]
  Amersol (Can)
  Anacin® [OTC]
  Anaprox®
  Ansaid® Oral
  APF (Can)
  Apo®-ASA (Can)
  Apo®-Diclo (Can)
  Apo®-Diflunisal (Can)
  Apo®-Flurbiprofen (Can)
  Apo®-Ibuprofen (Can)
  Apo®-Indomethacin (Can)
  Apo®-Keto (Can)
  Apo®-Keto-E (Can)
  Apo®-Nabumetone (Can)
  Apo®-Napro-Na (Can)
  Apo®-Naproxen (Can)
  Apo®-Piroxicam (Can)
  Apo®-Sulin (Can)
  Argesic®-SA
  Artha-G®
  Arthrisin (Can)

Arthropan® [OTC]
Artria (Can)
A.S.A. [OTC]
Asadrine (Can)
Asaphen (Can)
Ascriptin® [OTC]
aspirin
Aspirin Plus Stomach Guard (Can)
Back-Ese M (Can)
Bayer® Aspirin [OTC]
Bufferin® [OTC]
Cataflam® Oral
Children's Advil® Suspension
Children's Motrin® Suspension
  [OTC]
choline magnesium trisalicylate
choline salicylate
Clinoril®
Coryphen (Can)
Daypro™
diclofenac
diflunisal
Disalcid®
Doan's Backache Pills (Can)
Doan's®, Original [OTC]
Dolobid®
Easprin®
Ecotrin® [OTC]
Empirin® [OTC]
Entrophen® (Can)
Excedrin® IB [OTC]
Extra Strength Doan's® [OTC]
Feldene®
fenoprofen
flurbiprofen
Froben® (Can)
Froben-SR® (Can)
Genpril® [OTC]
Halfprin® [OTC]
Haltran® [OTC]
Headache Tablets (Can)
Herbogesic (Can)
Ibuprin® [OTC]

ibuprofen
Ibuprohm® [OTC]
Ibu-Tab®
Indocid® (Can)
Indocid PDA (Can)
Indocin® Oral
Indocin® SR Oral
Indocollyre (Can)
indomethacin
Indotec (Can)
Junior Strength Motrin® [OTC]
ketoprofen
Magan®
magnesium salicylate
Magsal®
Marthritic®
Measurin® [OTC]
meclofenamate
Medipren® [OTC]
Menadol® [OTC]
Midol® IB [OTC]
Mobidin®
Mono-Gesic®
Motrin®
Motrin® IB [OTC]
MSD® Enteric Coated ASA (Can)
nabumetone
Nalfon®
Naprelan®
Naprosyn®
naproxen
Naxen® (Can)
Novasen (Can)
Novo-Difenac-K (Can)
Novo-Difenac®-SR (Can)
Novo-Diflunisal (Can)
Novo-Flurprofen (Can)
Novo-Keto (Can)
Novo-Keto-EC (Can)
Novo-Methacin (Can)
Novo-Naprox (Can)
Novo-Pirocam (Can)
Novo-Piroxicam (Can)

Novo-Profen® (Can)
Novo-Sundac (Can)
Novo-Tolmetin (Can)
Nu-Diclo (Can)
Nu-Diflunisal (Can)
Nu-Flurprofen (Can)
Nu-Ibuprofen (Can)
Nu-Indo (Can)
Nu-Ketoprofen (Can)
Nu-Ketoprofen-E (Can)
Nu-Naprox (Can)
Nu-Pirox (Can)
Nuprin® [OTC]
Ocufen® Ophthalmic
Orafen (Can)
Orudis®
Orudis® KT [OTC]
Oruvail®
oxaprozin
Pamprin IB® [OTC]
Pedia-Profen™
piroxicam
PMS-Ketoprofen (Can)
Pro-Indo® (Can)
Pro-Piroxicam® (Can)
Relafen®
Rhodacine (Can)
Rhodis® (Can)
Rhodis-EC® (Can)
Rhovail (Can)
Sal (Can)
Saleto-200® [OTC]
Saleto-400®
Salflex®
Salgesic®
salsalate
Salsitab®
sulindac
Supasa (Can)
Surgam® (Can)
Surgam® SR (Can)
Synflex (Can)
Teejel (Can)

tiaprofenic acid (Canada only)
Tolectin®
Tolectin® DS
tolmetin
Trendar® [OTC]
Trilisate®
Uni-Pro® [OTC]
Vofenal™ (Can)
Voltaren® Oral
Voltaren Rapide® (Can)
Voltaren®-XR Oral
ZORprin®
Nonsteroidal Anti-inflammatory Drug
  (NSAID), COX-2 Selective
  Celebrex™
  celecoxib

BEHCET SYNDROME
Immunosuppressant Agent
  azathioprine
  cyclosporine
  Imuran®
  Neoral®
  Sandimmune®
  SangCya™

BITES (SNAKE)
Antivenin
  antivenin (Crotalidae) polyvalent
  antivenin (Micrurus fulvius)

BITES (SPIDER)
Antivenin
  antivenin (Latrodectus mactans)
Electrolyte Supplement, Oral
  calcium gluconate
  H-F Antidote (Can)
  Kalcinate®
Skeletal Muscle Relaxant
  methocarbamol
  Robaxin®

BULLOUS SKIN DISEASE
Antibacterial, Topical
  Dermazin® (Can)

Flamazine® (Can)
Silvadene®
silver sulfadiazine
SSD® AF
SSD® Cream
Thermazene®
Gold Compound
Aurolate®
aurothioglucose
gold sodium thiomalate
Myochrysine (Can)
Solganal®
Immunosuppressant Agent
azathioprine
Imuran®

BURNS

Antibacterial, Topical
Dermazin® (Can)
Flamazine® (Can)
Furacin® Topical
mafenide
nitrofurazone
Silvadene®
silver sulfadiazine
SSD® AF
SSD® Cream
Sulfamylon® Topical
Thermazene®
Protectant, Topical
A and D™ Ointment [OTC]
Aquasol A & D (Can)
Nutrol A D (Can)
vitamin A and vitamin D
zinc oxide, cod liver oil, and talc

CANDIDIASIS

Antifungal Agent
Abelcet™
Absorbine® Antifungal [OTC]
Absorbine® Antifungal Foot Powder
    [OTC]
Absorbine® Jock Itch [OTC]
Absorbine Jr.® Antifungal [OTC]

Aftate® [OTC]
Amphotec®
amphotericin B cholesteryl sulfate
    complex
amphotericin B (conventional)
amphotericin B lipid complex
Ancobon®
Ancotil® (Can)
Apo®-Fluconazole (Can)
AVC™ Cream
AVC™ Suppository
Breezee® Mist Antifungal [OTC]
butoconazole
Candistatin (Can)
Canesten (Can)
ciclopirox
Clotrimaderm (Can)
clotrimazole
Desenex® [OTC]
Diflucan®
econazole
Ecostatin® (Can)
Exelderm® Topical
Femizol-M® [OTC]
fluconazole
flucytosine
Fungizone®
Fungoid® Creme
Fungoid® Solution
Fungoid® Tincture
Genaspor® [OTC]
Gynazole•1®
Gynecure (Can)
Gyne-Lotrimin® [OTC]
Gyne-Lotrimin® 3 [OTC]
Gyno-Trosyd (Can)
itraconazole
ketoconazole
Lamisil® Cream
Loprox®
Lotrimin®
Lotrimin® AF Cream [OTC]
Lotrimin® AF Lotion [OTC]

Lotrimin® AF Powder [OTC]
Lotrimin® AF Solution [OTC]
Lotrimin® AF Spray Liquid [OTC]
Lotrimin® AF Spray Powder [OTC]
Maximum Strength Desenex®
　Antifungal Cream [OTC]
Mestatin® (Can)
Micatin® Topical [OTC]
miconazole
Mitrazol® [OTC]
Monazole-7® (Can)
Monistat-Derm™ Topical
Monistat i.v.™ Injection
Monistat™ Vaginal
Mycelex®
Mycelex®-7
Mycelex®-G
Myclo-Derm (Can)
Myclo-Gyne (Can)
Mycostatin®
M-Zole® 7 Dual Pack [OTC]
Nadostine® (Can)
naftifine
Naftin®
Neo-Zol (Can)
Nilstat®
Nizoral®
Nizoral® A-D Shampoo [OTC]
Novo-Ketoconazole (Can)
NP-27® [OTC]
Nu-Ketocon (Can)
Nyaderm (Can)
nystatin
Nystat-Rx®
Nystex®
Ony-Clear® Spray
O-V Staticin®
oxiconazole
Oxistat® Topical
Pedi-Dri® Topical Powder
Pitrex (Can)
PMS-Nystatin (Can)
Prescription Strength Desenex® [OTC]

Scholl Athlete's Foot Preparations
　(Can)
Spectazole™
Sporanox®
sulconazole
sulfanilamide
Terazol® Vaginal
terbinafine (topical)
terconazole
Tinactin® [OTC]
tioconazole
tolnaftate
Tritin (Can)
Trivagizole 3™ [OTC]
Trosyd (Can)
Vagistat®-1 Vaginal [OTC]
Vagitrol®
Zeasorb-AF® [OTC]
Zeasorb-AF® Powder [OTC]
Antifungal Agent, Systemic
　AmBisome®
　amphotericin B liposomal
Antifungal/Corticosteroid
　Mycogen II Topical
　Mycolog®-II Topical
　Myconel® Topical
　Myco-Triacet® II
　Mytrex® F Topical
　N.G.T.® Topical
　nystatin and triamcinolone
　Tri-Statin® II Topical

CANKER SORE
Anti-infective Agent, Oral
　carbamide peroxide
　Gly-Oxide® Oral [OTC]
　Orajel® Perioseptic® [OTC]
　Proxigel® Oral [OTC]
Anti-inflammatory Agent, Locally
　Applied
　amlexanox
　Aphthasol™
Local Anesthetic

Americaine® [OTC]
Anbesol® [OTC]
Anbesol Baby (Can)
Anbesol® Maximum Strength [OTC]
Babee® Teething® [OTC]
Baby Liquid (Can)
Baby Nighttime (Can)
Baby Orajel (Can)
benzocaine
Benzocol® [OTC]
Benzodent® [OTC]
Cylex® [OTC]
Maximum Strength Anbesol® [OTC]
Maximum Strength Orajel® [OTC]
Numzitdent® [OTC]
Numzit Teething® [OTC]
Orabase®-B [OTC]
Orabase®-O [OTC]
Orajel® Maximum Strength [OTC]
Orasept® [OTC]
Orasol® [OTC]
Spec-T® [OTC]
Tanac® [OTC]
Protectant, Topical
gelatin, pectin, and methylcellulose
Orabase® Plain [OTC]

CHOLERA
Vaccine, Inactivated Bacteria
cholera vaccine

CHROMOBLASTOMYCOSIS
Antifungal Agent
ketoconazole
Nizoral®
Novo-Ketoconazole (Can)
Nu-Ketocon (Can)

COLD SORE
Antiviral Agent
Denavir™
penciclovir

COLLAGEN DISORDERS
Adrenal Corticosteroid

Acthar®
Actharn (Can)
Adlone® Injection
Ak-Tate (Can)
Amcort® Injection
A-methaPred® Injection
Apo®-Prednisone (Can)
Aristocort® Forte Injection
Aristocort® Intralesional Injection
Aristocort® Oral
Aristospan® Intra-articular Injection
Aristospan® Intralesional Injection
Atolone® Oral
Balpred (Can)
betamethasone (systemic)
Celestone® Oral
Celestone® Phosphate Injection
Celestone® Soluspan®
Cel-U-Jec® Injection
Cortef®
corticotropin
cortisone acetate
Cortone® Acetate
Decadron® Injection
Decadron®-LA
Decadron® Oral
Decaject®
Decaject-LA®
Delta-Cortef® Oral
Deltasone®
depMedalone® Injection
Depoject® Injection
Depo-Medrol® Injection
Depopred® Injection
dexamethasone (systemic)
Dexasone®
Dexasone® L.A.
Dexone®
Dexone® LA
Diopred (Can)
D-Med® Injection
Duralone® Injection
Haldrone®

Hexadrol®
H.P. Acthar® Gel
hydrocortisone (systemic)
Hydrocortone® Acetate
Inflamase (Can)
Jaa-Prednisone® (Can)
Kenacort® Oral
Kenaject® Injection
Kenalog® Injection
Key-Pred® Injection
Key-Pred-SP® Injection
Liquid Pred®
Medralone® Injection
Medrol® Oral
Medrol Veriderm (Can)
methylprednisolone
Meticorten®
M-Prednisol® Injection
Novo-Prednisolone (Can)
Orasone®
paramethasone acetate
Pediapred® Oral
PMS-Dexamethasone (Can)
Prednicen-M®
prednisolone (systemic)
Prednisol® TBA Injection
prednisone
Prelone® Oral
RO-Predphate (Can)
Scheinpharm Triamcine-A (Can)
Solu-Cortef®
Solu-Medrol® Injection
Solurex L.A.®
Stemex®
Tac™-3 Injection
Tac™-40 Injection
Triam-A® Injection
triamcinolone (systemic)
Triam Forte® Injection
Triamonide® Injection
Tri-Kort® Injection
Trilog® Injection
Trilone® Injection

Trisoject® Injection
Ultracortenol (Can)
Winpred (Can)

CONDYLOMA ACUMINATA
Immune Response Modifier
Aldara™
imiquimod

CONDYLOMA ACUMINATUM
Antiviral Agent
interferon alfa-2b and ribavirin
combination pack
Rebetron™
Biological Response Modulator
Alferon® N
interferon alfa-2a
interferon alfa-2b
interferon alfa-2b and ribavirin
combination pack
interferon alfa-n3
Intron® A
Rebetron™
Roferon-A®
Keratolytic Agent
Condyline (Can)
Condylox®
Pod-Ben-25®
Podocon-25™
Podofilm® (Can)
podofilox
Podofin®
podophyllin and salicylic acid
podophyllum resin
Verrex-C&M®
Wartec (Can)

CONJUNCTIVITIS (SEASONAL ALLERGIC)
Corticosteroid, Ophthalmic
Alrex™
Lotemax®
loteprednol

CONJUNCTIVITIS (VERNAL)
Adrenal Corticosteroid
  HMS Liquifilm®
  medrysone
Mast Cell Stabilizer
  Alomide® Ophthalmic
  lodoxamide tromethamine

DANDRUFF
Antiseborrheic Agent, Topical
  Anti-Acne Formula for Men (Can)
  Anti-Dandruff Shampoo (Can)
  AquaTar® [OTC]
  Avant Garde Shampoo (Can)
  Aveeno® Cleansing Bar [OTC]
  Balnetar® [OTC]
  Capitrol®
  chloroxine
  coal tar
  coal tar and salicylic acid
  coal tar, lanolin, and mineral oil
  Dandruff Treatment Shampoo (Can)
  Dan-Gard (Can)
  Denorex® [OTC]
  DHS® Tar [OTC]
  DHS Zinc® [OTC]
  Doak-Oil (Can)
  Duplex® T [OTC]
  Estar® [OTC]
  Exsel® Shampoo
  Fostex® [OTC]
  Fototar® [OTC]
  Hair and Scalp (Can)
  Head & Shoulders® [OTC]
  Ionil-T (Can)
  Ionil-T Plus (Can)
  Keep Clear Anti-Dandruff Shampoo (Can)
  Lander Dandruff Control (Can)
  Mazon Medicated Soap (Can)
  Metasep® [OTC]
  Meted (Can)
  Neutrogena® T/Derm
  Neutrogena T/Gel (Can)
  Night Cast R (Can)
  No-Name Dandruff Treatment (Can)
  Out of Africa (Can)
  parachlorometaxylenol
  Pentrax® [OTC]
  Pernox® [OTC]
  Pert Plus (Can)
  Polytar® [OTC]
  psoriGel® [OTC]
  P & S Plus (Can)
  pyrithione zinc
  SAStid® Plain Therapeutic Shampoo and Acne Wash [OTC]
  Satinique Anti-Dandruff (Can)
  Sebcur/T (Can)
  Sebulex (Can)
  Sebulon (Can)
  selenium sulfide
  Selsun Blue® Shampoo [OTC]
  Selsun® Shampoo
  Shaklee Dandruff Control (Can)
  Shampooing Anti-Pelliculaire (Can)
  Spectro Tar (Can)
  sulfur and salicylic acid
  Sulsal (Can)
  Tardan (Can)
  Tar Distillate (Can)
  Tar Doak (Can)
  Targel (Can)
  Targel SA (Can)
  Tegrin (Can)
  Tersa-Tar (Can)
  T/Gel® [OTC]
  Theraplex Z® [OTC]
  Versel (Can)
  X-seb® T [OTC]
  Zetar® [OTC]
  Zincon® Shampoo [OTC]
  ZNP® Bar [OTC]
  ZP 11 (Can)

DECUBITUS ULCERS

Enzyme
  Biozyme-C®
  collagenase
  Santyl®
Enzyme, Topical Debridement
  Accuzyme™
  papain and urea
Protectant, Topical
  Granulex
  trypsin, balsam Peru, and castor oil
Topical Skin Product
  Accuzyme™
  Debrisan® [OTC]
  dextranomer
  papain and urea

DERMATOLOGIC DISORDERS

Adrenal Corticosteroid
  Acthar®
  Actharn (Can)
  Adlone® Injection
  Aeroseb-Dex®
  Ak-Tate (Can)
  Amcort® Injection
  A-methaPred® Injection
  Apo®-Prednisone (Can)
  Aristocort® Forte Injection
  Aristocort® Intralesional Injection
  Aristocort® Oral
  Aristospan® Intra-articular Injection
  Aristospan® Intralesional Injection
  Atolone® Oral
  Balpred (Can)
  betamethasone (systemic)
  Celestone® Oral
  Celestone® Phosphate Injection
  Celestone® Soluspan®
  Cel-U-Jec® Injection
  Colocort™
  Cortef®
  corticotropin

cortisone acetate
Cortone® Acetate
Decadron® Injection
Decadron®-LA
Decadron® Oral
Decadron® Phosphate
Decaject®
Decaject-LA®
Delta-Cortef® Oral
Deltasone®
depMedalone® Injection
Depoject® Injection
Depo-Medrol® Injection
Depopred® Injection
dexamethasone (systemic)
dexamethasone (topical)
Dexasone®
Dexasone® L.A.
Dexone®
Dexone® LA
Diopred (Can)
D-Med® Injection
Duralone® Injection
Haldrone®
Hexadrol®
H.P. Acthar® Gel
hydrocortisone (systemic)
Hydrocortone® Acetate
Inflamase (Can)
Jaa-Prednisone® (Can)
Kenacort® Oral
Kenaject® Injection
Kenalog® Injection
Key-Pred® Injection
Key-Pred-SP® Injection
Liquid Pred®
Medralone® Injection
Medrol® Oral
Medrol Veriderm (Can)
methylprednisolone
Meticorten®
M-Prednisol® Injection
Novo-Prednisolone (Can)

Orasone®
paramethasone acetate
Pediapred® Oral
PMS-Dexamethasone (Can)
Prednicen-M®
prednisolone (systemic)
Prednisol® TBA Injection
prednisone
Prelone® Oral
RO-Predphate (Can)
Scheinpharm Triamcine-A (Can)
Solu-Cortef®
Solu-Medrol® Injection
Solurex L.A.®
Stemex®
Tac™-3 Injection
Tac™-40 Injection
Triam-A® Injection
triamcinolone (systemic)
Triam Forte® Injection
Triamonide® Injection
Tri-Kort® Injection
Trilog® Injection
Trilone® Injection
Trisoject® Injection
Ultracortenol (Can)
Winpred (Can)

DERMATOMYCOSIS

Antifungal Agent
   Absorbine® Antifungal Foot Powder
     [OTC]
   Breezee® Mist Antifungal [OTC]
   Femizol-M® [OTC]
   Fulvicin (Can)
   Fulvicin® P/G
   Fulvicin-U/F®
   Fungoid® Creme
   Fungoid® Tincture
   Grifulvin® V
   Grisactin®
   Grisactin® Ultra
   griseofulvin

Grisovin®-FP (Can)
Gris-PEG®
ketoconazole
Lotrimin® AF Powder [OTC]
Lotrimin® AF Spray Liquid [OTC]
Lotrimin® AF Spray Powder [OTC]
Maximum Strength Desenex®
   Antifungal Cream [OTC]
Micatin® Topical [OTC]
miconazole
Mitrazol® [OTC]
Monazole-7® (Can)
Monistat-Derm™ Topical
Monistat i.v.™ Injection
Monistat™ Vaginal
M-Zole® 7 Dual Pack [OTC]
naftifine
Naftin®
Nizoral®
Nizoral® A-D Shampoo [OTC]
Novo-Ketoconazole (Can)
Nu-Ketocon (Can)
Ony-Clear® Spray
oxiconazole
Oxistat® Topical
Prescription Strength Desenex®
   [OTC]
Zeasorb-AF® Powder [OTC]

DERMATOSIS

Anesthetic/Corticosteroid
   Lida-Mantle HC® Topical
   lidocaine and hydrocortisone
Corticosteroid, Topical
   Aclovate® Topical
   Acticort® Topical
   Aeroseb-HC® Topical
   Ala-Cort® Topical
   Ala-Scalp® Topical
   alclometasone
   Alocort (Can)
   Alphatrex® Topical
   amcinonide

Anusol® HC-1 Topical [OTC]
Anusol® HC-2.5% Topical [OTC]
Aquacort® (Can)
Aristocort® A Topical
Aristocort® Topical
Bactine® Hydrocortisone [OTC]
Barriere-HC (Can)
Beben (Can)
Betacort (Can)
Betaderm (Can)
Betagel (Can)
Betalene® Topical
betamethasone (topical)
Betatrex® Topical
Beta-Val® Topical
Betnesol® (Can)
Betnovate (Can)
CaldeCort® Anti-Itch Topical Spray
CaldeCort® Topical [OTC]
Carmol-HC® Topical
Celestoderm (Can)
Cetacort® Topical
clobetasol
Clocort® Maximum Strength [OTC]
clocortolone
Cloderm® Topical
Cordran®
Cordran® SP
Cormax® Ointment
Cortacet (Can)
CortaGel® Topical [OTC]
Cortaid® Maximum Strength Topical
    [OTC]
Cortaid® with Aloe Topical [OTC]
Cortate (Can)
Cort-Dome® Topical
Cortef® Feminine Itch Topical
Cortizone®-5 Topical [OTC]
Cortizone®-10 Topical [OTC]
Cortoderm (Can)
Cutivate™
Cyclocort® Topical
Delcort® Topical

Delta-Tritex® Topical
Dermacort® Topical
Dermaflex HC (Can)
Dermarest Dricort® Topical
Derma-Smoothe/FS® Topical
Dermasone (Can)
Dermatop®
Dermolate® Topical [OTC]
Dermovate (Can)
Dermtex® HC with Aloe Topical
    [OTC]
Desocort (Can)
desonide
DesOwen® Topical
desoximetasone
diflorasone
Diprolene® AF Topical
Diprolene® Glycol (Can)
Diprolene® Topical
Diprosone (Can)
Diprosone® Topical
Drenison (Can)
Ectosone (Can)
Eldecort® Topical
Elocom® (Can)
Elocon®
Emo-Cort (Can)
Florone®
Florone E®
fluocinolone
fluocinonide
Fluoderm (Can)
Fluonid® Topical
flurandrenolide
Flurosyn® Topical
Flutex® Topical
fluticasone (topical)
Flutone (Can)
FS Shampoo® Topical
Gynecort® Topical [OTC]
halcinonide
halobetasol
Halog®

Halog®-E
Hi-Cor-1.0® Topical
Hi-Cor-2.5® Topical
Hycort
Hycort® Topical
Hyderm (Can)
hydrocortisone (topical)
Hydrocort® Topical
Hydrosone (Can)
Hydro-Tex® Topical [OTC]
Hytone® Topical
Kenalog® in Orabase®
Kenalog® Topical
Kenonel® Topical
LactiCare-HC® Topical
Lanacort® Topical [OTC]
Lidemol (Can)
Lidex®
Lidex-E®
Locoid® Topical
Lyderm (Can)
Maxiflor®
Maxivate® Topical
mometasone furoate
Nasonex®
Novobetamet (Can)
Nutracort® Topical
Orabase® HCA Topical
Penecort® Topical
prednicarbate
Prevex B (Can)
Prevex HC (Can)
Psorcon™
Psorion® Topical
Rholosone (Can)
Rhoprolene (Can)
Rhoprosone (Can)
Rivasone (Can)
Sarna HC (Can)
Scalpicin® Topical
Sential (Can)
S-T Cort® Topical
Synacort® Topical

Synalar-HP® Topical
Synalar® Topical
Synemol® Topical
Taro-Desoximetasone (Can)
Taro-Sone (Can)
Tegrin®-HC Topical [OTC]
Teladar® Topical
Temovate®
Texacort® Topical
Tiamol (Can)
Ti-U-Lac HC (Can)
Topactin (Can)
Topicort®
Topicort®-LP
Topilene (Can)
Topisone (Can)
Topsyn (Can)
Triacet™ Topical
Triaderm (Can)
triamcinolone (topical)
Tridesilon® Topical
U-Cort™ Topical
Ultravate™
Unicort (Can)
urea and hydrocortisone
Uremol-HC (Can)
Valisone® Topical
Westcort® Topical

DIAPER RASH
Antifungal Agent
   Caldesene® Topical [OTC]
   Cruex (Can)
   Fungoid® AF Topical Solution
     [OTC]
   Pedi-Pro Topical [OTC]
   undecylenic acid and derivatives
Dietary Supplement
   methionine
   Pedameth®
Protectant, Topical
   A and D™ Ointment [OTC]
   Aquasol A & D (Can)

Desitin® [OTC]
Nutrol A D (Can)
vitamin A and vitamin D
zinc oxide, cod liver oil, and talc
Topical Skin Product
Babys Own Ointment (Can)
Diaparene® [OTC]
Diaper Rash (Can)
Herisan (Can)
Infazinc (Can)
methylbenzethonium chloride
Neoderm (Can)
Pate d'Unna (Can)
Perineal Skin Cleanser (Can)
Prevex Diaper Rash Cream (Can)
Puri-Clens™ [OTC]
Sween Cream® [OTC]
Zinaderm (Can)
Zincoderm (Can)
Zincofax (Can)
zinc oxide

DISCOID LUPUS ERYTHEMATOSUS (DLE)

Aminoquinoline (Antimalarial)
Aralen® Phosphate
chloroquine phosphate
hydroxychloroquine
Plaquenil®
Corticosteroid, Topical
Aclovate® Topical
Acticort® Topical
Aeroseb-HC® Topical
Ala-Cort® Topical
Ala-Scalp® Topical
alclometasone
Alocort (Can)
Alphatrex® Topical
amcinonide
Aquacort® (Can)
Aristocort® A Topical
Aristocort® Topical
Bactine® Hydrocortisone [OTC]

Barriere-HC (Can)
Beben (Can)
Betacort (Can)
Betaderm (Can)
Betagel (Can)
Betalene® Topical
betamethasone (topical)
Betatrex® Topical
Beta-Val® Topical
Betnesol® (Can)
Betnovate (Can)
CaldeCort® Anti-Itch Topical Spray
CaldeCort® Topical [OTC]
Carmol-HC® Topical
Celestoderm (Can)
Cetacort® Topical
clobetasol
Clocort® Maximum Strength [OTC]
clocortolone
Cloderm® Topical
Cordran®
Cordran® SP
Cormax® Ointment
Cortacet (Can)
CortaGel® Topical [OTC]
Cortaid® Maximum Strength Topical [OTC]
Cortaid® with Aloe Topical [OTC]
Cortate (Can)
Cort-Dome® Topical
Cortef® Feminine Itch Topical
Cortizone®-5 Topical [OTC]
Cortizone®-10 Topical [OTC]
Cortoderm (Can)
Cutivate™
Cyclocort® Topical
Delcort® Topical
Delta-Tritex® Topical
Dermacort® Topical
Dermaflex HC (Can)
Dermarest Dricort® Topical
Derma-Smoothe/FS® Topical
Dermasone (Can)

Dermatop®
Dermolate® Topical [OTC]
Dermovate (Can)
Dermtex® HC with Aloe Topical [OTC]
Desocort (Can)
desonide
DesOwen® Topical
desoximetasone
diflorasone
Diprolene® AF Topical
Diprolene® Glycol (Can)
Diprolene® Topical
Diprosone (Can)
Diprosone® Topical
Drenison (Can)
Ectosone (Can)
Eldecort® Topical
Elocom® (Can)
Elocon®
Emo-Cort (Can)
Florone®
Florone E®
fluocinolone
fluocinonide
Fluoderm (Can)
Fluonid® Topical
flurandrenolide
Flurosyn® Topical
Flutex® Topical
fluticasone (topical)
Flutone (Can)
FS Shampoo® Topical
Gynecort® Topical [OTC]
halcinonide
halobetasol
Halog®
Halog®-E
Hi-Cor-1.0® Topical
Hi-Cor-2.5® Topical
Hycort
Hycort® Topical
Hyderm (Can)

hydrocortisone (topical)
Hydrocort® Topical
Hydrosone (Can)
Hydro-Tex® Topical [OTC]
Hytone® Topical
Kenalog® Topical
Kenonel® Topical
LactiCare-HC® Topical
Lanacort® Topical [OTC]
Lidemol (Can)
Lidex®
Lidex-E®
Locoid® Topical
Lyderm (Can)
Maxiflor®
Maxivate® Topical
mometasone furoate
Nasonex®
Novobetamet (Can)
Nutracort® Topical
Orabase® HCA Topical
Penecort® Topical
prednicarbate
Prevex B (Can)
Prevex HC (Can)
Psorcon™
Psorion® Topical
Rholosone (Can)
Rhoprolene (Can)
Rhoprosone (Can)
Rivasone (Can)
Sarna HC (Can)
Scalpicin® Topical
Sential (Can)
S-T Cort® Topical
Synacort® Topical
Synalar-HP® Topical
Synalar® Topical
Synemol® Topical
Taro-Desoximetasone (Can)
Taro-Sone (Can)
Tegrin®-HC Topical [OTC]
Teladar® Topical

Temovate®
Texacort® Topical
Tiamol (Can)
Ti-U-Lac HC (Can)
Topactin (Can)
Topicort®
Topicort®-LP
Topilene (Can)
Topisone (Can)
Topsyn (Can)
Triacet™ Topical
Triaderm (Can)
triamcinolone (topical)
Tridesilon® Topical
U-Cort™ Topical
Ultravate™
Unicort (Can)
urea and hydrocortisone
Uremol-HC (Can)
Valisone® Topical
Westcort® Topical

DRACUNCULIASIS
Amebicide
Apo®-Metronidazole (Can)
Flagyl® Oral
Metrocream (Can)
Metro I.V.® Injection
metronidazole
Neo-Metric (Can)
NidaGel (Can)
Noritate (Can)
Novo-Nidazol (Can)
Protostat® Oral
Trikacide (Can)

DRY SKIN
Topical Skin Product
Aquacare® Topical [OTC]
Calmurid (Can)
camphor, menthol, and phenol
Carmol® Topical [OTC]
Dermaflex (Can)
Gormel® Creme [OTC]

Lac-Hydrin®
lactic acid and sodium-PCA
lactic acid with ammonium
    hydroxide
LactiCare® [OTC]
Lanaphilic® Topical [OTC]
lanolin, cetyl alcohol, glycerin, and
    petrolatum
Lubriderm® [OTC]
Nutraplus® Topical [OTC]
Onyvul® (Can)
Rea-Lo® [OTC]
Rhodurea (Can)
Sarna [OTC]
Ti-U-Lac (Can)
Ultra Mide® Topical
urea
Ureacin®-20 Topical [OTC]
Ureaphil® Injection
Uree (Can)
Uremol® (Can)
Urisec® (Can)
Velvelan® (Can)
Vitamin, Topical
Amino-Opti-E® [OTC]
Aquasol E® [OTC]
E-Complex-600® [OTC]
E-Vitamin® [OTC]
Novo E (Can)
Organex (Can)
Vita-E (Can)
vitamin E
Vita-Plus® E Softgels® [OTC]
Vitec® [OTC]
Vite E® Creme [OTC]

ERYTHROPOIETIC PROTOPORPHYRIA (EPP)
Vitamin, Fat Soluble
A-Caro-25®
B-Caro-T®
beta-carotene
Biotene®

Caroguard®
Lumitene®

EYELID INFECTION

Antibiotic, Ophthalmic
  mercuric oxide
  Ocu-Merox®
Pharmaceutical Aid
  boric acid
  Borofax® Topical [OTC]
  Dri-Ear® Otic [OTC]
  RO-Eyewash (Can)
  Swim-Ear® Otic [OTC]

FUNGUS (DIAGNOSTIC)

Diagnostic Agent
  Candida albicans (Monilia)
  coccidioidin skin test
  Dermatophytin®
  Dermatophytin-O
  Histolyn-CYL®
  histoplasmin
  Spherulin®
  Trichophyton skin test

GENITAL HERPES

Antiviral Agent
  famciclovir
  Famvir™
  valacyclovir
  Valtrex®

GENITAL WART

Immune Response Modifier
  Aldara™
  imiquimod

GOUT

Antigout Agent
  colchicine
  colchicine and probenecid
Nonsteroidal Anti-inflammatory Drug
    (NSAID)
  Aches-N-Pain® [OTC]
  Actiprofen® (Can)

Advil® [OTC]
Aleve® [OTC]
Amersol (Can)
Anaprox®
Apo®-Diclo (Can)
Apo®-Ibuprofen (Can)
Apo®-Indomethacin (Can)
Apo®-Napro-Na (Can)
Apo®-Naproxen (Can)
Apo®-Sulin (Can)
Cataflam® Oral
Children's Advil® Suspension
Children's Motrin® Suspension
    [OTC]
Clinoril®
diclofenac
Excedrin® IB [OTC]
Genpril® [OTC]
Haltran® [OTC]
Ibuprin® [OTC]
ibuprofen
Ibuprohm® [OTC]
Ibu-Tab®
Indocid® (Can)
Indocid PDA (Can)
Indocin® Oral
Indocin® SR Oral
Indocollyre (Can)
indomethacin
Indotec (Can)
Junior Strength Motrin®
    [OTC]
Medipren® [OTC]
Menadol® [OTC]
Midol® IB [OTC]
Motrin®
Motrin® IB [OTC]
Naprelan®
Naprosyn®
naproxen
Naxen® (Can)
Novo-Difenac-K (Can)
Novo-Difenac®-SR (Can)

Novo-Methacin (Can)
Novo-Naprox (Can)
Novo-Profen® (Can)
Novo-Sundac (Can)
Nu-Diclo (Can)
Nu-Ibuprofen (Can)
Nu-Indo (Can)
Nu-Naprox (Can)
Nuprin® [OTC]
Oxybutazone (Can)
oxyphenbutazone
Pamprin IB® [OTC]
Pedia-Profen™
Pro-Indo® (Can)
Rhodacine (Can)
Saleto-200® [OTC]
Saleto-400®
sulindac
Synflex (Can)
Trendar® [OTC]
Uni-Pro® [OTC]
Vofenal™ (Can)
Voltaren® Oral
Voltaren Rapide® (Can)
Voltaren®-XR Oral
Uricosuric Agent
Antazone® (Can)
Anturan® (Can)
Anturane®
Apo®-Sulfinpyraz (Can)
Benemid (Can)
Benuryl® (Can)
Novo-Pyrazone (Can)
probenecid
sulfinpyrazone
Xanthine Oxidase Inhibitor
Alloprim™ Injection
Alloprin (Can)
allopurinol
Apo®-Allopurinol (Can)
Novo-Purol (Can)
Purinol® (Can)

Zyloprim®

GRAFT VS HOST DISEASE
Immunosuppressant Agent
Atgam®
CellCept®
cyclosporine
lymphocyte immune globulin
muromonab-CD3
mycophenolate
Neoral®
Orthoclone® OKT3
Prograf®
Sandimmune®
SangCya™
tacrolimus

HARTNUP DISEASE
Vitamin, Water Soluble
niacinamide
Papulex (Can)

HAY FEVER
Adrenergic Agonist Agent
Afrin® Children's Nose Drops [OTC]
Afrin® Nasal Solution [OTC]
Allerest® 12 Hour Nasal Solution
[OTC]
Chlorphed®-LA Nasal Solution
[OTC]
Dristan® Long Lasting Nasal
Solution [OTC]
Drixoral® (Can)
Duramist Plus® [OTC]
Duration® Nasal Solution [OTC]
Nafrine (Can)
Neo-Synephrine® 12 Hour Nasal
Solution [OTC]
Nostrilla® [OTC]
NTZ® Long Acting Nasal Solution
[OTC]
OcuClear® Ophthalmic [OTC]
oxymetazoline

Sinarest® 12 Hour Nasal Solution
Sinex® Long-Acting [OTC]
Twice-A-Day® Nasal Solution [OTC]
Vicks® Sinex (Can)
Visine® L.R. Ophthalmic [OTC]
Visine® Workplace (Can)
4-Way® Long Acting Nasal Solution
   [OTC]
Antihistamine
   Allegra®
   fexofenadine
Antihistamine/Decongestant
   Combination
   acrivastine and pseudoephedrine
   Actagen® Syrup [OTC]
   Actagen® Tablet [OTC]
   Actifed 12 Hour (Can)
   Actifed (Can)
   Allercon® Tablet [OTC]
   Allerest® Maximum Strength [OTC]
   Allerfrin® Syrup [OTC]
   Allerfrin® Tablet [OTC]
   Allerphed® Syrup [OTC]
   Anamine® Syrup [OTC]
   Anaplex® Liquid [OTC]
   Aprodine® Syrup [OTC]
   Aprodine® Tablet [OTC]
   Benylin® Cold (Can)
   Cenafed® Plus Tablet [OTC]
   Chlorafed® Liquid [OTC]
   chlorpheniramine and
      pseudoephedrine
   Chlor-Trimeton® 4 Hour Relief
      Tablet [OTC]
   Chlor-Tripolon Decongestant (Can)
   Co-Pyronil® 2 Pulvules® [OTC]
   Deconamine® SR
   Deconamine® Syrup [OTC]
   Deconamine® Tablet [OTC]
   Fedahist® Tablet [OTC]
   Genac® Tablet [OTC]
   Hayfebrol® Liquid [OTC]

Klerist-D® Tablet [OTC]
Pseudo-Gest Plus® Tablet [OTC]
Rhinosyn® Liquid [OTC]
Rhinosyn-PD® Liquid [OTC]
Ryna® Liquid [OTC]
Semprex®-D
Silafed® Syrup [OTC]
Sudafed® Plus Tablet [OTC]
Triofed® Syrup [OTC]
Triposed® Syrup [OTC]
Triposed® Tablet [OTC]
Triprofed (Can)
triprolidine and pseudoephedrine
Vasofrinic (Can)

HERPES SIMPLEX
Antiviral Agent
   acyclovir
   Avirax® (Can)
   Cytovene®
   famciclovir
   Famvir™
   foscarnet
   Foscavir®
   ganciclovir
   trifluridine
   vidarabine
   Vira-A® Ophthalmic
   Viroptic® Ophthalmic
   Vitrasert®
   Zovirax®

HERPES ZOSTER
Analgesic, Topical
   Axsain (Can)
   capsaicin
   Capsin® [OTC]
   Capzasin-P® [OTC]
   Dolorac™ [OTC]
   No Pain-HP® [OTC]
   R-Gel® [OTC]
   Zostrix® [OTC]

Zostrix®-HP [OTC]

Antiviral Agent
  acyclovir
  Avirax® (Can)
  famciclovir
  Famvir™
  valacyclovir
  Valtrex®
  vidarabine
  Vira-A® Ophthalmic
  Zovirax®

HOOKWORMS

Anthelmintic
  albendazole
  Albenza®
  Antiminth® [OTC]
  Combantrin (Can)
  Jaa Pyral® (Can)
  mebendazole
  Pin-Rid® [OTC]
  Pin-X® [OTC]
  pyrantel pamoate
  Reese's® Pinworm Medicine [OTC]
  Vermox®

HYPERHIDROSIS

Topical Skin Product
  aluminum chloride hexahydrate
  Drysol™

HYPERPIGMENTATION

Topical Skin Product
  African Gold (Can)
  Ambi® Skin Tone [OTC]
  Banishing Cream (Can)
  Eldopaque® [OTC]
  Eldopaque Forte®
  Eldoquin® [OTC]
  Eldoquin® Forte®
  Esoterica® Facial [OTC]
  Esoterica® Regular [OTC]
  Esoterica® Sensitive Skin Formula
    [OTC]

Esoterica® Sunscreen [OTC]
hydroquinone
Jouvence (Can)
Lustra®
Lustra-AF®
Melanex®
Nadinola (Can)
Neostrata® HQ (Can)
Porcelana® [OTC]
Porcelana® Sunscreen [OTC]
Solaquin® [OTC]
Solaquin Forte®
Ultraquin® (Can)
Ultraquin Plain (Can)

HYPERSENSITIVITY SKIN TESTING (DIAGNOSTIC)

Diagnostic Agent
  Multitest CMI®
  skin test antigens, multiple

HYPODERMOCLYSIS

Antidote
  Hyalase (Can)
  hyaluronidase
  Wydase®

ICHTHYOSIS

Keratolytic Agent
  Duofilm® Solution
  Keralyt® Gel
  salicylic acid and lactic acid
  salicylic acid and propylene glycol
  Soluver Plus (Can)
  Tiacid (Can)

IMMUNODEFICIENCY

Enzyme
  Adagen™
  pegademase (bovine)
Immune Globulin
  Gamimune® N
  Gammagard® S/D
  Gammar®-P I.V.

immune globulin (intravenous)
Polygam® S/D
Sandoglobulin®
Venoglobulin®-I
Venoglobulin®-S

IMPETIGO

Antibiotic, Topical
  bacitracin, neomycin, and
    polymyxin B
  Bactroban®
  Medi-Quick® Topical Ointment
    [OTC]
  mupirocin
  Mycitracin® Topical [OTC]
  Neomixin® Topical
  Neosporin® Topical Ointment [OTC]
  Neotopic (Can)
  Ocutricin® Topical Ointment
  Septa® Topical Ointment [OTC]
  Triple Antibiotic® Topical
Penicillin
  Apo®-Pen VK (Can)
  Ayercillin® (Can)
  Crysticillin® A.S.
  Nadopen-V® (Can)
  Novo-Pen-VK® (Can)
  Nu-Pen-VK (Can)
  penicillin G procaine
  penicillin V potassium
  Truxcillin®
  Veetids®
  Wycillin®

INFLAMMATION (NONRHEUMATIC)

Adrenal Corticosteroid
  Acthar®
  Actharn (Can)
  Adlone® Injection
  Ak-Tate (Can)
  Amcort® Injection
  A-methaPred® Injection

Apo®-Prednisone (Can)
Aristocort® Forte Injection
Aristocort® Intralesional Injection
Aristocort® Oral
Aristospan® Intra-articular Injection
Aristospan® Intralesional Injection
Atolone® Oral
Balpred (Can)
betamethasone (systemic)
Celestone® Oral
Celestone® Phosphate Injection
Celestone® Soluspan®
Cel-U-Jec® Injection
Cortef®
corticotropin
cortisone acetate
Cortone® Acetate
Decadron® Injection
Decadron®-LA
Decadron® Oral
Decaject®
Decaject-LA®
Delta-Cortef® Oral
Deltasone®
depMedalone® Injection
Depoject® Injection
Depo-Medrol® Injection
Depopred® Injection
dexamethasone (systemic)
Dexasone®
Dexasone® L.A.
Dexone®
Dexone® LA
Diopred (Can)
D-Med® Injection
Duralone® Injection
Haldrone®
Hexadrol®
H.P. Acthar® Gel
hydrocortisone (systemic)
Hydrocortone® Acetate
Inflamase (Can)
Jaa-Prednisone® (Can)

Kenacort® Oral
Kenaject® Injection
Kenalog® Injection
Key-Pred® Injection
Key-Pred-SP® Injection
Liquid Pred®
Medralone® Injection
Medrol® Oral
Medrol Veriderm (Can)
methylprednisolone
Meticorten®
M-Prednisol® Injection
Novo-Prednisolone (Can)
Orasone®
paramethasone acetate
Pediapred® Oral
PMS-Dexamethasone (Can)
Prednicen-M®
prednisolone (systemic)
Prednisol® TBA Injection
prednisone
Prelone® Oral
RO-Predphate (Can)
Scheinpharm Triamcine-A (Can)
Solu-Cortef®
Solu-Medrol® Injection
Solurex L.A.®
Stemex®
Tac™-3 Injection
Tac™-40 Injection
Triam-A® Injection
triamcinolone (systemic)
Triam Forte® Injection
Triamonide® Injection
Tri-Kort® Injection
Trilog® Injection
Trilone® Injection
Trisoject® Injection
Ultracortenol (Can)
Winpred (Can)

KAPOSI SARCOMA

Antineoplastic Agent

Alkaban-AQ®
daunorubicin citrate (liposomal)
DaunoXome®
Doxil®
doxorubicin (liposomal)
paclitaxel
Paxene®
Taxol®
Velban®
Velbe (Can)
vinblastine
Antineoplastic Agent, Miscellaneous
alitretinoin
Panretin™
Biological Response Modulator
interferon alfa-2a
interferon alfa-2b
Intron® A
Roferon-A®
Retinoic Acid Derivative
alitretinoin
Panretin™

KAWASAKI DISEASE

Immune Globulin
Gamimune® N
Gammabulin Immuno (Can)
Gammagard® S/D
Gammar®-P I.V.
immune globulin (intramuscular)
immune globulin (intravenous)
Polygam® S/D
Sandoglobulin®
Venoglobulin®-I
Venoglobulin®-S

LEPROSY

Immunosuppressant Agent
Contergan®
Distaval®
Kevadon®
thalidomide
Thalomid®
Leprostatic Agent

clofazimine
Lamprene®
Sulfone
Avlosulfon®
dapsone

LICE

Scabicides/Pediculicides
A-200™ Shampoo [OTC]
Acticin® Cream
Barc™ Liquid [OTC]
Elimite™ Cream
End Lice® Liquid [OTC]
GBH (Can)
G-well®
Hexit® (Can)
Kwellada® (Can)
Lice-Enz® Shampoo [OTC]
lindane
malathion
Nix™ Creme Rinse
Ovide™ Topical
permethrin
PMS-Lindane (Can)
Prioderm (Can)
Pronto® Shampoo [OTC]
pyrethrins and piperonyl butoxide
Pyrinex® Pediculicide Shampoo
    [OTC]
Pyrinyl II® Liquid [OTC]
Pyrinyl Plus® Shampoo [OTC]
R & C® Shampoo [OTC]
RID® Mousse [OTC]
RID® Shampoo [OTC]
Tisit® Blue Gel [OTC]
Tisit® Liquid [OTC]
Tisit® Shampoo [OTC]
Triple X® Liquid [OTC]

LICHEN SIMPLEX CHRONICUS

Topical Skin Product
doxepin
Zonalon® Topical Cream

LYME DISEASE

Antibiotic, Penicillin
pivampicillin (Canada only)
Pondocillin® (Can)
Cephalosporin (Third Generation)
ceftriaxone
Rocephin®
Macrolide (Antibiotic)
AK-Mycin®
Apo®-Erythro E-C (Can)
Diomycin (Can)
E.E.S.®
E-Mycin®
E-Mycin-E®
Erybid® (Can)
Eryc®
Ery-Tab®
Erythro-Base® (Can)
Erythrocin®
erythromycin (systemic)
Ilosone® Pulvules®
Ilotycin®
Novo-Rythro Encap (Can)
PCE®
PMS-Erythromycin (Can)
Wyamycin® S
Penicillin
amoxicillin
Amoxil®
ampicillin
Ampicin (Can)
Ampicin® Sodium (Can)
Ampilean (Can)
Apo®-Amoxi (Can)
Apo®-Ampi (Can)
Apo®-Pen VK (Can)
Gen-Amoxicillin (Can)
Jaa Amp® (Can)
Marcillin®
Nadopen-V® (Can)
Novamoxin® (Can)
Novo-Pen-VK® (Can)
Nu-Amoxi (Can)

Nu-Ampi (Can)
Nu-Pen-VK (Can)
Omnipen®
Omnipen®-N
penicillin V potassium
Principen®
Pro-Amox® (Can)
Totacillin®
Trimox®
Truxcillin®
Veetids®
Wymox®
Tetracycline Derivative
Achromycin® Ophthalmic
Achromycin® Topical
Achromycin V (Can)
Apo®-Doxy Tabs (Can)
Apo®-Tetra (Can)
Bio-Tab®
Doryx®
Doxy-200®
Doxy-Caps®
Doxychel®
Doxycin (Can)
doxycycline
Doxy-Tabs®
Doxytec (Can)
Monodox®
Nor-tet® Oral
Novo-Doxylin (Can)
Novo-Tetra (Can)
Nu-Doxycycline (Can)
Nu-Tetra (Can)
Panmycin® Oral
Robitet® Oral
Sumycin® Oral
Tetracap® Oral
tetracycline
Tetracyn (Can)
Topicycline® Topical
Vibramycin®
Vibra-Tabs®
Vaccine

Lyme disease vaccine
LYMErix™

MASTOCYTOSIS

Histamine H_2 Antagonist
Apo®-Cimetidine (Can)
Apo®-Famotidine (Can)
Apo®-Ranitidine (Can)
cimetidine
famotidine
Gaviscon Prevent (Can)
Maalox H2 Acid Controller (Can)
Novo-Cimetine (Can)
Novo-Famotidine (Can)
Novo-Ranidine (Can)
Nu-Cimet (Can)
Nu-Famotidine (Can)
Nu-Ranit (Can)
Pepcid®
Pepcid® AC Acid Controller [OTC]
Pepcid RPD®
Peptol® (Can)
ranitidine hydrochloride
Tagamet®
Tagamet-HB® [OTC]
Zantac®
Zantac® 75 [OTC]
Mast Cell Stabilizer
Crolom®
cromolyn sodium
Gastrocrom®
Intal®
Nalcrom (Can)
Nasalcrom® [OTC]
Novo-Cromolyn (Can)
Opticrom®
PMS-Sodium Cromoglycate (Can)
Rynacrom® (Can)
Vistacrom (Can)

MEASLES (RUBELLA)

Vaccine, Live Virus
measles and rubella vaccines,
combined

MoRu-Viraten (Can)
M-R-VAX® II

MEASLES (RUBEOLA)

Immune Globulin
  Gammabulin Immuno (Can)
  immune globulin (intramuscular)
Vaccine, Live Virus
  measles and rubella vaccines,
    combined
  MoRu-Viraten (Can)
  M-R-VAX® II

MELANOMA

Antineoplastic Agent
  Blenoxane®
  bleomycin
  CeeNU®
  cisplatin
  Cosmegen®
  dacarbazine
  dactinomycin
  Droxia™
  DTIC-Dome®
  Hydrea®
  hydroxyurea
  lomustine
  Platinol®
  Platinol®-AQ
  teniposide
  Vumon
Antiviral Agent
  interferon alfa-2b and ribavirin
    combination pack
  Rebetron™
Biological Response Modulator
  interferon alfa-2a
  interferon alfa-2b
  interferon alfa-2b and ribavirin
    combination pack
  Intron® A
  Rebetron™
  Roferon-A®

MUMPS (DIAGNOSTIC)

Diagnostic Agent
  MSTA® Mumps
  mumps skin test antigen

MYCOBACTERIUM AVIUM-INTRACELLULARE

Antibiotic, Aminoglycoside
  streptomycin
Antibiotic, Miscellaneous
  Mycobutin®
  rifabutin
  Rifadin® Injection
  Rifadin® Oral
  rifampin
  Rimactane® Oral
  Rofact® (Can)
Antimycobacterial Agent
  ethambutol
  Etibi® (Can)
  Myambutol®
Antitubercular Agent
  streptomycin
Carbapenem (Antibiotic)
  imipenem and cilastatin
  meropenem
  Merrem® I.V.
  Primaxin®
Leprostatic Agent
  clofazimine
  Lamprene®
Macrolide (Antibiotic)
  azithromycin
  Biaxin®
  Biaxin® XL
  clarithromycin
  Zithromax™
Quinolone
  Cipro®
  ciprofloxacin

OILY SKIN

Antiseborrheic Agent, Topical

Anti-Acne Formula for Men (Can)
Aveeno® Cleansing Bar [OTC]
Fostex® [OTC]
Meted (Can)
Night Cast R (Can)
Pernox® [OTC]
SAStid® Plain Therapeutic Shampoo
and Acne Wash [OTC]
Sebulex (Can)
sulfur and salicylic acid
Sulsal (Can)

ONYCHOMYCOSIS
Antifungal Agent
Fulvicin (Can)
Fulvicin® P/G
Fulvicin-U/F®
Grifulvin® V
Grisactin®
Grisactin® Ultra
griseofulvin
Grisovin®-FP (Can)
Gris-PEG®
Lamisil® Oral
terbinafine (oral)

ORGAN REJECTION
Immunosuppressant Agent
daclizumab
Zenapax®

ORGAN TRANSPLANT (SEE ALSO TISSUE GRAFT, GRAFT VS HOST DISEASE)
Immunosuppressant Agent
basiliximab
CellCept®
cyclosporine
muromonab-CD3
mycophenolate
Neoral®
Orthoclone® OKT3
Prograf®
Rapamune®

Sandimmune®
SangCya™
Simulect®
sirolimus
tacrolimus

PAIN (SKIN GRAFT HARVESTING)
Analgesic, Topical
EMLA®
lidocaine and prilocaine

PAPILLOMA
Keratolytic Agent
podophyllin and salicylic acid
Verrex-C&M®

PARACOCCIDIOIDO-MYCOSIS
Antifungal Agent
ketoconazole
Nizoral®
Novo-Ketoconazole (Can)
Nu-Ketocon (Can)

PERIANAL WART
Immune Response Modifier
Aldara™
imiquimod

PINWORMS
Anthelmintic
Antiminth® [OTC]
Combantrin (Can)
Jaa Pyral® (Can)
mebendazole
Pin-Rid® [OTC]
Pin-X® [OTC]
pyrantel pamoate
Reese's® Pinworm Medicine [OTC]
Vermox®

PITYRIASIS (ROSEA)
Corticosteroid, Topical
Aclovate® Topical

Acticort® Topical
Aeroseb-HC® Topical
Ala-Cort® Topical
Ala-Scalp® Topical
alclometasone
Alocort (Can)
Alphatrex® Topical
amcinonide
Anusol® HC-1 Topical [OTC]
Anusol® HC-2.5% Topical [OTC]
Aquacort® (Can)
Aristocort® A Topical
Aristocort® Topical
Bactine® Hydrocortisone [OTC]
Barriere-HC (Can)
Beben (Can)
Betacort (Can)
Betaderm (Can)
Betagel (Can)
Betalene® Topical
betamethasone (topical)
Betatrex® Topical
Beta-Val® Topical
Betnesol® (Can)
Betnovate (Can)
CaldeCort® Anti-Itch Topical Spray
CaldeCort® Topical [OTC]
Carmol-HC® Topical
Celestoderm (Can)
Cetacort® Topical
clobetasol
Clocort® Maximum Strength [OTC]
clocortolone
Cloderm® Topical
Cordran®
Cordran® SP
Cormax® Ointment
Cortacet (Can)
CortaGel® Topical [OTC]
Cortaid® Maximum Strength Topical
 [OTC]
Cortaid® with Aloe Topical [OTC]
Cortate (Can)

Cort-Dome® Topical
Cortef® Feminine Itch Topical
Cortizone®-5 Topical [OTC]
Cortizone®-10 Topical [OTC]
Cortoderm (Can)
Cutivate™
Cyclocort® Topical
Delcort® Topical
Delta-Tritex® Topical
Dermacort® Topical
Dermaflex HC (Can)
Dermarest Dricort® Topical
Derma-Smoothe/FS® Topical
Dermasone (Can)
Dermatop®
Dermolate® Topical [OTC]
Dermovate (Can)
Dermtex® HC with Aloe Topical
 [OTC]
Desocort (Can)
desonide
DesOwen® Topical
desoximetasone
diflorasone
Diprolene® AF Topical
Diprolene® Glycol (Can)
Diprolene® Topical
Diprosone (Can)
Diprosone® Topical
Drenison (Can)
Ectosone (Can)
Eldecort® Topical
Elocom® (Can)
Elocon®
Emo-Cort (Can)
Florone®
Florone E®
fluocinolone
fluocinonide
Fluoderm (Can)
Fluonid® Topical
flurandrenolide
Flurosyn® Topical

Flutex® Topical
fluticasone (topical)
Flutone (Can)
FS Shampoo® Topical
Gynecort® Topical [OTC]
halcinonide
halobetasol
Halog®
Halog®-E
Hi-Cor-1.0® Topical
Hi-Cor-2.5® Topical
Hycort
Hycort® Topical
Hyderm (Can)
hydrocortisone (topical)
Hydrocort® Topical
Hydrosone (Can)
Hydro-Tex® Topical [OTC]
Hytone® Topical
Kenalog® in Orabase®
Kenalog® Topical
Kenonel® Topical
LactiCare-HC® Topical
Lanacort® Topical [OTC]
Lidemol (Can)
Lidex®
Lidex-E®
Locoid® Topical
Lyderm (Can)
Maxiflor®
Maxivate® Topical
mometasone furoate
Nasonex®
Novobetamet (Can)
Nutracort® Topical
Orabase® HCA Topical
Penecort® Topical
prednicarbate
Prevex B (Can)
Prevex HC (Can)
Psorcon™
Psorion® Topical
Rholosone (Can)

Rhoprolene (Can)
Rhoprosone (Can)
Rivasone (Can)
Sarna HC (Can)
Scalpicin® Topical
Sential (Can)
S-T Cort® Topical
Synacort® Topical
Synalar-HP® Topical
Synalar® Topical
Synemol® Topical
Taro-Desoximetasone (Can)
Taro-Sone (Can)
Tegrin®-HC Topical [OTC]
Teladar® Topical
Temovate®
Texacort® Topical
Tiamol (Can)
Ti-U-Lac HC (Can)
Topactin (Can)
Topicort®
Topicort®-LP
Topilene (Can)
Topisone (Can)
Topsyn (Can)
Triacet™ Topical
Triaderm (Can)
triamcinolone (topical)
Tridesilon® Topical
U-Cort™ Topical
Ultravate™
Unicort (Can)
urea and hydrocortisone
Uremol-HC (Can)
Valisone® Topical
Westcort® Topical

PLANTARIS
Keratolytic Agent
Duofilm® Solution
Keralyt® Gel
salicylic acid and lactic acid
salicylic acid and propylene glycol

Soluver Plus (Can)
Tiacid (Can)
Topical Skin Product
Dey-Drop® Ophthalmic Solution
silver nitrate

POISON IVY
Protectant, Topical
bentoquatam
IvyBlock®

POISON OAK
Protectant, Topical
bentoquatam
IvyBlock®

POISON SUMAC
Protectant, Topical
bentoquatam
IvyBlock®

PROTOZOAL INFECTIONS
Antiprotozoal
Apo®-Metronidazole (Can)
Flagyl® Oral
furazolidone
Furoxone®
Metrocream (Can)
MetroGel® Topical
MetroGel®-Vaginal
Metro I.V.® Injection
metronidazole
NebuPent™ Inhalation
Neo-Metric (Can)
NidaGel (Can)
Noritate (Can)
Novo-Nidazol (Can)
Pentacarinat® Injection
Pentam-300® Injection
pentamidine
Pneumopent (Can)
Protostat® Oral
Trikacide (Can)

PSEUDOGOUT
Antigout Agent
colchicine
Nonsteroidal Anti-inflammatory Drug
(NSAID)
Apo®-Indomethacin (Can)
Indocid® (Can)
Indocid PDA (Can)
Indocin® Oral
Indocin® SR Oral
Indocollyre (Can)
indomethacin
Indotec (Can)
Novo-Methacin (Can)
Nu-Indo (Can)
Pro-Indo® (Can)
Rhodacine (Can)

PSORIASIS
Antibiotic/Corticosteroid, Topical
Neo-Cortef® Ophthalmic
neomycin and hydrocortisone
Antineoplastic Agent
Folex® PFS™
methotrexate
Rheumatrex®
Antipsoriatic Agent
AquaTar® [OTC]
Balnetar® [OTC]
calcipotriene
coal tar
coal tar and salicylic acid
coal tar, lanolin, and mineral oil
Denorex® [OTC]
DHS® Tar [OTC]
Doak-Oil (Can)
Dovonex®
Duplex® T [OTC]
Estar® [OTC]
etretinate
Fototar® [OTC]
Ionil-T (Can)
Ionil-T Plus (Can)

Mazon Medicated Soap (Can)
Neutrogena® T/Derm
Neutrogena T/Gel (Can)
Pentrax® [OTC]
Polytar® [OTC]
psoriGel® [OTC]
P & S Plus (Can)
Sebcur/T (Can)
Spectro Tar (Can)
Tardan (Can)
Tar Distillate (Can)
Tar Doak (Can)
Targel (Can)
Targel SA (Can)
Tegison®
Tegrin (Can)
Tersa-Tar (Can)
T/Gel® [OTC]
X-seb® T [OTC]
Zetar® [OTC]
Corticosteroid, Topical
Aclovate® Topical
Acticort® Topical
Aeroseb-HC® Topical
Ala-Cort® Topical
Ala-Scalp® Topical
alclometasone
Alocort (Can)
Alphatrex® Topical
amcinonide
Anusol® HC-1 Topical [OTC]
Anusol® HC-2.5% Topical [OTC]
Aquacort® (Can)
Aristocort® A Topical
Aristocort® Topical
Bactine® Hydrocortisone [OTC]
Barriere-HC (Can)
Beben (Can)
Betacort (Can)
Betaderm (Can)
Betagel (Can)
Betalene® Topical
betamethasone (topical)

Betatrex® Topical
Beta-Val® Topical
Betnesol® (Can)
Betnovate (Can)
CaldeCort® Anti-Itch Topical Spray
CaldeCort® Topical [OTC]
Carmol-HC® Topical
Celestoderm (Can)
Cetacort® Topical
clobetasol
Clocort® Maximum Strength [OTC]
clocortolone
Cloderm® Topical
Cordran®
Cordran® SP
Cormax® Ointment
Cortacet (Can)
CortaGel® Topical [OTC]
Cortaid® Maximum Strength Topical
  [OTC]
Cortaid® with Aloe Topical [OTC]
Cortate (Can)
Cort-Dome® Topical
Cortef® Feminine Itch Topical
Cortizone®-5 Topical [OTC]
Cortizone®-10 Topical [OTC]
Cortoderm (Can)
Cutivate™
Cyclocort® Topical
Delcort® Topical
Delta-Tritex® Topical
Dermacort® Topical
Dermaflex HC (Can)
Dermarest Dricort® Topical
Derma-Smoothe/FS® Topical
Dermasone (Can)
Dermatop®
Dermolate® Topical [OTC]
Dermovate (Can)
Dermtex® HC with Aloe Topical
  [OTC]
Desocort (Can)
desonide

DesOwen® Topical
desoximetasone
diflorasone
Diprolene® AF Topical
Diprolene® Glycol (Can)
Diprolene® Topical
Diprosone (Can)
Diprosone® Topical
Drenison (Can)
Ectosone (Can)
Eldecort® Topical
Elocom® (Can)
Elocon®
Emo-Cort (Can)
Florone®
Florone E®
fluocinolone
fluocinonide
Fluoderm (Can)
Fluonid® Topical
flurandrenolide
Flurosyn® Topical
Flutex® Topical
fluticasone (topical)
Flutone (Can)
FS Shampoo® Topical
Gynecort® Topical [OTC]
halcinonide
halobetasol
Halog®
Halog®-E
Hi-Cor-1.0® Topical
Hi-Cor-2.5® Topical
Hycort
Hycort® Topical
Hyderm (Can)
hydrocortisone (topical)
Hydrocort® Topical
Hydrosone (Can)
Hydro-Tex® Topical [OTC]
Hytone® Topical
Kenalog® in Orabase®
Kenalog® Topical

Kenonel® Topical
LactiCare-HC® Topical
Lanacort® Topical [OTC]
Lidemol (Can)
Lidex®
Lidex-E®
Locoid® Topical
Lyderm (Can)
Maxiflor®
Maxivate® Topical
mometasone furoate
Nasonex®
Novobetamet (Can)
Nutracort® Topical
Orabase® HCA Topical
Penecort® Topical
prednicarbate
Prevex B (Can)
Prevex HC (Can)
Psorcon™
Psorion® Topical
Rholosone (Can)
Rhoprolene (Can)
Rhoprosone (Can)
Rivasone (Can)
Sarna HC (Can)
Scalpicin® Topical
Sential (Can)
S-T Cort® Topical
Synacort® Topical
Synalar-HP® Topical
Synalar® Topical
Synemol® Topical
Taro-Desoximetasone (Can)
Taro-Sone (Can)
Tegrin®-HC Topical [OTC]
Teladar® Topical
Temovate®
Texacort® Topical
Tiamol (Can)
Ti-U-Lac HC (Can)
Topactin (Can)
Topicort®

Topicort®-LP
Topilene (Can)
Topisone (Can)
Topsyn (Can)
Triacet™ Topical
Triaderm (Can)
triamcinolone (topical)
Tridesilon® Topical
U-Cort™ Topical
Ultravate™
Unicort (Can)
urea and hydrocortisone
Uremol-HC (Can)
Valisone® Topical
Westcort® Topical
Keratolytic Agent
  Acnex (Can)
  Acnomel Acne Mask (Can)
  Anthra-Derm®
  Anthraforte® (Can)
  anthralin
  Anthranol® (Can)
  Anthrascalp® (Can)
  Anti-Acne Control Formula (Can)
  Anti-Acne Spot Treatment (Can)
  Blemish Control (Can)
  Callus Salve (Can)
  Clean & Clear Deep Cleaning
    Astringent (Can)
  Clean & Clear Invisible Clearasil
    Clearstick (Can)
  Clearasil® Pads (Can)
  Clear Away® Disc [OTC]
  Clear Pore Treatment (Can)
  Compound W (Can)
  Compound W Plus (Can)
  Drithocreme®
  Drithocreme® HP 1%
  Dritho-Scalp®
  Duoforte (Can)
  Fostex® Medicated Cleansing (Can)
  Freezone® Solution [OTC]
  Gordofilm® Liquid

Ionil (Can)
Keralyt (Can)
Keralyt® Gel
Mediplast® Plaster [OTC]
Micanol® Cream
Mosco (Can)
Mudd Acne (Can)
Neutrogena® Healthy Scalp Anti-
  Dandruff (Can)
Nova Perfecting Lotion (Can)
Occlusal (Can)
Occlusal®-HP Liquid
Off-Ezy® (Can)
Oil-Free Acne Wash (Can)
Oxy Control (Can)
Oxy Deep Pore (Can)
Oxy Medicated Pads (Can)
Oxy Night Watch (Can)
Oxy Power Pads (Can)
Panscol® Lotion [OTC]
Panscol® Ointment [OTC]
PediaPatch Transdermal Patch [OTC]
Propa PH (Can)
P&S® Shampoo [OTC]
Salac (Can)
Salacid® Ointment
Sal-Acid® Plaster
salicylic acid
salicylic acid and propylene glycol
Salseb (Can)
Scholl 2-Drop Corn Remedy (Can)
Scholl Corn, Callus Plaster
  Preparation (Can)
Scholl Corn Salve (Can)
Scholl Wart Remover (Can)
Scholl Zino (Can)
Sebcur (Can)
Soluver (Can)
tazarotene
Tazorac®
Ten-O-Six (Can)
Trans-Plantar® Transdermal Patch
  [OTC]

Trans-Ver-Sal® Transdermal Patch [OTC]
Vergogel® Gel [OTC]
Verukan® Solution
Wart Remover (Can)
X-Seb® (Can)
Psoralen
methoxsalen
Oxsoralen (Can)
Oxsoralen-Ultra®
Ultramop (Can)
Retinoid-like Compound
acitretin
Soriatane™

PURPURA

Immune Globulin
Gamimune® N
Gammagard® S/D
Gammar®-P I.V.
immune globulin (intravenous)
Polygam® S/D
Sandoglobulin®
Venoglobulin®-I
Venoglobulin®-S
Immunosuppressant Agent
azathioprine
Imuran®

PURPURA (THROMBOCYTOPENIC)

Antineoplastic Agent
Oncovin®
Vincasar® PFS™
vincristine

RATTLESNAKE BITE

Antivenin
antivenin (Crotalidae) polyvalent

RENAL ALLOGRAFT REJECTION

Immunosuppressant Agent
antithymocyte globulin (rabbit)

Thymoglobulin®

RHEUMATIC DISORDERS

Adrenal Corticosteroid
Acthar®
Actharn (Can)
Adlone® Injection
Ak-Tate (Can)
Amcort® Injection
A-methaPred® Injection
Apo®-Prednisone (Can)
Aristocort® Forte Injection
Aristocort® Intralesional Injection
Aristocort® Oral
Aristospan® Intra-articular Injection
Aristospan® Intralesional Injection
Atolone® Oral
Balpred (Can)
betamethasone (systemic)
Celestone® Oral
Celestone® Phosphate Injection
Celestone® Soluspan®
Cel-U-Jec® Injection
Cortef®
corticotropin
cortisone acetate
Cortone® Acetate
Decadron® Injection
Decadron®-LA
Decadron® Oral
Decaject®
Decaject-LA®
Delta-Cortef® Oral
Deltasone®
depMedalone® Injection
Depoject® Injection
Depo-Medrol® Injection
Depopred® Injection
dexamethasone (systemic)
Dexasone®
Dexasone® L.A.
Dexone®
Dexone® LA

Diopred (Can)
D-Med® Injection
Duralone® Injection
Haldrone®
Hexadrol®
H.P. Acthar® Gel
hydrocortisone (systemic)
Hydrocortone® Acetate
Inflamase (Can)
Jaa-Prednisone® (Can)
Kenacort® Oral
Kenaject® Injection
Kenalog® Injection
Key-Pred® Injection
Key-Pred-SP® Injection
Liquid Pred®
Medralone® Injection
Medrol® Oral
Medrol Veriderm (Can)
methylprednisolone
Meticorten®
M-Prednisol® Injection
Novo-Prednisolone (Can)
Orasone®
paramethasone acetate
Pediapred® Oral
PMS-Dexamethasone (Can)
Prednicen-M®
prednisolone (systemic)
Prednisol® TBA Injection
prednisone
Prelone® Oral
RO-Predphate (Can)
Scheinpharm Triamcine-A (Can)
Solu-Cortef®
Solu-Medrol® Injection
Solurex L.A.®
Stemex®
Tac™-3 Injection
Tac™-40 Injection
Triam-A® Injection
triamcinolone (systemic)
Triam Forte® Injection

Triamonide® Injection
Tri-Kort® Injection
Trilog® Injection
Trilone® Injection
Trisoject® Injection
Ultracortenol (Can)
Winpred (Can)

RHEUMATIC FEVER
Nonsteroidal Anti-inflammatory Drug
  (NSAID)
  Argesic®-SA
  Artha-G®
  Arthropan® [OTC]
  choline magnesium trisalicylate
  choline salicylate
  Disalcid®
  Herbogesic (Can)
  Magan®
  magnesium salicylate
  Magsal®
  Marthritic®
  Mobidin®
  Mono-Gesic®
  Salflex®
  Salgesic®
  salsalate
  Salsitab®
  Teejel (Can)
  Trilisate®
Penicillin
  Bicillin® C-R
  Bicillin® C-R 900/300
  penicillin G benzathine and procaine
    combined

RHINITIS
Adrenal Corticosteroid
  AeroBid®-M Oral Aerosol Inhaler
  AeroBid® Oral Aerosol Inhaler
  Alti-Flunisoline (Can)
  Apo®-Beclomethasone (Can)
  Beclodisk® (Can)
  Becloforte® (Can)

beclomethasone
Beclovent® Oral Inhaler
Beconase AQ® Nasal Inhaler
Beconase® Nasal Inhaler
Bronalide® (Can)
budesonide
Decadron® Injection
Decadron®-LA
Decadron® Oral
Decaject®
Decaject-LA®
Dexacort® Phosphate Turbinaire®
dexamethasone (nasal)
dexamethasone (systemic)
Dexasone®
Dexasone® L.A.
Dexone®
Dexone® LA
Entocort® (Can)
Flonase®
flunisolide
fluticasone (nasal)
Gen-Beclo (Can)
Hexadrol®
Nasalide® Nasal Aerosol
Nasarel™ Nasal Spray
Nu-Beclomethasone (Can)
PMS-Dexamethasone (Can)
Propaderm® (Can)
Pulmicort® Turbuhaler®
Rhinalar® (Can)
Rhinaris®-F (Can)
Rhinocort®
Solurex L.A.®
Syn-Flunisolide (Can)
Vancenase® AQ 84 mcg
Vancenase® AQ Inhaler
Vancenase® Nasal Inhaler
Vanceril® 84 mcg Double Strength
Vanceril® Oral Inhaler
Adrenergic Agonist Agent
  Actifed® Allergy Tablet (Day) [OTC]
  Afrin® Children's Nose Drops [OTC]

Afrin® Nasal Solution [OTC]
Afrinol® [OTC]
Allerest® 12 Hour Nasal Solution
  [OTC]
Balminil® Decongestant (Can)
Benylin Decongestant (Can)
Cenafed® [OTC]
Certified Decongestant (Can)
Children's Silfedrine® [OTC]
Chlorphed®-LA Nasal Solution
  [OTC]
Collyrium Fresh® Ophthalmic [OTC]
Congestac ND (Can)
Congest Aid (Can)
Congest-Eze (Can)
Contac Cold Nondrowsy (Can)
Decofed® Syrup [OTC]
Decongestant Nasal Spray (Can)
Decongestant Nose Drops (Can)
Decongestant Tablets (Can)
Dristan® Long Lasting Nasal
  Solution [OTC]
Drixoral® (Can)
Drixoral® Non-Drowsy [OTC]
Durafedrin (Can)
Duramist Plus® [OTC]
Duration® Nasal Solution [OTC]
Efidac/24® [OTC]
Eltor® (Can)
ephedrine
Kondon's Nasal® [OTC]
Mallazine® Eye Drops [OTC]
Maxenal (Can)
Nafrine (Can)
Nasal & Sinus Relief (Can)
Neofed® [OTC]
Neo-Synephrine® 12 Hour Nasal
  Solution [OTC]
Nostrilla® [OTC]
NTZ® Long Acting Nasal Solution
  [OTC]
Ornex Cold (Can)
Otrivin® Nasal [OTC]

oxymetazoline
PediaCare® Oral
Phenoxine® [OTC]
Phenyldrine® [OTC]
phenylpropanolamine
Plus Sinus™ (Can)
PMS-Pseudoephedrine (Can)
Pretz-D® [OTC]
Propagest® [OTC]
pseudoephedrine
Pseudofrin (Can)
Robidrine® (Can)
RO-Eye Drops (Can)
Sinarest® 12 Hour Nasal Solution
Sinex® Long-Acting [OTC]
Sudafed® [OTC]
Sudafed® 12 Hour [OTC]
Sudodrin (Can)
Sufedrin® [OTC]
Tantafed (Can)
tetrahydrozoline
Tetrasine® Extra Ophthalmic [OTC]
Tetrasine® Ophthalmic [OTC]
Triaminic® AM Decongestant
    Formula [OTC]
Twice-A-Day® Nasal Solution [OTC]
Tyzine® Nasal
Unitrol® [OTC]
Vaporisateur Nasal Decongestionnant
    (Can)
Vicks® Sinex (Can)
Visine® Workplace (Can)
4-Way® Long Acting Nasal Solution
    [OTC]
xylometazoline
Antihistamine
    Allegra®
    Aller-Chlor® Oral [OTC]
    Allergy Relief (Can)
    AL-Rr® Oral [OTC]
    Antihist-1® [OTC]
    Apo®-Cetirizine (Can)
    azatadine

Bromarest® [OTC]
Brombay® [OTC]
Bromphen® [OTC]
brompheniramine
Brotane® [OTC]
cetirizine
Chlo-Amine® Oral [OTC]
Chlorate® Oral [OTC]
Chlorphed® [OTC]
chlorpheniramine
Chlor-Pro® Injection
Chlor-Trimeton® Injection
Chlor-Trimeton® Oral [OTC]
Chlor-Tripolon (Can)
Claritin®
Claritin® RediTab®
clemastine
Contac Allergy Formula (Can)
Cophene-B®
cyproheptadine
Dexchlor®
dexchlorpheniramine
Diamine T.D.® [OTC]
Dimetane® Extentabs® [OTC]
fexofenadine
Gen-Cyproterone (Can)
Histalon (Can)
Klorominr® Oral [OTC]
loratadine
Nasahist B®
ND-Stat®
Nolahist® [OTC]
Novo-Pheniram (Can)
Optimine®
Periactin®
phenindamine
PMS-Cyproheptadine (Can)
Poladex®
Polaramine®
Pyribenzamine (Can)
Reactine (Can)
Tavist®
Tavist®-1 [OTC]

Telachlor® Oral
Teldrin® Oral [OTC]
terfenadine
tripelennamine
Vaginex (Can)
Zyrtec®
Antihistamine/Decongestant/Analgesic
phenyltoloxamine,
phenylpropanolamine, and
acetaminophen
Sinubid®
Sinutab® SA (Can)
Antihistamine/Decongestant/
Antitussive
Cerose-DM® [OTC]
chlorpheniramine, phenylephrine,
and codeine
chlorpheniramine, phenylephrine,
and dextromethorphan
Pediacof®
Pedituss®
Antihistamine/Decongestant
Combination
Actifed® Allergy Tablet (Night)
[OTC]
Allegra-D™
Antihist-D®
Banophen® Decongestant Capsule
[OTC]
Benadryl® Decongestant Allergy
Tablet [OTC]
Benylin® for Allergies (Can)
Brofed® Elixir [OTC]
Bromaline® Elixir [OTC]
Bromanate® Elixir [OTC]
Bromatapp® [OTC]
Bromfed® Syrup [OTC]
Bromfed® Tablet [OTC]
Bromfenex®
Bromfenex® PD
brompheniramine and phenylephrine
brompheniramine and
phenylpropanolamine

brompheniramine and
pseudoephedrine
Bromphen® Tablet [OTC]
chlorpheniramine, phenylephrine,
and phenylpropanolamine
chlorpheniramine, phenylephrine,
and phenyltoloxamine
chlorpheniramine, phenyltoloxamine,
phenylpropanolamine, and
phenylephrine
chlorpheniramine, pyrilamine,
phenylephrine, and
phenylpropanolamine
Chlor-Tripolon® N.D. (Can)
Claritin-D®
Claritin-D® 24-Hour
Claritin® Extra (Can)
clemastine and phenylpropanolamine
Cold & Allergy® Elixir [OTC]
Comhist®
Comhist® LA
Dimaphen® Elixir [OTC]
Dimaphen® Tablets [OTC]
Dimedrine (Can)
Dimetane® Decongestant Elixir
[OTC]
Dimetapp® 4-Hour Liqui-Gel
Capsule [OTC]
Dimetapp® Chewables (Can)
Dimetapp® Clear (Can)
Dimetapp® Elixir [OTC]
Dimetapp® Extentabs® [OTC]
Dimetapp® Tablet [OTC]
diphenhydramine and
pseudoephedrine
Drixoral® Syrup [OTC]
fexofenadine and pseudoephedrine
Genatap® Elixir [OTC]
Histalet Forte® Tablet
Hista-Vadrin® Tablet
Iofed®
Iofed® PD
loratadine and pseudoephedrine

Naldecon®
Naldelate®
Nalgest®
Nalspan®
New Decongestant®
Par Decon®
pheniramine, phenylpropanolamine,
    and pyrilamine
Tamine® [OTC]
Tavist-D®
Tri-Phen-Chlor®
Tri-P® Oral Infant Drops
Uni-Decon®
Vicks® DayQuil® Allergy Relief 4
    Hour Tablet [OTC]
Cold Preparation
phenyltoloxamine,
    phenylpropanolamine, pyrilamine,
    and pheniramine
Poly-Histine-D® Capsule
Corticosteroid, Intranasal
Elocom® (Can)
Elocon®
mometasone furoate
Nasonex®
Corticosteroid, Topical
Nasacort®
Nasacort® AQ
triamcinolone (inhalation, nasal)
Decongestant/Analgesic
Advil® Cold & Sinus Caplets [OTC]
Dayquil Sinus with Pain Relief (Can)
Dimetapp® Sinus Caplets [OTC]
Dristan® Sinus Caplets [OTC]
Motrin® IB Sinus [OTC]
pseudoephedrine and ibuprofen
Sine-Aid® IB [OTC]
Mast Cell Stabilizer
Crolom®
cromolyn sodium
Gastrocrom®
Intal®
Nalcrom (Can)

Nasalcrom® [OTC]
Novo-Cromolyn (Can)
Opticrom®
PMS-Sodium Cromoglycate (Can)
Rynacrom® (Can)
Vistacrom (Can)
Phenothiazine Derivative
Histantil (Can)
Phenazine® Injection
Phenergan® Injection
Phenergan® Oral
Phenergan® Rectal
promethazine
Prorex® Injection

RHINORRHEA
Anticholinergic Agent
Apo®-Ipravent (Can)
Atrovent®
Gen-Ipratropium (Can)
ipratropium

ROUNDWORMS
Anthelmintic
Antiminth® [OTC]
Combantrin (Can)
Jaa Pyral® (Can)
mebendazole
Pin-Rid® [OTC]
Pin-X® [OTC]
pyrantel pamoate
Reese's® Pinworm Medicine [OTC]
Vermox®

SCABIES
Scabicides/Pediculicides
A-200™ Shampoo [OTC]
Acticin® Cream
Barc™ Liquid [OTC]
crotamiton
Elimite™ Cream
End Lice® Liquid [OTC]
Eurax® Topical
GBH (Can)

G-well®
Hexit® (Can)
Kwellada® (Can)
Lice-Enz® Shampoo [OTC]
lindane
Nix™ Creme Rinse
permethrin
PMS-Lindane (Can)
Pronto® Shampoo [OTC]
pyrethrins and piperonyl butoxide
Pyrinex® Pediculicide Shampoo [OTC]
Pyrinyl II® Liquid [OTC]
Pyrinyl Plus® Shampoo [OTC]
R & C® Shampoo [OTC]
RID® Mousse [OTC]
RID® Shampoo [OTC]
Tisit® Blue Gel [OTC]
Tisit® Liquid [OTC]
Tisit® Shampoo [OTC]
Triple X® Liquid [OTC]

SCLERODERMA
Aminoquinoline (Antimalarial)
Aralen® Phosphate
chloroquine phosphate
Chelating Agent
Cuprimine®
Depen®
penicillamine

SEBORRHEIC DERMATITIS
Antiseborrheic Agent, Topical
Anti-Acne Formula for Men (Can)
Anti-Dandruff Shampoo (Can)
AquaTar® [OTC]
Avant Garde Shampoo (Can)
Aveeno® Cleansing Bar [OTC]
Balnetar® [OTC]
Capitrol®
chloroxine
coal tar
coal tar and salicylic acid
coal tar, lanolin, and mineral oil

Dandruff Treatment Shampoo (Can)
Dan-Gard (Can)
Denorex® [OTC]
DHS® Tar [OTC]
DHS Zinc® [OTC]
Doak-Oil (Can)
Duplex® T [OTC]
Estar® [OTC]
Exsel® Shampoo
Fostex® [OTC]
Fototar® [OTC]
Hair and Scalp (Can)
Head & Shoulders® [OTC]
Ionil-T (Can)
Ionil-T Plus (Can)
Keep Clear Anti-Dandruff Shampoo (Can)
Lander Dandruff Control (Can)
Mazon Medicated Soap (Can)
Meted (Can)
Neutrogena® T/Derm
Neutrogena T/Gel (Can)
Night Cast R (Can)
No-Name Dandruff Treatment (Can)
Novacet® Topical
Out of Africa (Can)
Pentrax® [OTC]
Pernox® [OTC]
Pert Plus (Can)
Polytar® [OTC]
psoriGel® [OTC]
P & S Plus (Can)
pyrithione zinc
SAStid® Plain Therapeutic Shampoo and Acne Wash [OTC]
Satinique Anti-Dandruff (Can)
Sebcur/T (Can)
Sebulex (Can)
Sebulon (Can)
selenium sulfide
Selsun Blue® Shampoo [OTC]
Selsun® Shampoo
Shaklee Dandruff Control (Can)

Shampooing Anti-Pelliculaire (Can)
Spectro Tar (Can)
Sulfacet-R® Topical
sulfur and salicylic acid
sulfur and sulfacetamide
Sulsal (Can)
Tardan (Can)
Tar Distillate (Can)
Tar Doak (Can)
Targel (Can)
Targel SA (Can)
Tegrin (Can)
Tersa-Tar (Can)
T/Gel® [OTC]
Theraplex Z® [OTC]
Versel (Can)
X-seb® T [OTC]
Zetar® [OTC]
Zincon® Shampoo [OTC]
ZNP® Bar [OTC]
ZP 11 (Can)
Keratolytic Agent
Acnex (Can)
Acnomel Acne Mask (Can)
Anti-Acne Control Formula (Can)
Anti-Acne Spot Treatment (Can)
Blemish Control (Can)
Callus Salve (Can)
Clean & Clear Deep Cleaning
  Astringent (Can)
Clean & Clear Invisible Clearasil
  Clearstick (Can)
Clearasil® Pads (Can)
Clear Away® Disc [OTC]
Clear Pore Treatment (Can)
Compound W (Can)
Compound W Plus (Can)
Duoforte (Can)
Fostex® Medicated Cleansing (Can)
Freezone® Solution [OTC]
Gordofilm® Liquid
Ionil (Can)
Keralyt (Can)

Mediplast® Plaster [OTC]
Mosco (Can)
Mudd Acne (Can)
Neutrogena® Healthy Scalp Anti-
  Dandruff (Can)
Nova Perfecting Lotion (Can)
Occlusal (Can)
Occlusal®-HP Liquid
Off-Ezy® (Can)
Oil-Free Acne Wash (Can)
Oxy Control (Can)
Oxy Deep Pore (Can)
Oxy Medicated Pads (Can)
Oxy Night Watch (Can)
Oxy Power Pads (Can)
Panscol® Lotion [OTC]
Panscol® Ointment [OTC]
PediaPatch Transdermal Patch
  [OTC]
Propa PH (Can)
P&S® Shampoo [OTC]
Salac (Can)
Salacid® Ointment
Sal-Acid® Plaster
salicylic acid
Salseb (Can)
Scholl 2-Drop Corn Remedy (Can)
Scholl Corn, Callus Plaster
  Preparation (Can)
Scholl Corn Salve (Can)
Scholl Wart Remover (Can)
Scholl Zino (Can)
Sebcur (Can)
Soluver (Can)
Ten-O-Six (Can)
Trans-Plantar® Transdermal Patch
  [OTC]
Trans-Ver-Sal® Transdermal Patch
  [OTC]
Vergogel® Gel [OTC]
Verukan® Solution
Wart Remover (Can)
X-Seb® (Can)

SKIN ULCER

Enzyme
Biozyme-C®
collagenase
Santyl®
Topical Skin Product
Debrisan® [OTC]
dextranomer

SOLAR LENTIGINES

Retinoic Acid Derivative
mequinol and tretinoin
Solagé™ Topical Solution

SUN OVEREXPOSURE

Sunscreen
Active Dry Lotion (Can)
Big V (Can)
Coppertone Lipkote (Can)
Coppertone® Oil-Free (Can)
Coppertone® Skin Selects (Can)
Coppertone® Sport (Can)
Coppertone® Sunscreen (Can)
Coppertone® Waterproof Sunblock
(Can)
Faces Only (Can)
Fruit of the Earth Moisturizing Aloe
(Can)
Fruit of the Earth Moisturizing Aloe
Sport (Can)
Hawaiian Tropic® Herbal (Can)
Herbal Answer (Can)
Huile Solaire Bronzage (Can)
Labello Active (Can)
London Drugs Sport (Can)
London Drugs Sunblock (Can)
London Drugs Sunscreen (Can)
Marcelle Sunblock (Can)
methoxycinnamate and oxybenzone
NO-AD Sunscreen (Can)
Ponds Prevent (Can)
PreSun® 29 [OTC]
Shade (Can)
Shaklee Sunscreen (Can)
Shiseido Sunblock (Can)
Sun Defense Lip Block (Can)
Sun Defense Sunscreen (Can)
Sun Management Lip Protection
(Can)
Sun Management Sensible Protection
(Can)
Sunseekers (Can)
Ti-Screen® [OTC]
Ti-UVA-B (Can)
Vaseline Lip Therapy (Can)
Water Babies (Can)

SYSTEMIC LUPUS ERYTHEMATOSUS (SLE)

Aminoquinoline (Antimalarial)
hydroxychloroquine
Plaquenil®
Antineoplastic Agent
cyclophosphamide
Cytoxan®
Neosar®
Procytox® (Can)

TAPEWORM INFESTATION

Amebicide
Humatin®
paromomycin
Anthelmintic
Biltricide®
praziquantel

TETANUS (PROPHYLAXIS)

Antitoxin
tetanus antitoxin

TINEA

Antifungal Agent
Absorbine® Antifungal [OTC]
Absorbine® Antifungal Foot Powder
[OTC]
Absorbine® Jock Itch [OTC]
Absorbine Jr.® Antifungal [OTC]
Aftate® [OTC]

benzoic acid and salicylic acid
Breezee® Mist Antifungal [OTC]
butenafine
Caldesene® Topical [OTC]
Canesten (Can)
carbol-fuchsin solution
ciclopirox
clioquinol
Clotrimaderm (Can)
clotrimazole
Cruex (Can)
Desenex® [OTC]
econazole
Ecostatin® (Can)
Exelderm® Topical
Femizol-M® [OTC]
Fulvicin (Can)
Fulvicin® P/G
Fulvicin-U/F®
Fungoid® AF Topical Solution [OTC]
Fungoid® Creme
Fungoid® Solution
Fungoid® Tincture
Genaspor® [OTC]
Grifulvin® V
Grisactin®
Grisactin® Ultra
griseofulvin
Grisovin®-FP (Can)
Gris-PEG®
Gyne-Lotrimin® [OTC]
Gyne-Lotrimin® 3 [OTC]
haloprogin
Halotex®
ketoconazole
Lamisil® Cream
Loprox®
Lotrimin®
Lotrimin® AF Cream [OTC]
Lotrimin® AF Lotion [OTC]
Lotrimin® AF Powder [OTC]
Lotrimin® AF Solution [OTC]

Lotrimin® AF Spray Liquid [OTC]
Lotrimin® AF Spray Powder [OTC]
Maximum Strength Desenex®
Antifungal Cream [OTC]
Mentax®
Micatin® Topical [OTC]
miconazole
Mitrazol® [OTC]
Monazole-7® (Can)
Monistat-Derm™ Topical
Monistat i.v.™ Injection
Monistat™ Vaginal
Mycelex®
Mycelex®-7
Mycelex®-G
Myclo-Derm (Can)
Myclo-Gyne (Can)
M-Zole® 7 Dual Pack [OTC]
naftifine
Naftin®
Neo-Zol (Can)
Nizoral®
Nizoral® A-D Shampoo [OTC]
Novo-Ketoconazole (Can)
NP-27® [OTC]
Nu-Ketocon (Can)
Ony-Clear® Nail
Ony-Clear® Spray
oxiconazole
Oxistat® Topical
Pedi-Pro Topical [OTC]
Pitrex (Can)
Prescription Strength Desenex® [OTC]
Scholl Athlete's Foot Preparations (Can)
sodium thiosulfate
Spectazole™
sulconazole
terbinafine (topical)
Tinactin® [OTC]
Tinver® [OTC]
tolnaftate

triacetin
Tritin (Can)
Trivagizole 3™ [OTC]
undecylenic acid and derivatives
Versiclear™
Vioform® [OTC]
Whitfield's Ointment [OTC]
Zeasorb-AF® [OTC]
Zeasorb-AF® Powder [OTC]
Antifungal/Corticosteroid
betamethasone and clotrimazole
Lotriderm® (Can)
Lotrisone®
Antiseborrheic Agent, Topical
Exsel® Shampoo
selenium sulfide
Selsun Blue® Shampoo [OTC]
Selsun® Shampoo
Versel (Can)
Disinfectant
sodium hypochlorite solution

TISSUE GRAFT

Immunosuppressant Agent
CellCept®
cyclosporine
muromonab-CD3
mycophenolate
Neoral®
Orthoclone® OKT3
Prograf®
Sandimmune®
SangCya™
tacrolimus

TRANSFUSION REACTION

Antihistamine
Aller-Aide (Can)
Aller-Chlor® Oral [OTC]
Allerdryl® (Can)
Allergy Elixir (Can)
Allergy Relief (Can)
Allergy Tablets (Can)
AllerMax® Oral [OTC]
Allernix® (Can)
AL-Rr® Oral [OTC]
Antihist-1® [OTC]
Anxanil® Oral
Apo®-Hydroxyzine (Can)
Atarax® Oral
Atozine® Oral
azatadine
Banophen® Oral [OTC]
Belix® Oral [OTC]
Benadryl® Injection
Benadryl® Oral [OTC]
Benadryl® Topical
Ben-Allergin-50® Injection
Bromarest® [OTC]
Brombay® [OTC]
Bromphen® [OTC]
brompheniramine
Brotane® [OTC]
Calmex (Can)
Chlo-Amine® Oral [OTC]
Chlorate® Oral [OTC]
Chlorphed® [OTC]
chlorpheniramine
Chlor-Pro® Injection
Chlor-Trimeton® Injection
Chlor-Trimeton® Oral [OTC]
Chlor-Tripolon (Can)
Claritin®
Claritin® RediTab®
Clear Caladryl Spray (Can)
clemastine
Contac Allergy Formula (Can)
Cophene-B®
cyproheptadine
Dexchlor®
dexchlorpheniramine
Diamine T.D.® [OTC]
Dihyrex® Injection
Dimetane® Extentabs® [OTC]
Diphenacen-50® Injection [OTC]
Diphen® Cough [OTC]
Diphenhist [OTC]

diphenhydramine
Genahist® Oral
Gen-Cyproterone (Can)
Histalon (Can)
Hydramyn® Syrup [OTC]
hydroxyzine
Hy-Pam® Oral
Hyrexin-50® Injection
Hyzine-50® Injection
Klorominr® Oral [OTC]
loratadine
Maximum Strength Nytol® [OTC]
Nasahist B®
ND-Stat®
Neucalm-50® Injection
Nolahist® [OTC]
Nordryl® Injection
Nordryl® Oral
Novo-Pheniram (Can)
Optimine®
Periactin®
Phendry® Oral [OTC]
phenindamine
PMS-Cyproheptadine (Can)
Poladex®
Polaramine®
Pyribenzamine (Can)
Tavist®
Tavist®-1 [OTC]
Telachlor® Oral
Teldrin® Oral [OTC]
tripelennamine
Vistaril® Injection
Vistaril® Oral
Vistazine® Injection
Phenothiazine Derivative
Histantil (Can)
Phenazine® Injection
Phenergan® Injection
Phenergan® Oral
Phenergan® Rectal
promethazine
Prorex® Injection

ULCER, DIABETIC FOOT OR LEG
Topical Skin Product
becaplermin
Regranex®

VARICELLA
Antiviral Agent
acyclovir
Avirax® (Can)
foscarnet
Foscavir®
Zovirax®
Immune Globulin
Gammabulin Immuno (Can)
immune globulin (intramuscular)

VARICELLA-ZOSTER
Vaccine, Live Virus
varicella virus vaccine
Varivax®

VARICOSE ULCERS
Protectant, Topical
Granulex
trypsin, balsam Peru, and castor oil

VENEREAL WARTS
Biological Response Modulator
Alferon® N
interferon alfa-n3

VITILIGO
Psoralen
methoxsalen
Oxsoralen (Can)
Oxsoralen-Ultra®
trioxsalen
Trisoralen®
Ultramop (Can)
Topical Skin Product
Benoquin®
monobenzone

WHIPWORMS
Anthelmintic
  mebendazole
  Vermox®

WORMS
Anthelmintic

Biltricide®
Mintezol®
oxamniquine
praziquantel
thiabendazole
Vansil™

Transplant Organizations

ORGAN PROCUREMENT ORGANIZATIONS

Organ Procurement Organizations (OPOs) coordinate the procurement of organs in designated service areas; these service areas may cover complete states or portions of states. For each state below, please find a list of the OPOs that provide services within its boundaries.

Alabama
Alabama Organ Center
301 South 20th Street, Suite 1001
Birmingham, AL 35233
Phone: (205)731–9200/(800)252–3677
Web: www.uab.edu/aoc

Alaska
LifeCenter Northwest
1407 116th Avenue, NE, Suite E210
Bellevue, WA 98004
Phone: (425)201–6563
Web: www.lcnw.org

Arizona
Donor Network of Arizona
201 West Coolidge
Phoenix, AZ 85013
Phone: (602)222–2200/(800)943–6667
Web: www.dnaz.org

Arkansas
Arkansas Regional Organ Recovery
   Agency
1100 N. University Avenue, Suite 200
Little Rock, AR 72207
Phone: (501)224–2623
Web: www.arora.org

Mid-America Transplant Services
1139 Olivette Executive Parkway
St. Louis, MO 63132
Phone: (314)991–1661/(800)87-Donor
Web: www.mts.stl.org

Mid-South Transplant Foundation
   (Eastern AR)
910 Madison Avenue, Suite 1002
Memphis, TN 38103
Phone: (901)326–4438
Web: www.midsouthtransplant.org

Southwest Transplant Alliance
3710 Rawlins #1100
Dallas, TX 75219
Phone: (214)522–0255
Web: www.organ.org

California
California Transplant Donor Network
1611 Telegraph Avenue, Suite 600
Oakland, CA 94612-2149
Phone: (510)444–8500
Web: www.ctdn.org

Golden State Donor Service
1760 Creekside Oaks Drive, Suite 160
Sacramento, CA 95833
Phone: (916)567–1600
Web: www.gsds.org

Life Sharing Community Organ
  Donation
3465 Camino Del Rio S., Suite 410
San Diego, CA 92108
Phone: (619)521–1983
Web: www.lifesharing.org

One Legacy
2200 West 3rd Street, 2nd Floor
Los Angeles, CA 90057
Phone: (213)413–6219
Web: http://pages.pages.prodigy.com/
  scope

Colorado
Donor Alliance, Inc.
3773 Cherry Creek North Drive,
  Suite 601
Denver, CO 80209
Phone: (303)329–4747/(888)686–4747
Web: www.donoralliance. org

Connecticut
Northeast OPO & Tissue Bank Hartford
  Hospital
80 Seymour Street, P.O. Box 5037
Hartford, CT 06102-5037
Phone: (806)545–6104
Fax: (860)545–4143
Web: www.harthosp.org/NEOPO

New England Organ Bank
One Gateway Center
Washington Street at Newton Center
Newton, MA 02458-2803
Phone: (800)446-NEOB
Web: www.neob.org

Delaware
Gift of Life Donor Program
2000 Hamilton Street, Suite 201
Philadelphia, PA 19130-3813
Phone: (215)557–8090
Web: www.donors1.org

District of Columbia
Washington Regional Transplant
  Consortium
8110 Gatehouse Road, Suite 101-West
Falls Church, VA 22042
Phone: (703)641–0100/(202)223–8229
Web: www.donors1.org

Florida
LifeLink of Florida
409 Bayshore Boulevard
Tampa, FL 33606
Phone: (813)348–6308
Web: www.lifelinkfound.org

LifeQuest, Organ Recovery Services
720 SW 2nd Avenue, Suite 570
Gainesville, FL 32601
Phone: (352)338–7133

TransLife/Florida Hospital
2501 North Orange Avenue, Suite 40
Orlando, FL 32804
Phone: (407)303–2474
Fax: (407)303–2473

University of Miami OPO
1150 Northwest 14th Street, Suite 208
Miami, FL 33136
Phone: (305)243–7622
Web: www.med.miami.edu/OPO

Georgia

Alabama Organ Center
301 South 20th Street, Suite 1001
Birmingham, AL 35233
Phone: (205)731–9200/(800)252–3677
Web: www.uab.edu/aoc

LifeLink of Georgia
3715 Northside Parkway
Bldg 100 Northcreek, Suite 300
Atlanta, GA 30327
Phone: (404)266–8884
Web: ww.lifelinkfound.org/georgia/ga.
html

Hawaii

Organ Donor Center of Hawaii
900 Fort Street Mall, Suite 1140
Honolulu, HI 96813
Phone: (808)599–7630
Fax: (808)599–7631

Idaho

Intermountain Organ Recovery System
(SE Idaho)
230 South 500 East, Suite 290
Salt Lake City, UT 84102
Phone: (801)521–1755
Web: www.iors.com

LifeCenter Northwest (No. Idaho)
1407 116th Avenue, NE, Suite 210
Bellevue, WA 98004
Phone: (425)210–6563
Web: www.lcnw.org

Pacific Northwest Transplant Bank
2611 Southwest 3rd Avenue, Suite 320
Portland, OR 97201-4952
Phone: (503)494–5560
Web: www.pntb.org

Illinois

Mid-America Transplant Association
1139 Olivette Executive Parkway
St. Louis, MO 63132
Phone: (800)87-DONOR/
(314)991–1661
Web: www.mts-stl.org

Regional Organ Bank of Illinois, Inc.
800 South Wells Street, Suite 190
Chicago, IL 60607-4529
Phone: (312)431–3600/
(800)545-GIFT (4438)
Web: www.robi.org

Indiana

Indiana Organ Procurement
Organization, Inc.
429 N. Pennsylvania Street, Suite 201
Indianapolis, IN 46204
Phone: (317)685–0389/(888)ask-iopo
Web: www.iopo.org

Kentucky Organ Donor Affiliates
106 East Broadway
Louisville, KY 40202
Phone: (502)581–9511
Web: www.kodaorgan.com

Ohio Valley Life Center (SE Indiana)
2925 Vernon Place, Suite 300
Cincinnati, OH 45219
Phone: (513)558–5555 or
(800)981-LIFE
Web: www.lifecnt.org

Regional Organ Bank of Illinois, Inc.
800 South Wells Street, Suite 190
Chicago, IL 60607-4529
Phone: (312)431–3600/
(800)545-GIFT (4438)
Web: www.robi.org

Iowa

Iowa Donor Network
2732 Northgate Drive
Iowa City, IA 52245
Phone: (319)337–7515
Web: www.iadn.org

Nebraska Organ Retrieval System
 (W. Iowa)
5725 F Street
Omaha, NE 68117
Phone: (402)733–4000

Kansas

Midwest Organ Bank, Inc.
1900 West 47th Place, Suite 400
Westwood, KS 66205
Phone: (913)262–1666
Web: www.mwob.org/

Kentucky

Kentucky Organ Donor Affiliates
106 East Broadway
Louisville, KY 40202
Phone: (502)581–9511
Web: www.kodaorgan.com

Indiana Organ Procurement
 Organization, Inc.
429 N. Pennsylvania Street, Suite 201
Indianapolis, IN 46204
Phone: (317)685–0389/(888)ask-iopo
Web: www.iopo.org

Tennessee Donor Services
1714 Hayes Street
Nashville, TN 37203
Phone: (615)234–5251
Web: www.kornet.org/donors

Louisiana

Louisiana Organ Procurement Agency
3501 North Causeway Boulevard,
 Suite 940
Metarie, LA 70002-3626
Phone: (504) 837–3355
Web: www.lopa.org

Maine

New England Organ Bank
Washington Street at Newton Corner
Newton, MA 02158-2803
Phone: (617)244–8000
Web: www.info@neob.org

Maryland

Transplant Resource Center of Maryland
1540 Caton Center Drive, Suite R
Baltimore, MD 21227
Web: www.mdtransplant.org

Washington Regional Transplant
 Consortium
8110 Gatehouse Road, Suite 101-West
Falls Church, VA 22042
Phone: (703)641–0100
Web: www.wrtc.org

Massachusetts

New England Organ Bank
Washington Street at Newton Corner
Newton, MA 02158-2803
Phone: (617)244–8000
Web: www.info@neob.org

Michigan

Transplantation Society of Michigan
2203 Platt Road
Ann Arbor, MI 48104
Phone: (734)973–1577
Web: www.tsm-giftoflife.com

University of Wisconsin OPO
Department of Surgery
600 Highland Avenue
Madison, WI 53792
Phone: (608)263–1341
*Web: www.surgery.wisc.edu/patient/
patient_txopoindex.html*

Minnesota

LifeSource, Upper Midwest Organ
Procurement Organization, Inc.
2550 University Avenue West, Suite 315
South St. Paul, MN 55114-1904
Phone: (612)603–7800
Web: www.life-source.org

Mississippi

Mississippi Organ Recovery Agency
12 River Bend Place, Suite B
Jackson, MS 39208
Phone: (601)933–1000
Web: www.msora.org

Missouri

Mid-America Transplant Services
1139 Olivette Executive Parkway
St. Louis, MO 63132
Phone: (314)991–1661
Web: www.mts-stl.org

Midwest Organ Bank, Inc.
1900 West 47th Place, Suite 400
Westwood, KS 66205
Phone: (913)262–1666
Web: www.mwob.org/

Nebraska

Nebraska Organ Retrieval System
5725 F Street
Omaha, NE 68117
Phone: (402)733–4000

Iowa Donor Network
2732 Northgate Drive
Iowa City, IA 52245
Phone: (319)337–7515
Web: www.iadn.org

Nevada

Nevada Donor Network, Inc.
4580 South Eastern Avenue, Suite 33
Las Vegas, NV 89119-6105
Phone: (702)796–9600

California Transplant Donor Network
1611 Telegraph Avenue, Suite 600
Oakland, CA 94612-2149
Phone: (510)444–8500
Web: www.ctdn.org

New Hampshire

New England Organ Bank
Washington Street at Newton Corner
Newton, MA 02158-2803
Phone: (617)244–8000
Web: www.info@neob.org

New Jersey

New Jersey Organ & Tissue Sharing
  Network
841 Mountain Avenue
Springfield, NJ 07081
Phone: (973)379–4535
Web: www.sharenj.org

Gift of Life Donor Program
2000 Hamilton Street, Suite 201
Philadelphia, PA 19130-3813
Phone: (215)557–8090/(610)543–6391
Web: www.donors1.org

New Mexico

New Mexico Donor Services
2715 Broadbent Parkway, Suite JNE
Albuquerque, NM 87107
Phone: (505)843–7672

New York

Center for Donation and Transplant
218 Great Oaks Boulevard
Albany, NY 12203
Phone: (518)262–5606
Web: www.centerfordonation.com

Center for Organ Recovery & Education
204 Sigma Drive, RIDC Park
Pittsburgh, PA 15238
Phone: (800)366–6777
Web: www.core.org

New York Organ Donor Network, Inc.
475 Riverside Drive, Suite 1244
New York, NY 10115-1244
Phone: (212)870–2240
Web: www.nyodn.org

Upstate New York Transplant Services,
  Inc.
165 Genesse Street, Suite 102
Buffalo, NY 14203
Phone: (716)853–6667
Web: www.donorrecovery.org

Finger Lakes Donor Recovery Network
Corporate Woods of Brighton
Building 30, Suite 220
Rochester, NY 14623
Phone: (716)272–4930
Web: www.donorrecovery.org

North Carolina

Carolina Organ Procurement Agency
702 John Hopkins Drive
Greenville, NC 27834
Phone: (919)757–0090
Web: www.copanc.org

LifeShare of the Carolinas
P.O. Box 32861
Charlotte, NC 28232-2861
Phone: (704)548–6850
Web: www.lifesharecarolinas.org

Ohio

LifeBanc
20600 Chagrin Boulevard, Suite 350
Cleveland, OH 44122-5343
Phone: (216)752–5433
Web: www.lifebanc.org

Life Connection of Ohio
1545 Holland Road, Suite C
Maumee, OH 43537-1694
Phone: (419)893–4891
Web: www.lifeconnectionofohio.org

Lifeline of Ohio Organ Procurement
Agency
770 Kinnear Road, Suite 200
Columbus, OH 43212
Phone: (614)291–5667
Web: www.lifelinofohio.org

Ohio Valley Life Center
2925 Vernon Place, Suite 300
Cincinnati, OH 45219-2425
Phone: (513)558–5555 or (800)981–5433
Web: www.lifecnt.org

Kentucky Organ Donor Affiliates
106 East Broadway
Louisville, KY 40202
Phone: (502)581–9511
Web: www.kodaorgan.com

Oklahoma

Oklahoma Organ Sharing Network
5801 North Broadway, Suite 200
Oklahoma City, OK 73118
Phone: (405)840–5551
Web: www.oosn.com

Oregon

LifeCenter Northwest
1407 116th Avenue, NE, Suite 210
Bellevue, WA 98004
Phone: (425)201–6563
Web: www.lcnw.org

Pacific Northwest Transplant Bank
2611 Southwest 3rd Avenue, Suite 320
Portland, OR 97201-4952
Phone: (503)494–5560
Web: www.pntb.org

Pennsylvania

The Center for Organ Recovery &
Education
204 Sigma Drive
Pittsburgh, PA 15238
Phone: (800)366–6777/(412)963–3550
Web: www.core.org

Gift of Life Donor Program
2000 Hamilton Street, Suite 201
Philadelphia, PA 19130-3813
Phone: (215)557–8090/(610)543–6391
Web: www.donors1.org

Puerto Rico

LifeLink of Puerto, Compaq Center,
Suite 402
Street 1, No. 3 Metro Office Park
Guaynaba, PR 00968
Phone: (787)227–0900
Web: www.lifelinkfound.org/pr/pr.html

Rhode Island

New England Organ Bank
Washington Street at Newton Corner
Newton, MA 02158-2803
Phone: (617)244–8000
Web: www.neob.org

South Carolina

South Carolina Organ Procurement
Agency
1064 Gardner Road, Suite 105
Charleston, SC 29407
Phone: (843)763–7755
*Web: www.midnet.sc.edu/scopa/scopa.
htm*

Tennessee

Mid-South Transplant Foundation
910 Madison Avenue, Suite 805
Memphis, TN 38103
Phone: (901)448–4588
Web: www.midsouthtransplant.org

Tennessee Donor Services
1714 Hayes Street
Nashville, TN 37203
Phone: (615)234–5251
Web: www.kornet.org/donors

Texas

LifeGift Organ Donation Center
5615 Kirby Drive, Suite 900
Houston, TX 77005
Phone: (713)523–4438
Web: www.lifegift.org

Texas Organ Sharing Alliance
8122 Datapoint Drive, Suite 1150
San Antonio, TX 78229
Phone: (210)614–7030

Southwest Transplant Alliance
3710 Rawlins #1100
Dallas, TX 75219
Phone: (214)522–0255
Web: www.organ.org

Utah

Intermountain Organ Recovery Systems
230 South 500 East, Suite 290
Salt Lake City, UT 84102
Phone: (801)521–1755
Web: www.iors.com

Vermont

Center for Donation and Transplant
218 Great Oaks Boulevard
Albany, NY 12203
Phone: (518)262–5606
Web: www.centerfordonation.com

New England Organ Bank
Washington Street at Newton Corner
Newton, MA 02158-2803
Phone: (617)244–8000
Web: www.info@neob.org

Virginia

LifeNet
5809 Ward Court
Virginia Beach, VA 23455
Phone: (757)464–4761
Web: www.lifenet.org/index.html

Washington Regional Transplant
    Consortium
8110 Gatehouse Road, Suite 101-West
Falls Church, VA 22042
Phone: (703)641–0100
Web: www.wrtc.org

Carolina Organ Procurement Agency
702 John Hopkins Drive
Greenville, NC 27834
Phone: (919)757–0090
Web: www.copanc.org

Washington

LifeCenter Northwest
1407 116th Avenue, NE, Suite 210
Bellevue, WA 98004
Phone: (425)201–6563
Web: www.lcnw.org

West Virginia

The Center for Organ Recovery &
  Education
204 Sigma Drive
Pittsburgh, PA 15238
Phone: (800)366–6777/(412)963–3550
Web: www.core.org

Kentucky Organ Donor Affiliates
106 East Broadway
Louisville, KY 40202
Phone: (502)581–9511
Web: www.kodaorgan.com

Wisconsin

Wisconsin Donor Network
9200 West Wisconsin Avenue
Milwaukee, WI 53226
Phone: (414)805–2024

University of Wisconsin OPO
Department of Surgery
600 Highland Avenue
Madison, WI 53792
Phone: (608)263–1341
*Web: www.surgery.wisc.edu/patient/
  patient_txopoindex.html*

Wyoming

Intermountain Organ Recovery Systems
230 South 500 East, Suite 290
Salt Lake City, UT 84102
Phone: (801)521–1755
Web: www.iors.com

Donor Alliance, Inc.
3773 Cherry Creek North Drive,
  Suite 601
Denver, CO 80209
Phone: (303)329–4747/(888)686–4747
Web: www.donoralliance.org

ORGAN AND TISSUE ORGANIZATIONS

American Association of Tissue Banks

Richard J. Kagan, President
P. Robert Rigney, Chief Executive Officer
1350 Beverly Road, Suite 220-A
McLean, VA 22101
Phone: (703)827–9582
Fax: (703)356–2198

American Red Cross National Tissue Services

Henry Korent, Chief Operating Office
1621 North Kent Street
Arlington, VA 22209
Phone: (703)248–4280
Fax: (703)248–4128

Coalition on Donation

Charles McClusky
c/o Life Quest Organ Recovery Services
720 SW 2nd Avenue
North Tower, Suite 570
Gainesville, FL 32601
(352)338–7133
(352)338–7135

David Fleming, Executive Director
1100 Boulders Parkway, Suite 500
Richmond, VA 23225-8770
Phone: (804)330–8620
Fax: (804)330–8593

Eye Bank Association of America

Patricia Aiken-Neill, President & CEO
1015 18th Street, Suite 1010
Washington, DC 20036-5504
Phone: (202)775–4999
Fax: (202)429–6036

Lifenet

Bill Anderson, CEO
5809 Ward Court
Virginia Beach, VA 23455
Phone: (800)847–7831

James Redford Institute for Transplant Awareness

President and Founder
Annie Aft, Executive Director
10573 West Pico Blvd., #214
Los Angeles, CA 90064
Phone: (310)441–4906
Fax: (310)441–9506

Mickey Mantle Foundation

Roy True
8080 Central, Suite 800
Dallas, TX 75206-1877
Phone: (214)987–7977
Fax: (214)691–0418

Musculoskeletal Transplant Foundation

Martha Anderson, Vice President
  Donor Services
Edison Corporate Center
125 May Street, Suite 300
Edison, NJ 08837
Phone: (732)661–0202
Fax: (732)662–2297

National Donor Family Council

Vicki Crosier, Chair
c/o National Kidney Foundation
30 East 33rd Street
New York, NY 10016
Phone: (212)889–2210
Fax: (212)689–9261

National Minority Organ and Tissue Transplant Education Program

Patrice Miles, Executive Director
Clive O. Callender, M.D., F.A.C.S.
Founder and Principal Investigator
2041 Georgia Avenue, Suite 3100
Washington, DC 20060
Phone: (202)856–4888
Fax: (202)865–4880

National Transplant Action Committee

Craig Irwin, President
Box 5357
Aloha, OR 97006
Phone: (503)690–8265
Fax: (503)629–8199

Tissue Banks International

Gerald Cole, CEO
815 Park Avenue
Baltimore, MD 21201
Phone: (410)752–3800
Fax: (410)783–0183

Transplant Recipients International Organizations

Bruce Weir, President
Transplant Recipients International
  Organization
835 Brick Mill Run
Westlake, OH 44145
Phone: (440)331–0559 or (800)TRIO-386
Fax: (440)356–0270

Lisa Kory, R.N., B.S.N., C.P.T.C.
Executive Director
1000 16th Street, NW, Suite 602
Washington, DC 20036-5705
Phone: (202)293–0980
Fax: (202)293–0973

Wendy Marx Foundation

Jeffrey Marx
Wendy Marx Foundation for Organ
  Donor Awareness
322 South Carolina Avenue, SE, Suite 201
Washington, DC 20003
Phone: (202)546–7270
Fax: N/A